SNELL'S CLINICAL
NEUROANATOMY

EIGHTH EDITION

IN MEMORIAM

Richard S. Snell, MRCS, LRCP, MB, MD, PhD
1925–2015

Clinical Anatomy by Regions
Clinical Anatomy by Systems
Clinical Neuroanatomy

SNELL'S CLINICAL NEUROANATOMY

EIGHTH EDITION

RYAN SPLITTGERBER, PhD

Associate Professor, Department of Surgery
Vanderbilt University Medical Center
Office of Health Sciences Education
Vanderbilt University School of Medicine
Nashville, Tennessee

Formerly CQuence Distinguished Professor
Assistant Dean
College of Allied Health Professions
University of Nebraska Medical Center
Omaha, Nebraska

Philadelphia • Baltimore • New York • London
Buenos Aires • Hong Kong • Sydney • Tokyo

Senior Acquisitions Editor: Crystal Taylor
Development Editor: Andrea Vosburgh, Kelly Horvath
Editorial Coordinator: John Larkin
Marketing Manager: Michael McMahon
Production Project Manager: Marian Bellus
Design Coordinator: Teresa Mallon
Manufacturing Coordinator: Margie Orzech
Prepress Vendor: Aptara, Inc.

Eighth edition

Copyright © 2019 Wolters Kluwer.

9 8 7 6 5 4 3 2 1

Printed in China

Library of Congress Cataloging-in-Publication Data

Names: Splittgerber, Ryan, author. ⏐ Preceded by (work): Snell, Richard S.
    Clinical neuroanatomy.
Title: Snell's clinical neuroanatomy / Ryan Splittgerber.
Other titles: Clinical neuroanatomy
Description: Eighth edition. ⏐ Philadelphia : Wolters Kluwer, [2019] ⏐
    Preceded by: Clinical neuroanatomy / Richard S. Snell. 7th ed.
    Philadelphia : Wolters Kluwer Lippincott Williams & Wilkins, c2010. ⏐
    Includes index.
Identifiers: LCCN 2018033967 ⏐ ISBN 9781496346759 (paperback)
Subjects: ⏐ MESH: Nervous System–anatomy & histology
Classification: LCC QM451 ⏐ NLM WL 101 ⏐ DDC 616.8–dc23
LC record available at https://lccn.loc.gov/2018033967

shop.lww.com

RRS1808

The trip has been long and the cost has been high . . . but no great thing was attained easily. A long tale, like a tall Tower, must be built a stone at a time.

—Stephen King

To my wife, Brienne
For providing more love and support than I deserve.
To my boys, Carter and Caden
For providing inspiration and humor…a lot of humor.

To my students
May you find your Tower.

Preface

This book contains the basic neuroanatomical facts necessary for the practice of medicine. It is suitable for medical students, dental students, nurses, and allied health students. Residents find this book useful during their rotations.

The functional organization of the nervous system has been emphasized and indicates how injury and disease can result in neurologic deficits. **The amount of factual information has been strictly limited to that which is clinically important.**

In this edition, authorship has transitioned from the late Dr. Richard Snell, who, with brilliance and dedication, fathered the previous seven editions and provided the framework for the eighth. The content of each chapter has been reviewed and edited to be more straightforward and concise. The traditional artwork has been recolored and updated to enhance the clarity and to provide additional information to each image. High-quality magnetic resonance images and histologic photomicrographs have been updated to provide greater visual details.

Each chapter introduces the relevance of neuroanatomy through a short case report.

- **Clinical Example.** A short case report that serves to dramatize the relevance of neuroanatomy introduces each chapter.
- **Chapter Objectives.** This section details the material that is most important to learn and understand in each chapter.
- **Basic Neuroanatomy.** This section provides basic information on neuroanatomical structures that are of clinical importance. Numerous examples of normal radiographs, CT scans, MRIs, and PET scans are also provided. Many cross-sectional diagrams have been included to stimulate students to think in terms of three-dimensional anatomy, which is so important in the interpretation of CT scans and MR images.
- **Clinical Notes.** This section provides the practical application of neuroanatomical facts that are essential in clinical practice. It emphasizes the structures that the clinician will encounter when making a diagnosis and treating a patient. It also provides the information necessary to understand many procedures and techniques and notes the anatomical "pitfalls" commonly encountered.
- **NEW! Key Concepts.** These quick, bulleted reviews of key topics and information are provided at the end of each chapter.
- **Clinical Problem Solving.** This section provides the student with many examples of clinical situations in which a knowledge of neuroanatomy is necessary to solve clinical problems and to institute treatment; solutions to the problems are provided at the end of the chapter.
- **Review Questions.** The purpose of the questions is threefold: to focus attention on areas of importance, to enable students to assess their areas of weakness, and to provide a form of self-evaluation when questions are answered under examination conditions. Some of the questions are centered around a clinical problem that requires a neuroanatomical answer. Solutions to the problem are provided at the end of each chapter.

An interactive **Review Test**, including over 450 questions, is provided online.

The book is extensively illustrated. The majority of the figures have been kept simple and are in color. As in the previous edition, a concise **Color Atlas** of the dissected brain is included prior to the text. This small but important group of colored plates enables the reader to quickly relate a particular part of the brain to the whole organ.

R.S.
R.S.S.

Acknowledgments

Starting with the first edition of Clinical Neuroanatomy published in 1980, many people have provided their expertise and should be recognized for their contributions. First and foremost, thanks to Richard S. Snell whose shoulders we stand upon to advance our own intellectual progress.

Throughout this text and in previous editions, the following individuals provided valuable contributions and are gratefully acknowledged: N. Cauna, L. Clerk, D. O. Davis, H. Dey, M. Feldman, T. M. J. Fitzgerald, I. Grunther, J. M. Kerns, T. McCarthy, A. Peters, G. Sze, and L. Wener.

EIGHTH EDITION

I am greatly indebted to the staff of Wolters Kluwer, including Crystal Taylor, who brought me in and provided me with this wonderful opportunity, as well as Andrea Vosburgh, development editor, and John Larkin, editorial coordinator. Thanks also to freelance development editor Kelly Horvath, who provided invaluable direction and patience with me throughout the entire process.

SPi Global is gratefully acknowledged for their brilliant art recoloring and enhancing the personality of this textbook.

My special thanks to Stephanie Vas, Program Director of the Magnetic Resonance Imaging Program at the University of Nebraska Medical Center, who produced exceptional MR images for this edition.

I would like to extend my gratitude to my students, colleagues, and mentors for their encouragement and wisdom—especially, Sabra Peetz, Art Dalley, Cathy Pettepher, Lillian Nanney, and Kyle Meyer.

R.S.

Contents

Preface vii

Acknowledgments ix

Color Atlas of Brain xix

CHAPTER 1   Introduction and Organization of the Nervous System   1

Central and Peripheral Nervous Systems   1
Major Divisions of the Central Nervous System   2
Major Divisions of the Peripheral Nervous System   12
Early Development of the Nervous System   14
Clinical Notes   16
Clinical Problem Solving   27
Answers and Explanations to Clinical Problem Solving   28
Review Questions   29
Answers and Explanations to Review Questions   31

CHAPTER 2   Neurons and Neuroglia   33

Neurons   33
Neuroglia   54
Extracellular Space   60
Clinical Notes   62
Clinical Problem Solving   65
Answers and Explanations to Clinical Problem Solving   66
Review Questions   67
Answers and Explanations to Review Questions   69

CHAPTER 3   Nerve Fibers and Peripheral Innervation   71

Nerve Fibers   71
Peripheral Nerves   80
Receptor Endings   84
Effector Endings   93
Segmental Innervation of Skin   98
Segmental Innervation of Muscles   100
Muscle Tone and Muscle Action   101
Motor Unit Summation   102
Muscle Fatigue   102
Posture   102
Clinical Notes   105
Clinical Problem Solving   119
Answers and Explanations to Clinical Problem Solving   122
Review Questions   125
Answers and Explanations to Review Questions   128

CHAPTER 4   **Spinal Cord and Ascending, Descending, and Intersegmental Tracts**   131

Brief Review of the Vertebral Column   131
Spinal Cord   136
Ascending Tracts   142
Descending Tracts   152
Intersegmental Tracts   160
Renshaw Cells and Lower Motor Neuron Inhibition   162
Clinical Notes   163
Clinical Problem Solving   175
Answers and Explanations to Clinical Problem Solving   177
Review Questions   180
Answers and Explanations to Review Questions   182

CHAPTER 5   **Brainstem**   185

Skull Anatomy   185
Cranial Cavity   191
Introduction to the Brainstem   195
Medulla Oblongata   196
Pons   204
Midbrain   209
Clinical Notes   215
Clinical Problem Solving   219
Answers and Explanations to Clinical Problem Solving   220
Review Questions   222
Answers and Explanations to Review Questions   226

CHAPTER 6   **Cerebellum and Its Connections**   229

Gross Appearance   229
Structures   231
Cerebellar Cortical Mechanisms   234
Cerebellar Afferent Fibers   236
Cerebellar Efferent Fibers   239
Functions of the Cerebellum   240
Clinical Notes   241
Clinical Problem Solving   244
Answers and Explanations to Clinical Problem Solving   244
Review Questions   245
Answers and Explanations to Review Questions   247

CHAPTER 7   **Cerebrum**   249

Subdivisions   249
Diencephalon   249
General Appearance of the Cerebral Hemispheres   255
Main Sulci   256
Cerebral Hemisphere Lobes   258
Internal Structure of the Cerebral Hemispheres (Atlas Plates 4 and 5)   260
Clinical Notes   267
Clinical Problem Solving   273
Answers and Explanations to Clinical Problem Solving   274
Review Questions   275
Answers and Explanations to Review Questions   277

CHAPTER 8   The Structure and Functional Localization of the Cerebral Cortex   279

Structure   279
Cortical Mechanisms   283
Cortical Areas   283
Cerebral Dominance   289
Clinical Notes   290
Clinical Problem Solving   293
Answers and Explanations to Clinical Problem Solving   294
Review Questions   295
Answers and Explanations to Review Questions   297

CHAPTER 9   Reticular Formation and Limbic System   299

Reticular Formation   299
Limbic System   301
Clinical Notes   306
Clinical Problem Solving   307
Answers and Explanations to Clinical Problem Solving   307
Review Questions   307
Answers and Explanations to Review Questions   308

CHAPTER 10   Basal Nuclei (Basal Ganglia)   310

Terminology   310
Corpus Striatum   310
Amygdaloid Nucleus   311
Substantia Nigra and Subthalamic Nuclei   312
Claustrum   312
Connections of the Corpus Striatum and Globus Pallidus   312
Basal Nuclei Functions   314
Clinical Notes   315
Clinical Problem Solving   319
Answers and Explanations to Clinical Problem Solving   319
Review Questions   320
Answers and Explanations to Review Questions   321

CHAPTER 11   Cranial Nerve Nuclei   323

Cranial Nerves   323
Cranial Nerve Organization   323
Olfactory Nerves (Cranial Nerve I)   326
Optic Nerve (Cranial Nerve II)   327
Oculomotor Nerve (Cranial Nerve III)   331
Trochlear Nerve (Cranial Nerve IV)   331
Trigeminal Nerve (Cranial Nerve V)   332
Abducens Nerve (Cranial Nerve VI)   335
Facial Nerve (Cranial Nerve VII)   337
Vestibulocochlear Nerve (Cranial Nerve VIII)   339
Glossopharyngeal Nerve (Cranial Nerve IX)   341
Vagus Nerve (Cranial Nerve X)   343
Accessory Nerve (Cranial Nerve XI)   345
Hypoglossal Nerve (Cranial Nerve XII)   347
Clinical Notes   348
Clinical Problem Solving   356
Answers and Explanations to Clinical Problem Solving   357
Review Questions   358
Answers and Explanations to Review Questions   361

CHAPTER 12   Thalamus   363

General Appearance   363
Subdivisions   363
Connections   366
Function   367
Clinical Notes   369
Clinical Problem Solving   370
Answers and Explanations to Clinical Problem Solving   370
Review Questions   370
Answers and Explanations to Review Questions   372

CHAPTER 13   Hypothalamus   373

Hypothalamus   373
Hypothalamic Nuclei   375
Hypothalamic Lines of Communication   376
Functions   380
Clinical Notes   382
Clinical Problem Solving   383
Answers and Explanations to Clinical Problem Solving   384
Review Questions   384
Answers and Explanations to Review Questions   385

CHAPTER 14   Autonomic Nervous System   387

Organization   387
Large Autonomic Plexuses   390
Autonomic Ganglia   390
Preganglionic Transmitters   392
Fast, Slow, and Inhibitory Synaptic Potentials   392
Ganglion-Stimulating Agents   392
Ganglion-Blocking Agents   392
Postganglionic Nerve Endings   393
Postganglionic Transmitters   393
Other Postganglionic Transmitters   394
Cholinergic Receptor Blockade   394
Adrenergic Receptor Blockade   394
Higher Control   394
Enteric Nervous System   394
Functions   395
Differences Between Sympathetic and Parasympathetic Systems   395
Autonomic Innervations   396
Ans Physiologic Reflexes   406
Clinical Notes   406
Clinical Problem Solving   411
Answers and Explanations to Clinical Problem Solving   412
Review Questions   413
Answers and Explanations to Review Questions   416

CHAPTER 15   Meninges   418

Brain Meninges   418
Spinal Cord Meninges   425
Clinical Notes   428
Clinical Problem Solving   432
Answers and Explanations to Clinical Problem Solving   433
Review Questions   434
Answers and Explanations to Review Questions   435

CHAPTER 16   Ventricular System and Cerebrospinal Fluid   436

Ventricular System   436
Subarachnoid Space   447
Cerebrospinal Fluid   448
Blood–Brain and Blood–Cerebrospinal Fluid Barriers   452
Clinical Notes   455
Clinical Problem Solving   458
Answers and Explanations to Clinical Problem Solving   459
Review Questions   460
Answers and Explanations to Review Questions   462

CHAPTER 17   Blood Supply of the Brain and Spinal Cord   464

Arteries of the Brain   464
Veins of the Brain   469
Brain Capillaries   470
Cerebral Circulation   470
Spinal Cord Arteries   471
Spinal Cord Veins   472
Clinical Notes   472
Clinical Problem Solving   480
Answers and Explanations to Clinical Problem Solving   482
Review Questions   484
Answers and Explanations to Review Questions   486

CHAPTER 18   Nervous System Development   488

Spinal Cord   488
Brain   490
Clinical Notes   498
Clinical Problem Solving   502
Answers and Explanations to Clinical Problem Solving   503
Review Questions   503
Answers and Explanations to Review Questions   504

APPENDIX   Neuroanatomical Data of Clinical Significance and Clinical
Neuroanatomy Techniques   507

Index   513

SNELL'S CLINICAL NEUROANATOMY

EIGHTH EDITION

Color Atlas of Brain

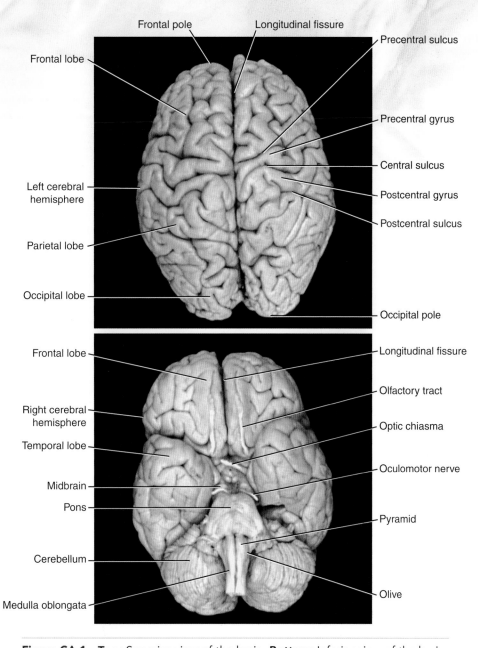

Figure CA-1 **Top:** Superior view of the brain. **Bottom:** Inferior view of the brain.

Longitudinal fissure

Right cerebral hemisphere

Superior frontal gyrus

Frontal pole

Pons

Temporal pole

Medulla oblongata

Left cerebral hemisphere

Parieto-occipital sulcus

Occipital pole

Occipital lobe

Horizontal fissure of cerebellum

Vermis of cerebellum

Cavity of fourth ventricle

Left cerebellar hemisphere

Inferior cerebellar peduncle

Gracile tubercle

Medulla oblongata

Cuneate tubercle

Figure CA-2   **Top:** Anterior view of the brain. **Bottom:** Posterior view of the brain.

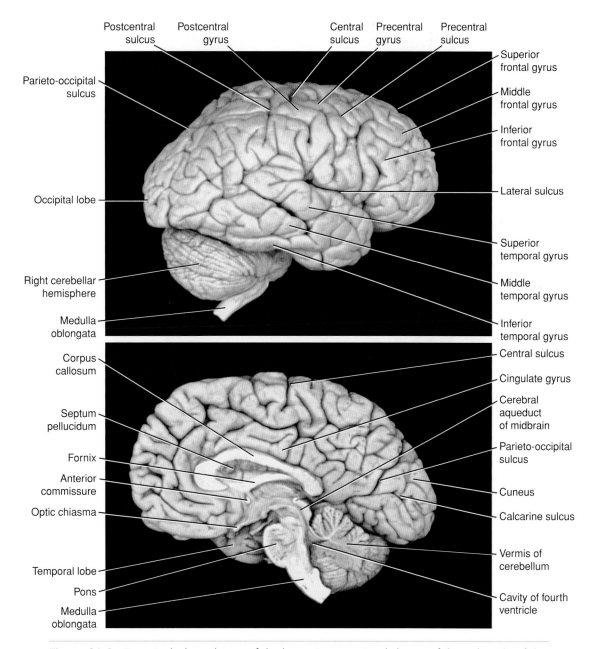

Figure CA-3 **Top:** Right lateral view of the brain. **Bottom:** Medial view of the right side of the brain following median sagittal section.

Figure CA-4   Coronal sections of the brain passing through the anterior horn of the lateral ventricle **(top)**, the mammillary bodies **(middle)**, and the pons **(bottom)**.

Figure CA-5 **Top:** Horizontal section of the cerebrum showing the lentiform nucleus, the caudate nucleus, the thalamus, and the internal capsule. **Bottom:** Oblique coronal section of the brain.

Figure CA-6 **Top:** Inferior view of the brain showing cranial nerves. The abducens and facial nerves cannot be seen. **Bottom:** Enlarged inferior view of the central part of the brain.

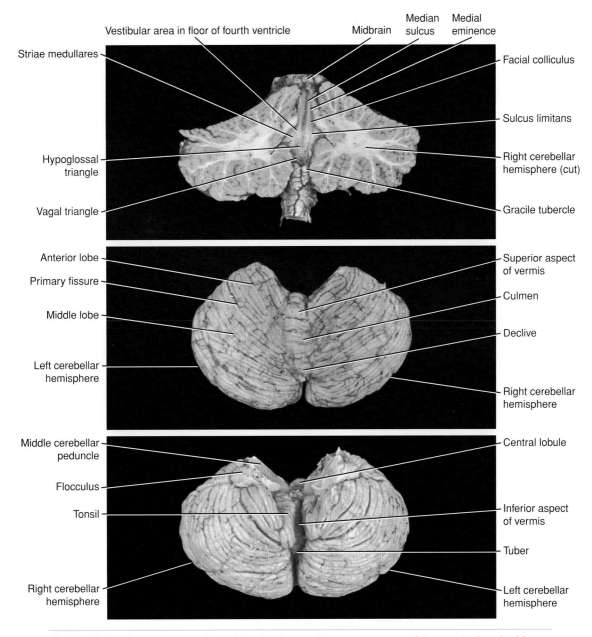

Figure CA-7   **Top:** Posterior view of the brainstem. The greater part of the cerebellum had been removed to expose the floor of the fourth ventricle. **Middle:** Superior view of the cerebellum showing the vermis and right and left cerebellar hemispheres. **Bottom:** Inferior view of the cerebellum showing the vermis and right and left cerebellar hemispheres.

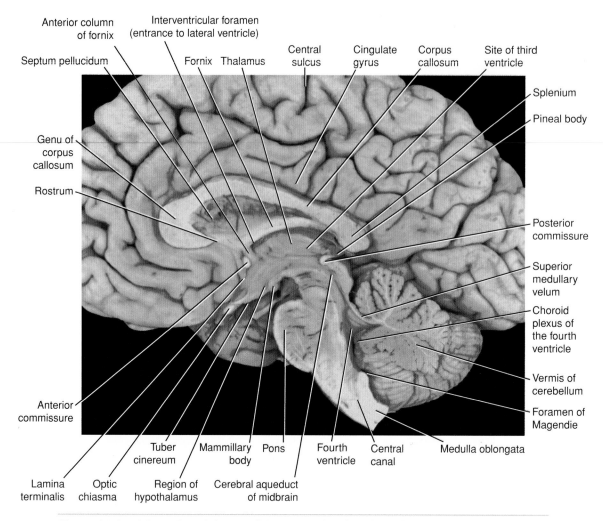

Figure CA-8 Enlarged medial view of the right side of the brain following median sagittal section, showing the continuity of the central canal, fourth ventricle, cerebral aqueduct, and the third ventricle and entrance into the lateral ventricle through the interventricular foramen.

1 Introduction and Organization of the Nervous System

CHAPTER OBJECTIVES

- To understand the basic organization of the main structures that form the nervous system

- To gain a three-dimensional appreciation of the parts of the brain and their relative positions to one another

A 23-year-old student is driving home from a party and crashes his car head-on into a tree. On examination in the emergency department of the local hospital, he has a fracture dislocation of the 7th thoracic vertebra, with signs and symptoms of severe damage to the spinal cord. Later, he is found to have paralysis of the left leg. Testing of cutaneous sensibility reveals a band of cutaneous hyperesthesia (increased sensitivity) extending around the abdominal wall on the left side at the level of the umbilicus. Just below this, he has a narrow band of anesthesia and analgesia. On the right side, he has total analgesia, thermoanesthesia, and partial loss of touch sensation of the skin of the abdominal wall below the level of the umbilicus and involving the whole of the right leg.

With knowledge of anatomy, a clinician knows that a fracture dislocation of the 7th thoracic vertebra can result in severe damage to the 10th thoracic segment of the spinal cord. Because of the small size of the vertebral foramen in the thoracic region, such an injury inevitably results in damage to the spinal cord. Knowledge of the vertebral levels of the various segments of the spinal cord enables the clinician to determine the likely neurologic deficits. The unequal sensory and motor losses on the two sides indicate a left hemisection of the cord. The band of anesthesia and analgesia was caused by the destruction of the cord on the left side at the level of the 10th thoracic

segment; all afferent nerve fibers entering the cord at that point were interrupted. The loss of pain and thermal sensibilities and the loss of light touch below the level of the umbilicus on the right side were caused by the interruption of the lateral and anterior spinothalamic tracts on the left side of the cord.

To comprehend what has happened to this patient, the relationship between the spinal cord and its surrounding vertebral column must be understood. The various neurologic deficits will be easier to understand after the reader has learned how the nervous pathways pass up and down the spinal cord. This information will be discussed in Chapter 4.

The nervous system and the endocrine system control the functions of the body. The nervous system is composed basically of specialized cells, whose function is to receive sensory stimuli and to transmit them to effector organs, whether muscular or glandular. The sensory stimuli that arise either outside or inside the body are correlated within the nervous system, and the efferent impulses are coordinated so that the effector organs work harmoniously together for the well-being of the individual. In addition, the nervous system of higher species has the ability to store sensory information received during past experiences. This information, when appropriate, is integrated with other nervous impulses and channeled into the common efferent pathway.

CENTRAL AND PERIPHERAL NERVOUS SYSTEMS

As shown in Figure 1-1, the nervous system is divided into two main parts, for purposes of description: the **central nervous system** (**CNS**), which consists of the brain and spinal cord, and the **peripheral nervous system** (**PNS**), which consists of the cranial and spinal nerves and their associated ganglia.

In the CNS, the brain and spinal cord are the main centers where correlation and integration of nervous information occur. Both the brain and spinal cord are covered with a system of membranes (**meninges**) and are suspended in **cerebrospinal fluid** (**CSF**). Meninges are further protected by the bones of the skull and the vertebral column (Fig. 1-2).

The CNS is composed of large numbers of **neurons**, which are excitable nerve cells, and their processes,

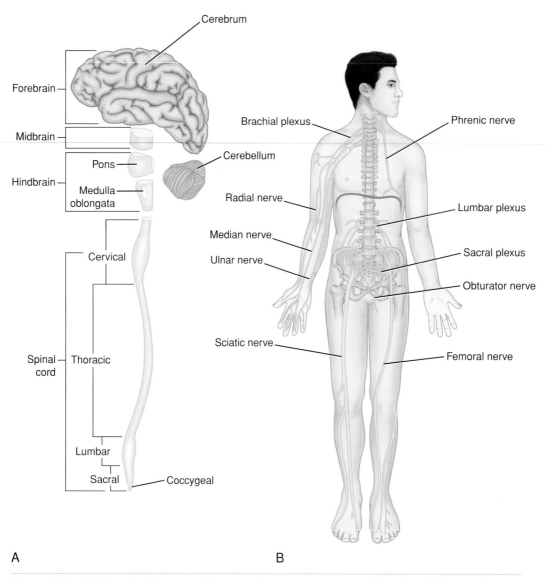

Figure 1-1 **A:** The main divisions of the central nervous system. **B:** The parts of the peripheral nervous system (the cranial nerves have been omitted).

known as **axons** or **nerve fibers**. Neurons are supported by specialized tissue called **neuroglia** (Fig. 1-3).

The CNS interior is organized into gray and white matter. **Gray matter**, which is gray in color, consists of nerve cells embedded in neuroglia. **White matter** consists of nerve fibers embedded in neuroglia and is white in color because of the presence of lipid material in nerve fiber myelin sheaths.

In the PNS, the cranial and spinal nerves, which consist of bundles of nerve fibers (or axons), conduct information to and from the CNS. Although the nerves are surrounded by fibrous sheaths as they run to different parts of the body, they are relatively unprotected and are commonly damaged by trauma.

Autonomic Nervous System

The autonomic nervous system (ANS) is the part of the nervous system that innervates the body's involuntary structures, such as the heart, smooth muscle, and glands. It is distributed throughout the CNS and PNS and is divided into two parts, the **sympathetic** and the **parasympathetic**, both containing afferent and efferent nerve fibers. The activities of the sympathetic part of the ANS prepare the body for an emergency, whereas those of the parasympathetic part are aimed at conserving and restoring energy.

MAJOR DIVISIONS OF THE CENTRAL NERVOUS SYSTEM

Before proceeding to a detailed description of the spinal cord and brain, understanding the main features of these structures and their general relationship to one another is essential (Table 1-1).

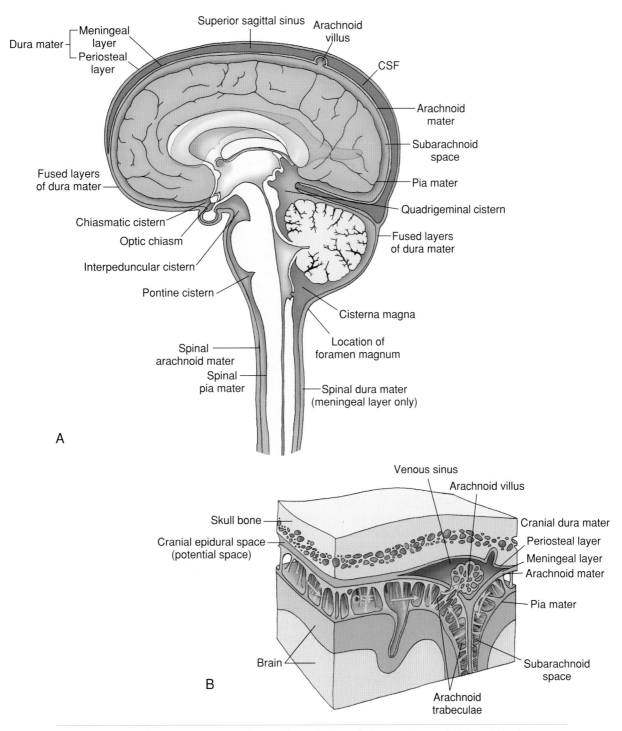

Figure 1-2   A: The protective covering of the spinal cord, the meninges, is formed by dura, arachnoid, and pia mater. The space between the arachnoid and pial membranes is called the subarachnoid space and contains cerebrospinal fluid (CSF). The subarachnoid space is enlarged at the cisterna magna and chiasmatic cistern. **B:** In the cranium, the dura consists of fused periosteal and meningeal layers that separate to form dural sinuses. Arachnoid mater projects into the dural venous sinuses to drain CSF from the subarachnoid space. (From Siegel, A., & Sapru, H. N. [2015]. *Essential neuroscience* [3rd ed.]. Baltimore, MD: Wolters Kluwer.)

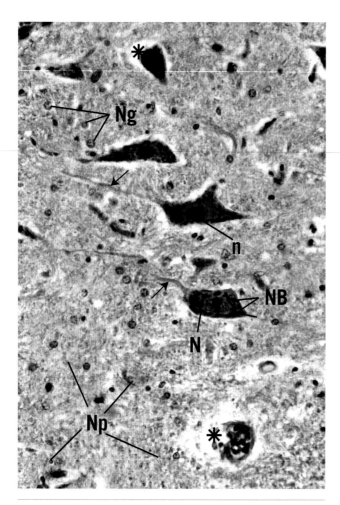

Figure 1-3 Photomicrograph of several large nerve cells with surrounding neuroglia. N, Neuron; n, nucleus; Ng, neuroglia; Np, neuropili; arrows, neurites. (From Gartner, L. P. [2017]. *Color atlas and text of histology* [7th ed.]. Baltimore, MD: Wolters Kluwer.)

Spinal Cord

The spinal cord is situated within the **vertebral canal** of the vertebral column and is surrounded by three meninges (Figs. 1-4 and 1-5): the **dura mater,** the **arachnoid mater,** and the **pia mater.** Further protection is provided by the **CSF,** which surrounds the spinal cord in the **subarachnoid space.**

The spinal cord is roughly cylindrical and begins superiorly at the foramen magnum in the skull, where it is continuous with the **medulla oblongata** of the brain. It terminates inferiorly in the lumbar region. Below, the spinal cord tapers off into the **conus medullaris,** from the apex of which the **filum terminale** (a prolongation of the pia mater) descends to attach to the back of the coccyx (see Fig. 1-4B).

Along the entire length of the spinal cord, 31 pairs of spinal nerves are attached by the **anterior** or **motor roots** and the **posterior** or **sensory roots** (Fig. 1-6; also see Fig. 1-5). Each root is attached to the cord by a series of rootlets, which extend the whole length of the corresponding segment of the cord. Each posterior

| Table 1-1 | Major Divisions of the Central and Peripheral Nervous Systems |

Central Nervous System

Brain
  Forebrain
    Cerebrum
    Diencephalon (between brain)
  Midbrain
  Hindbrain
    Medulla oblongata
    Pons
    Cerebellum
Spinal cord
  Cervical segments
  Thoracic segments
  Lumbar segments
  Sacral segments
  Coccygeal segments

Peripheral Nervous System

Cranial nerves and their ganglia—12 pairs that exit the skull through the foramina
Spinal nerves and their ganglia—31 pairs that exit the vertebral column through the intervertebral foramina
  8 Cervical
  12 Thoracic
  5 Lumbar
  5 Sacral
  1 Coccygeal

nerve root possesses a **posterior root ganglion,** the cells of which give rise to peripheral and central nerve fibers.

Spinal Cord Structure

The spinal cord is composed of an inner core of **gray matter,** which is surrounded by an outer covering of **white matter.** The gray matter is seen on cross section as an H-shaped pillar with **anterior** and **posterior gray columns,** or **horns,** united by a thin **gray commissure** containing the small **central canal.** The white matter, for purposes of description, is divided into **anterior, lateral,** and **posterior white columns** (see Fig. 1-6).

Brain

The brain (Fig. 1-7) lies in the cranial cavity and is continuous with the spinal cord through the foramen magnum (see Fig. 1-5A). As shown in Figure 1-2, it is surrounded by the **dura mater,** the **arachnoid mater,** and the **pia mater.** These three meninges are continuous with the corresponding meninges of the spinal cord. The CSF surrounds the brain in the subarachnoid space.

The brain is conventionally divided into three major divisions: the **hindbrain,** the **midbrain,** and the **forebrain** in ascending order from the spinal cord (see Fig. 1-1A). The **brainstem** (a collective term for the

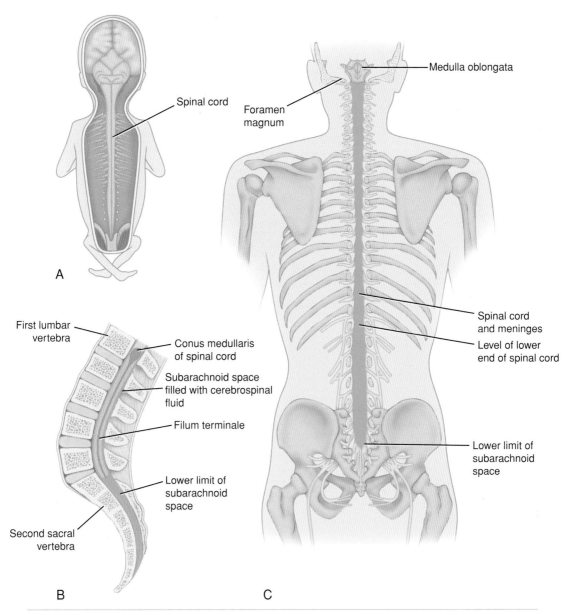

Figure 1-4   A: Fetus with the brain and spinal cord exposed on the posterior surface. Note that the spinal cord extends the full length of the vertebral column. **B:** Sagittal section of the vertebral column in an adult showing the spinal cord terminating inferiorly at the level of the lower border of the 1st lumbar vertebra. **C:** Adult spinal cord and covering meninges showing the relationship to surrounding structures.

medulla oblongata, pons, and midbrain) is what remains after the cerebral hemispheres and cerebellum (see below) are removed.

Hindbrain

The hindbrain comprises the **medulla oblongata**, the **pons**, and the **cerebellum**.

Medulla Oblongata

The medulla oblongata is conical in shape and connects the pons superiorly to the spinal cord inferiorly (Fig. 1-8). It contains many collections of neurons, called **nuclei**,

and serves as a conduit for ascending and descending nerve fibers.

Pons

The pons is situated on the anterior surface of the cerebellum, inferior to the midbrain and superior to the medulla oblongata (Fig. 1-9; also see Fig. 1-8). The pons, or bridge, derives its name from the large number of transverse fibers on its anterior aspect connecting the two cerebellar hemispheres. It also contains many nuclei and ascending and descending nerve fibers.

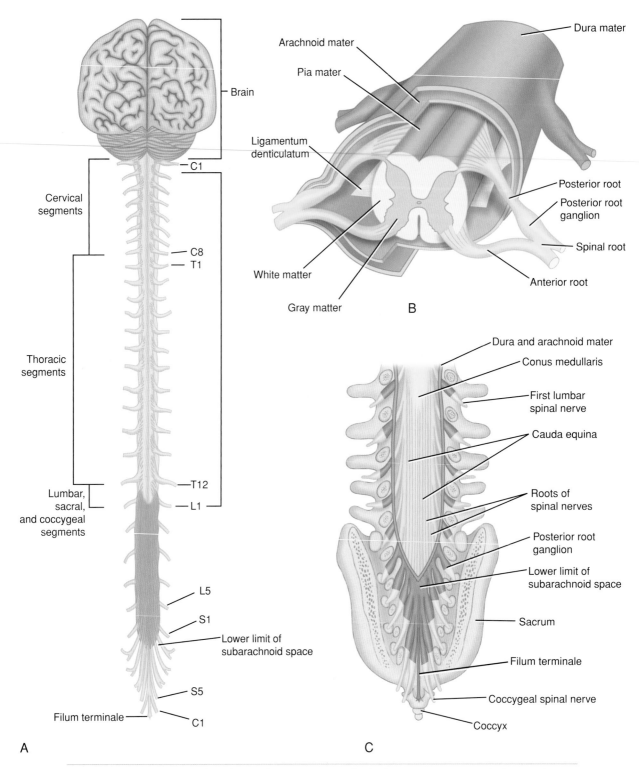

Figure 1-5   A: Brain, spinal cord, spinal nerve roots, and spinal nerves as seen on their posterior aspect. **B:** Transverse section through the thoracic region of the spinal cord showing the anterior and posterior roots of a spinal nerve and the meninges. **C:** Posterior view of the lower end of the spinal cord and cauda equina showing their relationship with the lumbar vertebrae, sacrum, and coccyx.

White matter

One segment of spinal cord

Posterior rootlets of spinal nerve

Posterior root of spinal nerve

Posterior root ganglion

Spinal nerve

Central canal

Posterior ramus of spinal nerve

Anterior ramus of spinal nerve

Anterior root of spinal nerve

Gray matter

A

Anterior rootlets of spinal nerve

Posterior median sulcus

Posterior median septum

Posterior white column

Posterior gray column

Lateral white column

Gray commissure

Posterior root ganglion

Central canal

Anterior gray column

Spinal nerve

B

Anterior median fissure

Anterior white column

Figure 1-6 **A:** Transverse section through the lumbar part of the spinal cord, oblique view. **B:** Transverse section through the lumbar part of the spinal cord, face view, showing the anterior and posterior roots of a spinal nerve.

Parietal bone

Central sulcus

Frontal bone

Parietal lobe

Frontal lobe

Occipital bone

Occipital lobe

Cerebellum

Lateral fissure

Temporal bone

Temporal lobe

Figure 1-7 Lateral view of the brain within the skull.

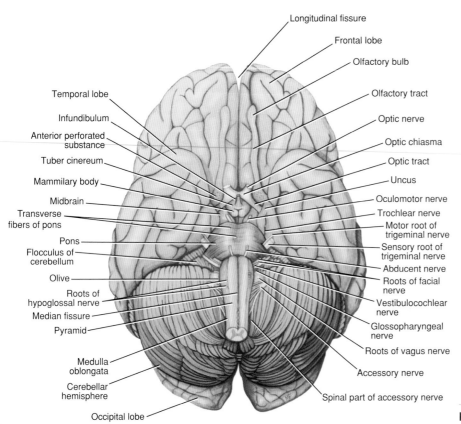

Figure 1-8   Inferior view of the brain.

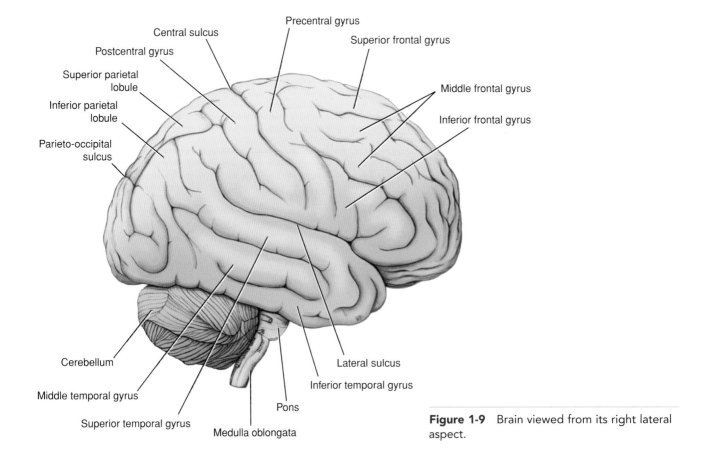

Figure 1-9   Brain viewed from its right lateral aspect.

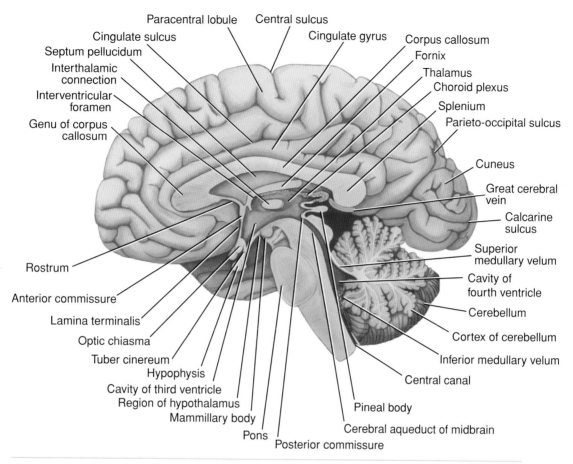

Figure 1-10 Median sagittal section of the brain to show the third ventricle, the cerebral aqueduct, and the fourth ventricle.

Cerebellum

The cerebellum lies within the posterior cranial fossa of the skull (see Figs. 1-7 to 1-9), posterior to the pons and the medulla oblongata. It consists of two laterally placed hemispheres connected by a median portion, the **vermis**. The cerebellum is connected to the midbrain by the **superior cerebellar peduncles**, to the pons by the **middle cerebellar peduncles**, and to the medulla by the **inferior cerebellar peduncles** (see Fig. 6-9). The peduncles are composed of large bundles of nerve fibers connecting the cerebellum to the remainder of the nervous system.

The surface layer of each cerebellar hemisphere is called the **cortex** and is composed of gray matter (Fig. 1-10). The cerebellar cortex is thrown into folds, or folia, separated by closely set transverse fissures. Certain masses of gray matter are found in the interior of the cerebellum, embedded in the white matter; the largest of these is known as the **dentate nucleus** (see Fig. 6-7).

The medulla oblongata, the pons, and the cerebellum surround a cavity filled with CSF, called the **fourth ventricle.** This is connected superiorly to the third ventricle by the **cerebral aqueduct**; inferiorly, it is continuous with the central canal of the spinal cord (Fig. 1-11). It communicates with the subarachnoid space through

three openings in the inferior part of the roof. Through these openings, the CSF within the CNS can enter the subarachnoid space.

Midbrain

The midbrain is the narrow part of the brain that connects the forebrain to the hindbrain (see Figs. 1-1A and 1-10). The narrow cavity of the midbrain is the **cerebral aqueduct,** which connects the third and fourth ventricles. The midbrain contains many nuclei and bundles of ascending and descending nerve fibers.

Forebrain

The forebrain comprises the **diencephalon** (between brain), which is the central part of the forebrain, and the **cerebrum**.

Diencephalon

The diencephalon is almost completely hidden from the surface of the brain. It consists of a dorsal **thalamus** and a ventral **hypothalamus** (see Fig. 1-10). The thalamus is a large, egg-shaped mass of gray matter that lies on either side of the third ventricle. The anterior end of the thalamus forms the posterior boundary of the **interventricular foramen**, the

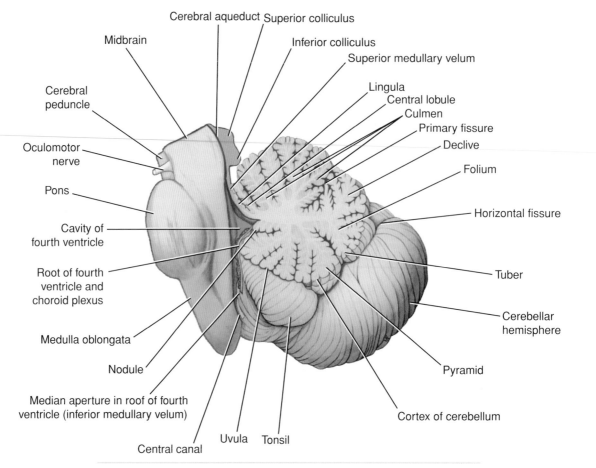

Figure 1-11   Sagittal section through the brainstem and the cerebellum.

opening between the third and lateral ventricles. The hypothalamus forms the lower part of the lateral wall and floor of the third ventricle.

Cerebrum

The cerebrum, the largest part of the brain, consists of two cerebral hemispheres, which are connected by a mass of white matter called the **corpus callosum** (see Figs. 1-9 and 1-10). Each hemisphere extends from the frontal to the occipital bones in the skull, superior to the anterior and middle cranial fossae; posteriorly, the cerebrum lies above the tentorium cerebelli (see Fig. 15-3). The hemispheres are separated by a deep cleft, the **longitudinal fissure**, into which projects the **falx cerebri** (see Fig. 15-1).

The surface layer of each hemisphere, the **cortex**, is composed of gray matter. The cerebral cortex is thrown into folds (**gyri**) separated by fissures, or **sulci** (see Fig. 1-9). This arrangement greatly increases the surface area of the cortex. A number of the large sulci are conveniently used to subdivide the surface of each hemisphere into **lobes**, which are named from the bones of the cranium they lie under.

Within the hemisphere is a central core of white matter containing several large masses of gray matter,

the **basal nuclei or ganglia**. A fan-shaped collection of nerve fibers, the **corona radiata** (Fig. 1-12), passes in the white matter to and from the cerebral cortex to the brainstem. The corona radiata converges on the basal nuclei and passes between them as the **internal capsule**. The tailed nucleus situated on the medial side of the internal capsule is the **caudate nucleus** (Fig. 1-13), and the lens-shaped nucleus on the lateral side of the internal capsule is the **lentiform nucleus**.

Within each cerebral hemisphere is a cavity called the **lateral ventricle** (see Figs. 16-2 and 16-3). The lateral ventricles communicate with the third ventricle through the **interventricular foramina**.

During the process of development, the cerebrum becomes enormously enlarged and overhangs the diencephalon, the midbrain, and the hindbrain.

Brain Structure

Unlike the spinal cord, the brain is composed of an inner core of white matter, which is surrounded by an outer covering of gray matter. However, as mentioned previously, certain important masses of gray matter are situated deeply within the white matter: the gray cerebellar nuclei in the cerebellum and the gray thalamic, caudate, and lentiform nuclei in the cerebrum.

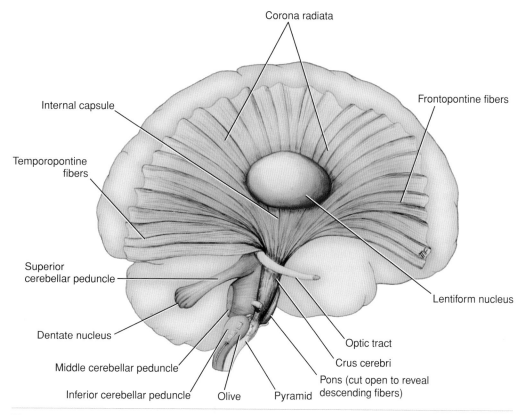

Corona radiata

Internal capsule

Frontopontine fibers

Temporopontine fibers

Superior cerebellar peduncle

Lentiform nucleus

Dentate nucleus

Optic tract

Middle cerebellar peduncle

Crus cerebri

Inferior cerebellar peduncle   Olive   Pyramid

Pons (cut open to reveal descending fibers)

Figure 1-12 Right lateral view showing continuity of the corona radiata, the internal capsule, and the crus cerebri of the cerebral peduncles. Note the position of the lentiform nucleus lateral to the internal capsule.

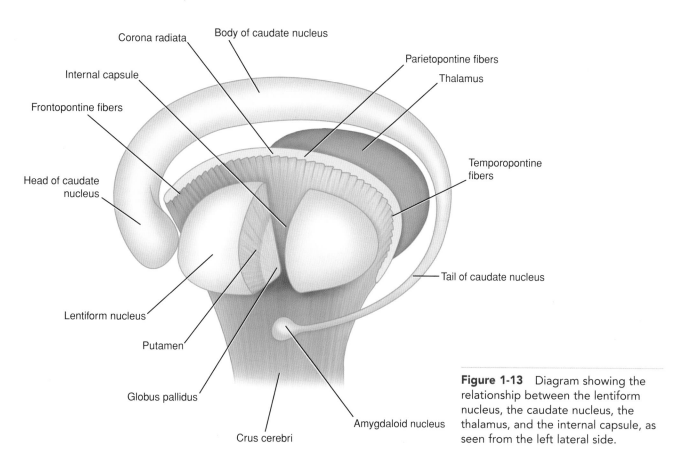

Corona radiata   Body of caudate nucleus

Internal capsule

Parietopontine fibers

Frontopontine fibers

Thalamus

Head of caudate nucleus

Temporopontine fibers

Lentiform nucleus

Tail of caudate nucleus

Putamen

Globus pallidus

Amygdaloid nucleus

Crus cerebri

Figure 1-13 Diagram showing the relationship between the lentiform nucleus, the caudate nucleus, the thalamus, and the internal capsule, as seen from the left lateral side.

MAJOR DIVISIONS OF THE PERIPHERAL NERVOUS SYSTEM

The PNS comprises the cranial and spinal nerves and their associated ganglia.

Cranial and Spinal Nerves

The cranial and spinal nerves are made up of bundles of nerve fibers supported by connective tissue.

The 12 pairs of **cranial nerves** (see Fig. 1-8) leave the brain and pass through foramina in the skull. The 31 pairs of **spinal nerves** (see Fig. 1-5) leave the spinal cord and pass through intervertebral foramina in the vertebral column. The spinal nerves are associated with regions of the spinal cord: 8 **cervical**, 12 **thoracic**, 5 **lumbar**, 5 **sacral**, and 1 **coccygeal**. Note that there are 8 cervical nerves yet only 7 cervical vertebrae and that there is 1 coccygeal nerve but 4 coccygeal vertebrae.

Each spinal nerve is connected to the spinal cord by two roots: the **anterior root** and the **posterior root** (see Fig. 1-5B). The anterior root consists of bundles of nerve fibers carrying nerve impulses *away* from the CNS—**efferent fibers**. Those that go to skeletal muscles and cause them to contract are **motor fibers**. Their cells of origin lie in the anterior gray horn of the spinal cord.

The posterior root consists of bundles of **afferent fibers** that carry nervous impulses *to* the CNS. Because these fibers convey information about sensations of touch, pain, temperature, and vibration, they are called **sensory fibers**. The cell bodies of these nerve fibers are situated in a swelling on the posterior root called the **posterior root ganglion**.

The spinal nerve roots pass from the spinal cord to the level of their respective intervertebral foramina, where they unite to form a **spinal nerve** (Fig. 1-14). Here, the motor and sensory fibers mix together; thus, a spinal nerve comprises both motor and sensory fibers.

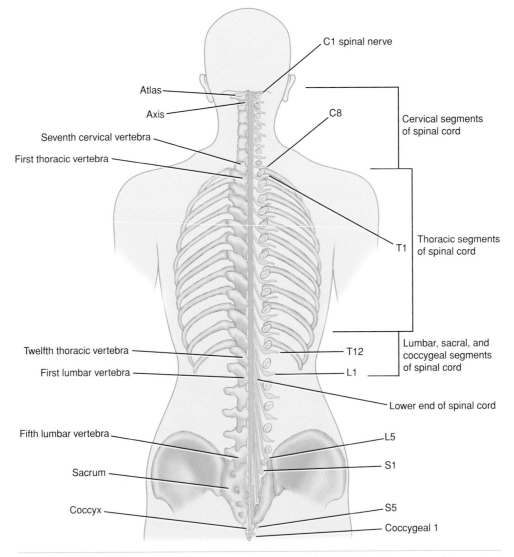

Figure 1-14   Posterior view of the spinal cord showing the origins of the roots of the spinal nerves and their relationship to the different vertebrae. On the right, the laminae have been removed to expose the right half of the spinal cord and the nerve roots.

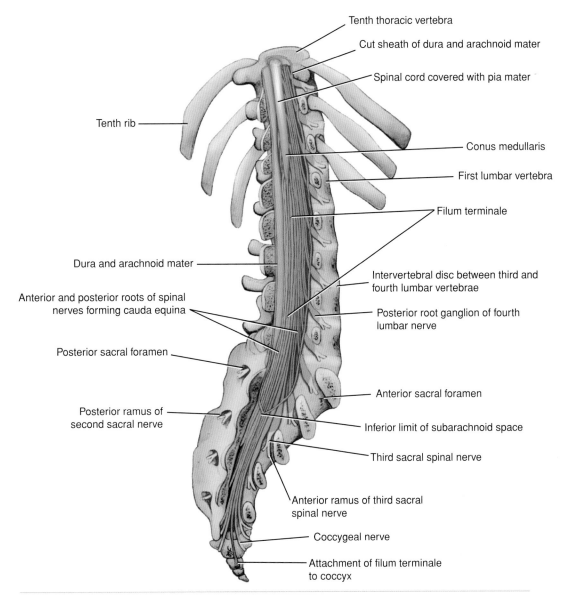

Tenth thoracic vertebra

Cut sheath of dura and arachnoid mater

Spinal cord covered with pia mater

Tenth rib

Conus medullaris

First lumbar vertebra

Filum terminale

Dura and arachnoid mater

Intervertebral disc between third and fourth lumbar vertebrae

Anterior and posterior roots of spinal nerves forming cauda equina

Posterior root ganglion of fourth lumbar nerve

Posterior sacral foramen

Anterior sacral foramen

Posterior ramus of second sacral nerve

Inferior limit of subarachnoid space

Third sacral spinal nerve

Anterior ramus of third sacral spinal nerve

Coccygeal nerve

Attachment of filum terminale to coccyx

Figure 1-15 Oblique posterior view of the lower end of the spinal cord and the cauda equina. On the right, the laminae have been removed to expose the right half of the spinal cord and the nerve roots.

Because of the disproportionate growth in length of the vertebral column during development, compared with that of the spinal cord, the length of the roots increases progressively from above downward (see Fig. 1-15). In the upper cervical region, the spinal nerve roots are short and run almost horizontally, but the roots of the lumbar and sacral nerves below the level of the termination of the cord (lower border of the 1st lumbar vertebra in the adult) form a vertical leash of nerves around the **filum terminale** (Fig. 1-15). Together, these lower nerve roots are called the **cauda equina**.

After emerging from the intervertebral foramen, each spinal nerve immediately divides into a large **anterior ramus** and a smaller **posterior ramus**, each containing both motor and sensory fibers. The posterior ramus passes posteriorly around the vertebral column to supply the muscles and skin of the back. The anterior ramus continues anteriorly to supply the muscles and skin over the anterolateral body wall and all the muscles and skin of the limbs.

The anterior rami join one another at the root of the limbs to form complicated **nerve plexuses** (see Fig. 1-1B). The **cervical and brachial plexuses** are found at the root of the upper limbs, and the **lumbar and sacral plexuses** are found at the root of the lower limbs.

Ganglia

Ganglia can be divided into sensory ganglia of spinal nerves (posterior root ganglia) and cranial nerves and autonomic ganglia.

Sensory Ganglia

Sensory ganglia are fusiform swellings (see Fig. 1-5) on the posterior root of each spinal nerve just proximal to the root's junction with a corresponding anterior root. They are referred to as **posterior root ganglia**. Similar ganglia found along the course of cranial nerves V, VII, VIII, IX, and X are the **sensory ganglia** of these nerves.

Autonomic Ganglia

Autonomic ganglia, which are often irregular in shape, are situated along the course of efferent nerve fibers of the ANS. They are found in the paravertebral sympathetic chains (see Figs. 14-1 and 14-2) around the roots of the great visceral arteries in the abdomen and close to, or embedded within, the walls of various viscera.

EARLY DEVELOPMENT OF THE NERVOUS SYSTEM

Before the formation of the nervous system in the embryo, three main cell layers differentiate. The innermost layer, the **entoderm**, gives rise to the gastrointestinal tract, the lungs, and the liver. The **mesoderm** gives rise to the muscle, connective tissues, and the vascular system. The third and outermost layer, the **ectoderm**, formed of columnar epithelium, gives rise to the entire nervous system.

During the third week of development, the ectoderm on the dorsal surface of the embryo between the primitive knot and the buccopharyngeal membrane thickens to form the **neural plate**. The plate, which is pear shaped and wider cranially, develops a longitudinal **neural groove**. The groove now deepens so that it is bounded on either side by **neural folds** (Fig. 1-16).

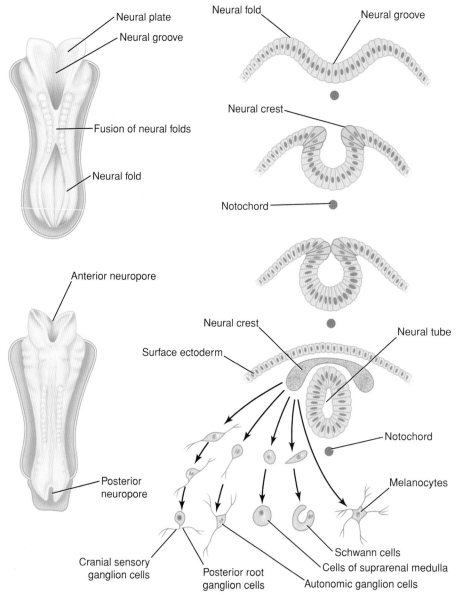

Figure 1-16 Formation of the neural plate, neural groove, and neural tube. The cells of the neural crest differentiate into the cells of the posterior root ganglia, the sensory ganglia of cranial nerves, autonomic ganglia, neurilemmal cells (Schwann cells), the cells of the suprarenal medulla, and melanocytes.

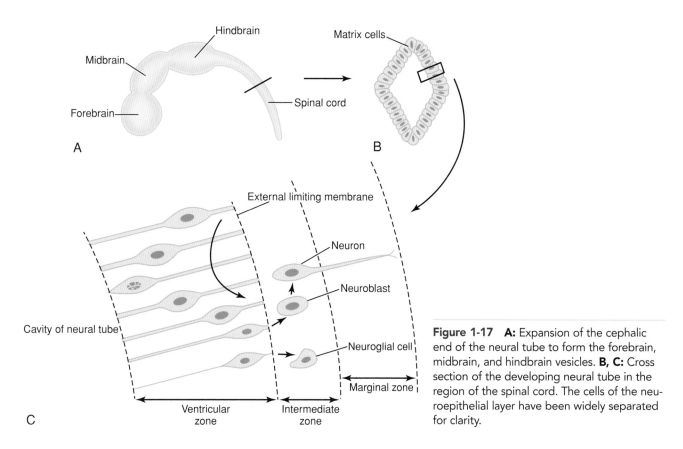

Figure 1-17 A: Expansion of the cephalic end of the neural tube to form the forebrain, midbrain, and hindbrain vesicles. **B, C:** Cross section of the developing neural tube in the region of the spinal cord. The cells of the neuroepithelial layer have been widely separated for clarity.

With further development, the neural folds fuse, converting the neural groove into a **neural tube**. Fusion starts at about the midpoint along the groove and extends cranially and caudally so that, in the earliest stage, the cavity of the tube remains in communication with the amniotic cavity through the **anterior** and **posterior neuropores**. The anterior neuropore closes first and the posterior neuropore 2 days later. Thus, normally, the neural tube closure is complete within 28 days. Meanwhile, the neural tube has sunk beneath the surface ectoderm.

During the invagination of the neural plate to form the neural groove, the cells forming the lateral margin of the plate do not become incorporated in the neural tube but instead form a strip of ectodermal cells that lie between the neural tube and the covering ectoderm, the **neural crest** (Fig. 1-16). Subsequently, this group of cells will migrate ventrolaterally on each side around the neural tube. Ultimately, the neural crest cells will differentiate into the cells of the **posterior root ganglia**, the **sensory ganglia of the cranial nerves**, **autonomic ganglia**, the **cells of the suprarenal medulla**, and the **melanocytes**. These cells also probably give rise to mesenchymal cells in the head and neck.

Meanwhile, the proliferation of cells at the cephalic end of the neural tube causes it to dilate and form **three primary brain vesicles**: the **forebrain**, **midbrain**, and **hindbrain vesicles** (Fig. 1-17) (Table 1-2). The rest of the tube elongates and remains smaller in diameter; it will form the **spinal cord.**

Table 1-2   The Primary Divisions of the Developing Brain

Primary Vesicle	Primary Division	Subdivision	Adult Structures
Forebrain vesicle	Prosencephalon (forebrain)	Telencephalon	Cerebral hemisphere, basal ganglia, hippocampus
		Diencephalon	Thalamus, hypothalamus, pineal body, infundibulum
Midbrain vesicle	Mesencephalon (midbrain)	Mesencephalon (midbrain)	Tectum, tegmentum, crus cerebri
Hindbrain vesicle	Rhombencephalon (hindbrain)	Metencephalon	Pons, cerebellum
		Myelencephalon	Medulla oblongata

The subsequent differentiation of cells in the neural tube is brought about by the inductive interactions of one group of cells with another. The inducing factors influence the control of the gene expression in the target cells. Ultimately, the simplest progenitor cell will differentiate into neurons and neuroglial cells. Interestingly, excessive numbers of neurons and neuroglial cells develop, and many (nearly half of the developing neurons) will be programmed to die by a process known as **programmed cell death**. Research into the identification of neurotrophic factors that promote the development and survival of neurons is of great importance, as the results could possibly be applied to the problem of regeneration of the spinal cord neurons following trauma or the inhibition of degenerative diseases such as Alzheimer disease.

The further development of the nervous system will be fully described in Chapter 18 following the description of the different parts of the nervous system and their neuronal connections.

 Clinical Notes

Relationship of Spinal Cord Segments to Vertebral Numbers

Because the spinal cord is shorter than the vertebral column, the spinal cord segments do not correspond numerically with the vertebrae that lie at the same level (see Fig. 1-14). The following table will help a clinician determine which spinal segment is related to a given vertebral body (Table 1-3).

Examination of a patient's back shows that the spinous processes lie approximately at the same level as the vertebral bodies. In the lower thoracic region, however, because of the length and extreme obliquity of the spinous processes, the tips of the spines lie at the level of the vertebral body below.

Spinal Cord and Brain Injuries

The spinal cord and brain are well protected. Both are suspended in **cerebrospinal fluid** (**CSF**) and are surrounded by the bones of the vertebral column and skull (see Chapters 4 and 5). However, with enough force, these protective structures can be damaged, with consequent injury to the delicate underlying nervous tissue. Moreover, the cranial and spinal nerves and blood vessels are also likely to be injured.

Spinal Cord Injuries

The degree of spinal cord injury at different vertebral levels is determined largely by anatomical factors. In the cervical region, dislocation or fracture dislocation is common, but the large size of the vertebral canal usually prevents severe injury to the spinal cord. However, with considerable displacement of the bones or bone fragments, the cord is sectioned. Respiration ceases if the cord is completely severed above the segmental origin of the phrenic nerves (C3–C5) because the intercostal muscles and the diaphragm are paralyzed, resulting in death.

In fracture dislocations of the thoracic region, displacement can be considerable. The small size of the vertebral canal results in severe injury to this region of the spinal cord.

In fracture dislocations of the lumbar region, two anatomic facts help prevent substantial nerve injury. First, the spinal cord in the adult extends down only as far as the level of the lower border of the 1st lumbar vertebra (see Fig. 1-15). Second, the large size of the vertebral foramen in this region gives the roots of the cauda equina ample room.

Injury to the spinal cord may produce partial or complete loss of function at the level of the lesion and partial or complete loss of function of afferent and efferent nerve tracts below the level of the lesion. The symptoms and signs of such injuries are discussed after the detailed structure of the spinal cord, and the ascending and descending tracts are discussed in Chapter 4.

Spinal Nerve Injuries

The intervertebral foramina (Fig. 1-18) transmit the spinal nerves and the small segmental arteries and veins, all of which are embedded in areolar tissue. Each foramen is bounded superiorly and inferiorly by the pedicles of adjacent vertebrae, anteriorly by the lower part of the vertebral body and the intervertebral disc, and posteriorly by the articular processes and the joint between them. In this situation, the spinal nerve is very vulnerable and may be pressed on or irritated by disease of the surrounding structures. Herniation of the intervertebral disc, fractures of the vertebral bodies, and osteoarthritis involving the joints of the articular processes or the joints between the vertebral bodies may all result in pressure, stretching, or edema of the emerging spinal nerve. Such pressure would give rise to dermatomal pain, muscle weakness, and diminished or absent reflexes.

HERNIATED INTERVERTEBRAL DISCS

Herniation of the intervertebral discs occurs most commonly in areas of the vertebral column where a mobile part joins a relatively immobile part—for example, the cervicothoracic and lumbosacral junctions. In these areas, the

Table 1-3	Relationship of Spinal Cord Segments to Vertebral Numbers
Vertebrae	**Spinal Segment**
Cervical vertebrae	Add 1
Upper thoracic vertebrae	Add 2
Lower thoracic vertebrae (7–9)	Add 3
10th thoracic vertebra	L1–L2 cord segments
11th thoracic vertebra	L3–L4 cord segments
12th thoracic vertebra	L5 cord segment
1st lumbar vertebra	Sacral and coccygeal cord segments

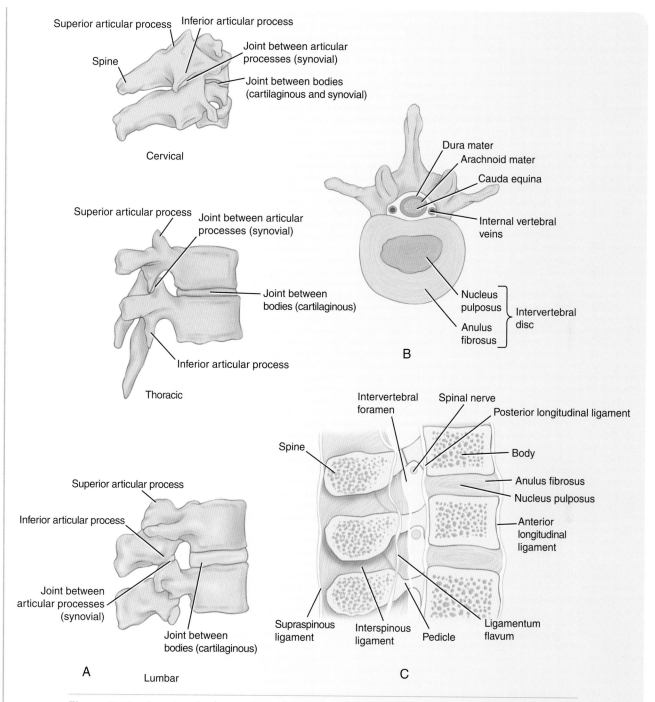

Figure 1-18   A: Joints in the cervical, thoracic, and lumbar regions of the vertebral column. **B:** Third lumbar vertebra seen from above showing the relationship between the intervertebral disc and the cauda equina. **C:** Sagittal section through three lumbar vertebrae showing the ligaments and the intervertebral discs. Note the relationship between the emerging spinal nerve in an intervertebral foramen and the intervertebral disc.

posterior part of the anulus fibrosus of the disc ruptures, and the central nucleus pulposus is forced posteriorly like toothpaste out of a tube. This herniation of the nucleus pulposus may result either in a central protrusion in the midline under the posterior longitudinal ligament of the vertebrae or in a lateral protrusion at the side of the posterior ligament close to the intervertebral foramen (Fig. 1-19).

Cervical disc herniations are less common than herniations in the lumbar region. The discs most susceptible are those between the 5th and 6th and the 6th and 7th cervical vertebrae. Lateral protrusions cause pressure on a spinal nerve or its roots. Each spinal nerve emerges above the corresponding vertebra; thus, the protrusion of the disc between the 5th and 6th cervical vertebrae

Figure 1-19 A, B: Posterior views of the vertebral bodies in the cervical and lumbar regions showing the relationship that might exist between a herniated nucleus pulposus and spinal nerve roots. Note there are eight cervical spinal nerves and only seven cervical vertebrae. In the lumbar region, for example, the emerging L4 nerve roots pass out laterally close to the pedicle of the 4th lumbar vertebra and are not related to the intervertebral disc between the 4th and 5th lumbar vertebrae. **C:** Posterolateral herniation of the nucleus pulposus of the intervertebral disc between the 5th lumbar vertebra and the 1st sacral vertebra showing pressure on the S1 nerve root. **D:** An intervertebral disc that has herniated its nucleus pulposus posteriorly. **E:** Pressure on the L5 motor nerve root produces weakness of dorsiflexion of the ankle; pressure on the S1 motor nerve root produces weakness of plantar flexion of the ankle joint.

may compress the C6 spinal nerve or its roots. Pain is felt near the lower part of the back of the neck and shoulder and along the area in the distribution of the spinal nerve involved. Central protrusions may press on the spinal cord and the anterior spinal artery and involve the various spinal tracts.

Lumbar disc herniations are more common than cervical disc herniations. The discs usually affected are those between the 4th and 5th lumbar vertebrae and between the 5th lumbar vertebra and the sacrum. In the lumbar region, the roots of the cauda equina run posteriorly over a number of intervertebral discs. A lateral herniation may press on one or two roots and commonly involves the nerve root going to the intervertebral foramen just below. The nucleus pulposus occasionally herniates directly backward, and if it is a large herniation, the whole cauda equina may be compressed, causing paraplegia.

In lumbar disc herniations, pain is referred down the leg and foot in the distribution of the affected nerve. Because the sensory posterior roots most commonly pressed on are the 5th lumbar and 1st sacral, pain is usually felt down the back and lateral side of the leg, radiating to the sole of the foot, a condition known as **sciatica**. In severe cases, paresthesia or actual sensory loss may occur.

Pressure on the anterior motor roots causes muscle weakness. Involvement of the 5th lumbar motor root weakens dorsiflexion of the ankle, whereas pressure on the 1st sacral motor root causes plantar flexion weakness. The ankle jerk reflex may be diminished or absent (see Fig. 1-19E).

A large, centrally placed protrusion may give rise to bilateral pain and muscle weakness in both legs. Acute retention of urine may also occur.

Spinal Tap

Spinal tap (lumbar puncture) may be performed to withdraw a sample of CSF for microscopic or bacteriologic examination or to inject drugs to combat infection or induce anesthesia. Fortunately, the spinal cord terminates inferiorly at the level of the lower border of the 1st lumbar vertebra in adults (in infants, it may reach inferiorly to the 3rd lumbar vertebra). The subarachnoid space extends inferiorly as far as the lower border of the 2nd sacral vertebra. The lower lumbar part of the vertebral canal is thus occupied by the subarachnoid space, which contains the lumbar and sacral nerve roots and the filum terminale (the cauda equina). A needle inserted into the subarachnoid space in this region usually pushes the nerve roots to one side without causing damage.

With the patient lying on his or her side or in the upright sitting position, with the vertebral column well flexed, the space between adjoining laminae in the lumbar region is opened to a maximum (Fig. 1-20). An imaginary line joining the highest points on the iliac crests passes over the 4th lumbar spine. Using a careful aseptic technique and local anesthesia, the clinician passes the lumbar puncture needle fitted with a stylet into the vertebral canal above or below the 4th lumbar spine. The needle will pass through the following anatomical structures before it enters the subarachnoid space: (a) skin, (b) superficial fascia, (c) supraspinous ligament, (d) interspinous ligament, (e) ligamentum flavum, (f) areolar tissue containing the internal vertebral venous plexus, (g) dura mater, and (h) arachnoid mater. The depth to which the needle will have to pass will vary from 1 in (2.5 cm) or less in a child to as much as 4 in (10 cm) in an obese adult.

As the stylet is withdrawn, a few drops of blood may escape. This usually indicates that the point of the needle is in one of the veins of the internal vertebral plexus and has not yet reached the subarachnoid space. If the needle stimulates one of the nerve roots of the cauda equina, the patient will experience a fleeting discomfort in one of the dermatomes or a muscle will twitch, depending on whether a sensory or a motor root was affected.

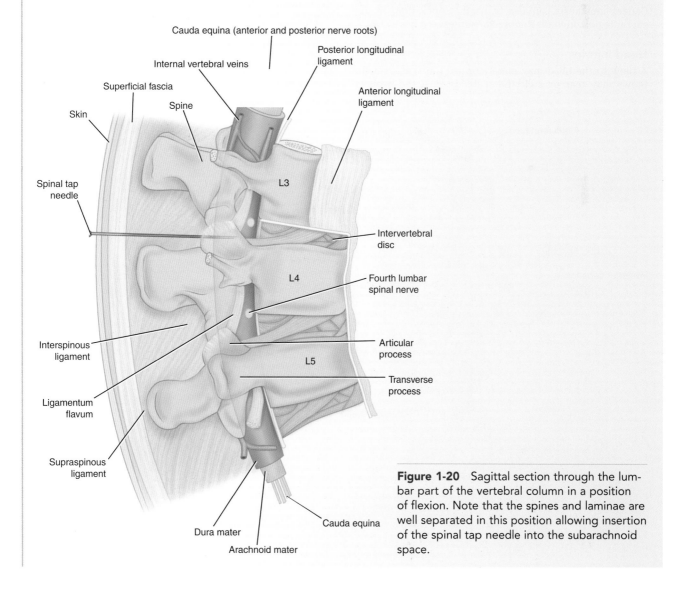

Figure 1-20 Sagittal section through the lumbar part of the vertebral column in a position of flexion. Note that the spines and laminae are well separated in this position allowing insertion of the spinal tap needle into the subarachnoid space.

CSF pressure can be measured by attaching a manometer to the needle. When the patient is in the recumbent position, the **normal pressure is about 60 to 150 mm** of water. The pressure shows oscillations corresponding to the movements of respiration and the arterial pulse.

A block of the subarachnoid space in the vertebral canal, which may be caused by a tumor of the spinal cord or the meninges, can be detected by compressing the internal jugular veins in the neck. This raises the cerebral venous pressure and inhibits the absorption of CSF in the arachnoid granulations, thereby increasing the manometer reading of the CSF pressure. If this rise does not occur, the subarachnoid space is blocked, and the patient exhibits a positive **Queckenstedt sign**.

Caudal Anesthesia

Anesthetic solutions may be injected into the sacral canal through the sacral hiatus. The solutions pass upward in the loose connective tissue and bathe the spinal nerves as they emerge from the dural sheath (Fig. 1-21). Obstetricians use this method of nerve block to relieve the pains of the first and second stages of labor because anesthetic administered by this method does not affect the infant. Caudal anesthesia can also be used in operations in the sacral region, including anorectal surgery.

Head Injuries

A blow to the head may merely bruise the scalp; severe blows may tear or split the scalp. Even if the head is protected by a helmet, the brain can be severely damaged without clinical evidence of scalp injury.

Skull Fractures

Severe blows to the head can change the shape of the skull at the point of impact. Small objects may penetrate the skull and lacerate the brain. Larger objects applied with great force may shatter the skull and drive fragments of bone into the brain at the site of impact.

In the adult, fractures of the skull are common, but they are less common in the young child. In the infant, the skull bones are more resilient, and they are separated by fibrous sutural ligaments. In the adult, the inner table of the skull is particularly brittle. Moreover, the sutural ligaments begin to ossify during middle age.

The type of fracture that occurs in the skull will depend on the age of the patient, the severity of the blow, and the area of the skull receiving the trauma. The **adult skull** resembles an eggshell, with limited resilience. A severe, localized blow will cause a local indentation, commonly with bone splintering. Blows to the vault can result in a series of linear fractures, which radiate out through the thin areas of the bone. The petrous parts of the temporal bones and the occipital crests (see Fig. 5-6) strongly reinforce the base of the skull and tend to deflect linear fractures.

The **young child's skull** resembles a ping-pong ball, because a localized blow produces a depression without splintering. This common type of circumscribed lesion is known as a "pond" fracture.

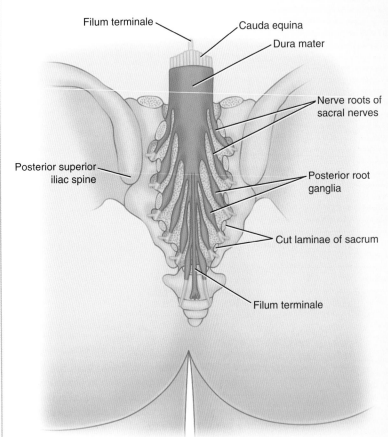

Figure 1-21 Posterior view of the sacrum. Laminae have been removed to show the sacral nerve roots lying within the sacral canal.

Figure 1-22 **A:** Mechanisms of acute cerebral injury when a blow is applied to the lateral side of the head. **B:** Varieties of intracranial hemorrhage. **C:** Mechanism of cerebral trauma following a blow on the chin. The movement of the brain within the skull can also tear the cerebral veins.

Brain Injuries

Brain injuries are caused by displacement and distortion of the neuronal tissues at the moment of impact (Fig. 1-22). The brain, which is incompressible, is like a water-soaked log suspended in water. The brain is floating in the CSF in the subarachnoid space and is capable of a certain amount of anteroposterior and lateral gliding movement. The anteroposterior movement is limited by the attachment of the superior cerebral veins to the superior sagittal sinus. Lateral displacement of the brain is limited by the falx cerebri. The tentorium cerebelli and the falx cerebelli also restrict displacement of the brain.

Thus, blows on the front or back of the head lead to displacement of the brain, which may cause severe cerebral damage, stretching and distortion of the brainstem, and stretching and even tearing of brain commissures. Blows to the side of the head cause less cerebral displacement, and the injuries to the brain consequently tend to be less severe. However, the falx cerebri is a tough structure and may cause considerable damage to the softer brain tissue in cases of a severe blow to the side of the head. Furthermore, remember that glancing blows to the head may cause considerable brain rotation, with shearing strains and brain distortion, particularly in areas where further rotation is prevented by bony prominences in the anterior and middle cranial fossae. Brain lacerations are very likely to occur when the brain is forcibly thrown against the sharp edges of bone within the skull (see pp. 191–192)—the lesser wings of the sphenoid, for example.

When the brain moves suddenly within the skull, the part of the brain that moves away from the skull wall is subjected to diminished pressure because the CSF has not had time to accommodate to the brain movement. This results in a suction effect on the brain surface, with rupture of surface blood vessels.

A sudden severe blow to the head, as in an automobile accident, may result in damage to the brain at two sites: at the point of impact and at the pole of the brain opposite the point of impact, where the brain is thrown against the skull wall. This is referred to as **contrecoup injury**.

The movement of the brain within the skull at the time of head injuries not only is likely to cause avulsion of cranial nerves but commonly leads to rupture of tethering blood vessels. Fortunately, the large arteries found at the base of the brain are tortuous, and this, coupled with their strength, explains why they are rarely torn. The thin-walled cortical veins, which drain into the large dural venous sinuses, are very vulnerable and can cause severe subdural or subarachnoid hemorrhage.

Traumatic Brain Injury Following an Explosion or Blast

Deployed soldiers are frequently exposed to explosive devices, which may result in extensive injuries to the limbs, eyes, and ears. Open injuries to the skull, where shrapnel has entered the brain, are clearly visible and are dealt with accordingly.

However, in closed injuries, in which the skull remains intact, the underlying brain may be damaged but left untreated. In these cases, the explosion produces a blast of air that strikes the skull and shakes up the brain, resulting in multiple injuries to the soft brain tissue as it is driven against the hard bony projections within the skull. The symptoms and signs will depend on the extent of the neurologic damage and will be mild, moderate, or severe. Although the moderate and severe cases are quickly recognized by medical personnel, the mild cases may be missed, and patients may later develop headaches, nausea, mood changes, and memory loss. Early diagnosis is imperative as studies of these patients have shown that mild neurologic damage can be successfully treated. Individuals who have been exposed to explosive devices should undergo computed tomography (CT) scan or magnetic resonance imaging (MRI) before returning to civilian life.

Intracranial Hemorrhage

Although the brain is cushioned by the surrounding CSF in the subarachnoid space, any severe hemorrhage within the relatively rigid skull will ultimately exert pressure on the brain.

Four types of intracranial hemorrhage may result from trauma or cerebral vascular lesions (see Fig. 1-22).

Epidural (extradural) **hemorrhage** results from injuries to the meningeal arteries (commonly the anterior division of the middle meningeal artery) or veins (see Fig. 15-6). A comparatively minor blow to the side of the head, resulting in fracture of the skull in the region of the anterior–inferior portion of the parietal bone, may sever the artery (see Fig. 1-22). Arterial or venous injury is especially likely to occur if the vessels enter a bony canal in this region. Bleeding occurs and strips the meningeal layer of dura from the internal surface of the skull. The intracranial pressure (ICP) rises, and the enlarging blood clot exerts local pressure on the underlying precentral gyrus (motor area). Blood may also pass laterally through the fracture line to form a soft swelling on the side of the head. To stop the hemorrhage, the torn artery must be ligated or plugged. The burr hole through the skull wall should be placed about 1.5 in (4 cm) above the midpoint of the zygomatic arch.

Subdural hemorrhage results from tearing of the superior cerebral veins where they enter the superior sagittal sinus (see Figs. 15-1 and 17-5). The cause is usually a blow to the front or back of the head resulting in excessive anteroposterior displacement of the brain within the skull. This condition, which is much more common than middle meningeal hemorrhage, can be caused by a sudden minor blow. Once the vein is torn, blood under low pressure begins to accumulate in the potential space between the dura and the arachnoid. The condition is rarely bilateral.

Acute and chronic forms occur depending on the speed of accumulation of fluid in the subdural space. For example, if the patient starts to vomit, the venous pressure will rise as the result of a rise in the intrathoracic pressure. Under these circumstances, the subdural blood clot will rapidly increase in size, causing acute symptoms. In the chronic form, over a course of several months, the small blood clot will attract fluid by osmosis, in which case a hemorrhagic cyst forms and gradually expands, causing pressure symptoms. In both forms, the blood clot must be removed through burr holes in the skull.

Subarachnoid hemorrhage results from nontraumatic leakage or rupture of a congenital aneurysm on the cerebral arterial circle (circle of Willis) or, less commonly, from an arteriovenous malformation. Sudden onset of severe headache, neck stiffness, and loss of consciousness occurs. The diagnosis is established by CT or MRI or by withdrawing heavily blood-stained CSF through a lumbar puncture.

With **cerebral hemorrhage**, **spontaneous intracerebral hemorrhage** (see Fig. 1-22) is most common in patients with hypertension. It is generally due to rupture of the thin-walled **lenticulostriate artery** (see Fig. 17-11), a branch of the middle cerebral artery (see Fig. 17-4). The hemorrhage involves important descending nerve fibers in the internal capsule and causes hemiplegia on the contralateral side. The patient immediately loses consciousness, and paralysis is evident when consciousness is regained. The diagnosis is established by brain CT or MRI.

Shaken Baby Syndrome

Inflicted head injury is the most common cause of traumatic death in infancy. Sudden deceleration, which occurs when an infant is held by the arms or trunk and shaken or the head is forcefully struck against a hard surface, is believed to be responsible for the brain injuries. Biomechanical studies have shown that the rotation of the floating brain around its center of gravity causes diffuse brain injuries, including diffuse axonal injury and subdural hematoma. In shaken baby syndrome, major rotational forces have to occur that clearly exceed those encountered in normal child play activities.

Most cases of shaken baby syndrome take place during the first year of life, and they are usually restricted to infants under 3 years of age. Common symptoms include lethargy, irritability, seizures, altered muscle tone, and symptoms indicating raised ICP, such as impaired consciousness, vomiting, breathing abnormalities, and apnea. In severe cases, the baby may be unresponsive, the fontanelles are bulging, and the child may have retinal hemorrhages. Spinal tap may reveal blood in the CSF. Subdural or subarachnoid hemorrhages can be readily detected on CT or MRI scans. Autopsy findings commonly include localized subdural hemorrhage in the parietal–occipital region and subarachnoid blood, associated with massive cerebral swelling and widespread neuronal loss.

Space-Occupying Lesions Within the Skull

Space-occupying or expanding lesions within the skull include tumor, hematoma, and abscess. Because the skull is a rigid container of fixed volume, these lesions will add to the normal bulk of the intracranial contents.

An expanding lesion is first accommodated by the expulsion of CSF from the cranial cavity. Later, the veins become compressed, interference with the circulation of blood and CSF begins, and the ICP starts to rise. The venous congestion results in increased production and diminished absorption of CSF, the CSF volume begins to rise, and thus, a vicious circle is established.

The position of the tumor within the brain may have a dramatic effect on the signs and symptoms. For example, a tumor that obstructs the outflow of CSF or directly presses on the great veins will cause a rapid increase in ICP. The signs and symptoms that enable the clinician to localize the lesion will depend on the degree of interference with brain function and nervous tissue destruction. Severe headache, possibly due to the stretching of the dura mater, and vomiting, due to pressure on the brainstem, are common complaints.

A spinal tap should not be performed in patients with suspected intracranial tumor. The withdrawal of CSF may lead to a sudden displacement of the cerebral hemisphere through the notch in the tentorium cerebelli into the posterior cranial fossa (Fig. 1-23) or herniation of the medulla oblongata and cerebellum through the foramen magnum. CT scans or MRIs are used in diagnosis.

Computed Tomography

CT is used for the detection of intracranial lesions. The procedure is quick, safe, and accurate. The total dose of irradiation is no greater than for a conventional skull radiograph.

CT relies on the same physics as conventional radiographs, in that structures are distinguished from one another by their ability to absorb energy from x-rays. The x-ray tube emits a narrow beam of radiation as it passes in a series of scanning movements through an arc of 180 degrees around the patient's head. The x-rays having passed through the head are collected by a special x-ray detector. The information is fed to a computer that processes the information, which is then displayed as a reconstructed picture on a screen. Essentially, the observer sees an image of a thin slice through the head, which may then be photographed for later examination (Fig. 1-24).

The sensitivity is such that small differences in x-ray absorption can be easily displayed. The gray matter of the cerebral cortex, white matter, internal capsule, corpus callosum, ventricles, and subarachnoid spaces can all be recognized. An iodine-containing medium can be injected intravascularly, which enhances greatly the contrast between tissues having a different blood flow.

Because a CT scan can be performed in 5 to 10 minutes, it is the method of choice in an emergency situation with patients with head trauma or suspected intracranial hemorrhage.

Magnetic Resonance Imaging

MRI uses the magnetic properties of the hydrogen nucleus excited by radiofrequency radiation transmitted by a coil surrounding the head. The excited hydrogen nuclei emit a signal that is detected as induced electric currents in a receiver coil. MRI is absolutely safe to the patient, and

Falx cerebri

Expanding cerebral tumor

Distortion and displacement of ventricles

Tentorium cerebelli

Herniation of part of cerebrum through tentorial notch

Cerebellum

Figure 1-23 Sudden displacement of the cerebral hemispheres through the tentorial notch into the posterior cranial fossa following a lumbar puncture; the cerebral tumor is situated in the right cerebral hemisphere. CT or MRI should be used rather than lumbar puncture when investigating a cerebral tumor.

Figure 1-24 CT scan showing the structure of the brain. **A, B:** Horizontal cuts (axial sections).

because it provides better differentiation between gray and white matter, MRI can be more revealing than CT. The reason for this is that gray matter contains more hydrogen in the form of water than white matter, and the hydrogen atoms are less bound in fat (Fig. 1-25). MRI is the best imaging method for detecting low-contrast lesions such as brain tumors or small multiple sclerosis plaques. It is also capable of showing clear images of the brainstem, cerebellum, and the pituitary fossa, which, in the case of a CT scan, are overshadowed by the dense bones of the base of the skull.

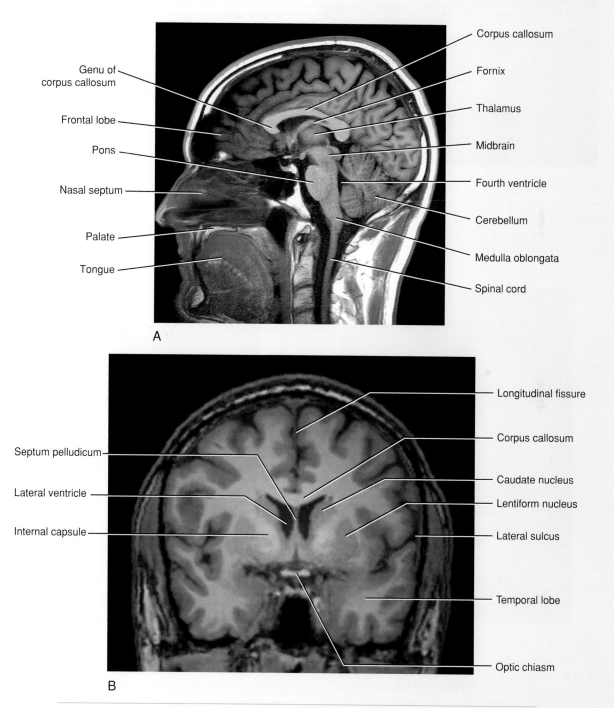

Figure 1-25 MRI showing the structure of the brain. **A:** Sagittal. **B:** Coronal. Compare with Figure 1-24. Note the better differentiation between gray and white matter.

Figure 1-26 Axial (horizontal) PET scan of a normal brain following the injection of 18-fluorodeoxyglucose. Regions of active metabolism (*yellow areas*) are seen in the cerebral cortex. The lateral ventricles are also demonstrated. (Courtesy Dr. Holley Dey.)

The spinal cord structure is much more clearly visualized with MRI.

Unfortunately, an MRI takes longer and costs two-thirds more than a CT scan.

Positron Emission Tomography

Positron emission tomography (PET) uses radioactive isotopes that decay with the emission of positively charged electrons (positrons) to map the biochemical, physiologic, and pharmacologic processes taking place in the brain.

The appropriate isotope is incorporated into molecules of known biochemical behavior in the brain and then is injected into the patient. The metabolic activity of the compound can then be studied by making cross-sectional tomographic images of the brain using the same principles as in CT (Fig. 1-26). Making a series of time-lapse images at different anatomical sites allows variations in brain metabolism to be studied at these sites. This technique has been used to study the distribution and activity of neurotransmitters, variations in oxygen utilization, and cerebral blood flow.

PET has been successfully used in the evaluation of patients with brain tumors (Figs. 1-27 and 1-28), movement disorders, seizures, and schizophrenia.

Figure 1-27 Axial (horizontal) PET scan of a 62-year-old male patient with a malignant glioma in the left parietal lobe following the injection of 18-fluorodeoxyglucose. A high concentration of the compound (*circular yellow area*) is seen in the region of the tumor. (Courtesy Dr. Holley Dey.)

Figure 1-28 Coronal PET scan of a 62-year-old male patient with a malignant glioma in the left parietal lobe following the injection of 18-fluorodeoxyglucose (same patient as in Fig. 1-25). A high concentration of the compound (*circular yellow area*) is seen in the region of the tumor. (Courtesy Dr. Holley Dey.)

Key Concepts

Central and Peripheral Nervous Systems

- The nervous system comprises the central nervous system (CNS) and peripheral nervous system (PNS).
- The CNS consists of the brain and the spinal cord, both of which are surrounded by the meninges and the cerebrospinal fluid (CSF).
- The PNS consists of all other nerves in the body.
- The autonomic nervous system (ANS) is concerned with involuntary structures and distributed throughout both CNS and PNS.

Major Divisions of the Central Nervous System

- The brain has three major divisions: hindbrain, midbrain, and forebrain.
- The hindbrain can be subdivided into the medulla oblongata, the pons, and the cerebellum; the forebrain into the diencephalon and the cerebrum.
- The cerebrum is the largest component of the brain and consists of two hemispheres, covered by cerebral cortex, which is made up of a series of folds and fissures called gyri and sulci.
- The spinal cord is a cylindrical structure continuous with the medulla oblongata of the brainstem.
- Along the length of the spinal cord, 31 pairs of spinal nerves are attached.

Major Divisions of the Peripheral Nervous System

- Motor and sensory roots connect the spinal nerve to the spinal cord.
- The spinal nerves divide into anterior and posterior rami, both containing motor and sensory fibers.
- The posterior rami are distributed to the muscles and skin of the back.
- Anterior rami supply the muscles and skin of the limbs and the anterolateral body wall.
- Ganglia are collections of neuronal cell bodies that result in fusiform swellings within the dorsal roots, or as irregular swellings within the ANS.

Early Development of the Nervous System

- During development, the embryo differentiates into three layers, entoderm, mesoderm, and ectoderm.
- The ectoderm gives rise to the entire nervous system, initially forming the neural plate, then neural folds, and subsequently fusing into the neural tube.
- The leading edge of the neural folds contains neural crest cells which differentiate into ganglion cells, Schwann cells, melanocytes, and cells of the suprarenal medulla.

? Clinical Problem Solving

1. A 45-year-old woman is examined by her physician and found to have carcinoma of the thyroid gland. Apart from swelling in the neck, the patient also complains of back pain in the lower thoracic region, with a burning soreness radiating around the right side of her thorax over the 10th intercostal space. Although the back pain can be relieved by changing posture, it is worsened by coughing and sneezing. A lateral radiograph of the thoracic part of the vertebral column reveals a secondary carcinomatous deposit in the 10th thoracic vertebral body. Further physical examination reveals muscular weakness of both legs. Using your knowledge of neuroanatomy, explain the following: (a) the pain in the back, (b) the soreness over the right 10th intercostal space, (c) the muscular weakness of both legs, and (d) which segments of the spinal cord lie at the level of the 10th thoracic vertebral body.

2. A 35-year-old coal miner is crouching down at the mine face to inspect a drilling machine. A large rock suddenly dislodges from the roof of the mine shaft and strikes the miner on the upper part of his back. Examination shows an obvious forward displacement of the 8th thoracic vertebra. What anatomical factors in the thoracic region determine the degree of injury that may occur to the spinal cord?

3. A 20-year-old man with a long history of tuberculosis of the lungs is examined by an orthopedic surgeon because of the sudden development of a humpback (kyphosis). He also has symptoms of a stabbing pain radiating around both sides of

his thorax intensified by coughing or sneezing. A diagnosis of tuberculous osteitis of the 5th thoracic vertebra is made, with the collapse of the vertebral body responsible for the kyphosis. Using your knowledge of neuroanatomy, explain why the collapse of the 5th thoracic vertebral body should cause pain in the distribution of the 5th thoracic segmental nerve on both sides.

4. A 50-year-old man wakes up one morning with a severe pain near the lower part of the back of his neck and left shoulder. The pain is also referred along the outer side of the left upper arm. Movement of the neck causes an increase in the intensity of the pain, which is also accentuated by coughing. A lateral radiograph of the neck shows a slight narrowing of the space between the 5th and 6th cervical vertebral bodies. A magnetic resonance imaging (MRI) shows disruption of the intervertebral disc between the 5th and 6th cervical vertebrae. Using your knowledge of anatomy, state which nerve root was involved. Also, state the nature of the disease.

5. A medical student offers to help a fellow student straighten out the bumper of a car. He has just finished his course in neuroanatomy and is in poor physical shape. Undaunted, he attempts to lift the end of the bumper while his friend stands on the other end. Suddenly, he feels an acute pain in the back that extends down the back and outer side of his right leg. Later, he is examined by an orthopedic surgeon, who finds that the pain is accentuated by coughing. A lateral radiograph of the lumbar vertebral column reveals nothing abnormal. A magnetic resonance imaging (MRI) taken in the sagittal plane shows a small posterior prolapse of the nucleus pulposus in the disc between the 5th lumbar and the 1st sacral vertebrae. A diagnosis of herniation of the intervertebral disc between the 5th lumbar and 1st sacral vertebrae is made. Using your knowledge of neuroanatomy, explain the symptoms of this disease. Which spinal nerve roots were pressed on?

6. A 5-year-old child is seen in the emergency department, and a diagnosis of acute meningitis is made.

The resident decides to perform a lumbar puncture in order to confirm the diagnosis. Using your knowledge of neuroanatomy, where would you perform a lumbar puncture? Name, in order, the structures pierced when a lumbar puncture needle is inserted into the subarachnoid space.

7. A pregnant young woman tells her friends that she hates the idea of going through the pain of childbirth but that she equally detests the thought of having a general anesthetic. Is there a specialized local analgesic technique that will alleviate labor pains?

8. While crossing the road, a pedestrian is struck on the right side of his head by a passing car. He falls to the ground but does not lose consciousness. After resting for an hour and then getting up, he appears to be confused and irritable. Later, he staggers and falls to the floor. On questioning, he is seen to be drowsy, and twitching of the lower left half of his face and left arm is noted. A diagnosis of epidural hemorrhage is made. Which artery is likely to have been damaged? What is causing the drowsiness and muscle twitching?

9. A 45-year-old woman is examined by a neurologist and found to have an intracranial tumor. She complains of severe headaches, which occur during the night and early morning. She describes the pain as "bursting" in nature, and although at first, 6 months ago, the headaches were intermittent, they are now more or less continuous. Coughing, stooping, and straining during defecation make the pain worse. The pain is accompanied by vomiting on three recent occasions. What is the sequence of events that occurs within the skull as the intracranial pressure (ICP) rises? Would you perform a routine lumbar puncture on every patient you suspected of having an intracranial tumor?

10. While examining an unconscious 18-year-old man admitted to the emergency room following a motorcycle accident, the neurosurgeon asks the attending medical student what happens to the brain in an accident in which it is suddenly decelerated within the skull. How would you answer the inquiry? What is the value of wearing a helmet?

 Answers and Explanations to Clinical Problem Solving

1. Carcinoma of the thyroid, breast, kidney, lung, and prostate commonly gives rise to metastases in bone. (a) The pain in the back was caused by the carcinoma invading and destroying the 10th thoracic vertebral body. (b) Compression of the posterior nerve root of the 10th thoracic spinal nerve by the carcinoma of the vertebral column caused the hyperesthesia and hyperalgesia over the right 10th intercostal space. (c) Muscular weakness of the legs was caused by pressure on the descending motor nerve fibers in the spinal cord by the carcinoma's invasion of the vertebral canal. (d) Although disproportionate growth in length of the vertebral column occurs during development compared with that of

the spinal cord, the upper cervical segments of the spinal cord still lie posterior to the vertebral bodies of the same number. However, the spinal cord in the adult terminates inferiorly at the level of the lower border of the 1st lumbar vertebra, and therefore, the 1st and 2nd lumbar segments of the spinal cord lie at the level of the 10th thoracic vertebral body.

2. This patient had a severe fracture dislocation between the 7th and 8th thoracic vertebrae. The vertical arrangement of the articular processes and the low mobility of this region because of the thoracic cage mean that a dislocation can occur in this region only if the articular processes are fractured by a great force. The small circular vertebral canal

leaves little space around the spinal cord; thus, severe cord injuries are certain.

3. Each spinal nerve is formed by the union of a posterior sensory root and an anterior motor root and leaves the vertebral canal by traveling through an intervertebral foramen. Each foramen is bounded superiorly and inferiorly by the pedicles of adjacent vertebrae, anteriorly by the lower part of the vertebral body and by the intervertebral disc, and posteriorly by the articular processes and the joint between them. In this patient, the 5th thoracic vertebral body had collapsed and the intervertebral foramina on both sides had been considerably reduced in size, causing compression of the posterior sensory roots and the spinal nerves. The consequent irritation of the sensory fibers was responsible for the pain.

4. This patient had symptoms suggestive of irritation of the left 6th cervical posterior nerve root. The radiograph revealed narrowing of the space between the 5th and 6th cervical vertebral bodies, suggesting a herniation of the nucleus pulposus of the intervertebral disc at this level. MRI showed the nucleus pulposus extending posteriorly beyond the anulus fibrosus, thus confirming the diagnosis.

5. The herniation occurred on the right side and was relatively small. The pain occurred in the distribution of the 5th lumbar and 1st sacral segments of the spinal cord, and the posterior sensory roots of these segments of the cord were pressed on the right side.

6. In a 5-year-old child, the spinal cord terminates inferiorly at about the level of the 2nd lumbar vertebra (certainly no lower than the 3rd lumbar vertebra). With the child lying on his side and with the operator using an aseptic technique, the skin is anesthetized in the midline just below the 4th lumbar spine. The 4th lumbar spine lies on an imaginary line joining the highest points on the iliac crests. The lumbar puncture needle fitted with a stylet is then passed carefully into the vertebral canal. The needle will pass through the skin, superficial fascia, supraspinous and interspinous ligaments, ligamentum flavum, areolar tissue containing the internal vertebral venous plexus, and the dura and arachnoid mater before entering the subarachnoid space.

7. Caudal analgesia (anesthesia) is very effective in labor if it is performed skillfully. The anesthetic solutions are introduced into the sacral canal through the sacral hiatus. Sufficient solution is given so that the nerve roots up as far as T11–T12 and L1 are blocked. This will make the uterine contractions painless during the first stage of labor. If the nerve fibers of S2–S4 are also blocked, the perineum will be anesthetized.

8. A blow on the side of the head can fracture the thin anterior part of the parietal bone. The anterior branch of the middle meningeal artery commonly enters a bony canal in this region and is sectioned at the time of the fracture. The resulting hemorrhage causes gradual accumulation of blood under high pressure outside the meningeal layer of the dura mater. The pressure is exerted on the underlying brain as the blood clot enlarges, and the symptoms of confusion and irritability become apparent. This is followed later by drowsiness. Pressure on the lower end of the motor area of the cerebral cortex (the right precentral gyrus) causes facial muscle twitching and, later, left arm muscle twitching. As the blood clot progressively enlarges, the intracranial pressure (ICP) rises and the patient's condition deteriorates.

9. A detailed account of the various changes that occur in the skull in patients with an intracranial tumor is given on page 23. A patient suspected of having an intracranial tumor should *not* undergo a spinal tap. The withdrawal of cerebrospinal fluid (CSF) may lead to a sudden displacement of the cerebral hemisphere through the opening in the tentorium cerebelli into the posterior cranial fossa or herniation of the medulla oblongata and cerebellum through the foramen magnum. CT scans or MRIs are now used in making the diagnosis.

10. The brain is floating in the cerebrospinal fluid (CSF) within the skull, so a blow to the head or sudden deceleration leads to displacement of the brain. This may produce severe cerebral damage; stretching or distortion of the brainstem; avulsion of cranial nerves; and, commonly, rupture of tethering cerebral veins. A helmet helps to protect the brain by cushioning the blow and thus slowing the rate of brain deceleration.

 Review Questions

Directions: Each of the incomplete statements in this section is followed by completions of the statement. Select the ONE lettered completion that is BEST in each case.

1. The spinal cord has
   (a) an outer covering of gray matter and an inner core of white matter.
   (b) an enlargement below that forms the conus medullaris.
   (c) anterior and posterior roots of a single spinal nerve attached to a single segment.
   (d) cells in the posterior gray horn that give rise to efferent fibers that supply skeletal muscles.
   (e) a central canal that is situated in the white commissure.

2. The medulla oblongata has
    (a) a tubular shape.
    (b) the fourth ventricle lying posterior to its lower part.
    (c) the midbrain directly continuous with its upper border.
    (d) no central canal in its lower part.
    (e) the spinal cord directly continuous with its lower end in the foramen magnum.
3. The midbrain has
    (a) a cavity called the cerebral aqueduct.
    (b) a large size.
    (c) no cerebrospinal fluid (CSF) around it.
    (d) a cavity that opens above into the lateral ventricle.
    (e) a location in the middle cranial fossa of the skull.

Directions: Each of the numbered items in this section is followed by answers. Select the ONE lettered answer that is CORRECT.

4. The following statements concern the cerebellum:
    (a) It lies within the middle cranial fossa.
    (b) The cerebellar cortex is composed of white matter.
    (c) The vermis is the name given to that part joining the cerebellar hemispheres together.
    (d) The cerebellum lies anterior to the fourth ventricle.
    (e) The dentate nucleus is a mass of white matter found in each cerebellar hemisphere.
5. The following statements concern the cerebrum:
    (a) The cerebral hemispheres are separated by a fibrous septum called the tentorium cerebelli.
    (b) The bones of the vault of the skull are named for the lobes of the cerebral hemisphere they lie over.
    (c) The corpus callosum is a mass of gray matter lying within each cerebral hemisphere.
    (d) The internal capsule is an important collection of nerve fibers, which has the caudate nucleus and the thalamus on its medial side and the lentiform nucleus on its lateral side.
    (e) The cavity present within each cerebral hemisphere is called the cerebral ventricle.
6. The following statements concern the peripheral nervous system:
    (a) There are 10 pairs of cranial nerves.
    (b) There are 8 pairs of cervical spinal nerves.
    (c) The posterior root of a spinal nerve contains many efferent motor nerve fibers.
    (d) A spinal nerve is formed by the union of an anterior and a posterior ramus in an intervertebral foramen.
    (e) A posterior root ganglion contains the cell bodies of autonomic nerve fibers leaving the spinal cord.
7. The following statements concern the central nervous system:
    (a) A computed tomography (CT) brain scan cannot distinguish between white matter and gray matter.
    (b) The lateral ventricles are in direct communication with the fourth ventricle.
    (c) A magnetic resonance imaging (MRI) of the brain uses the magnetic properties of the hydrogen nucleus excited by radiofrequency radiation transmitted by a coil surrounding the patient's head.
    (d) Following trauma and sudden movement of the brain within the skull, the large arteries at the base of the brain are commonly torn.
    (e) The movement of the brain at the time of head injuries is unlikely to damage the small 6th cranial nerve.
8. The following statements concern the cerebrospinal fluid (CSF):
    (a) The CSF in the central canal of the spinal cord is unable to enter the fourth ventricle.
    (b) With the patient in the recumbent position, the normal pressure is about 60 to 150 mm of water.
    (c) It plays only a minor role in the protection of the brain and spinal cord from traumatic injury.
    (d) Compression of the internal jugular veins in the neck lowers the CSF pressure.
    (e) The subdural space is filled with CSF.
9. The following statements concern the vertebral levels and the spinal cord segmental levels:
    (a) The 1st lumbar vertebra lies opposite the L3–L4 segments of the cord.
    (b) The 3rd thoracic vertebra lies opposite the 3rd thoracic spinal cord segment.
    (c) The 5th cervical vertebra lies opposite the 7th cervical spinal cord segment.
    (d) The 8th thoracic vertebra lies opposite the 9th thoracic spinal cord segment.
    (e) The 3rd cervical vertebra lies opposite the 4th cervical spinal cord segment.

Directions: Each case history is followed by questions. Select the ONE BEST lettered answer.

A 23-year-old woman was unconscious when admitted to the emergency department. While crossing the road, she had been hit on the side of the head by a bus. Within an hour, she was found to have a large, dough-like swelling over the right temporal region. She also had signs of muscular paralysis on the left side of the body. A lateral radiograph of the skull showed a fracture line running downward and forward across the anterior–inferior angle of the right parietal bone. Her coma deepened, and she died 5 hours after the accident.

10. Select the most likely cause of the swelling over the right temporal region in this patient.
    (a) Superficial bruising of the skin
    (b) Hemorrhage from a blood vessel in the temporalis muscle
    (c) Rupture of the right middle meningeal vessels
    (d) Edema of the skin
    (e) Hemorrhage from a blood vessel in the superficial fascia

11. Select the most likely cause of the muscular paralysis of the left side of the body in this patient.
    (a) Laceration of the right side of the cerebral hemisphere
    (b) Right-sided epidural hemorrhage
    (c) Left-sided epidural hemorrhage
    (d) Injury to the cerebral cortex on the left side of the brain
    (e) Injury to the right cerebellar hemisphere

A 69-year-old man was admitted to the neurology unit complaining of severe discomfort of the lower back. Radiologic examination of the lumbar region of the vertebral column revealed significant narrowing of the spinal canal caused by advanced osteoarthritis.

12. Explain the discomfort in the lower back experienced by this patient.
    (a) Muscle fatigue
    (b) Prolapsed intervertebral disc
    (c) Torn ligament in the joints of the lumbar region of the spine
    (d) Compression of the cauda equina
    (e) Bad posture

Later, in this same patient, the back pain became more severe and now radiated down the back of the left leg; the patient was also experiencing difficulty walking. Examination of the patient revealed weakness and some wasting of the muscles of the left leg. Radiologic examination showed that the osteoarthritic changes had spread to involve the boundaries of many of the lumbar intervertebral foramina.

13. Explain the change in the symptoms and signs found in this patient.
    (a) The sciatic nerve was compressed in the pelvis by a spreading rectal cancer.
    (b) The patient had developed advanced atherosclerosis of the arteries of the right lower limb.
    (c) The osteoarthritic process had produced osteophytes that encroached on the intervertebral foramina, compressing the segmental spinal nerve roots.
    (d) Neuritis had developed in the sciatic nerve trunk.
    (e) The patient was experiencing psychiatric problems.

 Answers and Explanations to Review Questions

1. C is correct. Anterior and posterior roots of a single spinal nerve are attached to a single spinal cord segment. A. The spinal cord has an outer covering of white matter and an inner core of gray matter (see Fig. 1-5). B. The spinal cord tapers off below to form the conus medullaris. D. The cells in the posterior gray horn of the spinal cord are associated with sensory function (see p. 139). E. The central canal of the spinal cord is situated in the gray commissure (see Fig. 1-6).

2. E is correct. The lower end of the medulla oblongata is directly continuous with the spinal cord in the foramen magnum (see Fig. 1-4). A. The medulla oblongata is conical in shape (see Fig. 1-8). B. The medulla oblongata has the fourth ventricle lying posterior to its upper part. C. The medulla oblongata has the pons directly continuous with its upper border. D. The medulla oblongata has a central canal in its lower part that is continuous with that of the spinal cord.

3. A is correct. The midbrain has a cavity called the cerebral aqueduct. B. The midbrain is of small size (see Fig. 1-1). C. The midbrain is completely surrounded with CSF in the subarachnoid space (see Fig. 1-2A). D. The midbrain has a cavity called the cerebral aqueduct, which opens above into the third ventricle (see Fig. 1-10). E. The midbrain is located in the posterior cranial fossa.

4. C is correct. The vermis is the name given to that part of the cerebellum joining the cerebellar hemispheres together (see Fig. 6-2). A. The cerebellum lies in the posterior cranial fossa (see Fig. 1-7). B. The cerebellar cortex is composed of gray matter (see Fig. 1-10). D.

The cerebellum lies posterior to the fourth ventricle (see Fig. 1-10). E. The dentate nucleus is a mass of gray matter found in each cerebellar hemisphere (see Fig. 6-7).

5. D is correct. The internal capsule is an important collection of ascending and descending nerve fibers, which has the caudate nucleus and the thalamus on its medial side and the lentiform nucleus on its lateral side (see Fig. 1-13). A. The cerebral hemispheres are separated by a vertical, sagittally placed fibrous septum called the falx cerebri. The tentorium cerebelli is horizontally placed and roofs over the posterior cranial fossa and separates the cerebellum from the occipital lobes of the cerebrum (see Fig. 15-1). B. The lobes of the cerebral hemisphere are named for the skull bones they lie under. C. The corpus callosum is a mass of white matter lying within each cerebral hemisphere (see Fig. 1-10). E. The cavity present within each cerebral hemisphere is called the lateral ventricle.

6. B is correct. There are 8 pairs of cervical spinal nerves (only 7 cervical vertebrae). A. There are 12 pairs of cranial nerves. C. The posterior root of a spinal nerve contains afferent nerve fibers. D. A spinal nerve is formed by the union of an anterior and a posterior root in an intervertebral foramen. E. A posterior root ganglion contains the cell bodies of sensory nerve fibers entering the spinal cord.

7. C is correct. An MRI of the brain uses the magnetic properties of the hydrogen nucleus excited by radiofrequency radiation transmitted by a coil surrounding the patient's head (see p. 23). A. A CT brain

scan can distinguish between white and gray matter (see Fig. 1-22). B. The lateral ventricles communicate indirectly with the fourth ventricle through the interventricular foramen, the third ventricle, and the cerebral aqueduct of the midbrain (see Fig. 1-10). D. Following trauma and sudden movement of the brain within the skull, the large arteries at the base of the brain are rarely torn. E. The movement of the brain at the time of head injuries may stretch and damage the small delicate 6th cranial nerve (the small 4th cranial nerve may also be injured).

8. B is correct. With the patient in the recumbent position, the normal pressure of CSF is 60 to 150 mm of water. A. The CSF in the central canal of the spinal cord is able to enter the fourth ventricle through the central canal of the lower part of the medulla oblongata (see Fig. 1-2A). C. The CSF is important in protecting the brain and spinal cord from traumatic injury by dissipating the force (compare with the role of the amniotic fluid in protecting the fetus in the pregnant uterus). D. Compression of the internal jugular vein in the neck raises the CSF pressure by inhibiting its absorption into the venous system. E. The subarachnoid space is filled with CSF; the potential subdural space contains only tissue fluid.

9. E is correct. The 3rd cervical vertebra lies opposite the 4th cervical spinal cord segment (see Table 1-3, p. 16). A. The 1st lumbar vertebra lies opposite the sacral and coccygeal spinal cord segments. B. The 3rd thoracic vertebra lies opposite the 5th thoracic spinal cord segment. C. The 5th cervical vertebra lies opposite the 6th cervical spinal cord segment. D. The 8th thoracic vertebra lies opposite the 11th thoracic spinal cord segment.

10. C is correct. The swelling over the right temporal region and the radiologic finding of a linear fracture over the anterior–inferior angle of the right parietal bone would strongly suggest that the right middle meningeal artery had been damaged and an epidural (extradural) hemorrhage had occurred. Blood had spread through the fracture line into the overlying temporalis muscle and soft tissue.

11. B is correct. The left-sided paralysis (left hemiplegia) was due to pressure exerted by the right-sided epidural hemorrhage on the precentral gyrus of the right cerebral hemisphere.

12. D is correct. In persons in whom the spinal canal was originally small, significant narrowing of the canal in the lumbar region can lead to neurologic compression of the cauda equina with pain radiating to the back, as in this patient.

13. C is correct. One of the complications of osteoarthritis of the vertebral column is the growth of osteophytes, which commonly encroach on the intervertebral foramina, causing pain along the distribution of the segmental nerve. In this patient, the segmental nerves L4–L5 and S1–S3, which form the important sciatic nerve, were involved. This would explain the pain radiating down the left leg and the atrophy of the leg muscles.

2 Neurons and Neuroglia

CHAPTER OBJECTIVES

- To define the neuron and name its processes
- To learn the varieties of neurons and identify them in different parts of the nervous system
- To review the cell biology of a neuron and understand the function of a nerve cell and its processes
- To review the structure of the plasma membrane as it is related to its physiology
- To learn the transport of materials from the cell body to the axon terminals
- To understand the structure and function of synapses and neurotransmitters
- To review the supporting function of the neuroglial cells for nerve cells and the possible role that they play in neuronal metabolism, function, and neuronal death

A 38-year-old man with a history of involuntary movements, personality changes, and mental deterioration is referred to a neurologist. The symptoms started insidiously 8 years ago and are getting progressively worse. The first symptoms are involuntary, abrupt, and purposeless movements of the upper limbs associated with clumsiness and dropping things. At presentation, the patient has difficulty walking, speaking, and swallowing. Associated with these movement defects are memory impairment and loss of intellectual capacity. Impulsive behavior and bouts of depression also occur. Close questioning of the patient and his wife reveals that the patient's father and his older brother had similar symptoms before they died. A diagnosis of Huntington disease is made.

Huntington disease is an autosomal-dominant disorder with the defect localized to the short arm of chromosome 4. Histologically, the caudate nucleus and the putamen show extensive degeneration, mainly involving the acetylcholine and γ-aminobutyric acid (GABA)-producing neurons; the dopamine neurons are unaffected. Secondary degeneration of the cerebral cortex also occurs. This case is an example of a hereditary disorder that mainly involves a particular group of neurons.

The purpose of this chapter is to help students understand how the basic excitable cell—the neuron—communicates with other neurons. It also considers certain injuries to the neuron and the effects of drugs on the mechanism by which neurons communicate with one another.

NEURONS

Neuron is the name given to the nerve cell and all its processes (Fig. 2-1). Neurons are excitable cells that are specialized for the reception of stimuli and the conduction of the nerve impulse. They vary considerably in size and shape, but each possesses a **cell body** from which one or more processes called **neurites** project (Fig. 2-2). Neurites responsible for receiving information and conducting it toward the cell body are **dendrites**. The single long tubular neurite that conducts impulses away from the cell body is the **axon**. Dendrites and axons are commonly referred to as **nerve fibers**.

Neurons are found in the brain and spinal cord and in ganglia. Unlike most other cells in the body, normal neurons in the mature individual do not undergo division and replication.

Neuron Types

Although the cell body of a neuron may be as small as 5 μm or as large as 135 μm in diameter, the processes or neurites may extend over a distance of more than 1 m. Neurons can be classified morphologically based on the number, length, and mode of branching of their neurites (Fig. 2-3).

Unipolar neurons have a single neurite that divides a short distance from the cell body into two branches, one proceeding to some peripheral structure and the other entering the central nervous system (CNS). The

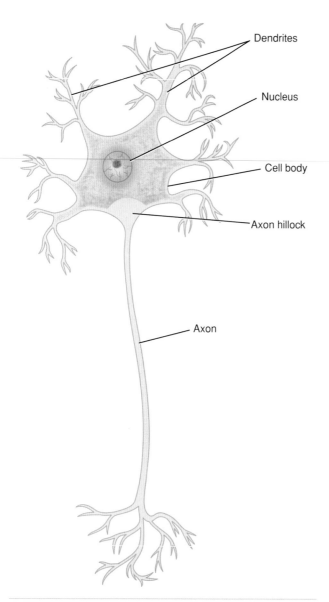

Dendrites

Nucleus

Cell body

Axon hillock

Axon

Figure 2-1   A neuron.

Figure 2-2   Photomicrograph of a smear preparation of the spinal cord showing a neuron with its cell body and its processes or neurites.

branches of this single neurite have the structural and functional characteristics of an axon. In this type of neuron, the fine terminal branches found at the peripheral end of the axon at the receptor site are often referred to as the dendrites. Examples of this form of neuron are found in the posterior root ganglion.

Bipolar neurons have an elongated cell body, with a single neurite emerging from each end. Examples of this type of neuron are found in the retinal bipolar cells and the cells of the sensory cochlear and vestibular ganglia.

Multipolar neurons have a number of neurites arising from the cell body. With the exception of the long process, the axon, the remainder of the neurites are dendrites. Most neurons of the brain and spinal cord are of this type.

Neurons may also be classified according to size. **Golgi type I neurons** have a long axon that can stretch

1 m or more in length in extreme cases (Figs. 2-4 to 2-6). The axons of these neurons form the long fiber tracts of the brain and spinal cord and the nerve fibers of peripheral nerves. The pyramidal cells of the cerebral cortex, the Purkinje cells of the cerebellar cortex, and the motor cells of the spinal cord are good examples.

Golgi type II neurons have a short axon that terminates in the neighborhood of the cell body or is entirely absent (Figs. 2-5 and 2-6). They greatly outnumber the Golgi type I neurons. The short dendrites that arise from these neurons give them a star-shaped appearance. These neurons are numerous in the cerebral and cerebellar cortex and are often inhibitory in function. Table 2-1 summarizes neuronal classification.

Neuronal Structure

A neuron's cell body, like that of other cells, consists essentially of a mass of cytoplasm in which a nucleus is embedded (Figs. 2-7 and 2-8), bounded externally by a plasma membrane.

Nerve Cell Body

Interestingly, the volume of cytoplasm within the nerve cell body is often far less than the total volume of cytoplasm in the neurites. The cell bodies of the small

Figure 2-3 The classification of neurons according to the number, length, and mode of branching of the neurites.

Figure 2-4 Photomicrograph of a silver-stained section of the cerebellar cortex showing two Purkinje cells. These are examples of Golgi type I neurons. De, dendrite; PC, Purkinje cell; N, Nucleus. (From Gartner, L. P. (2018). *Color atlas and text of histology* (7th ed). Baltimore, MD: Wolters Kluwer.)

Figure 2-5 Photomicrograph of a silver-stained section of the cerebral cortex. Note the presence of large pyramidal cells, which are examples of Golgi type I neurons, and numerous Golgi type II neurons. (From Bear, M. F., Connors, B. W., & Paradiso, M. A. (2016). *Neuroscience: Exploring the brain* (4th ed). Baltimore, MD: Wolters Kluwer.)

Stellate cell—
cerebellar cortex

Granule cell—
cerebellar cortex

Lower motor neuron—
spinal cord

Pyramidal cell
(upper motor neuron)—
cerebral cortex

Purkinje cell—
cerebellar cortex

Figure 2-6 Different types of neurons.

Table 2-1   Neuron Classification

Morphologic Classification	Arrangement of Neurites	Location
Number, Length, and Mode of Branching of Neurites		
Unipolar	Single neurite divides a short distance from cell body	Posterior root ganglion
Bipolar	Single neurite emerges from either end of cell body	Retina, sensory cochlea, and vestibular ganglia
Multipolar	Many dendrites and one long axon	Fiber tracts of brain and spinal cord, peripheral nerves, and motor cells of spinal cord
Size of Neuron		
Golgi type I	Single long axon	Fiber tracts of brain and spinal cord, peripheral nerves, and motor cells of spinal cord
Golgi type II	Short axon that with dendrites resembles a star	Cerebral and cerebellar cortex

granular cells of the cerebellar cortex measure about 5 μm in diameter, whereas those of the large anterior horn cells may measure as much as 135 μm in diameter. The main structures of a nerve cell body are summarized in Table 2-2.

Nucleus

The nucleus, which stores the genes, is commonly centrally located within the cell body and is typically large and rounded. Do not confuse the term *nucleus* in cytology with the term *nucleus* in neuroanatomy, which refers to a discrete group of nerve cell bodies in the CNS. In mature neurons, the chromosomes no longer duplicate themselves and function only in gene expression. Therefore, the chromosomes are not arranged as compact structures but exist in an uncoiled state. Thus, the nucleus is pale, and the fine chromatin granules are widely dispersed (Figs. 2-6 and 2-7).

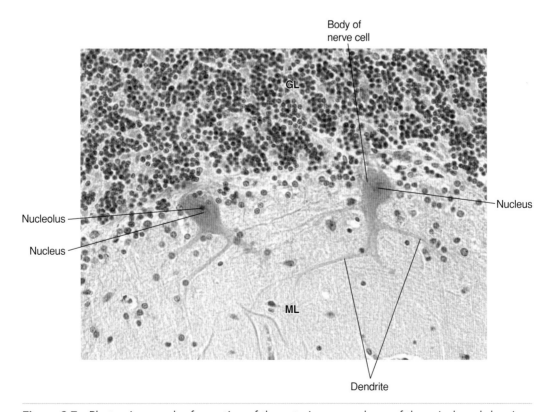

Figure 2-7 Photomicrograph of a section of the anterior gray column of the spinal cord showing two large motor nerve cells with nuclei. Note the prominent nucleolus in one of the nuclei. GL, granular layer; ML, molecular layer.

Figure 2-8 Diagrammatic representation of the fine structure of a neuron.

A single prominent nucleolus synthesizes ribosomal ribonucleic acid (rRNA) and assists with ribosome subunit assembly. The large size of the nucleolus probably is due to the high rate of protein synthesis, which is necessary to maintain the protein level in the large cytoplasmic volume that is present in the long neurites as well as in the cell body.

In the female, one of the two X chromosomes is compact and is known as the **Barr body**. It is composed of sex chromatin and sits at the inner surface of the nuclear envelope.

The **nuclear envelope** (Fig. 2-9; also see Fig. 2-8) is continuous with the cytoplasmic rough, or granular, endoplasmic reticulum (RER). The envelope is double layered and possesses fine **nuclear pores**, through which materials can diffuse into and out of the nucleus. Therefore, the substance in the nucleus and the cytoplasm can be considered as functionally continuous. Newly formed ribosomal subunits can be passed into the cytoplasm through the nuclear pores.

Cytoplasm

The cytoplasm is rich in rough (granular) and smooth (agranular) endoplasmic reticulum (Fig. 2-10; also see Fig. 2-9) and contains the following organelles and inclusions: (a) Nissl substance; (b) the Golgi complex; (c) mitochondria; (d) microfilaments; (e) microtubules; (f) lysosomes; (g) centrioles; and (h) lipofuscin, melanin, glycogen, and lipid.

Nissl substance consists of granules that are distributed throughout the cytoplasm of the cell body, except for the region close to the axon, called the **axon hillock** (Fig. 2-11). The granular material also extends into the proximal parts of the dendrites but is not present in the axon.

Electron micrographs show that the Nissl substance is composed of RER (Fig. 2-12) arranged in the form of broad cisternae stacked one on top of the other. Although many of the ribosomes are attached to the surface of the endoplasmic reticulum, many more lie free in the intervals between the cisternae. Because the ribosomes

Table 2-2   Main Structures in a Nerve Cell Body

Structure	Shape	Appearance	Location	Function
Nucleus	Large, rounded	Pale, chromatin widely scattered; single prominent nucleolus; Barr body present in female	Centrally placed, displaced to periphery in cell injury	Controls cell activity
Cytoplasmic organelles Nissl substance	Granules of rough endoplasmic reticulum	Broad cisternae; ribosomes are basophilic	Throughout cytoplasm and proximal part of dendrites, absent from axon hillock and axon, fatigue and injury result in concentration at periphery	Synthesizes protein
Golgi complex	Wavy threads; clusters of flattened cisternae and small vesicles	Smooth endoplasmic reticulum	Close to the nucleus	Adds carbohydrate to protein molecule; packages products for transport to nerve terminals; forms cell membranes
Mitochondria	Spherical, rod shaped	Double membrane with cristae	Scattered	Form chemical energy
Neurofibrils	Linear fibrils	Run parallel to each other; composed bundles of microfilaments, each 10 nm in diameter	Run from dendrites through cell body to axon	Determines the shape of the neuron
Microfilaments	Linear fibrils	Filaments 3–5 nm in diameter	Form a dense network beneath the plasma membrane	Role in formation and retraction of cell processes and in cell transport
Microtubules	Linear tubes	Run between neurofibrils, 25 nm in diameter	Run from dendrites through cell body to axon	Cell transport
Lysosomes	Vesicles	Diameter = 8 nm; three forms: primary, secondary, and residual bodies	Throughout cell	Cell scavengers
Centrioles	Paired hollow cylinders	Wall made up of bundles of microtubules	Confined to cytoplasm of cell body	Take part in cell division; maintain microtubules
Lipofuscin	Granules	Yellowish brown	Scattered through cytoplasm	Metabolic by product
Melanin	Granules	Yellowish brown	Substantia nigra of midbrain	Related to formation of dopamine

contain RNA, the Nissl substance is basophilic and can be well demonstrated by staining with toluidine blue or other basic aniline dyes (Fig. 2-11) and using the light microscope.

The Nissl substance is responsible for synthesizing protein, which flows along the dendrites and the axon and replaces the proteins that are broken down during cellular activity. Fatigue or neuronal damage causes the Nissl substance to move and become concentrated at the periphery of the cytoplasm. This phenomenon, which gives the impression that the Nissl substance has disappeared, is known as **chromatolysis**.

The **Golgi complex**, when seen with the light microscope after staining with a silver-osmium method, appears as a network of irregular wavy threads around the nucleus. In electron micrographs, it appears as clusters of flattened cisternae and small vesicles made up of smooth endoplasmic reticulum (SER) (Figs. 2-8 and 2-9).

The protein produced by the Nissl substance is transferred to the inside of the Golgi complex in transport

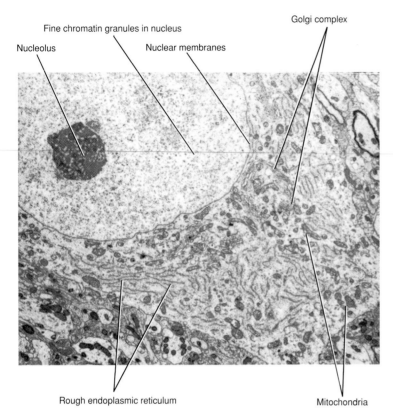

Nucleolus

Fine chromatin granules in nucleus

Nuclear membranes

Golgi complex

Rough endoplasmic reticulum

Mitochondria

Figure 2-9 Electron micrograph of a neuron showing the structure of the nucleus and a number of cytoplasmic organelles. (Courtesy Dr. J. M. Kerns.)

Cytoplasm of neuron

Nucleus

Plasma membrane

Nuclear membranes

Rough endoplasmic reticulum

Figure 2-10 Electron micrograph of a neuron showing nuclear and plasma membranes and cytoplasmic organelles. (Courtesy Dr. J. M. Kerns.)

Nissl substance

Axon hillock

Figure 2-11 Photomicrograph of a section of the anterior gray column of the spinal cord stained with toluidine blue. Note the presence of dark-staining Nissl substance in the cytoplasm of four neurons.

vesicles, where it is temporarily stored and where carbohydrate may be added to the protein to form glycoproteins. The proteins are believed to travel from one cisterna to another via transport vesicles. Each cisterna of the Golgi complex is specialized for different types of enzymatic reaction. At the *trans* side of the complex, the macromolecules are packaged in vesicles for transport to the nerve terminals. The Golgi complex is also thought to be active in lysosome production and in the synthesis of cell membranes. The latter function

is particularly important in the formation of synaptic vesicles at the axon terminals.

Mitochondria are found scattered throughout the cell body, dendrites, and axons (Figs. 2-8 and 2-9). They are spherical or rod shaped. In electron micrographs, the walls show a characteristic double membrane. The inner membrane is thrown into folds or cristae that project into the center of the mitochondrion. Mitochondria possess many enzymes, which are localized chiefly on the inner mitochondrial membrane. These enzymes

Nissl substance

Nissl substance

Figure 2-12 Electron micrograph of the cytoplasm of two neurons showing the structure of Nissl bodies (substance). (Courtesy Dr. J. M. Kerns.)

Figure 2-13 Photomicrograph of a silver-stained section of a neuron showing the presence of large numbers of neurofibrils in the cytoplasm of the cell body and the neurites.

take part in the tricarboxylic acid cycle and the cytochrome chains of respiration. Therefore, mitochondria are important in nerve cells, as in other cells, in the production of energy.

Neurofibrils, as seen with the light microscope after staining with silver, are numerous and run parallel to each other through the cell body into the neurites (Fig. 2-13). With the electron microscope, the neurofibrils resolve into bundles of **neurofilaments**—each filament measuring about 10 nm in diameter (Fig. 2-14). The neurofilaments form the main component of the cytoskeleton. Chemically, neurofilaments are very stable and belong to the cytokeratin family.

Microfilaments measure about 3 to 5 nm in diameter and are formed of actin. Microfilaments are concentrated at the periphery of the cytoplasm just beneath the plasma membrane where they form a dense network. Together with microtubules, microfilaments play a key role in the formation of new cell processes and the retraction of old ones. They also assist the microtubules in axon transport.

Microtubules are similar to those seen in other types of cells. They measure about 25 nm in diameter and are found interspersed among the neurofilaments (Fig. 2-14). They extend throughout the cell body and its processes. In the axon, all the microtubules are arranged in parallel, with one end pointing to the cell body and the other end pointing distally away from the cell body.

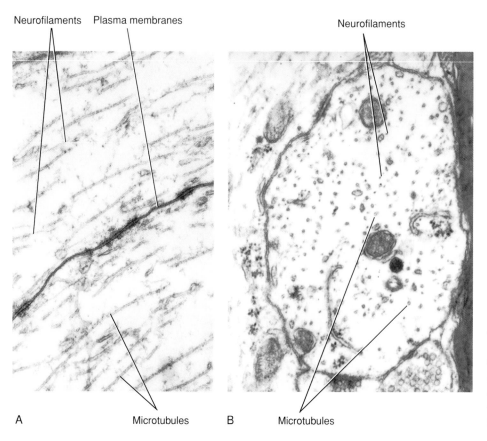

Figure 2-14 Electron micrograph of dendrites showing the presence of neurofilaments and microtubules within their cytoplasm. **A:** Longitudinal section of two adjacent dendrites. **B:** Transverse section of a dendrite. (Courtesy Dr. J. M. Kerns.)

Microtubules and microfilaments provide a stationary track that permits specific organelles to move by molecular motors. The stop-and-start movement is caused by the periodic dissociation of the organelles from the track or the collision with other structures.

Cell transport involves the movement of membrane organelles, secretory material, synaptic precursor membranes, large dense core vesicles, mitochondria, and SER.

Cell transport can take place in both directions in the cell body and its processes. **Rapid transport** (100 to 400 mm/day) is mediated by two motor proteins associated with the microtubule adenosine triphosphate (ATP)-ase sites. In *anterograde* (away from the cell) movement, **kinesin**-coated organelles are thought to move toward one end of the tubule, and, in *retrograde* (toward the cell) movement, dynein-coated organelles are thought to move toward the other end of the tubule. The direction and speed of the movement of an organelle can be brought about by the activation of one of the motor proteins or of both simultaneously.

Slow transport (0.1 to 3.0 mm/day) involves the bulk movement of the cytoplasm and includes the movement of mitochondria and other organelles. Slow axonal transport occurs only in the anterograde direction. The molecular motor has not been identified but is probably one of the kinesin families.

Lysosomes are membrane-bound vesicles measuring about 8 nm in diameter. They serve the cell by acting as intracellular scavengers and contain hydrolytic enzymes. They are formed by the budding off of the Golgi apparatus. Lysosomes exist in three forms: (1) **primary lysosomes**, which have just been formed; (2) **secondary lysosomes**, which contain partially digested material (myelin figures); and (3) **residual bodies**, in which the enzymes are inactive and the bodies have evolved from digestible materials such as pigment and lipid.

Centrioles are small, paired structures found in immature dividing nerve cells. Each centriole is a hollow cylinder whose wall is made up of microtubule bundles. They are associated with the formation of the spindle during cell division and in the formation of microtubules. Centrioles are also found in mature nerve cells, where they are likely involved in the maintenance of microtubules.

Lipofuscin (pigment material) occurs as yellowish-brown granules within the cytoplasm (Fig. 2-15). It probably forms as the result of lysosomal activity, and it represents a harmless metabolic byproduct. Lipofuscin accumulates with age.

Melanin granules are found in the cytoplasm of cells in certain parts of the brain (e.g., the substantia nigra of the midbrain). Their presence may be related to the catecholamine-synthesizing ability of these neurons, whose neurotransmitter is dopamine.

Plasma Membrane

The plasma membrane forms the continuous external boundary of the cell body and its processes, and, in the neuron, it is the site for the initiation and conduction of the nerve impulse (Figs. 2-10 and 2-14). The membrane is about 8 nm thick, which is too thin to be seen with the light microscope. When viewed under the electron

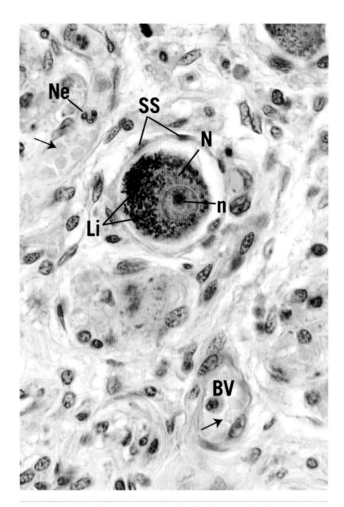

Figure 2-15 Photomicrograph of a longitudinal section of a posterior root ganglion showing the presence of lipofuscin granules within the cytoplasm of sensory neurons. Ne, neutrophil; arrow, red blood cell; SS, satellite cells; N, nucleus; n, nucleolus; Li, lipofuscin; BV, blood vessel.(From Gartner, L. P. (2018). *Color atlas and text of histology* (7th ed). Baltimore, MD: Wolters Kluwer.)

microscope, the plasma membrane appears as two dark lines with a light line between them.

The plasma membrane is composed of an inner and an outer layer of very loosely arranged protein molecules, each layer being about 2.5 nm thick, separated by a middle layer of lipid about 3 nm thick. The lipid layer is made up of two rows of phospholipid molecules arranged so that their hydrophobic ends are in contact with each other and their polar ends are in contact with the protein layers. Certain protein molecules lie within the phospholipid layer and span the entire width of the lipid layer. These molecules provide the membrane with hydrophilic channels through which inorganic ions may enter and leave the cell. Carbohydrate molecules are attached to the outside of the plasma membrane and are linked to the proteins or the lipids, forming what is known as the **cell coat** or **glycocalyx**.

The plasma membrane and the cell coat together form a semipermeable membrane that allows diffusion of certain ions through it but restricts others. In the

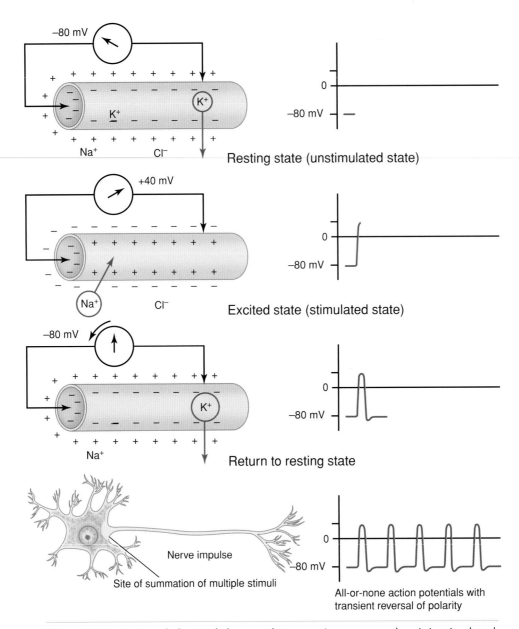

Figure 2-16 Ionic and electrical changes that occur in a neuron when it is stimulated.

resting state (unstimulated state), K⁺ ions diffuse through the plasma membrane from the cell cytoplasm to the tissue fluid (Fig. 2-16). The permeability of the membrane to K⁺ ions is much greater than that to Na⁺ ions; thus, the passive efflux of K⁺ is much greater than the influx of Na⁺. This results in a steady potential difference of about 280 mV, which can be measured across the plasma membrane because the inside of the membrane is negative with respect to the outside. This potential is known as the **resting potential**.

Membrane Excitation and Conduction

In the resting unstimulated state, a nerve fiber is polarized so that the interior is negative to the exterior; the potential difference across the plasma membrane (axolemma) is about –80 mV and is called the **resting membrane potential** (Fig. 2-17).

When the nerve cell is excited (stimulated) by electrical, mechanical, or chemical means, a rapid change in membrane permeability to Na⁺ ions takes place, and Na⁺ ions diffuse through the plasma membrane into the cell cytoplasm from the tissue fluid. This results in the membrane becoming progressively depolarized. The sudden influx of Na⁺ ions followed by the altered polarity produces an **action potential** (**AP**), which is approximately 140 mV. This potential is very brief, lasting about 5 msec. The increased membrane permeability for Na⁺ ions quickly ceases, and membrane permeability for K⁺ ions increases. Therefore, K⁺ ions start to flow from the cell cytoplasm and return the localized area of the cell to the resting state.

A nerve impulse (**AP**) starts at the initial segment of the axon and is a self-propagating wave of electrical negativity that passes rapidly along the surface of

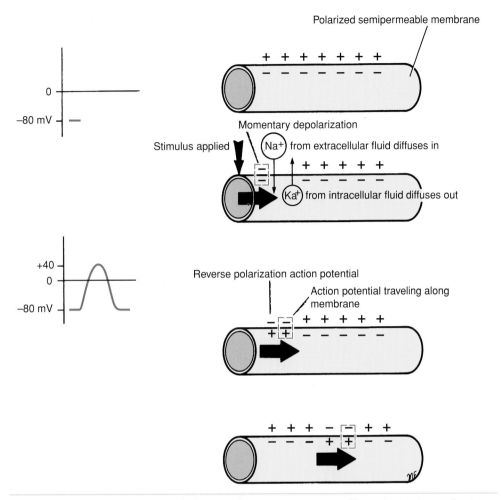

Polarized semipermeable membrane

0

−80 mV

Momentary depolarization

Stimulus applied

Na⁺ from extracellular fluid diffuses in

Ka⁺ from intracellular fluid diffuses out

+40
0
−80 mV

Reverse polarization action potential

Action potential traveling along membrane

Figure 2-17 Ionic and electrical changes that occur in a nerve fiber when it is conducting an impulse.

the axolemma. Once generated, the AP spreads away from the site of initiation and is conducted along neurites as the **nerve impulse**. The wave of electrical negativity is initiated by an adequate stimulus being applied to the surface of the neuron (Fig. 2-18). Under normal circumstances, this occurs at the initial segment of the axon, which is the most sensitive part of the neuron. The stimulus alters the permeability of the membrane to Na⁺ ions at the point of stimulation. Now, Na⁺ ions rapidly enter the axon (Fig. 2-17). The positive ions outside the axolemma quickly decrease to zero. Therefore, the membrane potential is reduced to zero and is said to be **depolarized**. A typical resting potential is −80 mV, with the outside of the membrane positive to the inside; the AP is about 140 mV, with the outside of the membrane negative to the inside. In small-diameter axons, the AP may not rise to as much as 40 mV.

The negatively charged point on the outside of the axolemma now acts as a stimulus to the adjacent positively charged axolemma, and, in less than 1 msec, the polarity of the adjacent resting potential is reversed. The AP now has moved along the axolemma from the point originally stimulated to the adjacent point on the

membrane. In this manner, the AP travels along the full length of a nerve fiber to its end.

As the AP moves along the nerve fiber, entry of the Na⁺ ions into the axon ceases, and the permeability of the axolemma to K⁺ ions increases. Now, K⁺ ions rapidly diffuse outside the axon because the concentration is much higher within the axon than outside so that the original resting membrane potential is restored. The permeability of the axolemma now decreases, and the status quo is restored by the active transport of the Na⁺ ions out of the axon and the K⁺ ions into the axon. The outer surface of the axolemma is again electrically positive compared with that of the inner surface. This is a simplistic description of the movements of the Na⁺ and K⁺ ions. (For further details on the voltage-gated Na⁺ and K⁺ channels, the Na⁺ and K⁺ pumps, and the Na⁺ and K⁺ leak channels, refer to a textbook of physiology.)

For a short time after the passage of a nerve impulse along a nerve fiber, while the axolemma is still depolarized, a second stimulus, however strong, is unable to excite the nerve. This period of time is called the **absolute refractory period**. The underlying reason for the refractory period is that the Na⁺ channels become inactivated, and no stimulation, however strong, will

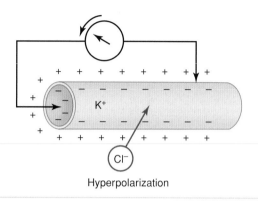

Figure 2-19 Ionic and electrical changes that occur in a neuron during hyperpolarization.

Figure 2-18 Creation of the action potential by the arrival of a stimulus from a single presynaptic terminal. Note that the action potential generated at the initial segment will only occur if the threshold for excitation is reached at the initial segment. (From Snell, R. S. *Clinical neuroanatomy: A review with questions and explanations* (3rd ed., p. 7). Baltimore, MD: Lippincott Williams & Wilkins.)

open the Na⁺ gates. This period is followed by a further short interval during which the excitability of the nerve gradually returns to normal. This latter period is called the **relative refractory period**. Therefore, the refractory period makes a continuous excitatory state of the nerve impossible and limits the frequency of the impulses.

The greater the strength of the initial stimulus, the larger the initial depolarization and the greater will be the spread into the surrounding areas of the plasma membrane. Multiple excitatory stimuli applied to a neuron's surface result in **summation**. For example, subthreshold stimuli may pass over the surface of the cell body and be summated at the origin of the axon and so initiate an AP. Inhibitory stimuli are believed to produce their effect by causing an influx of Cl⁻ ions through the plasma membrane into the neuron, thus producing hyperpolarization and reducing the excitatory state of the cell (Fig. 2-19).

The **conduction velocity** of a nerve fiber is proportional to the cross-sectional area of the axon, with the thicker fibers conducting more rapidly than those of smaller diameter. In the large motor fibers (α fibers), the rate may be as high as 70 to 120 m/s; the smaller sensory fibers have slower conduction rates (Table 2-3).

Table 2-3 Classification of Nerve Fibers by Speed of Conduction and Size

Fiber Type	Conduction Velocity (m/s)	Fiber Diameter (μm)	Functions	Myelin	Sensitivity to Local Anesthetics
A Fibers					
α	70–120	12–20	Motor, skeletal muscle	Yes	Least
β	40–70	5–12	Sensory, touch, pressure, vibration	Yes	
γ	10–50	3–6	Muscle spindle	Yes	
δ	6–30	2–5	Pain (sharp, localized), temperature, touch	Yes	
B Fibers	3–15	≤3	Preganglionic autonomic	Yes	
C Fibers	0.5–2.0	0.4–1.2	Pain (diffuse, deep), temperature, postganglionic autonomic	No	Most

Figure 2-20 Electrical changes that occur in stimulated myelinated axon (saltatory conduction) (**A**) and stimulated nonmyelinated axon (**B**).

In nonmyelinated fibers, the AP passes continuously along the axolemma, progressively exciting neighboring areas of membrane (Fig. 2-20). In myelinated fibers, the presence of a myelin sheath serves as an insulator, and few ions can flow through the sheath. Consequently, a myelinated nerve fiber can be stimulated only at the nodes of Ranvier, where the axon is naked and the ions can pass freely through the plasma membrane between the extracellular fluid and the axoplasm. In these fibers, the AP jumps from one node to the next. The AP at one node sets up a current in the surrounding tissue fluid, which quickly produces depolarization at the next node. This leaping of the AP from one node to the next is referred to as **saltatory conduction**. This is a more rapid mechanism than is found in nonmyelinated fibers (120.0 m/s in a large myelinated fiber compared with 0.5 m/s in a very small unmyelinated fiber).

Sodium and Potassium Channels

Sodium and potassium channels, through which the sodium and potassium ions diffuse through the plasma membrane, are formed of the protein molecules that extend through the full thickness of the plasma membrane (Fig. 2-21). Why a particular channel permits the passage of K^+ ions while excluding Na^+ ions is difficult to explain. The selectivity cannot be due to the diameter of the ions, insofar as the K^+ ion is larger than the Na^+ ion. However, the movement of ions in solution depends not only on the size of the ion but also on the size of the

shell of water surrounding it. K^+ ions have weaker electric fields than Na^+ ions; thus, K^+ ions attract less water than Na^+ ions. Therefore, K^+ ions behave as if they are smaller than Na^+ ions. However, this physicochemical explanation does not entirely account for why a channel is selective. The channels may have narrow regions along their length that act as sieves or molecular filters. The ions may also participate in electrostatic interactions with the amino acid residues lining the walls of the channel.

Ion channel proteins are relatively stable, but they exist in at least two conformational states, open and closed functional states. The mechanism responsible for the opening and closing of a channel is not understood but can be thought of as a gate. **Gating** may involve the twisting and distortion of the channel, thus creating a wider or narrower lumen. Gating appears to occur in response to such stimuli as voltage change, the presence of a ligand, or stretch or pressure.

In the nonstimulated state, potassium channel gates are open wider than sodium channel gates, which are nearly closed. This permits the K^+ ions to diffuse out of the cell cytoplasm more readily than the Na^+ ions can diffuse in. In the stimulated state, the sodium channel gates are at first wide open; then, the potassium channel gates are opened, and the sodium channel gates are nearly closed again. The opening and closing of these channels is thought to produce the depolarization and repolarization of the plasma membrane.

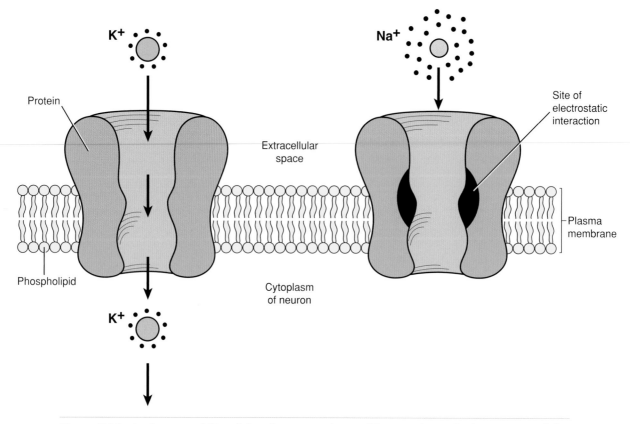

Figure 2-21   Ionic permeability of the plasma membrane. Diagram shows the interactions of the ions with water, the membrane lipid bilayer, and the ion channels.

Nerve Cell Processes

Neurites—the processes of a nerve cell—may be divided into dendrites and an axon.

Dendrites are the short processes of the cell body (Fig. 2-22). Their diameter tapers as they extend from the cell body, and they often branch profusely. In many neurons, the finer branches bear large numbers of small projections called **dendritic spines**. The cytoplasm of the dendrites closely resembles that of the cell body and contains Nissl granules, mitochondria, microtubules, microfilaments, ribosomes, and SER. Dendrites are extensions of the cell body to increase the surface area for the reception of axons from other neurons. Essentially, they conduct the nerve impulse toward the cell body.

During early embryonic development, dendrites are overproduced. Later, they are reduced in number and size in response to altered functional demand from afferent axons. Evidence shows that dendrites remain plastic throughout life and elongate and branch or contract in response to afferent activity.

The **axon** is the longest process of the cell body. It arises from a small conical elevation on the cell body, devoid of Nissl granules, called the **axon hillock** (Fig. 2-23; also see Fig. 2-8). Occasionally, an axon arises from the proximal part of a dendrite. An axon is tubular and is uniform in diameter; it tends to have a smooth surface.

Axons usually do not branch close to the cell body; collateral branches may occur along their length. Shortly before their termination, axons commonly branch profusely. The distal ends of the terminal branches of the axons are often enlarged; they are called **terminals** (Fig. 2-24). Some axons (especially those of autonomic nerves) show a series of swellings resembling a string of beads near their termination; these swellings are called **varicosities**.

Axons may be very short (0.1 mm), as seen in many neurons of the CNS, or extremely long (3.0 m), as seen when they extend from a peripheral receptor in the skin of the toe to the spinal cord and thence to the brain.

Axon diameter varies considerably with different neurons. Those of larger diameter conduct impulses rapidly, and those of smaller diameter conduct impulses very slowly.

The plasma membrane bounding the axon is called the **axolemma**; the cytoplasm of the axon is the **axoplasm**. Unlike the cytoplasm of the cell body, axoplasm lacks Nissl granules and a Golgi complex. The sites for the production of protein, namely RNA and ribosomes, are absent. Thus, axonal survival depends on the transport of substances from the cell bodies.

The **initial segment** of the axon is the first 50 to 100 μm after it leaves the axon hillock of the nerve cell body (Fig. 2-23). This is the most excitable part of the axon and is the site at which an AP originates.

Figure 2-22 **A:** Light photomicrograph of a motor neuron in the anterior gray column of the spinal cord showing the nerve cell body, two dendrites, and the surrounding neuropil. **B:** Electron micrograph of a dendrite showing axodendritic synapses. (Courtesy Dr. J. M. Kerns.)

Remember that, under normal conditions, an AP does not originate on the plasma membrane of the cell body but, instead, always at the initial segment.

An axon always conducts impulses away from the cell body. The axons of sensory posterior root ganglion cells are an exception; here, the long neurite, which is indistinguishable from an axon, carries the impulse toward the cell body. (See unipolar neurons, p. 33.)

Axon Transport

Materials are transported from the cell body to the axon terminals (**anterograde transport**) and to a lesser extent in the opposite direction (**retrograde transport**).

Fast anterograde transport of 100 to 400 mm/day refers to the transport of proteins and transmitter substances or their precursors. **Slow anterograde transport** of 0.1 to 3.0 mm/day refers to the transport

of axoplasm and includes the microfilaments and microtubules.

Retrograde transport explains how the cell bodies of nerve cells respond to changes in the distal end of the axons. For example, activated growth factor receptors can be carried along the axon to their site of action in the nucleus. Pinocytotic vesicles arising at the axon terminals can be quickly returned to the cell body. Worn-out organelles can be returned to the cell body for breakdown by the lysosomes.

Axon transport is brought about by microtubules assisted by the microfilaments.

Synapses

The nervous system consists of a large number of neurons that are linked together to form functional

Axon hillock

Initial segment of axon

Microtubules

Figure 2-23 Electron micrograph of a longitudinal section of a neuron from the cerebral cortex showing the detailed structure of the region of the axon hillock and the initial segment of the axon. Note the absence of Nissl substance (rough endoplasmic reticulum) in the axon hillock and the presence of numerous microtubules in the axoplasm. Note also the axon terminals (*arrows*) forming axoaxonal synapses with the initial segment of the axon. (Courtesy Dr. A. Peters.)

conducting pathways. The site where two neurons (or a neuron and a skeletal muscle or gland cell) come into close proximity and functional interneuronal communication occurs is referred to as a **synapse** (Fig. 2-25). Most neurons may make synapse with 1,000 or more other neurons and may receive up to 10,000 connections from other neurons. Communication at a synapse, under physiologic conditions, takes place in one direction only. Synapses occur in a number of forms. The most common type is that which occurs between an axon of one neuron and the dendrite or cell body of the second neuron. As the axon approaches the synapse, it may have a terminal expansion (bouton terminal), or it may have a series of expansions (bouton de passage), each of which makes synaptic contact. In other types

of synapses, the axon synapses on the initial segment of another axon—that is, proximal to where the myelin sheath begins—or synapses may exist between terminal expansions from different neurons. Depending on the site of the synapse, they are referred to as **axodendritic**, **axosomatic**, or **axoaxonic**.

How an axon terminates varies considerably in different parts of the nervous system. For example, a single axon may terminate on a single neuron, or a single axon may synapse with multiple neurons, as in the case of the parallel fibers of the cerebellar cortex synapsing with multiple Purkinje cells. In the same way, a single neuron may have synaptic junctions with axons of many different neurons. The arrangement of these synapses will determine the means by which a neuron can

Axon containing large number of presynaptic vesicles

Terminal expansion of axon (bouton terminal)

Axodendritic synapse

Dendrite

Axodendritic synapses

Figure 2-24   Electron micrograph showing multiple axodendritic synapses. Note the presence of large numbers of presynaptic vesicles within the axons. The definition has come to include the site at which a neuron comes into close proximity with a skeletal muscle cell and functional communication occurs. (Courtesy Dr. J. M. Kerns.)

be stimulated or inhibited. **Synaptic spines**, extensions of the surface of a neuron, form receptive sites for synaptic contact with afferent boutons.

Synapses are of two types: chemical and electrical. Most synapses are chemical, in which a chemical substance, the **neurotransmitter**, passes across the narrow space between the cells and becomes attached to a protein molecule in the postsynaptic membrane called the **receptor**.

In most chemical synapses, several neurotransmitters may be present. One neurotransmitter is usually the principal activator and acts directly on the postsynaptic membrane, while the other transmitters function as modulators and modify the activity of the principal transmitter.

Chemical Synapses

On examination with an electron microscope, synapses are seen to be areas of structural specialization (Fig. 2-26; also see Fig. 2-24). The apposed surfaces of the terminal axonal expansion and the neuron are called the **presynaptic** and **postsynaptic membranes**, respectively, and they are separated by a **synaptic cleft** measuring about 20 to 30 nm wide. The presynaptic and postsynaptic membranes are thickened, and the adjacent underlying cytoplasm shows increased density. On the presynaptic side, the dense cytoplasm is broken up into groups; on the postsynaptic side, the density often extends into a **subsynaptic web**. **Presynaptic vesicles**, mitochondria, and occasional lysosomes are present in the cytoplasm close to the presynaptic membrane (see Fig. 2-26). On the postsynaptic side, the cytoplasm often contains parallel cisternae. The synaptic cleft contains polysaccharides.

The presynaptic terminal contains many small presynaptic vesicles that contain the molecules of the neurotransmitter(s). The vesicles fuse with the presynaptic membrane and discharge the neurotransmitter(s) into the synaptic cleft by a process of exocytosis (Fig. 2-27).

When synapses are first formed in the embryo, they are recognized as small zones of density separated by a synaptic cleft. Later, they mature into well-differentiated structures. The presence of simple, undifferentiated synapses in the postnatal nervous system has led to the suggestion that synapses can be developed as required and possibly undergo atrophy when redundant. This plasticity of synapses may be of great importance in the process of learning and in the development and maintenance of memory.

Figure 2-25   A–D: Different types of chemical synapses.

Neurotransmitters

Presynaptic vesicles and mitochondria play a key role in the release of neurotransmitter substances at synapses. The vesicles contain the neurotransmitter substance that is released into the synaptic cleft; the mitochondria provide ATP for the synthesis of new transmitter substance.

Most neurons produce and release only one principal transmitter at all their nerve endings. For example, acetylcholine (ACh) is widely used as a transmitter by different neurons in the central and peripheral parts of the nervous system, whereas dopamine is released by neurons in the substantia nigra. Glycine, another transmitter, is found principally in synapses in the spinal cord.

The following chemical substances act as neurotransmitters (many more exist): ACh, norepinephrine, epinephrine, dopamine, glycine, serotonin, GABA, enkephalins, substance P, and glutamic acid.

Note that all skeletal neuromuscular junctions use only ACh as the transmitter, whereas synapses between neurons use a large number of different transmitters.

Axons near termination

Presynaptic vesicles

Dendrite

Terminal expansion of axon

Mitochondria

Synaptic sites

Microtubules interspersed among microfilaments

Figure 2-26 High-power electron micrograph of axodendritic synapses showing the thickening of the cell membranes at the synaptic sites, presynaptic vesicles, and the presence of mitochondria within the axons near their termination. (Courtesy Dr. J. M. Kerns.)

NEUROTRANSMITTER ACTION

All neurotransmitters are released from their nerve endings by the arrival of the nerve impulse (AP). This results in an influx of Ca^{2+} ions, which causes the synaptic vesicles to fuse with the presynaptic membrane. The neurotransmitters are then ejected into the extracellular fluid in the synaptic cleft. Once in the cleft, they diffuse across the gap to the postsynaptic membrane. There they achieve their objective by raising or lowering the resting potential of the postsynaptic membrane for a brief period of time.

The receptor proteins on the postsynaptic membrane bind the transmitter substance and undergo an immediate conformational change that opens the ion channel, generating an immediate but brief excitatory postsynaptic potential (EPSP) or an inhibitory postsynaptic potential (IPSP). The rapid excitation is seen with ACh (nicotinic) and L-glutamate, or the inhibition is seen with GABA (Table 2-4). Other receptor proteins bind the transmitter substance and activate a second-messenger system, usually through a molecular transducer, a G protein. These receptors have a longer latent period, and the duration of the response may last several minutes or longer. ACh (muscarinic), serotonin, histamine, neuropeptides, and adenosine are good examples of this type of transmitter, which is often referred to as a neuromodulator (see next section, Neuromodulators).

The excitatory and the inhibitory effects on the postsynaptic membrane of the neuron will depend on the summation of the postsynaptic responses at the different synapses. If the overall effect is one of depolarization, the neuron will be excited, an AP will be initiated at the initial segment of the axon, and a

Acetylcholine

Site of acetylcholinesterase

A

Catecholamines

Take-up process

B

Figure 2-27 Release of neurotransmitters. **A:** Acetylcholine. **B:** Catecholamines.

Table 2-4 Examples of Principal (Classic) Neurotransmitters and Neuromodulators at Synapses

Neuromediators[a]	Function	Receptor Mechanism	Ionic Mechanism	Location
Principal Neurotransmitters				
ACh (nicotinic), L-glutamate	Rapid excitation	Ion channel receptors	Opens cation channel (fast EPSP)	Main sensory and motor systems
GABA	Rapid inhibition		Opens anion channel for Cl⁻ (fast IPSP)	
Neuromodulators				
ACh (muscarinic), serotonin, histamine, adenosine	Modulation and modification of activity	G protein–coupled receptors	Opens or closes K^+ or Ca^{2+} channels (slow IPSP and slow EPSP)	Systems that control homeostasis

[a]Note that these are only a few examples of an ever-increasing number of known neuromediators.
ACh, acetylcholine; GABA, γ-aminobutyric acid; EPSP, excitatory postsynaptic potential; IPSP, inhibitory postsynaptic potential.

nerve impulse will travel along the axon. If, on the other hand, the overall effect is one of hyperpolarization, the neuron will be inhibited and no nerve impulse will arise.

NEUROTRANSMITTER DISTRIBUTION AND FATE
The distribution of the neurotransmitters varies in different parts of the nervous system. **ACh**, for example, is found at the neuromuscular junction, in autonomic ganglia, and at parasympathetic nerve endings. In the CNS, the motor neuron collaterals to the **Renshaw cells** are cholinergic. In the hippocampus, the ascending reticular pathways, and the afferent fibers for the visual and auditory systems, the neurotransmitters are also cholinergic.

Norepinephrine is found at sympathetic nerve endings. In the CNS, it is found in high concentration in the hypothalamus. **Dopamine** is found in high concentration in different parts of the CNS, such as in the basal nuclei (ganglia).

The effect produced by a neurotransmitter is limited by its destruction or reabsorption. For example, in the case of ACh, the effect is limited by the destruction of the transmitter in the synaptic cleft by the enzyme **acetylcholinesterase (AChE)** (Fig. 2-27). However, with the **catecholamines**, the effect is limited by the return of the transmitter to the presynaptic nerve ending.

Neuromodulators

Interestingly, in many synapses, certain substances other than the principal neurotransmitters are ejected from the presynaptic membrane into the synaptic cleft. These substances are capable of modulating and modifying the activity of the postsynaptic neuron and are called **neuromodulators**.

NEUROMODULATOR ACTION
Neuromodulators can coexist with the principal neurotransmitter at a single synapse. Usually, but not always, the neuromodulators are in separate presynaptic vesicles. Although the principal neurotransmitters have a rapid, brief effect on the postsynaptic membrane

on release into the synaptic cleft, neuromodulators do not have a direct effect on the postsynaptic membrane. Rather, they enhance, prolong, inhibit, or limit the principal neurotransmitter's effect on the postsynaptic membrane. Neuromodulators act through a second-messenger system, usually through a molecular transducer, such as a G protein, and alter the response of the receptor to the neurotransmitter. In a given area of the nervous system, many different afferent neurons can release several different neuromodulators that affect the postsynaptic neuron. Such an arrangement can lead to a wide variety of responses, depending on input from the afferent neurons.

Electrical Synapses

Electrical synapses are gap junctions containing channels that extend from the cytoplasm of the presynaptic neuron to that of the postsynaptic neuron: They are rare in the human CNS. The neurons communicate electrically; a chemical transmitter is not present. The bridging channels permit ionic current flow to take place from one cell to the other with a minimum of delay. In electrical synapses, the rapid spread of activity from one neuron to another ensures that a group of neurons performing an identical function act together. Electrical synapses also have the advantage that they are bidirectional; chemical synapses are not.

NEUROGLIA

The neurons of the CNS are supported by several varieties of nonexcitable cells, which together are called **neuroglia** (Fig. 2-28). Neuroglial cells are generally smaller than neurons and outnumber them by 5 to 10 times; they comprise about half the total volume of the brain and spinal cord.

The four types of neuroglial cells are (1) astrocytes, (2) oligodendrocytes, (3) microglia, and (4) ependyma. A summary of the structural features, location, and functions of the different neuroglial cells is provided in Table 2-5.

Figure 2-28 Diagrammatic representation of the arrangement of different types of neuroglial cells.

Labels in figure: Ependyma, Fibrous astrocyte, Protoplasmic astrocyte, Neuron, Capillary, Oligodendrocyte, Outer glial limiting membrane, Microglial cell, Cells of pia mater

Astrocytes

Astrocytes have small cell bodies with branching processes that extend in all directions. The two types of astrocytes include fibrous and protoplasmic.

Fibrous astrocytes are found mainly in the white matter, where their processes pass between the nerve fibers (Fig. 2-29). Each process is long, slender, smooth, and not much branched. The cell bodies and processes contain many filaments in their cytoplasm.

Protoplasmic astrocytes are found mainly in the gray matter, where their processes pass between the nerve cell bodies (Figs. 2-30 and 2-31). The processes are shorter, thicker, and more branched than those of the fibrous astrocyte, and their cytoplasm contains fewer filaments.

Many of the processes of astrocytes end in expansions on blood vessels (perivascular feet), where they form an almost complete covering on the external surface of capillaries. Large numbers of astrocytic processes are interwoven at the outer and inner surfaces of the CNS, where they form the **outer** and **inner glial limiting membranes**. Thus, the outer glial limiting membrane is found beneath the pia mater, and the inner glial limiting membrane lies beneath the ependyma lining the ventricles of the brain and the central canal of the spinal cord.

Astrocytic processes are also found in large numbers around the initial segment of most axons and in the bare segments of axons at the nodes of Ranvier. Axon terminals at many sites are separated from other nerve cells and their processes by an envelope of astrocytic processes.

Astrocyte Functions

Astrocytes, with their branching processes, form a supporting framework for the nerve cells and nerve fibers. Their processes are functionally coupled at gap junctions. In the embryo, they serve as a scaffolding

Table 2-5   Structural Features, Location, and Functions of Neuroglial Cells

Neuroglial Cell	Structure	Location	Function
Astrocytes			
Fibrous	Small cell bodies, long slender processes, cytoplasmic filaments, perivascular feet	White matter	Provide supporting framework, are electrical insulators, limit spread of neurotransmitters, take up K⁺ ions
Protoplasmic	Small cell bodies, short thick processes, many branches, few cytoplasmic filaments, perivascular feet	Gray matter	Store glycogen, have a phagocytic function, take place of dead neurons, are a conduit for metabolites or raw materials, produce trophic substances
Oligodendrocytes	Small cell bodies, few delicate processes, no cytoplasmic filaments	In rows along myelinated nerves, surrounding neuron cell bodies	Form myelin in CNS, influence biochemistry of neurons
Microglia	Smallest of neuroglial cells, wavy branches with spines	Scattered throughout CNS	Are inactive in normal CNS, proliferate in disease and phagocytosis, joined by blood monocytes
Ependyma			
Ependymocytes	Cuboidal or columnar in shape with cilia and microvilli, gap junctions	Line ventricles, central canal	Circulate CSF, absorb CSF
Tanycytes	Long basal processes with end feet on capillaries	Line floor of third ventricle	Transport substances from CSF to hypophyseal–portal system
Choroidal epithelial cells	Sides and bases thrown into folds, tight junctions	Cover surfaces of choroid plexuses	Produce and secrete CSF

CNS, central nervous system; CSF, cerebrospinal fluid.

Figure 2-29 A: Photomicrograph of a section of the gray matter of the spinal cord showing fibrous astrocytes. **B:** Electron micrograph showing an astrocyte. (Courtesy Dr. J. M. Kerns.)

Figure 2-30 Photomicrograph of a protoplasmic astrocyte in the cerebral cortex.

for the migration of immature neurons. By covering the synaptic contacts between neurons, they may serve as electrical insulators preventing axon terminals from influencing neighboring and unrelated neurons. They may even form barriers for the spread of neurotransmitter substances released at synapses. Astrocytes have been shown to be affected by GABA and glutamic acid secreted by the nerve terminals, thereby limiting the influence of these neurotransmitters. Astrocytes appear to be able to take up excess K^+ ions from the extracellular space so that they may have an important function during repetitive firing of a neuron. They store glycogen within their cytoplasm. The glycogen can be broken down into glucose and even further into lactate, both of which are released to surrounding neurons in response to norepinephrine.

Astrocytes may serve as phagocytes by taking up degenerating synaptic axon terminals. Following the death of neurons due to disease, astrocytes proliferate and fill in the spaces previously occupied by the neurons, a process called **replacement gliosis**. Astrocytes possibly serve as a conduit for the passage of metabolites or raw materials from blood capillaries to the neurons through their perivascular feet. Because astrocytes are linked together by gap junctions, they enable ions to pass from one cell to another without entering the extracellular space. Astrocytes may produce substances that have a trophic influence on neighboring neurons. Recent research has suggested that astrocytes secrete cytokines that regulate the activity of immune

Nucleus of astrocyte

Cell membrane

Dendrite

Golgi apparatus

Cytoplasm of astrocyte

Figure 2-31 Electron micrograph of a protoplasmic astrocyte in the cerebral cortex. (Courtesy Dr. A. Peters.)

Oligodendrocytes

A   B

Figure 2-32   A: Photomicrograph of a group of oligodendrocytes. **B:** Electron micrograph of two oligodendrocytes. (Courtesy Dr. J. M. Kerns.)

cells entering the nervous system in disease. Finally, astrocytes play an important role in the structure of the blood–brain barrier. Here, the astrocyte processes terminate as expanded feet at the basement membrane of blood vessels.

Oligodendrocytes

Oligodendrocytes have small cell bodies and a few delicate processes; their cytoplasm does not contain filaments. Oligodendrocytes are found in rows along myelinated nerve fibers and surround nerve cell bodies (Fig. 2-32). Electron micrographs show the processes of a single oligodendrocyte joining the myelin sheaths of several nerve fibers (Fig. 2-33). However, only one process joins the myelin between two adjacent nodes of Ranvier.

Oligodendrocyte Functions

Oligodendrocytes are responsible for the formation of the myelin sheath of nerve fibers in the CNS, much as the myelin of peripheral nerves is formed from Schwann cells. This formation and maintenance of myelin around many CNS axons provides them with an insulating coat

and greatly increases the speed of nerve conduction along them (see p. 47). Because oligodendrocytes have several processes, unlike Schwann cells, they can each form several internodal segments of myelin on the same or different axons. A single oligodendrocyte can form as many as 60 internodal segments. Note that, unlike Schwann cells in the peripheral nervous system (PNS), oligodendrocytes and their associated axons are *not* surrounded by a basement membrane. Myelination begins at about the 16th week of intrauterine life and continues postnatally until practically all the major nerve fibers are myelinated by the time the child is walking.

Oligodendrocytes also surround nerve cell bodies (satellite oligodendrocytes) and probably have a similar function to the satellite or capsular cells of peripheral sensory ganglia. They are thought to influence the biochemical environment of neurons.

Microglia

The microglial cells are embryologically unrelated to the other neuroglial cells and are derived from macrophages outside the nervous system. They are the

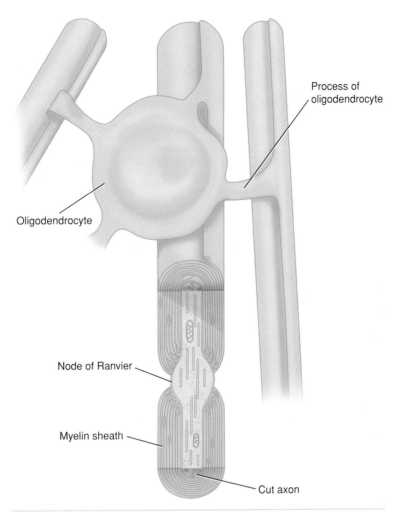

Process of
oligodendrocyte

Oligodendrocyte

Node of Ranvier

Myelin sheath

Cut axon

Figure 2-33   A single oligodendrocyte whose processes are continuous with the myelin sheaths of four nerve fibers within the central nervous system.

smallest of the neuroglial cells and are found scattered throughout the CNS (Fig. 2-34). Wavy branching processes arise from their small cell bodies that give off numerous spinelike projections. They closely resemble connective tissue macrophages. They migrate into the nervous system during fetal life. Microglial cells increase in number in the presence of damaged nervous tissue resulting from trauma and ischemic injury and in the presence of diseases including Alzheimer disease, Parkinson disease, multiple sclerosis, and AIDS. Many of these new cells are monocytes that have migrated from the blood.

Microglia Function

Microglial cells in the normal brain and spinal cord appear to be inactive and are sometimes called **resting microglial cells**. In inflammatory disease of the CNS, they become the immune effector cells. They retract their processes and migrate to the site of the lesion. Here, they proliferate and become antigen-presenting cells, which, together with the invading T lymphocytes, confront invading organisms. They are also actively phagocytic; their cytoplasm becomes filled with lipids and cell remnants. The microglial cells are joined by monocytes from neighboring blood vessels.

Ependyma

Ependymal cells line the cavities of the brain and the central canal of the spinal cord. They form a single layer of cells that are cuboidal or columnar in shape and possess microvilli and cilia (Fig. 2-35). The cilia are often motile, and their movements contribute to the flow of the cerebrospinal fluid (CSF). The bases of the ependymal cells lie on the internal glial limiting membrane.

Ependymal cells can be divided into three groups:

1. **Ependymocytes** line the ventricles of the brain and the central canal of the spinal cord and are in contact with the CSF. Their adjacent surfaces have gap junctions, but the CSF is in free communication with CNS intercellular spaces.
2. **Tanycytes** line the floor of the third ventricle overlying the median eminence of the hypothalamus.

Nucleus of microglial cell

Neuron

Golgi apparatus

Lipofuscin granules

Cytoplasm of microglial cell

Figure 2-34 Electron micrograph of a microglial cell in the cerebral cortex. (Courtesy Dr. A. Peters.)

These cells have long basal processes that pass between the cells of the median eminence and place endfeet on blood capillaries.

3. **Choroidal epithelial cells** cover the surfaces of the choroid plexuses. The sides and bases of these cells are thrown into folds; near their luminal surfaces, the cells are held together by tight junctions that encircle the cells. The presence of tight junctions prevents the leakage of CSF into the underlying tissues.

Ependymal Cell Functions

Ependymocytes assist in CSF circulation within the cavities of the brain and the central canal of the spinal cord by the movements of the cilia. The microvilli on the free surfaces of the ependymocytes indicate that they also have an absorptive function. Tanycytes are thought to transport chemical substances from the CSF to the hypophyseal portal system. In this manner, they may play a part in the control of the hormone production by the anterior lobe of the pituitary. Choroidal epithelial cells are involved in the production and secretion of CSF from the choroid plexuses.

EXTRACELLULAR SPACE

When nervous tissue is examined under an electron microscope, a very narrow gap separates the neurons and the neuroglial cells. These gaps are linked together and filled with tissue fluid; they are called the **extracellular space**. The extracellular space is in almost direct continuity with the CSF in the subarachnoid space externally and with the CSF in the ventricles of the brain and the central canal of the spinal cord internally. The extracellular space also surrounds the blood capillaries in the brain and spinal cord. (The CNS does not have lymphatic capillaries.)

The extracellular space thus provides a pathway for the exchange of ions and molecules between the blood and the neurons and glial cells. The plasma membrane of the endothelial cells of most capillaries is impermeable to many chemicals, and this forms the blood–brain barrier.

A

Cilia

Cavity of central canal of spinal cord

Processes of ependymal cells

Nuclei of ependymal cells

B   Microvilli

Cilia

Tight junctions

Cavity of ventricle

Ependymal cells

Figure 2-35   A: Photomicrograph of ependymal cells lining the central canal of the spinal cord. **B:** Electron micrograph of ependymal cells lining the cavity of the third ventricle. (Courtesy Dr. J. M. Kerns.)

Clinical Notes

General Considerations

The neuron is the basic functional unit of the nervous system. In the mature human, if it is destroyed by trauma or disease, it is not replaced. It is incapable of undergoing cell division.

The neuron consists of the cell body and its processes, the axons, and the dendrites. All three parts are concerned with the process of conduction. The cell body is necessary for the normal metabolism of all its processes. Should these processes become separated from the cell body as the result of disease or simple trauma, they will quickly degenerate. This would explain the necessity for the transport of macromolecules down the axon from the cell body and also emphasizes the dependence of the axon on the cell body. The rate of axoplasmic transport is insufficient to satisfy the release of transmitter substances at the nerve terminals. This problem is resolved in two ways. First, enzymes are present within the nerve terminals in order to synthesize the transmitters from amino acids derived from the extracellular fluid, and second, at some terminals, the transmitter is reabsorbed back into the terminal following its release. Clinically, drugs can influence this reuptake mechanism.

Neuroglial cells, in contrast to neurons, are nonexcitable and do not have axons; furthermore, axon terminals do not synapse on them. They are smaller than neurons and yet outnumber them 5 to 10 times. They comprise about half the total volume of the central nervous system (CNS).

Neuronal Reaction to Injury

The first reaction of a nerve cell to injury is loss of function. Whether the cell recovers or dies will depend on the severity and duration of the damaging agent. If death occurs quickly, such as in a few minutes from lack of oxygen, no morphologic changes would be immediately apparent. Morphologic evidence of cell injury requires a minimum of 6 to 12 hours of survival. The nerve cell becomes swollen and rounded off, the nucleus swells and is displaced toward the cell periphery, and the Nissl granules become dispersed toward the cytoplasm periphery. At this stage, the neuron could recover. If the kind of neuronal injury were not so severe as to cause death, the reparative changes would start to appear. The cell would resume its former size and shape, the nucleus would return to the center of the cell body, and the Nissl granules would take up their normal position.

When cell death is imminent or has just occurred, the cell cytoplasm stains dark with basic dyes (hyperchromatism), and the nuclear structure becomes unclear. The final stage occurs after cell death. The cytoplasm becomes vacuolated, and the nucleus and cytoplasmic organelles disintegrate. The neuron now is dissolved and removed by the activity of the phagocytes. In the CNS, this function is performed by the microglial cells; in the peripheral nervous system (PNS), this function is performed by local members of the reticuloendothelial system.

In chronic forms of injury, the size of the cell body is reduced, the nucleus and cytoplasm show hyperchromatism, and the nuclear membranes and those of the cytoplasmic organelles show irregularity.

Axonal Reaction and Axonal Degeneration

Axonal reaction and axonal degeneration are the changes that take place in a nerve cell when its axon is cut or injured. The changes start to appear within 24 to 48 hours after injury; the degree of change will depend on the severity of the injury to the axon and will be greater if the injury occurred close to the cell body. The nerve cell becomes rounded off and swollen, the nucleus swells and becomes eccentrically placed, and the Nissl granules disperse toward the cytoplasm periphery. These changes reach their maximum in about 12 days.

In the PNS, section of an axon is followed by attempts at regeneration, and reparative changes take place in the cell body.

In the CNS, degeneration is not followed by regeneration. If the corticospinal tracts, for example, are destroyed by disease, the nerve cells that give rise to these axons degenerate and disappear completely.

An important exception to the axonal reaction of nerve cells described above occurs in the nerve cells of the posterior root ganglia of the spinal nerves. If the peripheral axons are sectioned, the nerve cells show degenerative changes; if, however, the central axons are sectioned or destroyed by disease, such as tabes dorsalis, the nerve cells show no degenerative changes.

Axonal Transport and Disease Spread

Rabies, which is an acute viral disease of the CNS, is transmitted by the bite of an infected animal. The virus is present in the saliva of the infected animal; following a bite, it travels to the CNS by way of axonal transport in both sensory and motor nerves. The incubation period is related to the length of the peripheral nerve involved. The longer the nerve, the longer the duration of the incubation period. **Herpes simplex** and **herpes zoster** are viral diseases that also involve axonal transport to spread to different parts of the body. Axonal transport is also believed to play a role in the spread of the **poliomyelitis** virus from the gastrointestinal tract to the motor cells of the anterior gray horns of the spinal cord and the brainstem.

Neuron Tumors

Recall that the nervous system is made up of many different types of tissues: neurons, neuroglia, blood vessels, and meninges in the CNS and neurons, Schwann cells, connective tissue, and blood vessels in the PNS. Tumors of neurons in the CNS are rare, but tumors of peripheral neurons are not uncommon.

Neuroblastoma occurs in association with the suprarenal gland; it is highly malignant and occurs in infants and children. **Ganglioneuroma** occurs in the suprarenal medulla or sympathetic ganglia; it is benign and occurs in children and adults. **Pheochromocytoma** occurs in the suprarenal medulla; it is usually benign and gives rise to hypertension because it secretes norepinephrine and epinephrine.

Synaptic Blocking Agents

Transmission of a nervous impulse across a synapse is accomplished by the release of neurotransmitters into the synaptic cleft. Transmission occurs in one direction, and subthreshold stimulation of many synapses leads to summation. The released transmitter then exerts its effect on the postsynaptic membrane by increasing the permeability of the postsynaptic membrane to sodium and causing excitation or by increasing the permeability of the postsynaptic membrane to chloride and causing inhibition.

The synapse is a region in which transmission is easily blocked. As a general rule, long chains of neurons with multiple synapses are more easily blocked than shorter, simpler chains of neurons. General anesthetic agents are effective because they have the ability to block synaptic transmission.

At autonomic ganglia, preganglionic fibers enter the ganglia and synapse with the postganglionic sympathetic or parasympathetic neurons. The nerve impulse, on reaching the termination of the preganglionic nerve, brings about the release of **acetylcholine (ACh)**, which excites a nervous impulse in the postganglionic neuron.

Ganglionic blocking agents may be divided into three groups, depending on their mechanism of action. The first group of agents, which includes the **hexamethonium** and **tetraethylammonium salts**, resembles ACh at the postsynaptic membrane; thus, these agents inhibit transmission across a synapse. The second group of agents, which includes **nicotine**, has the same action as ACh on the postsynaptic membrane, but these agents are not destroyed by the cholinesterase. This results in a prolonged depolarization of the postsynaptic membrane; therefore, it is insensitive to further stimulation by ACh. Unfortunately, this depolarization block is associated with initial stimulation, so these drugs are not suitable for clinical use. The third group of agents, which includes **procaine**, inhibits the release of ACh from the preganglionic fibers.

In the CNS, demonstrating the release of a particular transmitter substance at specific synapses is difficult due to inaccessibility. For example, perfusing specific localized brain areas through their vascular system is impossible, and stimulating an isolated neuronal pathway within the brain or spinal cord is very difficult. The motor neuron collaterals to the Renshaw cells have been shown to liberate ACh at their endings. Many synapses in the CNS are also cholinergic. The development of monoclonal antibody techniques has opened a whole new approach to the identification and localization of chemical mediators in the CNS. Substance P, somatostatin, and cholecystokinin are a few examples of the neuropeptides that have been located here.

The nonuniform concentrations of norepinephrine in the CNS have led many investigators to believe that it might function as a central neurotransmitter. The concentrations are greater in gray matter than in white matter, and the highest concentrations are found in the hypothalamus. Dopamine is found in high concentrations in the CNS and is secreted by neurons that originate in the substantia nigra.

Many of the cholinergic blocking agents used in the PNS have little or no effect on CNS cholinergic synapses because they are unable to cross the blood–brain barrier in significant concentrations. **Atropine, scopolamine,** and **diisopropylphosphorofluoridate** (DPF) can effectively cross the barrier, and their effects on human behavior have been extensively studied. Similarly, many psychotropic drugs are believed to affect CNS activities by influencing the release of catecholamines at synaptic sites. The **phenothiazines**, for example, are thought to block dopamine receptors on postsynaptic neurons.

Treatment of Neurologic Disease by Neurotransmitter Manipulation

The increasing numbers of neurotransmitters being discovered in the CNS and the location of their site of action are raising the possibility that certain diseases can be modified by the administration of specific drugs. Huntington chorea, for example, involves loss of neurons that use GABA and

ACh as transmitters. GABA is unable to cross the blood–brain barrier, but physostigmine, a cholinesterase inhibitor, can cross the barrier, and its use has brought about some improvement. The use of L-dopa in the treatment of parkinsonism has been most successful; in this disease, it replaces the deficiency of dopamine, which is normally released to the basal ganglia by the neurons of the substantia nigra.

Drugs are now rapidly being developed to modify the process of synaptic transmission in a number of ways: (1) by interfering with the process of neurotransmitter synthesis, (2) by inhibiting the uptake of drugs by the postsynaptic membrane, (3) by binding the neurotransmitter at the receptor site on the postsynaptic membrane, and (4) by terminating the neurotransmitter action.

Neuroglial Reactions to Injury

The reaction of neuroglial cells to injury, whether caused by physical trauma or by vascular occlusion, is characterized by the hyperplasia and hypertrophy of the astrocytes, which become fibrous irrespective of their antecedent morphology. The proliferation of the astrocytes is referred to as **astrocytosis** or **gliosis**. The loss of neuronal tissue is not compensated for in volume by the glial hypertrophy. The cytoplasm of the enlarged astrocytes contains large numbers of fibrils and glycogen granules. The dense feltwork of astrocytic processes that occurs in the areas of neuronal degeneration produces the so-called **gliotic scar**. The degree of gliosis is much greater in the presence of residual damaged neuronal tissue as compared with a clean surgical excision in which no traumatized brain remains. This is why, in patients with focal epilepsy due to a large gliotic scar, the scar is excised surgically, leaving a minimal glial reaction.

Oligodendrocytes respond to injury by expanding and showing vacuolation of their cytoplasm; the nuclei also tend to become pyknotic. Severe damage to oligodendrocytes results in demyelination.

Microglial cells in inflammatory and degenerative lesions of the CNS retract their processes and migrate to the site of the lesion. Here, they proliferate and are actively phagocytic, and their cytoplasm becomes filled with lipids and cell remnants. They are joined in their scavenger activity by monocytes that migrate from the neighboring blood vessels.

Microglial cells are active in a number of diseases including multiple sclerosis, dementia in AIDS, Parkinson disease, and Alzheimer disease.

Neuroglia Neoplasms

Tumors of neuroglia account for 40% to 50% of intracranial tumors. Such tumors are referred to as **gliomas**. Tumors of astrocytes are those most commonly encountered and include **astrocytomas** and **glioblastomas**. Apart from the ependymomas, tumors of the neuroglia are highly invasive. This explains the difficulty in achieving complete surgical removal and the great possibility of recurrence after surgery. Another feature is that as these tumors infiltrate, they often do so without interfering with the function of neighboring neurons. As a result, the tumor can be very much larger than the symptoms and physical signs would indicate.

Multiple Sclerosis

Multiple sclerosis is one of the most common CNS diseases, affecting about 250,000 Americans. It is characterized by the appearance of patches of demyelination in CNS white matter, generally starting in the optic nerve, spinal cord, or cerebellum. The myelin sheaths degenerate, and the myelin is removed by microglial cells. Astrocytes proliferate, leading to the formation of a gliotic scar. As demyelination occurs, the conduction of the nerve impulses in the axons is impeded. Because raising the temperature shortens the duration of the action potential, one of the early signs of multiple sclerosis is that the symptoms and signs can be improved by cooling and made worse by heating by a hot bath. Most cases occur between the ages of 20 and 40 years. The cause of the disease is unknown, although an interplay between a viral infection and a host immune response may be responsible. For further discussion of this disease, see Chapter 4.

Cerebral Edema

Cerebral edema is a very common clinical condition that can follow head injuries, cerebral infections, or tumors. The resultant swelling of the brain may lead to flattening of the cerebral gyri, herniation of the brain through the tentorial notch or the foramen magnum, and even death.

Cerebral edema is an abnormal increase in the water content of CNS tissues and takes three forms. **Vasogenic edema** is the most common type and is due to the accumulation of tissue fluid in the extracellular space following damage to the vascular capillary walls or the presence of new capillaries without fully formed blood–brain barriers. It can result from infections, trauma, and tumors. **Cytotoxic edema** is due to the accumulation of fluid within the cells of nervous tissue (neurons and glial), resulting in cellular swelling. The cause may be toxic or metabolic and produces a failure in the plasma membrane ATP sodium pump mechanism. **Interstitial edema** occurs in obstructive hydrocephalus when the rise in cerebrospinal fluid (CSF) pressure forces the fluid out of the ventricular system into the extracellular space.

Two anatomical factors must always be remembered in cerebral edema: (1) the brain volume is restricted by the surrounding skull, and (2) the tissue fluid is drained primarily into the venous sinuses via cerebral veins because there is no lymphatic drainage.

Key Concepts

Neurons

- Neuron is the name given to the nerve cell and all its processes, including the cell body, dendrites, and axon.
- The number, length, and mode of branching allows for a morphologic method of classifying neurons.
- Unipolar neurons are those in which the cell body has a single neurite that divides into two branches, one on a peripheral structure and the other ending in the CNS.
- Bipolar neurons are those in which an elongated cell body has two neurites extending from each end.
- Multipolar neurons have many neurites arising from the cell body, only one of which is the axon.
- The neuron cell body is similar to other cells, consisting of a mass of cytoplasm in which a nucleus is embedded.
- The cytoplasm of a neuron contains Nissl substance, rough-surfaced endoplasmic reticulum arranged in the form of broad, stacked cisternae.
- Staining of the Nissl substance is often used to demonstrate neuronal cell bodies in histologic sections.
- Neurofilaments extend throughout the cell and form the cytoskeleton of the neuron.
- Microfilaments and microtubules are interspersed among the cytoskeleton and provide a stationary track for transport of organelles.

- Motor proteins, kinesin and dynein, move organelles through the neuron in a process called rapid transport.
- The plasma membrane of the cell forms a semipermeable membrane that allows diffusion of certain ions but restricts others, resulting in a steady negative potential inside the cell, compared to outside, called the resting potential.
- Excited cells, either by electrical, mechanical, or chemical means, will undergo a rapid change in permeability causing the negative membrane potential to rapidly depolarize, resulting in an action potential.
- The action potential will spread over the plasma membrane, away from the site of initiation, as a nerve impulse.

Neuroglia

- Neuroglia are small nonexcitable cells that greatly outnumber neurons.
- Neuroglia includes astrocytes, oligodendrocytes, microglia, and ependyma.

Astrocytes

- Fibrous and protoplasmic types form a supporting framework for nerve cells and nerve fibers.
- By covering the synaptic contacts between neurons, astrocytes serve as electrical insulators by preventing neighboring axons from influencing unrelated fibers.

Oligodendrocytes

- Oligodendrocytes are responsible for the formation of the myelin sheath of nerve fibers in the CNS.
- They have multiple processes and insulate fiber segments of multiple nerves.

Microglia

- Smallest of all the neuroglial types, microglia act as immune effector cells during inflammatory diseases.

Ependyma

- Ependyma is a single layer of columnar or cuboidal cells that assist in the circulation of the CSF within the cavities of the brain.
- Ependymocytes and tanycytes line the lateral and third ventricles, respectively. Choroidal epithelial cells cover the surface of the choroid plexus.

 ## Clinical Problem Solving

1. During an operation for the repair of a sectioned radial nerve in the arm, the neurosurgeon understands that he is operating on a large bundle of nerve fibers supported by connective tissue. He realizes that the nerve fibers are either axons or dendrites or the nerve is made up of a mixture of axons and dendrites. What is your understanding of the composition of the radial nerve?

2. A well-known textbook of neurosurgery makes the following statements regarding the prognosis following peripheral nerve repair: (a) the younger the patient, the better the return of function; (b) the more distal the injury to a nerve, the more effective the regeneration; (c) the closer a lesion is to the nerve cell body, the more profound the effect on this trophic center; and (d) sensory nerve cells are affected more by this retrograde phenomenon than are motor nerve cells. Comment on these statements.

3. An 18-year-old male patient is examined by a neurosurgeon, 12 months after injury to the right forearm in which the median nerve is severed. At the initial operation, shortly after the injury has occurred, debridement is performed, and the separated nerve ends are tagged with radiopaque sutures. Unfortunately, the wound is infected, and surgical repair of the nerve is deferred. Is it practical to consider repairing a peripheral nerve after a delay of 12 months?

4. While examining a pathology specimen of nervous tissue under a microscope, the pathologist is able to determine the sex of the individual from whom the tissue had been removed. How would you be able to do this?

5. Axoplasmic flow is involved in the transport of certain viruses in the nervous system. What structures present in the cytoplasm of the neuron take part in this process?

6. About 1% of all deaths are due to intracranial tumors. Many different tissues are present within the skull in addition to the nervous system. Moreover, the nervous system itself is composed of many different types of tissues. In fact, tumors that arise as neoplasms of nerve cells and fibers are rare. Name the different types of tissues that are found in the central nervous system (CNS) and in the peripheral nervous system (PNS).

7. When a nerve cell is stimulated, the permeability of the plasma membrane changes, permitting certain ionic movements to take place across the membrane. (a) What is the structure of the plasma membrane? (b) Is the permeability of the plasma membrane increased or decreased when the nerve cell is stimulated? (c) What is the action of local analgesics on the cell membrane?

8. The synapse is a region where nervous transmission is easily blocked. Clinically, the ganglion-blocking drugs used act by competing with acetylcholine (ACh) released from the nerve endings in the ganglia. Name two groups of drugs that have been used for this purpose and indicate the site at which they act.

9. A 2-year-old boy is taken to a pediatrician because his mother has noticed that his right eye is protruding (proptosis). When questioned, the mother states that she had first noticed this protrusion 1 month previously and that it has progressively worsened since that time. The child is otherwise perfectly fit. On physical examination, the child is observed to be healthy in every respect except for the marked proptosis of the right eye. A careful palpation of the abdomen, however, reveals a large, soft mass in the upper part of the abdomen that extends across the midline. X-ray examination, including a computed tomography (CT) body scan, reveal a large, soft tissue mass that displaces the right kidney downward. A diagnosis of malignant tumor of the suprarenal or neighboring sympathetic nervous tissue, with metastases in the right orbital cavity, is made, the latter being responsible for the right-side proptosis. Name a tumor of the suprarenal gland or sympathetic nervous tissue that occurs commonly in children and may metastasize in the bones of the orbit.

10. At an autopsy, a third-year medical student is handed a slice of the cerebrum and is asked what proportion of central nervous tissue is made up by neuroglia. How would you have answered that question? Which cells are present in the largest numbers—neurons or neuroglial cells?

11. A 23-year-old man received a penetrating gunshot wound to the left side of his head while serving in the army. At the operation, the neurosurgeon was able to remove the bullet from the left frontal lobe of his brain. Apart from a slight weakness of his right leg, the patient makes an uneventful recovery. Eighteen months later, the patient starts to have severe generalized attacks of convulsions, during which he loses consciousness. Since this time, the attacks have occurred irregularly at about monthly intervals. Each attack is preceded by a feeling of mental irritability, and twitching of the right leg occurs. A diagnosis of epilepsy is made by the examining neurologist. Is it possible that this patient's attacks of epilepsy are related to his gunshot wound? Is traumatic epilepsy a common condition? What treatment would you recommend?

12. A 42-year-old woman visits her physician because she is suffering from very severe headaches. Until 6 months ago, she experienced only an occasional mild headache. Since that time, her headaches gradually have become more severe, and their duration has increased. They now last 3 to 4 hours and are so intense that she has to lie down. She has felt sick on two occasions, but she vomited only once. The headaches are generalized in nature and are made worse by coughing or straining. A physical examination reveals swelling of both optic discs with congestion of the retinal veins and the presence of multiple retinal hemorrhages. Weakness of the lateral rectus muscle of the right eye also is detected. Anteroposterior (A/P) radiographs of the skull show displacement of the calcified pineal gland to the left side. A/P and lateral radiographs of the skull show some degree of calcification in a localized area in the right cerebral hemisphere. These findings, together with those obtained from CT scans of the brain and magnetic resonance imaging (MRI), make the diagnosis of a right-sided cerebral tumor certain. Surgical exploration confirms the presence of a large infiltrating tumor of the right parietal lobe. What is the most common type of tumor found in such a site in a middle-aged patient? How would you treat such a patient?

 Answers and Explanations to Clinical Problem Solving

1. The radial nerve is made up of nerve fibers derived from motor, sensory, and autonomic neurons. By definition, the nerve fibers, or nerve cell processes, are referred to as neurites (short ones are dendrites, and long ones are axons). Customarily, those that conduct the nervous impulse toward the cell body are referred to as the dendrites and those that conduct the impulses away from the cell body as the axons. However, in the case of the unipolar sensory neurons found in the posterior root ganglia, the neurite carrying nervous information toward the cell body has all the structural characteristics of an axon and is referred to as an axon. Thus, the radial nerve, which is composed of sensory and motor fibers, is made up of axons.

2. (a) As a general rule, all reparative phenomena throughout the body occur more readily in the young than in the old. (b) As the distal end of a peripheral nerve is approached, fewer branches remain, and thus there are fewer structures yet to innervate; consequently, fewer possibilities exist of nerve fibers innervating the wrong structure during the process of regeneration. Moreover, the more distal the injury, the less the metabolism of the proximal nerve cell body is affected by the injury. (c) This is a physiologic fact. A very severe nerve injury close to its nerve cell body may result in the death of the entire neuron. (d) The physiology of sensory neurons is more susceptible to change by retrograde phenomena than that of motor neurons.

3. If the wound is not infected, the best time to perform a nerve suture is about 3 weeks after the injury.

Satisfactory results have been obtained after a delay of as much as 14 months, provided that paralyzed muscles have not been overstretched and joint adhesions have been avoided by passive movements of the joints. In other words, the neuron still retains the ability to regenerate its processes even after 14 months, but the degree of recovery of function will depend a great deal on the care that the denervated structures receive in the intervening time.

4. In 1949, Barr and Bertram noticed the presence of a small, stainable body of chromatin (Barr body) situated at the inner surface of the nuclear envelope in the female that could not be seen in the cells of the male. It is one of the two X chromosomes present in the female. The presence or absence of the Barr body enables one to readily determine the sex of the individual from whom the tissue was removed.

5. An electron microscope allows visualization of both small tubules that measure about 25 nm in diameter within a neuron's cytoplasm as well as microfilaments measuring about 3 to 5 nm in diameter. The possible role that these structures play in cell transport is discussed on page 43.

6. The CNS comprises (a) neurons, (b) neuroglia, (c) blood vessels, and (d) meninges. The PNS is composed of (a) neurons, (b) Schwann cells, (c) connective tissue, and (d) blood vessels.

7. (a) The structure of the plasma membrane is described on page 43. (b) When a neuron is excited, the permeability of the plasma membrane to Na$^+$ ions is increased, and these diffuse from the tissue fluid

into the neuron cytoplasm. (c) Local analgesics act as membrane stabilizers and inhibit the increase in permeability to Na$^+$ ions in response to stimulation. How this stabilization is brought about is not understood. One theory is that the analgesic agent becomes attached to receptor sites on the protein layer of the plasma membrane, reducing the permeability to Na$^+$ ions and preventing depolarization from taking place. Small-diameter nerve fibers are more readily blocked than large fibers, and nonmyelinated fibers are more readily blocked than myelinated ones. For these reasons, nerve fibers that conduct pain and temperature are most easily blocked, and the large motor fibers are the least easily blocked. The small autonomic nerve fibers are blocked early and account for the rapid appearance of vasodilatation.

8. Tetraethylammonium salts and hexamethonium salts are the two groups of drugs. These salts closely resemble ACh in structure and compete with ACh at the postsynaptic membrane. By this means, they successfully block a ganglion, although the amount of ACh released is unaffected.

9. The neuroblastoma is a tumor of primitive neuroblasts and arises either in the suprarenal medulla or in the upper abdominal sympathetic ganglia. It is malignant and confined to children. The tumor metastasizes early, and the metastasis may be the reason why the child receives medical attention, as in this case. The bones of the orbit are a common site for metastasis of a neuroblastoma.

10. Neuroglia comprises about half the total volume of the central nervous system. Neuroglial cells outnumber neurons by 5 to 10 times.

11. The reaction of tissue of the central nervous system to injury is characterized by astrocyte hyperplasia and hypertrophy. Astrocyte proliferation is referred to as astrocytosis or gliosis. The degree of gliosis is much greater in the presence of residual damaged brain tissue than with a clean surgical incision. The resulting scar tissue, the gliotic scar, in the case of a penetrating gunshot wound, may be extensive and may give rise to focal or generalized epileptic attacks. The majority of such patients who become epileptic do so within 2 years. After careful examination of these patients, including the performance of radiography, CT brain scans, MRIs, and electroencephalography, the trauma site should be explored with a view to removing the gliotic scar. Such a scar will be replaced by a much smaller surgical scar. This operative intervention cures many of these patients.

12. A history of severe headaches and nausea and the finding of a choked optic disc (swelling of the optic disc, congestion of the retinal veins, and retinal hemorrhages) are not always diagnostic of a brain tumor. However, the finding of weakness of the lateral rectus muscle of the right eye owing to compression of the right sixth cranial nerve against the floor of the skull, together with the positive results on radiologic and other laboratory tests, made the diagnosis certain. The glioma (tumor of neuroglia) is the most common type of tumor found in such a patient. Unfortunately, gliomas tend to infiltrate the brain tissue and cannot be completely removed surgically. Biopsy is performed to establish the diagnosis, as much of the tumor is removed as is clinically feasible, and the area is treated by deep x-ray therapy postoperatively. Survival time may also be increased by the use of chemotherapy.

❓ Review Questions

Directions: Each of the numbered items in this section is followed by answers. Select the ONE lettered answer that is CORRECT.

1. The following statements concern the cytology of a neuron:
   (a) A unipolar neuron is one that gives rise to a single neurite that divides a short distance from the cell body into two branches, one proceeding to some peripheral structure and the other entering the central nervous system (CNS).
   (b) A bipolar neuron is one that has two neurites that emerge together from the cell body.
   (c) Nissl substance is found in the axon of a neuron.
   (d) The Golgi complex does not synthesize cell membranes.
   (e) Melanin granules are not found in the neurons of the substantia nigra.

2. The following statements concern the cytology of a neuron:
   (a) The protein molecules projecting from the surface of the microtubules take no part in rapid transport in axoplasm.
   (b) The protein molecules that extend through the full thickness of the plasma membrane of a neuron serve as sodium and potassium channels.
   (c) Strong experimental evidence suggests that the gates of the sodium and potassium channels are formed by actin molecules.
   (d) The size of the nucleolus in a neuron is unrelated to the volume of cytoplasm possessed by neurons.
   (e) A synapse is the site where two neurons come together and their membranes are in contact; interneuronal communication occurs.

3. The following statements concern the axon:
   (a) The initial segment of the axon is the first 500 μm after it leaves the axon hillock.
   (b) The nerve impulse generated by a neuron does not originate at the initial segment of an axon but on the dendrite.
   (c) The action potential is produced by the sudden influx of Na$^+$ ions into the cytoplasm.
   (d) Following the influx of Na$^+$ ions in the production of the action potential, the permeability for Na$^+$ ions increases further, and the permeability for K$^+$ ions ceases.
   (e) The spread of the action potential along the microtubules of the axon constitutes the nerve impulse.
4. The following statements concern a nerve impulse:
   (a) The refractory period is the duration of the non-excitable state of the plasma membrane following the passage of a wave of repolarization.
   (b) Subthreshold stimuli, when applied to the surface of a neuron, cannot be summated.
   (c) Inhibitory stimuli are believed to produce their effect by causing an influx of K$^+$ ions through the plasma membrane of the neuron.
   (d) Hyperpolarization can be produced by causing an influx of K$^+$ ions through the plasma membrane.
   (e) The axolemma is the site of nerve conduction.
5. The following statements concern the structure of a synapse:
   (a) Synapses may be axodendritic, axosomatic, or axoaxonic.
   (b) The synaptic cleft is the space between the presynaptic and postsynaptic membranes and measures about 200 nm.
   (c) The subsynaptic web lies beneath the presynaptic membrane.
   (d) Presynaptic vesicles do not contain the neurotransmitter substance.
   (e) All neurons produce and release several types of transmitter substances at all their nerve endings.
6. The following statements concern a neuron:
   (a) Nerve fibers are the dendrites and axons of a neuron.
   (b) The volume of cytoplasm within the nerve cell body always far exceeds that found in the neurites.
   (c) Golgi type I neurons have very short axons.
   (d) Golgi type II neurons have very long axons.
   (e) Golgi type II neurons form the Purkinje cells of the cerebellar cortex.
7. The following statements concern the neuron organelles and inclusions:
   (a) Centrioles are not found in mature nerve cells.
   (b) Lipofuscin granules tend to disappear with age.
   (c) The Nissl substance fills the axon hillock but is absent from other areas of the cytoplasm.
   (d) Microfilaments contain actin and do not assist in cell transport.
   (e) Mitochondria are found in the dendrites and axons.
8. The following statements concern dendrites:
   (a) A dendrite conveys a nerve impulse away from the nerve cell body.
   (b) Dendritic spines are small projections of the plasma membrane that increase the receptor surface area of the dendrite.
   (c) The cytoplasm of dendrites does not contain ribosomes and agranular endoplasmic reticulum.
   (d) Most dendrites expand in width as they extend from the nerve cell body.
   (e) Dendrites rarely branch.
9. The following statements concern neuromodulators:
   (a) Neuromodulators may coexist with the principal (classic) transmitter at a single synapse.
   (b) They often diminish and shorten the effect of the principal transmitter.
   (c) They never act through a second messenger.
   (d) They have a brief effect on the postsynaptic membrane.
   (e) Acetylcholine (ACh) (muscarinic) is not a good example of a neuromodulator.
10. The following statements concern the neurobiology of neuron structures:
    (a) A lysosome is a membrane-bound vesicle covered with ribosomes.
    (b) A terminal bouton is the postsynaptic part of an axon.
    (c) A receptor is a protein molecule on the postsynaptic membrane.
    (d) Nissl substance is formed of the smooth-surfaced endoplasmic reticulum.
    (e) Microtubules provide a mobile track that allows specific organelles to move by molecular motors.
11. The following statements concern neuroglia:
    (a) Fibrous astrocytes are located mainly in the gray matter of the central nervous system (CNS).
    (b) Replacement gliosis follows the death of neurons in the CNS and is due to the proliferation of astrocytes.
    (c) Astrocytes are not involved in the absorption of γ-aminobutyric acid (GABA) secreted by the nerve terminals.
    (d) Oligodendrocytes are responsible for the formation of the myelin of nerve fibers in the peripheral nervous system (PNS).
    (e) A single oligodendrocyte can form, by means of its processes, only one internodal segment of myelin on the same axon.
12. The following statements concern the microglial cells:
    (a) Microglial cells resemble connective tissue mast cells.
    (b) Microglial cells are larger than astrocytes or oligodendrocytes.
    (c) Microglial cells migrate into the central nervous system (CNS) during adult life.
    (d) In the presence of damaged neurons, microglial cells become branched.
    (e) In degenerative lesions of the CNS, the circulating blood contributes cells to the population of microglial cells.

13. The following statements concern the ependymal cells:
    (a) Choroidal epithelial cells do not secrete cerebrospinal fluid (CSF).
    (b) Ependymocytes line the ventricular system but do not permit the CSF to enter the extracellular spaces of the nervous tissue.
    (c) Tanycytes have short, unbranched basal processes, many of which have endfeet placed on the capillaries of the median eminence.
    (d) The ependymal cells form a single layer, and many possess microvilli and cilia.
    (e) Ependymal cells are incapable of absorbing substances from the CSF.
14. The following statements concern the extracellular space:
    (a) The space is formed by the gaps between the neurons and not the gaps between the neuroglial cells.
    (b) The space surrounds the lymphatic capillaries present in the brain and spinal cord.
    (c) The space is not continuous with the subarachnoid space.
    (d) The space is filled with tissue fluid.
    (e) The space is not continuous with the synaptic cleft between two neurons.
15. The following statements concern tumors of neuroglia:
    (a) They form about 5% of all intracranial tumors.
    (b) Apart from the ependymomas, tumors of neuroglia grow slowly and are not highly invasive.
    (c) They commonly infiltrate between neurons, causing the minimum disturbance of function.
    (d) They are nonmalignant and easily removed surgically.
    (e) As they expand, they raise the intracranial pressure.
16. The following statements concern neuroglial cells:
    (a) They tend to be larger than nerve cell bodies.
    (b) Heat increases the action potential in an axon and reduces the signs and symptoms in multiple sclerosis.
    (c) Oligodendrocytes are found some distance away from nerve cell bodies and their neurites.
    (d) Multiple sclerosis is a disease involving the oligodendrocyte.
    (e) Like Schwann cells, oligodendrocytes are surrounded by a basement membrane.
17. The following general statements concern the neuroglial cells:
    (a) Microglial cells have straight processes with spinelike projections.
    (b) Astrocytes form a scaffold for developing neurons.
    (c) Oligodendrocyte processes are not continuous with the myelin sheaths.
    (d) Ependymal cells have no cilia on their free borders.
    (e) *Macroglia* is the term used to distinguish the larger oligodendrocytes from the smaller astrocyte.

 Answers and Explanations to Review Questions

1. A is correct. A unipolar neuron is one that gives rise to a single neurite that divides a short distance from the cell body into two branches, one proceeding to some peripheral structure and the other entering the CNS (see Fig. 2-3). B. A bipolar neuron is one that gives rise to a neurite that emerges from each end of the cell body. The sensory ganglia of the vestibulocochlear nerve (eighth cranial nerve) possess bipolar neurons. C. Nissl substance is not found in the axon of a neuron but in the cell body of a neuron. D. The Golgi complex is important in the synthesis of cell membranes. E. Melanin granules are found in the neurons of the substantia nigra, and these neurons are responsible for the neurotransmitter dopamine.
2. B is correct. The protein molecules that extend through the full thickness of the plasma membrane of a neuron serve as sodium and potassium channels (see Fig. 2-21). A. The protein molecules projecting from the surface of the microtubules take part in rapid transport in axoplasm. C. The gates of the sodium and potassium channels are formed of protein molecules but not actin molecules. D. The large size of the nucleolus in a neuron is related to the very large volume of cytoplasm possessed by certain neurons. E. A synapse is the site where two neurons come into close proximity and where functional interneuronal communication occurs.
3. C is correct. The action potential within an axon is produced by the sudden influx of Na^+ ions into the cytoplasm (see Fig. 2-17). A. The initial segment of the axon is the first 50 to 100 μm after it leaves the axon hillock. B. The nerve impulse generated by a neuron does originate at the initial segment of an axon but not on the dendrite. D. Following the influx of Na^+ ions in the production of the action potential, the permeability for Na^+ ions ceases, and the permeability for K^+ ions increases; thus K^+ ions start to flow from the cell cytoplasm. E. The spread of the action potential along the plasma membrane of the axon constitutes the nerve impulse.
4. E is correct. The axolemma is the site of nerve conduction. A. The refractory period is the duration of the nonexcitable state of the plasma membrane following the passage of a wave of depolarization (see p. 45). B. Subthreshold stimuli, when applied to the surface of a neuron, can be summated. C. Inhibitory stimuli are believed to produce their effect by causing an influx of Cl^- ions through the plasma membrane of the neuron. D. Hyperpolarization can be produced by causing an influx of Cl^- ions through the plasma membrane.

5. A is correct. The synapses may be axodendritic, axosomatic, or axoaxonic (see Fig. 2-25). B. The synaptic cleft is the space between the presynaptic and postsynaptic membranes and measures about 20 nm. C. The subsynaptic web lies beneath the postsynaptic membrane. D. Presynaptic vesicles may contain the neurotransmitter substance (see Fig. 2-27). E. The majority of neurons produce and release only one principal transmitter at all their nerve endings.

6. A is correct. Nerve fibers are the dendrons and axons of a neuron. B. The volume of cytoplasm within the nerve cell body is often far less than the total volume of cytoplasm in the neurites. C. Golgi type I neurons have very long axons. D. Golgi type II neurons have very short axons. E. Golgi type I neurons form the Purkinje cells of the cerebellar cortex.

7. E is correct. Mitochondria are found in the dendrites and axons. A. Centrioles are found in mature nerve cells as well as in immature dividing nerve cells. B. Lipofuscin granules tend to accumulate with age. C. The Nissl substance is absent from the axon hillock. D. Microfilaments contain actin and probably assist in cell transport (see p. 42).

8. B is correct. Dendritic spines are small projections of the plasma membrane that increase the receptor surface area of the dendrite. A. A dendrite conveys a nerve impulse toward the nerve cell body (see p. 48). C. The cytoplasm of dendrites contains ribosomes and agranular endoplasmic reticulum as well as Nissl granules, microtubules, and microfilaments. D. Most dendrites taper in width as they extend from the nerve cell body. E. Dendrites often branch profusely.

9. A is correct. Neuromodulators may coexist with the principal (classic) transmitter at a single synapse (see p. 54). B. Neuromodulators often enhance and prolong the effect of the principal transmitter. C. Neuromodulators act through a second messenger. D. Neuromodulators may have a prolonged effect on the postsynaptic membrane. E. ACh (muscarinic) is a good example of a neuromodulator.

10. C is correct. A receptor is a protein molecule on the postsynaptic membrane. A. A lysosome is a membrane-bound vesicle that is not covered with ribosomes. B. A terminal bouton is the presynaptic part of an axon. D. Nissl substance is formed of the rough endoplasmic reticulum. E. Microtubules provide a stationary track that allows specific organelles to move by molecular motors.

11. B is correct. Replacement gliosis follows the death of neurons in the CNS and is due to the proliferation of astrocytes (see p. 57). A. Fibrous astrocytes are located mainly in the white matter of the CNS. C. Astrocytes are involved in the absorption of GABA as it is secreted by the nerve terminals. D. Oligodendrocytes are responsible for the formation and maintenance of the myelin of nerve fibers in the CNS (see p. 58). E. Unlike Schwann cells in the PNS, a single oligodendrocyte can form, by means of its many processes, several internodal segments of myelin on the same or different axons.

12. E is correct. In degenerative lesions of the CNS, the circulating blood contributes cells to the population of microglial cells. A. Microglial cells resemble connective tissue macrophages. B. Microglial cells are smaller than astrocytes or oligodendrocytes (Fig. 2-28). C. Microglial cells migrate into the CNS during fetal life. D. In the presence of damaged neurons, microglial cells round off, lose their branches, and increase in number.

13. D is correct. The ependymal cells form a single layer, and many possess microvilli and cilia (see p. 60). A. Choroidal epithelial cells secrete CSF. B. The ependymocytes line the ventricular system but permit CSF to enter the extracellular spaces of the nervous system. C. Tanycytes have long, branching basal processes, many of which have endfeet placed on the capillaries of the median eminence. E. Ependymal cells absorb substances from the CSF.

14. D is correct. The extracellular space is filled with tissue fluid. A. The extracellular space is formed by the gaps between the neurons and the neuroglial cells (see p. 60). B. The central nervous system does not have lymphatic vessels. C. The extracellular space is in almost direct continuity with the subarachnoid space. E. The extracellular space is continuous with the synaptic cleft between two neurons.

15. E is correct. As neuroglial tumors expand, they raise the intracranial pressure. A. Neuroglial tumors form about 40% to 50% of all intracranial tumors. B. Apart from the ependymomas, tumors of neuroglia are highly invasive. C. Neuroglial tumors commonly infiltrate between neurons, initially causing the minimum disturbance of function; later, they completely disrupt neuronal activities. D. Neuroglial tumors, apart from ependymomas, are highly malignant and difficult to remove surgically.

16. D is correct. Multiple sclerosis is a disease involving the oligodendrocyte (see pp. 63–64). A. Neuroglial cells tend to be smaller than nerve cell bodies. B. Heat reduces the action potential in an axon and accentuates the signs and symptoms in multiple sclerosis. C. Oligodendrocytes are found close to nerve cell bodies and their neurites. E. Unlike Schwann cells, oligodendrocytes are not surrounded by a basement membrane.

17. B is correct. Astrocytes form a scaffold for developing neurons. A. Microglial cells have wavy processes with spinelike projections. C. Oligodendrocyte processes are continuous with the myelin sheaths. D. Ependymal cells have cilia on their free borders. E. *Macroglia* is the collective term sometimes used to describe astrocytes and oligodendrocytes as distinct from the smaller microglial cells.

3 Nerve Fibers and Peripheral Innervation

CHAPTER OBJECTIVES

- To consider the basic structure and function of nerve fibers
- To understand the process of nerve degeneration and regeneration
- To review the special organs that lie at the ends of sensory and motor nerves
- To examine the different sensory modalities
- To learn the terms used in assessing skin sensory loss and abnormal muscle activity

A 45-year-old man is recovering from a mild upper respiratory tract infection when he suddenly notices weakness in both legs while walking upstairs. He also develops a numb sensation over the lower part of both legs and feet. Two days later, while shaving, he notices weakness of the muscles on the right side of his face.

On physical examination, the patient does not appear to be ill. He has no pyrexia. Examination of his leg muscles shows obvious signs of muscle weakness involving both legs, especially below the knees. Both ankle reflexes are absent, and the right knee jerk is diminished. He has sensory deficits for touch and pain sensations in the distribution of the stocking area of both feet and lower legs and a mild form of facial nerve palsy involving the right side of the face. Neurologic evidence of loss of function of the brain or spinal cord is not present.

The patient is suspected of having Guillain–Barré syndrome and is admitted to the hospital for observation. The cause of this disease is unknown, although it is believed to be viral and involves the immune system. Histologically, the peripheral nerves show focal scattered areas of demyelination with an accumulation of lymphocytes and macrophages. As the myelin is lost, the axons are left naked, and the Schwann cell bodies remain intact. In the majority of patients, recovery occurs in 2 to 4 weeks with nerve remyelination. Hospitalization is necessary in the early stages because the disease can spread rapidly to involve the intercostal and phrenic nerves, resulting in paralysis of the intercostal muscles and diaphragm. For the same reason, the coughing and swallowing reflexes should be watched carefully. A clinician would find this disease impossible to understand without knowledge of peripheral nerve structure.

In this chapter, the process of nerve degeneration and regeneration is described in detail because nerve lesions are very common in clinical practice and can be caused by a wide variety of diseases, including trauma, neoplasms, infection, metabolic dysfunction (diabetes), and chemical toxins such as lead. The process of nerve degeneration is fast and can take place in nerves in the central and peripheral nervous systems. The regeneration of nerves is slow and confined to the peripheral nervous system (PNS). Because so much research today is being devoted to investigating why regeneration in the central nervous system (CNS) ceases within 2 weeks, the histologic changes that occur must be learned.

The material in this chapter commonly forms the basis for examination questions.

NERVE FIBERS

Nerve fiber is the name given to an axon (or a dendrite) of a nerve cell. The structure of axons and dendrites is described on page 33–34. Bundles of nerve fibers found in the CNS are referred to as **nerve tracts** (Fig. 3-1); bundles of nerve fibers found in the PNS are called **peripheral nerves** (Fig. 3-2).

Two types of nerve fibers are present in the CNS and PNS: myelinated and nonmyelinated.

Myelinated Nerve Fibers

A myelinated nerve fiber is one that is surrounded by a myelin sheath. The myelin sheath is not part of the neuron but is formed by a supporting cell (Fig. 3-3;

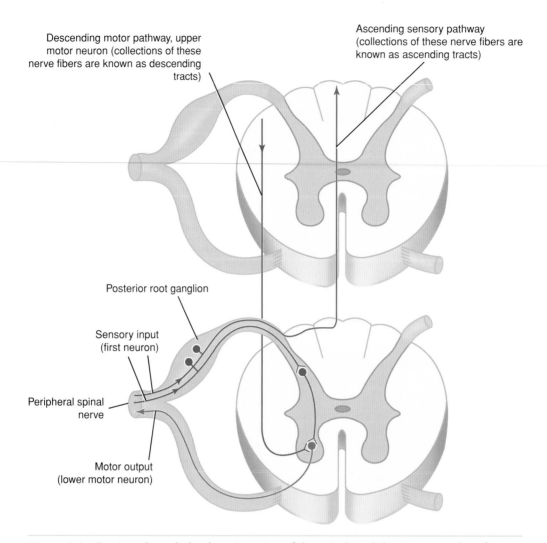

Descending motor pathway, upper motor neuron (collections of these nerve fibers are known as descending tracts)

Ascending sensory pathway (collections of these nerve fibers are known as ascending tracts)

Posterior root ganglion

Sensory input (first neuron)

Peripheral spinal nerve

Motor output (lower motor neuron)

Figure 3-1   Sections through the thoracic region of the spinal cord showing examples of nerve fibers entering or leaving the central nervous system; ascending and descending nerve fibers (tracts or pathways) are also shown.

also see Fig. 3-2). In the CNS, the supporting cell is called the **oligodendrocyte**; in the PNS, it is called the **Schwann cell**.

The myelin sheath is a segmented, discontinuous layer interrupted at regular intervals by the **nodes of Ranvier** (Figs. 3-4 and 3-5). Each segment of the myelin sheath measures approximately 0.5 to 1.0 mm in length. In the CNS, each oligodendrocyte may form and maintain myelin sheaths for as many as 60 nerve fibers (axons). In the PNS, only one Schwann cell maintains each segment of one nerve fiber.

Myelin Formation

Myelin sheaths begin to form before birth and during the first year postnatally. The process has been studied with the electron microscope (Fig. 3-6).

In the **peripheral nervous system** (**PNS**), the nerve fiber or axon first indents the side of a Schwann cell (Fig. 3-4). Later, as the axon sinks farther into the

Schwann cell, the external plasma membrane of the Schwann cell forms a **mesaxon**, which suspends the axon within the Schwann cell (Fig. 3-6A). Subsequently, the Schwann cell is believed to rotate on the axon so that the plasma membrane becomes wrapped around the axon in a spiral. The direction of the spiral is clockwise in some segments and counterclockwise in others. To begin with, the wrappings are loose, but gradually the cytoplasm between the layers of the cell membrane disappears, leaving cytoplasm near the surface and in the region of the nucleus. The wrappings become tight with maturation of the nerve fiber. The thickness of the myelin depends on the number of spirals of Schwann cell membrane. Some nerve fibers are surrounded by only a few turns of the membrane, while others have as many as 50 turns. In electron micrographs of cross sections of mature myelinated nerve fibers, the myelin is seen to be laminated. Each lamella measures 13 to 18 nm thick. The dark **major dense line**, about 2.5 nm thick, consists of two inner protein layers

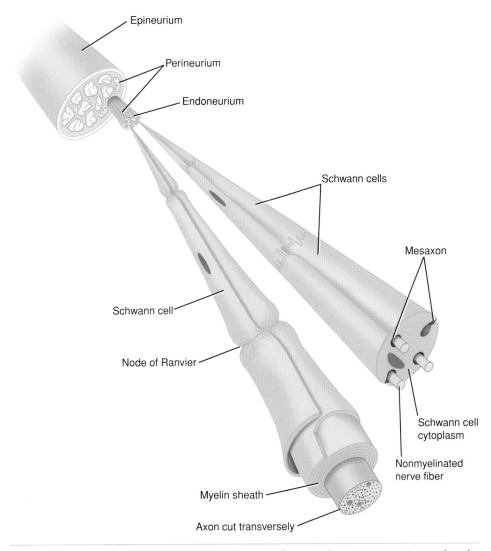

Figure 3-2 Exploded view of a peripheral nerve showing the connective tissue sheaths and the structure of myelinated and nonmyelinated nerve fibers.

of the plasma membrane that are fused together. The lighter **minor dense line**, about 10 nm thick, is formed by the approximation of the outer surfaces of adjacent plasma membranes and is made up of lipid. The fused outer protein layers of the plasma membranes are very thin and form a thin intraperiod line situated in the center of the lighter lipid layer. At the node of Ranvier, two adjacent Schwann cells terminate, and the myelin sheaths become thinner by the turning off of the lamellae (Fig. 3-5). At these regions, the plasma membrane of the axon, the axolemma, is exposed.

The **incisures of Schmidt–Lanterman** are seen on longitudinal sections of myelinated nerve fibers. They represent areas where the dark major dense line is not formed as a result of the localized persistence of Schwann cell cytoplasm (Fig. 3-7). This persistence of cytoplasm involves all the layers of the myelin, and thus, there is a continuous spiral of cytoplasm from the outermost region of the Schwann cell to the region of the axon. This spiral of cytoplasm may provide a pathway for the conduction of metabolites from the surface region of the Schwann cell to the axon.

In the **central nervous system** (**CNS**), oligodendrocytes are responsible for the formation of the myelin sheaths. The plasma membrane of the oligodendrocyte becomes wrapped around the axon, and the number of layers will determine the thickness of the myelin sheath (Fig. 3-3). The **nodes of Ranvier** are situated in the intervals between adjacent oligodendrocytes. A single oligodendrocyte may be connected to the myelin sheaths of as many as 60 nerve fibers. For this reason, the process of myelination in the CNS cannot take place by rotation of the oligodendrocyte on the axon, as did the Schwann cell in the PNS. Myelination in the CNS possibly occurs by the growth in length of the process of the oligodendrocyte, the process wrapping itself around the axon. Incisures of Schmidt–Lanterman exist in CNS nerve fibers. Table 3-1 provides a summary of facts concerning CNS and PNS myelination.

(*text continue on page 79*)

Figure 3-3 The relationship between an oligodendrocyte and myelinated nerve fibers in the central nervous system. Note the absence of a basement membrane.

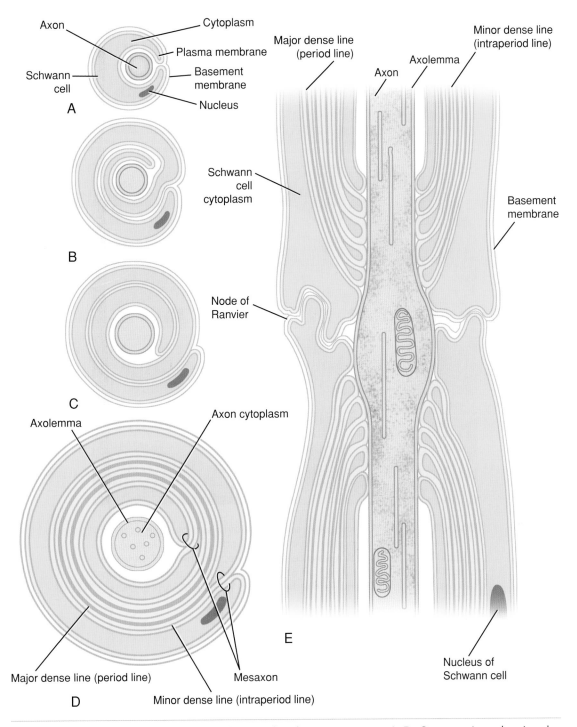

Figure 3-4 A myelinated nerve fiber in the peripheral nervous system. **A–D:** Cross sections showing the stages in the formation of the myelin sheath. **E:** A longitudinal section of a mature myelinated nerve fiber showing a node of Ranvier. Note the presence of a basement membrane.

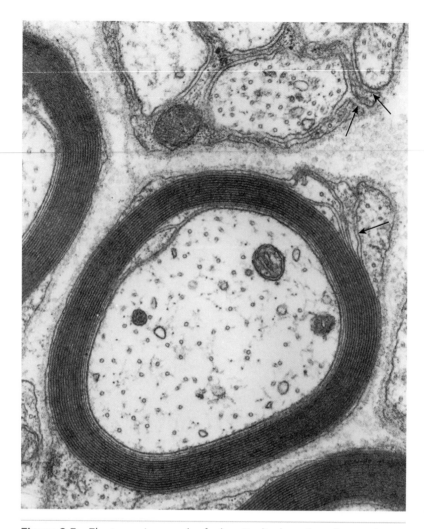

Figure 3-5 Electron micrograph of a longitudinal section of several myelinated axons showing the structure of a node of Ranvier (*arrow*). At the node, two adjacent Schwann cells terminate, and the myelin sheaths become thinner by the turning off of the lamellae. Note the many microtubules and microfilaments within the axons (×12,220). (Courtesy Dr. H. de F. Webster.)

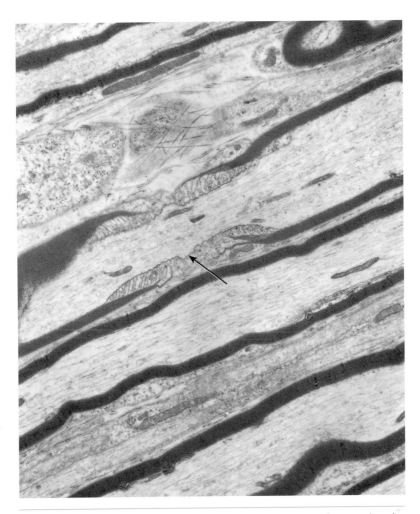

Figure 3-6 Electron micrograph of a transverse section of a peripheral nerve showing a myelinated axon with spiral myelin lamellae (**center**). Note the mesaxon (*arrow*). Parts of two other myelinated fibers are also shown. A number of nonmyelinated axons are enclosed in the peripheral cytoplasm of a Schwann cell (**top**). The mesaxons are indicated by *arrows* (×28,000). (Courtesy Dr. H. de F. Webster.)

Figure 3-7 Schmidt–Lanterman incisures in the myelin sheath of a peripheral nerve. **A:** Transverse section of a myelinated nerve fiber. **B:** Schematic diagram of a myelinated nerve fiber in which the myelin sheath has been unrolled.

Table 3-1   Classification of Neurons

Location	Cell Responsible	Number of Nerve Fibers Served by Cell	Nodes of Ranvier	Schmidt–Lanterman Incisures	Mesaxon
Peripheral nerve	Schwann cell	1	Present	Present	Present
CNS tract	Oligodendrocyte	Up to 60	Present	Present	Absent

CNS, central nervous system.

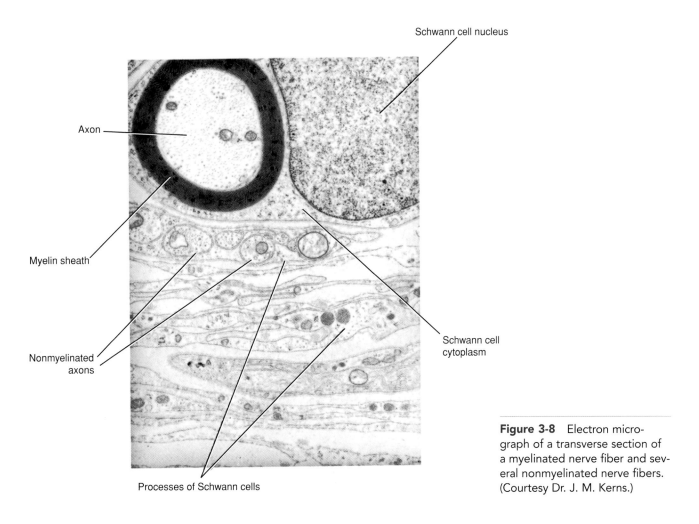

Schwann cell nucleus

Axon

Myelin sheath

Nonmyelinated
axons

Schwann cell
cytoplasm

Processes of Schwann cells

Figure 3-8 Electron micrograph of a transverse section of a myelinated nerve fiber and several nonmyelinated nerve fibers. (Courtesy Dr. J. M. Kerns.)

Nonmyelinated Nerve Fibers

The smaller axons of the CNS, the postganglionic axons of the autonomic part of the nervous system, and some fine sensory axons associated with the reception of pain are nonmyelinated.

In the **PNS**, each axon, which is usually less than 1 μm in diameter, indents the surface of the Schwann cell so that it lies within a trough (Fig. 3-2). As many as 15 or more axons may share a single Schwann cell, each lying within its own trough or sometimes sharing a trough. In some situations, the troughs are deep and the axons are embedded deep in the Schwann cells, forming a **mesaxon** from the Schwann cell plasma membrane (Fig. 3-8; also see Fig. 3-6). The Schwann cells lie close to one another along the length of the axons, and nodes of Ranvier do not exist.

In areas with synapses or where motor transmission occurs, the axon emerges from the trough of the Schwann cell for a short distance, thus exposing the active region of the axon (Fig. 3-9).

In the **CNS**, nonmyelinated nerve fibers run in small groups and are not particularly related to the oligodendrocytes.

Nonmyelinated axons   Schwann cell   Bare axon

Smooth muscle fiber

Figure 3-9 Autonomic neuromuscular junction between a nonmyelinated axon and a smooth muscle fiber.

Figure 3-10 Peripheral nerve. l.s. Paraffin section. ×270. This is a higher magnification of a region similar to the boxed area of Figure 1a. A distinguishing characteristic of longitudinal sections of peripheral nerves is that they appear to follow a zigzag course, particularly evident in this photomicrograph. The sinuous course of these fibers is accentuated by the presence of nuclei of Schwann cells (ScC), fibroblasts (F), and endothelial cells of capillaries belonging to the endoneurium. Many of these nerve fibers are myelinated (M) as corroborated by the presence of the nodes of Ranvier (NR) and myelin proteins around the axons (Ax). (From Gartner, L. P. *Color Atlas and Text of Histology*, 7e. Baltimore: Wolters Kluwer, 2018.)

PERIPHERAL NERVES

Peripheral nerves is a collective term for the cranial and spinal nerves. Each peripheral nerve consists of parallel bundles of nerve fibers, which may be efferent or afferent axons, may be myelinated or nonmyelinated, and are surrounded by connective tissue sheaths (Figs. 3-10 and 3-11).

The nerve trunk is surrounded by a dense connective tissue sheath called the **epineurium** (Fig. 3-12). Within the sheath are bundles of nerve fibers, each of which is surrounded by a connective tissue sheath called the **perineurium**. Between the individual nerve fibers is a loose, delicate connective tissue referred to as the **endoneurium**. The connective tissue sheaths serve to support the nerve fibers and their associated blood vessels and lymph vessels. Peripheral nerve fibers can be classified according to their speed of conduction and size (see Table 2-3).

Figure 3-11 Peripheral nerve sheaths and compartments. **A:** A low-power view of a transverse section of a normal sural nerve. The nerve fascicles with roughly circular outlines are surrounded by perineurium and embedded in the connective tissue of the epineurium. Epineurial blood vessels (A) are also cut in cross section and there is adherent adipose tissue. The 1 μm sections are stained with hematoxylin and eosin (×16). **B:** The endoneurial compartment containing myelinated and non-myelinated nerve fibers and their accompanying Schwann cells is surrounded by perineurium. Paraffin section stained with hematoxylin and eosin (×45). (From Mills, S. E. *Histology for Pathologists*, 4e. Philadelphia, PA: Wolters Kluwer, 2013.)

Spinal Nerves and Spinal Nerve Roots

The 31 pairs of spinal nerves leave the spinal cord and pass through intervertebral foramina in the vertebral column. (For details, see Fig. 1-5.) Each spinal nerve is connected to the spinal cord by **two roots**: the **anterior root** and the **posterior root** (Fig. 3-13). The anterior root consists of bundles of nerve fibers carrying nerve impulses *away from* the CNS, the **efferent fibers**. The **posterior root** consists of bundles of nerve fibers

Nerve fibers

Endoneurium

Perineurium

Epineurium

Figure 3-12 Structure of a peripheral nerve.

carrying nerve impulses *to* the CNS, the **afferent fibers**. Because these fibers are concerned with conveying information to the CNS, they are called **sensory fibers**. The cell bodies of these nerve fibers are situated in a swelling on the posterior root called the **posterior root ganglion**.

Cranial Nerves

The 12 pairs of cranial nerves (see Fig. 3-13) leave the brain and pass through foramina in the skull. Some of these nerves are composed entirely of afferent nerve fibers bringing sensations to the brain (olfactory, optic, and vestibulocochlear), others are composed entirely of efferent fibers (oculomotor, trochlear, abducent, accessory, and hypoglossal), while the remainder possess both afferent and efferent fibers (trigeminal, facial, glossopharyngeal, and vagus). The cranial nerves are described in detail in Chapter 11.

Sensory Ganglia

The sensory ganglia of the posterior spinal nerve roots and of the trunks of the trigeminal, facial, glossopharyngeal, and vagal cranial nerves have the same structure.

Each ganglion is surrounded by a layer of connective tissue that is continuous with the epineurium and perineurium of the peripheral nerve. The neurons are unipolar, possessing cell bodies that are rounded or oval in shape (Fig. 3-14). The cell bodies tend to be aggregated and separated by bundles of nerve fibers. A single nonmyelinated process leaves each cell body and, after a convoluted course, bifurcates at a T junction into peripheral and central branches. The former axon terminates in a series of dendrites in a peripheral sensory ending, and the latter axon enters the CNS. The nerve impulse, on reaching the T junction, passes directly from the peripheral axon to the central axon, thus bypassing the nerve cell body.

Each nerve cell body is closely surrounded by a layer of flattened cells called **capsular cells** or **satellite cells**. The capsular cells are similar in structure to Schwann cells and are continuous with these cells as they envelop the peripheral and central processes of each neuron.

Autonomic Ganglia

The autonomic ganglia (sympathetic and parasympathetic ganglia) are situated at a distance from the brain and spinal cord. They are found in the sympathetic trunks, in prevertebral autonomic plexuses (e.g., in the cardiac, celiac, and mesenteric plexuses), and as ganglia in or close to viscera. Each ganglion is surrounded by a layer of connective tissue that is continuous with the epineurium and perineurium of the peripheral nerve. The neurons are multipolar and possess cell bodies that are irregular in shape (Fig. 3-15). The dendrites of the neurons make synaptic connections with the myelinated axons of preganglionic neurons. The axons of the neurons are of small diameter (C fibers) and unmyelinated, and they pass to viscera, blood vessels, and sweat glands.

Just as with sensory ganglia, each nerve cell body is closely surrounded by **capsular cells** (or **satellite cells**). Unlike those of sensory ganglia, however, these capsular cells are similar in structure to Schwann cells and are continuous with them as they envelop the peripheral and central processes of each neuron.

Peripheral Nerve Plexuses

Peripheral nerves are composed of bundles of nerve fibers. In their course, peripheral nerves sometimes divide into branches that join neighboring peripheral nerves. If this occurs frequently, a network of nerves, called a **nerve plexus**, forms. Note that the formation of a nerve plexus allows individual nerve fibers to pass from one peripheral nerve to another, and **in most instances, branching of nerve fibers does not take place**. A plexus thus permits a redistribution of the nerve fibers within the different peripheral nerves.

At the root of the limbs, the anterior rami of the spinal nerves form complicated plexuses. The cervical and brachial plexuses are at the root of the upper limbs (Fig. 3-16), and the lumbar and sacral plexuses are at the root of the lower limbs. This allows the nerve fibers

Figure 3-13 A: Transverse section of the thoracic region of the spinal cord showing the formation of a spinal nerve from the union of an anterior and a posterior nerve root. **B:** Transverse section of the pons showing the sensory and motor roots of the trigeminal nerve.

Figure 3-14 Sensory ganglion. l.s. Human. Paraffin section. ×132. The dorsal root ganglion provides a good representative example of a sensory ganglion. It possesses a **vascular** (BV) connective tissue **capsule** (C), which also envelops its sensory root. The neurons of the dorsal root ganglion are pseudounipolar in morphology; therefore, their **somata** (So) appear spherical in shape. The **fibers** (f), many of which are myelinated, alternate with rows of cell bodies. Note that some somata are large (*arrow*), whereas others are small (*arrowhead*). Each soma is surrounded by neuroectodermally derived **capsule cells** (Cc). A region similar to the *boxed area* is presented at a high magnification in Figure 4. (From Gartner, L. P. *Color Atlas and Text of Histology,* 7e. Baltimore: Wolters Kluwer, 2018.)

Figure 3-15 Photomicrograph of a longitudinal section of a ganglion of the sympathetic trunk stained with hematoxylin and eosin (×300).

derived from different segments of the spinal cord to be arranged and distributed efficiently in different nerve trunks to the various parts of the upper and lower limbs.

Cutaneous nerves, as they approach their final destination, commonly form fine plexuses that again permit a rearrangement of nerve fibers before they reach their terminal sensory endings.

The autonomic nervous system also possesses numerous nerve plexuses that consist of preganglionic and postganglionic nerve fibers and ganglia.

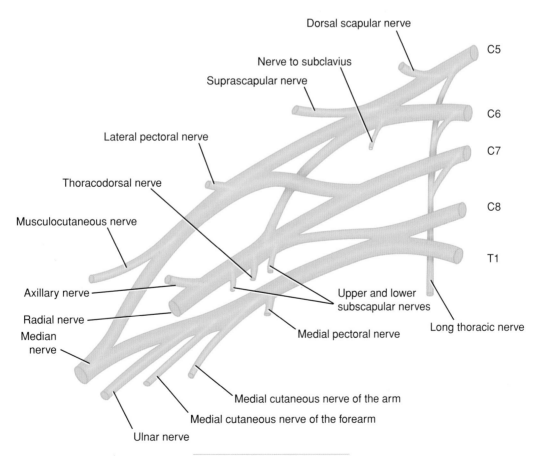

Figure 3-16 Brachial plexus.

RECEPTOR ENDINGS

An individual receives impressions from the outside world and from within the body by special sensory nerve endings or receptors.

Sensory receptors can be classified into five basic functional types:

Mechanoreceptors respond to mechanical deformation.

Thermoreceptors respond to changes in temperature; some receptors respond to cold and others to heat.

Nociceptors respond to any stimuli that bring about damage to the tissue.

Electromagnetic receptors, the rods and cones of the eyes, are sensitive to changes in light intensity and wavelength.

Chemoreceptors respond to chemical changes associated with taste and smell and oxygen and carbon dioxide concentrations in the blood.

Anatomical Types of Receptors

For convenience, the sensory endings can be classified, on a structural basis, into nonencapsulated and encapsulated receptors. Table 3-2 classifies and compares the receptor types.

Nonencapsulated Receptors

Free Nerve Endings

Free nerve endings are widely distributed throughout the body (Fig. 3-17). They are found between the epithelial cells of the skin, the cornea, and the alimentary tract, and in connective tissues, including the dermis, fascia, ligaments, joint capsules, tendons, periosteum, perichondrium, haversian systems of bone, tympanic membrane, and dental pulp; they are also present in muscle.

The afferent nerve fibers from the free nerve endings are either myelinated or nonmyelinated. The terminal endings are devoid of a myelin sheath as well as Schwann cells covering their tips.

Most of these endings detect pain, while others detect crude touch, pressure, and tickle sensations, and possibly cold and heat.

Merkel Discs

Merkel discs are found in hairless skin, for example, the fingertips (Figs. 3-18 and 3-19), and in hair follicles. The nerve fiber passes into the epidermis and terminates as a disc-shaped expansion that is applied closely to a dark-staining epithelial cell in the deeper part of the epidermis, called the **Merkel cell**. In hairy skin, clusters of Merkel discs, known as **tactile domes**, are found in the epidermis between the hair follicles.

Merkel discs are slowly adapting touch receptors that transmit information about the degree of pressure exerted on the skin, such as from holding a pen.

Hair Follicle Receptors

Nerve fibers wind around the follicle in its outer connective tissue sheath below the sebaceous gland. Some branches surround the follicle, while others run parallel to its long axis (Figs. 3-20 and 3-21). Many naked axon filaments terminate among the cells of the outer root sheath.

Table 3-2 Classification and Comparison of Receptor Types

Type of Receptor	Location	Stimulus	Sensory Modality	Adaptability	Fibers
Nonencapsulated Receptors					
Free nerve endings	Epidermis, cornea, gut, dermis, ligaments, joint capsules, bone, dental pulp, etc.	Mechanoreceptor	Pain (fast), pain (slow), touch (crude), pressure, heat and cold	Rapid	A δ, C
Merkel discs	Hairless skin	Mechanoreceptor	Touch	Slow	A β
Hair follicle receptors	Hairy skin	Mechanoreceptor	Touch	Rapid	A β
Encapsulated Receptors					
Meissner corpuscles	Dermal papillae of skin of palm and sole of foot	Mechanoreceptor	Touch	Rapid	A β
Pacinian corpuscles	Dermis, ligaments, joint capsules, peritoneum, external genitalia, etc.	Mechanoreceptor	Vibration	Rapid	A β
Ruffini corpuscles	Dermis of hairy skin	Mechanoreceptor	Stretch	Slow	A β
Neuromuscular spindles	Skeletal muscle	Mechanoreceptor	Stretch—muscle length	Fast	A α, A β
Neurotendinous spindles	Tendons	Mechanoreceptor	Compression—muscle tension	Fast	A α

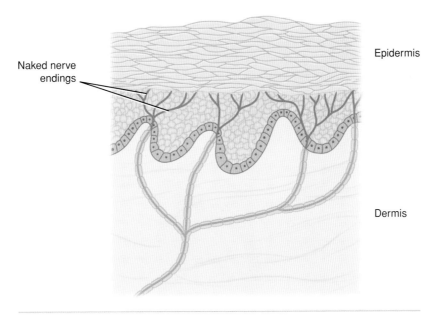

Figure 3-17   Free nerve endings in the skin. The nerve fibers in the epidermis are naked.

Bending of the hair stimulates the follicle receptor, which belongs to the rapidly adapting group of mechanoreceptors. While the hair remains bent, the receptor is silent, but when the hair is released, a further burst of nerve impulses is initiated.

Encapsulated Receptors

Encapsulated receptors show wide variations in size and shape, and the termination of the nerve is covered by a capsule.

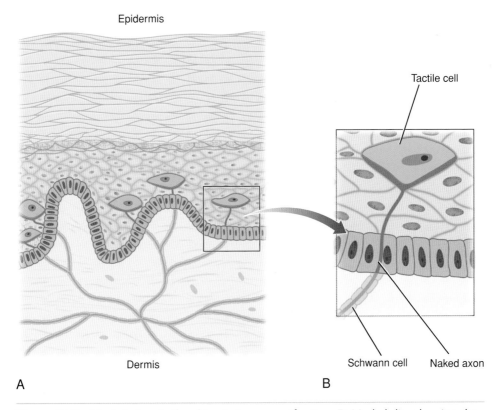

Figure 3-18   Merkel discs in the skin. **A:** Low magnification. **B:** Merkel disc showing the expanded ending of an axon with a stippled tactile cell.

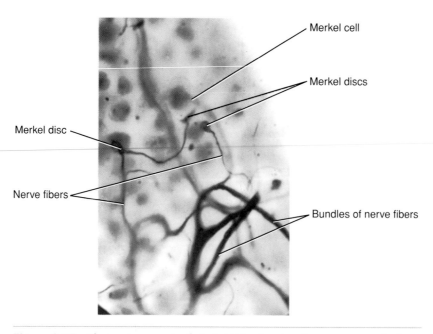

Figure 3-19   Photomicrograph of digital skin showing fine nerve terminals ending in Merkel discs, stained by the silver method. (Courtesy Dr. N. Cauna.)

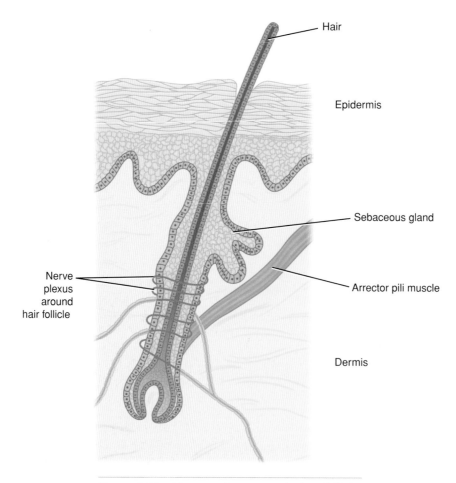

Figure 3-20   Nerve endings around a hair follicle.

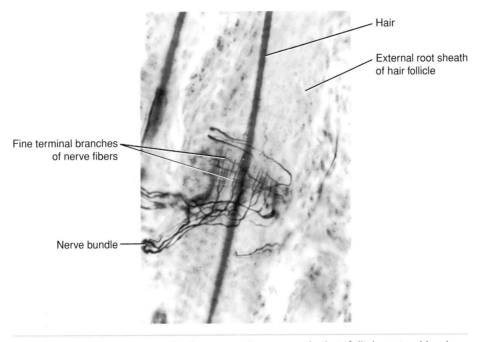

Figure 3-21 Photomicrograph of nerve endings around a hair follicle stained by the silver method. (Courtesy Dr. M. J. T. Fitzgerald.)

Meissner Corpuscles

Meissner corpuscles are located in the dermal papillae of the skin (Figs. 3-22 and 3-23), especially that of the palm of the hand and the sole of the foot. Many also are present in the skin of the nipple and the external genitalia. Each corpuscle is ovoid in shape and consists of a stack of

modified flattened Schwann cells arranged transversely across the long axis of the corpuscle. The corpuscle is enclosed by a capsule of connective tissue that is continuous with the endoneurium of the nerves that enter it. A few myelinated nerve fibers enter the deep end of the corpuscle; myelinated and unmyelinated branches

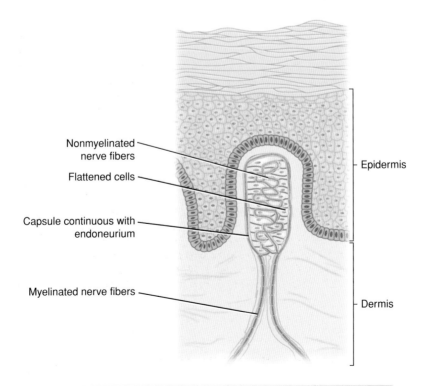

Figure 3-22 Detailed structure of a Meissner corpuscle in the skin.

SB

Ca — — N

NF

Figure 3-23 Photomicrograph of a Meissner corpuscle of the skin. (Courtesy Dr. N. Cauna.)

decrease in size and ramify among the Schwann cells. The number of Meissner corpuscles considerably diminishes between birth and old age.

Meissner corpuscles are very sensitive to touch and are rapidly adapting mechanoreceptors. They enable an individual to distinguish between two pointed structures when they are placed close together on the skin (two-point tactile discrimination).

Pacinian Corpuscles

Pacinian corpuscles (Figs. 3-24 and 3-25) are widely distributed throughout the body and are abundant in the dermis, subcutaneous tissue, ligaments, joint capsules, pleura, peritoneum, nipples, and external genitalia. Each corpuscle is ovoid in shape, measuring about 2 mm long and about 100 to 500 μm across. It consists of a capsule and a central core containing the nerve ending. The capsule consists of numerous concentric lamellae of flattened cells. A large myelinated nerve fiber enters the corpuscle and loses its myelin sheath and then its Schwann cell covering. The naked axon, surrounded by lamellae formed of flattened cells, passes through the center of the core and terminates in an expanded end.

The Pacinian corpuscle is a rapidly adapting mechanoreceptor that is particularly sensitive to vibration. It can respond to up to 600 stimuli per second.

Ruffini Corpuscles

Ruffini corpuscles are located in the dermis of hairy skin. Each corpuscle consists of several large unmyelinated nerve fibers ending within a bundle of collagen fibers and surrounded by a cellular capsule. These

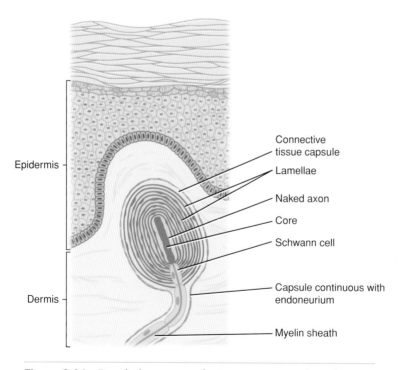

Epidermis

Dermis

Connective tissue capsule

Lamellae

Naked axon

Core

Schwann cell

Capsule continuous with endoneurium

Myelin sheath

Figure 3-24 Detailed structure of a Pacinian corpuscle in the skin.

Figure 3-25 Pacinian corpuscle. Paraffin section. 132.
Pacinian corpuscles, located in the dermis and hypodermis,
are mechanoreceptors. They are composed of a core with
an inner (IC) and an outer (OC) region, as well as a capsule
(Ca) that surrounds the core. The inner core invests the
afferent nerve fiber (NF), which loses its myelin sheath soon
after entering the corpuscle. The core cells are modified
Schwann cells, whereas the components of the capsule are
continuous with the endoneurium of the afferent nerve fiber.
Pacinian corpuscles are readily recognizable in section since
they resemble the cut surface of an onion. Observe the
presence of an arrector pili muscle (AP) and profiles of ducts
(d) of a sweat gland in the vicinity of, but not associated
with, the pacinian corpuscle. (From Gartner, L. P. *Color Atlas
and Text of Histology*, 7e. Baltimore: Wolters Kluwer, 2018.)

slowly adapting mechanoreceptors are stretch receptors, which respond when the skin is stretched.

Cutaneous Receptor Function

The different histologic types of receptors were previously thought to correspond to specific types of
sensation, until scientists pointed out that some areas
of the body have only one or two histologic types of
receptors and yet are sensitive to a variety of different
stimuli. Moreover, although the body has these different receptors, all nerves only transmit nerve impulses.
Now scientists generally agree that the type of sensation felt is determined by the specific area of the CNS
to which the afferent nerve fiber passes. For example, if

a pain nerve fiber is stimulated by heat, cold, touch, or
pressure, the individual will experience only pain.

Sensory Stimulus Transduction into Nerve Impulse

Transduction is the process by which one form of
energy (the stimulus) is changed into another form of
energy (electrochemical energy of the nerve impulse).
The stimulus, when applied to the receptor, brings about a
change in potential of the plasma membrane of the nerve
ending. Because this process takes place in the receptor,
it is referred to as the **receptor potential**. The amplitude
of the receptor potential is proportional to the intensity
of the stimulus. By opening more ion channels for a longer time, a stronger mechanical pressure, for example,
can produce a greater depolarization than does weak
pressure. With chemoreceptors and photoreceptors, the
receptor potential is produced by second messengers
activated when the stimulus agent binds to the membrane receptors coupled to G proteins. If large enough,
the receptor potential will generate an AP that will travel
along the afferent nerve fiber to the CNS.

Joint Receptors

Four types of sensory endings can be located in the
capsule and ligaments of synovial joints. Three of these
endings are encapsulated and resemble Pacinian, Ruffini, and tendon stretch receptors. They provide the
CNS with information regarding the position and movements of the joint. A fourth type of ending is nonencapsulated and is thought to be sensitive to excessive
movements and to transmit pain sensations.

Neuromuscular Spindles

Neuromuscular spindles, or muscular spindles (Figs. 3-26
and 3-27), are found in skeletal muscle and are most
numerous toward the tendinous attachment of the
muscle. They provide the CNS with sensory information
regarding the muscle length and the rate of change in
the muscle length. The CNS uses this information to
control muscle activity.

Each spindle measures about 1 to 4 mm in length
and is surrounded by a fusiform capsule of connective
tissue (Fig. 3-28). Within the capsule are 6 to 14 slender
intrafusal muscle fibers; the ordinary muscle fibers situated outside the spindles are referred to as **extrafusal
fibers**. The intrafusal fibers of the spindles are of two
types: the **nuclear bag** and **nuclear chain** fibers. The
nuclear bag fibers are recognized by the presence of
numerous nuclei in the equatorial region, which consequently is expanded; also, cross striations are absent in
this region. In the nuclear chain fibers, the nuclei form
a single longitudinal row or chain in the center of each
fiber at the equatorial region. The nuclear bag fibers
are larger in diameter than the nuclear chain fibers,
and they extend beyond the capsule at each end to be
attached to the endomysium of the extrafusal fibers.

The two types of sensory innervation of muscle spindles are annulospiral and flower spray. The **annulospiral**

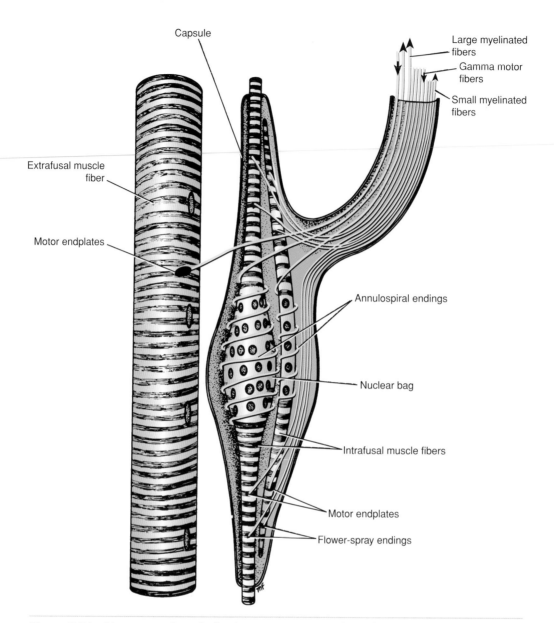

Figure 3-26 Neuromuscular spindle showing two types of intrafusal fibers: the nuclear bag and nuclear chain fibers.

endings are situated at the equator of the intrafusal fibers. As the large myelinated nerve fiber pierces the capsule, it loses its myelin sheath, and the naked axon winds spirally around the nuclear bag or chain portions of the intrafusal fibers.

The **flower-spray endings** are situated mainly on the nuclear chain fibers some distance away from the equatorial region. A myelinated nerve fiber slightly smaller than that for the annulospiral ending pierces the capsule and loses its myelin sheath, and the naked axon branches terminally and ends as varicosities; it resembles a spray of flowers.

Stretching (elongation) of the intrafusal fibers results in stimulation of the annulospiral and flower-spray endings, and nerve impulses pass to the spinal cord in the afferent neurons.

Motor innervation of the intrafusal fibers is provided by fine γ motor fibers. The nerves terminate in small motor endplates situated at both ends of the intrafusal fibers. Stimulation of the motor nerves causes both ends of the intrafusal fibers to contract and activate the sensory endings. The equatorial region, which lacks cross striations, is noncontractile. The extrafusal fibers of the remainder of the muscle receive their innervation in the usual way from large α-size axons.

Neuromuscular Spindle Function

Under resting conditions, the muscle spindles give rise to afferent nerve impulses all the time, and most of this information is not consciously perceived. When muscle activity occurs, either actively or passively, the

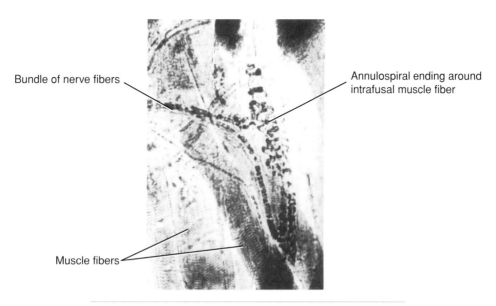

Figure 3-27 Photomicrograph of a neuromuscular spindle.

Figure 3-28 Muscle spindle. Mouse. Electron microscopy. ×6,300. Parts of the outer capsule (oC) may be observed at the corners of this electron micrograph. The periaxial space (PS) surrounds the slender inner capsule (iC), whose component cells form attenuated branches, subdividing the axial space (AS) into several compartments for the nuclear chain (NC) and nuclear bag (NB) intrafusal fibers and their corresponding sensory terminals (ST). Note that the attenuated processes of the inner capsule cells establish contact with each other (*arrows*). (From Ovalle, W., Dow, P. (1983). Comparative ultrastructure of the inner capsule of the muscle spindle and the tendon organ. *American Journal of Anatomy, 166,* 343–357.)

intrafusal fibers are stretched, and the rate of passage of nerve impulses to the spinal cord or brain increases in the afferent neurons. Similarly, if the intrafusal fibers are now relaxed due to the cessation of muscle activity, the result is a decrease in the rate of passage of nerve impulses. The neuromuscular spindle thus plays a very important role in keeping the CNS informed about the length of a muscle and the rate of change of its length, thereby indirectly influencing the control of voluntary muscle.

Stretch Reflex

The neurons of the spinal cord involved in the simple stretch reflex are as follows. Stretching a muscle results in elongation of the intrafusal fibers of the muscle spindle and stimulation of the annulospiral and flower-spray endings. The nerve impulses reach the spinal cord in the afferent neurons and synapse with the large α motor neurons situated in the anterior gray horns of the spinal cord. Nerve impulses now pass via the efferent motor nerves and stimulate the extrafusal muscle fibers, and the muscle contracts. This simple stretch reflex depends on a two-neuron arc consisting of an afferent neuron and an efferent neuron. Interestingly, the muscle spindle afferent impulses inhibit the α motor neurons supplying the antagonist muscles. This effect is called **reciprocal inhibition**.

Intrafusal Fiber Control

In the brain and spinal cord, certain centers give rise to tracts that synapse with γ motor neurons in the spinal cord. The reticular formation, the basal ganglia, and the cerebellum are examples of such centers. By these means, these centers can greatly influence voluntary muscle activity. The γ efferent motor fibers cause shortening of the intrafusal fibers, stretching the equatorial regions and stimulating the annulospiral and flower-spray endings. This, in turn, initiates the reflex contraction of the extrafusal fibers described previously.

Approximately one-third of all the motor fibers passing to a muscle are γ efferents; the remaining two-thirds are the large α motor fibers. The nuclear bag fibers are believed to be concerned with dynamic responses and are associated more with position and velocity of contraction, whereas the nuclear chain fibers are associated with slow static contractions of voluntary muscle.

Neurotendinous Spindles

Neurotendinous spindles (Golgi tendon organs) are present in tendons and are located near the junctions of tendons with muscles (Fig. 3-29). They provide the CNS with sensory information regarding the tension of muscles.

Each spindle consists of a fibrous capsule that surrounds a small bundle of loosely arranged tendon (collagen) fibers (intrafusal fibers). The tendon cells are

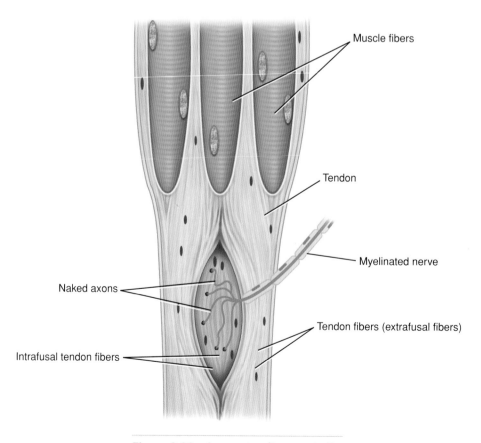

Figure 3-29 A neurotendinous spindle.

larger and more numerous than those found elsewhere in the tendon. One or more myelinated sensory nerve fibers pierce the capsule, lose their myelin sheath, branch, and terminate in club-shaped endings.

The nerve endings are activated by being squeezed by the adjacent tendon fibers within the spindle when tension develops in the tendon. Unlike the neuromuscular spindle, which is sensitive to changes in muscle length, the neurotendinous organ detects changes in muscle tension.

Neurotendinous Spindle Function

Increased muscle tension stimulates the neurotendinous spindles, and an increased number of nerve impulses reach the spinal cord through the afferent nerve fibers. These fibers synapse with the large α motor neurons situated in the anterior gray horns of the spinal cord. Unlike the muscle spindle reflex, this reflex is inhibitory and inhibits muscle contraction. In this manner, the tendon reflex prevents the development of too much tension in the muscle. Although this function is probably important as a protective mechanism, its main function is to provide the CNS with information that can influence voluntary muscle activity.

EFFECTOR ENDINGS

The PNS controls muscle and secretory cell functions. These axonal endings establish chemical synapses on nonneuronal cells such as skeletal, smooth, and cardiac muscle cells and to the cells of glandular tissue.

Skeletal Muscle Innervation

Skeletal muscle is innervated by one or more nerves. In the limbs and head and neck, the innervation is usually single, but, in the large muscles of the abdominal wall, the innervation is multiple, the latter muscles having retained their embryonic segmental nerve supply.

The nerve supply and blood supply to a muscle enter it at a more or less constant position called the **neurovascular** hilus. The nerve to a muscle contains motor and sensory fibers. The motor fibers are of three types: (1) large α myelinated fibers, (2) small γ myelinated fibers, and (3) fine unmyelinated C fibers. The large myelinated axons of the α anterior horn cells supply the extrafusal fibers that form the main mass of the muscle. The small γ myelinated fibers supply the intrafusal fibers of the neuromuscular spindles. The fine unmyelinated fibers are postganglionic autonomic efferents that supply the smooth muscle in the walls of blood vessels.

The sensory fibers are of three main types: (1) myelinated fibers that originate in annulospiral and flower-spray endings of the neuromuscular spindles, (2) myelinated fibers that originate in neurotendinous spindles; and (3) myelinated and nonmyelinated fibers that originate from a variety of sensory endings in muscle connective tissue.

Motor Unit

The motor unit may be defined as the single α motor neuron and the muscle fibers that it innervates (Fig. 3-30). The muscle fibers of a single motor unit are widely scattered throughout the muscle. Where

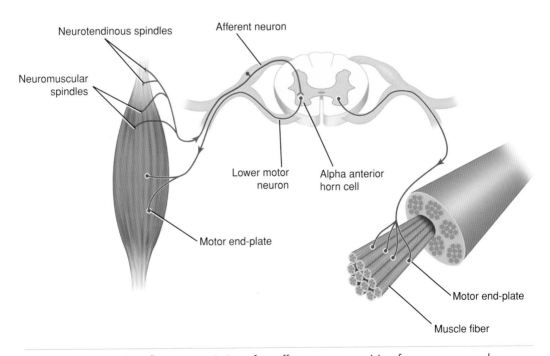

Figure 3-30 Simple reflex arc consisting of an afferent neuron arising from neuromuscular spindles and neurotendinous spindles and an efferent lower motor neuron whose cell body is an α anterior horn cell within the spinal cord. Note that the efferent neuron terminates on muscle fibers at motor endplates.

fine, precise muscle control is required, such as in the extraocular muscles or the small muscles of the hand, the motor units possess only a few muscle fibers. Where precise control is not necessary, however, as in a large limb muscle such as the gluteus maximus, a single motor nerve may innervate many hundreds of muscle fibers.

Skeletal Muscle Neuromuscular Junctions

Skeletal muscle fibers are innervated by large, α myelinated nerve fibers derived from large motor neurons in the anterior gray columns (horns) of the spinal cord or from cranial nerve motor nuclei. As each myelinated fiber enters a skeletal muscle, it branches many times. The number of branches depends on the size of the motor unit. A single branch then terminates on a muscle fiber at the **neuromuscular junction** or **motor endplate** (Figs. 3-31 and 3-32).

The great majority of muscle fibers are innervated by just one motor endplate. On reaching the muscle fiber, the nerve loses its myelin sheath and breaks up into a number of fine branches. Each branch ends as a naked axon and forms the **neural element** of the motor endplate (Fig. 3-33). The axon is expanded slightly and contains many mitochondria and vesicles (approximately 45 nm in diameter). At the site of the motor endplate, the surface of the muscle fiber is elevated slightly to form the **muscular element** of the plate, often referred to as the **sole plate** (see Fig. 3-31A). The elevation is due to the local accumulation of granular sarcoplasm beneath the sarcolemma and the presence of numerous nuclei and mitochondria, the latter providing the ATP, which is the energy source for acetylcholine (ACh) synthesis.

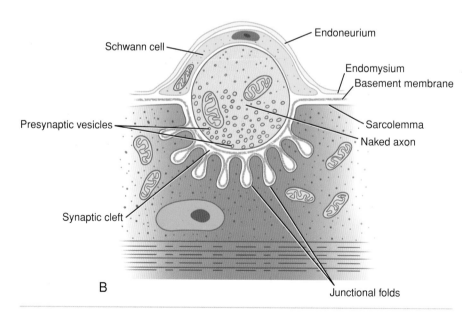

Figure 3-31 **A:** A skeletal neuromuscular junction. **B:** Enlarged view of a muscle fiber showing the terminal naked axon lying in the surface groove of the muscle fiber.

Nerve fibers and bundles of nerve fibers

Acetylcholinesterase at motor endplates

Figure 3-32   Photomicrograph showing nerve fibers terminating on skeletal muscle fibers at motor endplates, stained histochemically for acetylcholinesterase and counterstained with silver. (Courtesy Dr. M. J. T. Fitzgerald.)

Motor endplate

Muscle fiber

Schwann cell

Nerve fiber

Axon

Muscle fiber

A

B

Figure 3-33   A: Photomicrograph of a motor endplate showing terminal branching of a nerve fiber. **B:** Electron micrograph of a terminal axon at a motor endplate showing the axon lying in a groove on the surface of the muscle fiber. (Courtesy Dr. J. M. Kerns.)

Figure 3-34 Electron micrograph of a cross section of an axon at a motor endplate showing the axon lying in a groove of folded sarcolemma. (Courtesy Dr. J. M. Kerns.)

The expanded naked axon lies in a groove on the surface of the muscle fiber outside the plasma membrane (sarcolemma). Each groove is formed by the infolding of the plasma membrane. The groove may branch many times, with each branch containing a division of the axon. Importantly, the axons are truly naked; the Schwann cells merely serve as a cap or roof to the groove and never project into it. The floor of the groove is formed of the plasma membrane, which is thrown into numerous small folds, called **junctional folds**, which increase the surface area of the plasma membrane that lies close to the naked axon (Fig. 3-34).

The plasma membrane of the axon (the axolemma or presynaptic membrane) is separated, by a space about 30 to 50 nm wide, from the plasma membrane of the muscle fiber (the sarcolemma or postsynaptic membrane). This space constitutes the **synaptic cleft**. The synaptic cleft is filled with the basement membranes of the axon and the muscle fiber (see Fig. 3-31B). The motor endplate is strengthened by the connective tissue sheath of the nerve fiber (endoneurium), which becomes continuous with the connective tissue sheath of the muscle fiber (endomysium).

A nerve impulse (AP), on reaching the presynaptic membrane of the motor endplate, causes the opening of voltage-gated Ca^{2+} channels that allow Ca^{2+} ions to enter the axon. This stimulates the fusion of some of the synaptic vesicles with the presynaptic membrane and causes the release of ACh into the synaptic cleft. The ACh is thus discharged into the cleft by a process of **exocytosis** and diffuses rapidly across the cleft to reach

the nicotinic type of ACh receptors on the postsynaptic membrane of the junctional folds. The postsynaptic membrane possesses large numbers of ACh-gated channels.

Once the ACh-gated channels are opened, the postsynaptic membrane becomes more permeable to Na^+ ions, which flow into the muscle cell, and a local potential called the **endplate potential** is created. (The ACh-gated channels are also permeable to K^+ ions, which flow out of the cell but to a lesser extent.) If the endplate potential is large enough, the voltage-gated channels for Na^+ ions are opened, and an AP will be initiated and spread along the surface of the plasma membrane (sarcolemma). The wave of depolarization is carried into the muscle fiber to the contractile myofibrils through the system of T tubules. This leads to the release of Ca^{2+} ions from the sarcoplasmic reticulum, which, in turn, causes the muscle to contract.

The amount of ACh released at the motor endplate will depend on the number of nerve impulses arriving at the nerve terminal. Once the ACh crosses the synaptic cleft and triggers the ionic channels on the postsynaptic membrane, it immediately undergoes hydrolysis due to the presence of the enzyme **acetylcholinesterase (AChE)** (see Fig. 3-32). The enzyme adheres to the fine collagen fibrils of the basement membranes in the cleft; some of the ACh diffuses away from the cleft. The ACh remains in contact with the postsynaptic membrane for about 1 msec, and it is rapidly destroyed to prevent re-excitation of the muscle fiber. After the fall in concentration of ACh in the cleft, the ionic channels close and remain closed until more ACh arrives.

Skeletal muscle fiber contraction is thus controlled by the frequency of the nerve impulses that arrive at the motor nerve terminal. A resting muscle fiber shows small occasional depolarizations (endplate potentials) at the motor endplate, which are insufficient to cause an AP and make the fiber contract. These are believed to be due to the sporadic release of ACh into the synaptic cleft from a single presynaptic vesicle.

The sequence of events that takes place at a motor endplate on stimulation of a motor nerve can be briefly summarized as follows:

ACh → Nicotinic type of ACh receptor, ACh-gated channels opened → Na^+ influx → Endplate potential created

Endplate potential (if large enough) → Na^+-gated channels opened → Na^+ influx → AP created

AP → Increased release of Ca^{2+} → Muscle fiber contraction

Immediate hydrolysis of ACh by AChE → ACh-gated channels closed → Muscle fiber repolarization

If drugs having a similar chemical structure to ACh were to arrive at the receptor site of a motor endplate, they might bring about the same changes as ACh and mimic its action. Two examples of such drugs are **nicotine** and **carbamylcholine**. If, on the other hand, drugs having a similar chemical structure to ACh were to arrive at the receptor site of a motor endplate and were unable to bring about the sequence of changes normally induced by ACh, they would occupy the receptor site and block access of ACh. Such drugs would be competing with ACh and are called **competitive blocking agents**. An example of such a drug is **d-tubocurarine**, which causes skeletal muscle to relax and not contract by preventing the action of locally produced ACh (see p. 114).

Smooth Muscle Neuromuscular Junctions

In smooth muscle, where the action is slow and widespread, such as within the wall of the intestine, the autonomic nerve fibers branch extensively; thus, a single neuron exerts control over a large number of muscle fibers. In some areas (e.g., the longitudinal layer of smooth muscle in the intestine), only a few muscle fibers are associated with autonomic endings, the wave of contraction passing from one muscle cell to another by means of gap junctions (Fig. 3-35).

In smooth muscle, in which the action is fast and precision is required, such as in the iris, the branching of the nerve fibers is less extensive; thus, a single neuron exerts control over only a few muscle fibers.

Naked axons

Schwann cell

Smooth muscle fibers

Gap junctions

Figure 3-35 Autonomic neuromuscular junction. The exposed axons are close to the smooth muscle fibers.

Figure 3-36 Nerve fibers ending around glandular acini.

The autonomic nerve fibers, which are postganglionic, are nonmyelinated and terminate as a series of varicosed branches. An interval of 10 to 100 nm may exist between the axon and the muscle fiber. At the site where transmission is to occur, the Schwann cell is retracted so that the axon lies within a shallow groove on its surface. Therefore, part of the axon is naked, permitting free diffusion of the transmitter substance from the axon to the muscle cell. Here, the axoplasm contains numerous vesicles similar to those seen at the motor endplate of skeletal muscle.

Smooth muscle is innervated by sympathetic and parasympathetic parts of the autonomic system. Those nerves that are cholinergic liberate ACh at their endings by a process of exocytosis, with the ACh being present in the vesicles at the nerve ending. Those nerves that are noradrenergic liberate **norepinephrine (NE)** at their endings by a process of exocytosis, with the NE being present in dark-cored vesicles at the nerve endings. Both ACh and NE bring about depolarization of the muscle fibers innervated, which thereupon contract. The fate of these neurotransmitter substances differs. ACh is hydrolyzed in the presence of AChE in the synaptic cleft of the muscle fiber, and NE is taken up by the nerve endings. Notably, in some areas of the body (e.g., bronchial muscle), the NE liberated from postganglionic sympathetic fibers causes smooth muscle to relax and not contract.

Cardiac Muscle Neuromuscular Junctions

Nonmyelinated postganglionic sympathetic and parasympathetic autonomic nerves extend into the connective tissue between the muscle fibers and terminate in close proximity to the individual cardiac muscle fibers. At the site where transmission takes place, the axon becomes naked because of the retraction of the Schwann cell. This permits free diffusion of the neurotransmitter substance

from the axon to the muscle fiber. Because of the presence of intermittent desmosomes and gap junctions between abutting muscle fibers, excitation and contraction of one muscle fiber rapidly spread from fiber to fiber.

Nerve Endings on Secretory Cells of Glands

Nonmyelinated postganglionic autonomic nerves extend into the connective tissue of glands and branch close to the secretory cells (Fig. 3-36). In many glands, the nerve fibers have been found to innervate only the blood vessels.

SEGMENTAL INNERVATION OF SKIN

The area of skin supplied by a single spinal nerve and, therefore, a single segment of the spinal cord is called a **dermatome**. On the trunk, dermatomes extend round the body from the posterior to the anterior median plane. Adjacent dermatomes overlap considerably, so to produce a region of complete anesthesia, at least three contiguous spinal nerves have to be sectioned. Note that the area of tactile loss is always greater than the area of loss of painful and thermal sensations. The reason for this difference is that the degree of overlap of fibers carrying pain and thermal sensations is much more extensive than the overlap of fibers carrying tactile sensations. Dermatomal charts for the anterior and posterior surfaces of the body are shown in Figures 3-37 and 3-38.

In the limbs, the arrangement of the dermatomes is more complicated because of the embryologic rotation of the limbs as they grow out from the trunk.

In the face, the divisions of the trigeminal nerve supply a precise area of skin, with little or no overlap to the cutaneous area of another division.

Figure 3-37 Anterior aspect of the body showing the distribution of cutaneous nerves on the left side and dermatomes on the right side.

Figure 3-38   Posterior aspect of the body showing the distribution of cutaneous nerves on the left side and dermatomes on the right side.

SEGMENTAL INNERVATION OF MUSCLES

Skeletal muscle also receives a segmental innervation. Most of these muscles are innervated by more than one spinal nerve and, therefore, by the same number of segments of the spinal cord. Thus, to paralyze a muscle completely, sectioning several spinal nerves or destroying several segments of the spinal cord would be necessary.

Learning the segmental innervation of all the muscles of the body is an impossible task. Nevertheless, the segmental innervation of the following muscles should be known because testing them by eliciting simple muscle reflexes in the patient is possible (Fig. 3-39):

Biceps brachii tendon reflex C5–C6: Flexion of the elbow joint by tapping the biceps tendon

Triceps tendon reflex C6–C7 and C8: Extension of the elbow joint by tapping the triceps tendon

Brachioradialis tendon reflex C5–C6 and C7: Supination of the radioulnar joints by tapping the insertion of the brachioradialis tendon

Abdominal superficial reflexes: Contraction of underlying abdominal muscles by stroking the skin: upper abdominal skin T6–T7, middle abdominal skin T8–T9, lower abdominal skin T10–T12

Figure 3-39 Biceps brachii tendon reflex. Note that the reflex arc passes through the fifth and sixth cervical segments of the spinal cord. This is usually monosynaptic, and the internuncial neuron (*black*) is absent.

Patellar tendon reflex (knee jerk) L2, L3, and L4: Extension of knee joint on tapping the patellar tendon

Achilles tendon reflex (ankle jerk) S1 and S2: Plantar flexion of ankle joint on tapping the Achilles tendon (calcaneus tendon)

MUSCLE TONE AND MUSCLE ACTION

A **motor unit** consists of a motor neuron in the anterior gray column (horn) of the spinal cord and all the muscle fibers it supplies (Fig. 3-40). In a large buttock muscle, such as the gluteus maximus, where fine control is unnecessary, a given motor neuron may supply as many as 200 muscle fibers. In contrast, in the small muscles of the hand or the extrinsic muscles of the eyeball, where fine control is required, one nerve fiber supplies only a few muscle fibers.

Every skeletal muscle, while resting, is in a partial state of contraction, a condition referred to as **muscle tone**. With no intermediate stage, muscle fibers are either fully contracted or relaxed; therefore, a few muscle fibers within a muscle are fully contracted all the time. To bring about this state and to avoid fatigue, different groups of motor units and, thus, different groups of muscle fibers are activated at different times. This is accomplished by the asynchronous discharge of nervous impulses in the motor neurons in the anterior gray horn of the spinal cord.

Basically, muscle tone is dependent on the integrity of a simple monosynaptic reflex arc composed of two neurons in the nervous system (Fig. 3-41). The lengthening and shortening in a muscle are detected by sensitive sensory endings called **muscle spindles** (see p. 90), and the tension is detected by **tendon spindles** (see p. 92). The nervous impulses travel in the large afferent fibers to the spinal cord. There, they synapse with the motor neurons situated in the anterior gray column, which, in turn, send impulses down their axons to the muscle fibers. The muscle spindles themselves are innervated by small γ efferent fibers that regulate the response of the muscle spindles, acting synergically with external stretch. In this manner, muscle tone is maintained reflexly and adjusted to the needs of posture and movement.

Should the afferent or efferent pathways of the reflex arc be cut, the muscle would lose its tone immediately and become flaccid. A flaccid muscle, on palpation, feels like a mass of dough that has completely lost its resilience. It

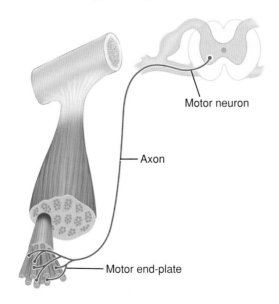

Motor neuron

Axon

Motor end-plate

Bundle of muscle fibers

Figure 3-40 Components of a motor unit.

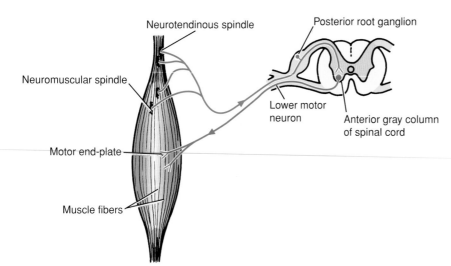

Figure 3-41 Simple reflex arc consisting of an afferent neuron arising from neuromuscular spindles and neurotendinous spindles and an efferent neuron whose cell body lies in the anterior gray column (horn) of the spinal cord. Note that for simplicity, the afferent fibers from the neurotendinous spindle and the neuromuscular spindle are shown as one pathway; in fact, the neurotendinous receptor is inhibitory and reduces tone, whereas the neuromuscular spindle is excitatory and increases tone.

quickly atrophies and becomes reduced in volume. The degree of activity of the motor anterior column cells and, therefore, the degree of muscle tone depends on the summation of the nerve impulses received by these cells from other neurons of the nervous system.

Muscle movement is accomplished by activating increasing numbers of motor units and, at the same time, reducing the activity of the motor units of muscles that will oppose or antagonize the movement. When the maximum effort is required, all the motor units of a muscle are active.

MOTOR UNIT SUMMATION

When a muscle begins to contract, the smaller motor units are stimulated first. This is because the smaller motor units are innervated by smaller neurons in the spinal cord and brainstem, and they have a lower threshold of excitability. As the contraction increases, progressively larger motor units are recruited. This phenomenon causes a gradual increase in muscle strength as the muscle contracts.

MUSCLE FATIGUE

The progressive loss of strength of a muscle with prolonged strong contraction is due to the reduction in the amounts of ATP within the muscle fibers. Nerve impulses continue to arrive at the neuromuscular junction, and normal depolarization of the plasma membrane of the muscle fiber occurs.

POSTURE

Posture is the position adopted by the individual within his or her environment. In the standing position, the

line of gravity passes through the odontoid process of the axis, behind the centers of the hip joints, and in front of the knee and ankle joints. In order to stabilize the body and prevent it from collapsing, humans have well-developed antigravity muscles that exhibit the greatest degree of tone. Therefore, posture depends on the degree and distribution of muscle tone, which, in turn, depends on the normal integrity of simple reflex arcs centered in the spinal cord.

An individual may assume a particular posture (sitting or standing) over long periods of time with little evidence of fatigue. The reason for this is that muscle tone is maintained through different groups of muscle fibers contracting in relays, with only a small number of muscle fibers within a muscle being in a state of contraction at any one time. The active muscle fiber groups are scattered throughout the muscle.

In order to maintain posture, the simple muscle reflex, on which muscle tone is dependent, must receive adequate nervous input from higher levels of the nervous system (Fig. 3-42). For example, impulses arising from the labyrinths and neck muscles, information arising from the cerebellum, midbrain, and cerebral centers, and general information arising from other muscle groups, joints, and even skin receptors will result in nervous impulses impinging on the large anterior gray column cells (i.e., the final common pathway) controlling the muscle fibers.

When an individual assumes a given posture, the tone of the muscles controlling that posture is constantly undergoing fine adjustments so that the posture is maintained. Normal posture thus depends not only on the integrity of the reflex arc but also on the summation of the nervous impulses received by the motor anterior gray column cells from other neurons of the nervous system (Fig. 3-43). The detail of the different nervous pathways involved in bringing the information to the anterior gray column cells is dealt with in Chapter 4.

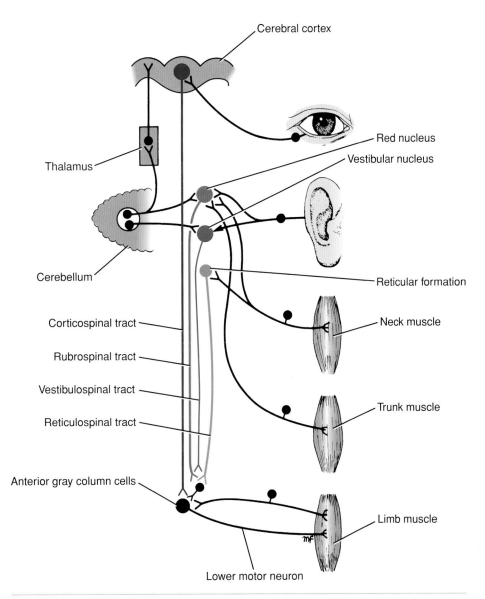

Figure 3-42 Nervous input from higher levels of the central nervous system, which can influence the activity of the anterior gray column (horn) cells of the spinal cord.

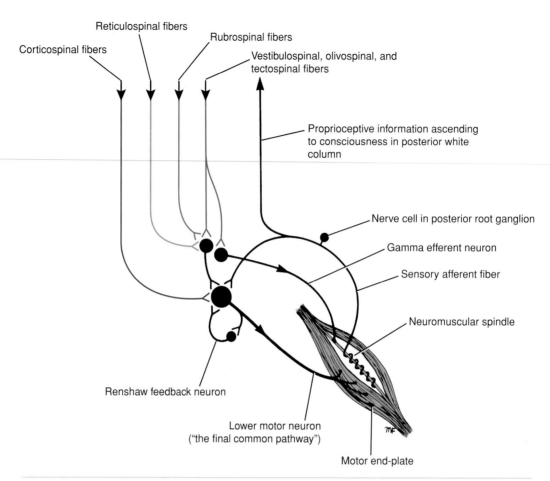

Figure 3-43 Normal postural tone of skeletal muscle is dependent not only on the integrity of the reflex arc but also on the summation of the nervous impulses received by the motor anterior gray column (horn) cells from other neurons of the nervous system.

Clinical Notes

Neuronal Response to Injury

The survival of a neuron's cytoplasm depends on its being connected, however indirectly, with the nucleus. The nucleus plays a key role in the synthesis of proteins, which pass into the cell processes and replace proteins that have been metabolized by cell activity. Thus, the cytoplasm of axons and dendrites will undergo degeneration quickly if these processes are separated from the nerve cell body.

Nerve Cell Body Injury

Severe damage of the nerve cell body due to trauma, interference with the blood supply, or disease may result in degeneration of the entire neuron, including its dendrites and synaptic endings. In the brain and spinal cord, the neuronal debris and the fragments of myelin (if the processes are myelinated) are engulfed and phagocytosed by the microglial cells. Later, the neighboring astrocytes proliferate and replace the neuron with scar tissue.

In the peripheral nervous system (PNS), the tissue macrophages remove the debris, and the local fibroblasts replace the neuron with scar tissue.

Nerve Cell Process Injury

If the axon of the nerve cell is divided, degenerative changes will take place in (1) the distal segment that is separated from the cell body, (2) a portion of the axon proximal to the injury, and (3) possibly the cell body from which the axon arises.

CHANGES IN THE DISTAL SEGMENT OF THE AXON

The changes spread distally from the site of the lesion (Fig. 3-44) and include its terminations; the process is referred to as **wallerian degeneration**. In the PNS, on the first

Figure 3-44   A–D: Degeneration and regeneration in a divided nerve.

A

B

Figure 3-45 Photomicrographs of motor neurons of the anterior gray column of the spinal cord. **A:** Nissl substance in normal neurons. **B:** Following section of anterior roots of spinal nerve, showing chromatolysis.

day, the axon becomes swollen and irregular; by the third or fourth day, the axon is broken into fragments, and the debris is digested by the surrounding Schwann cells and tissue macrophages. The entire axon is destroyed within a week.

Meanwhile, the myelin sheath slowly breaks down, and lipid droplets appear within the Schwann cell cytoplasm. Later, the droplets are extruded from the Schwann cell and subsequently phagocytosed by tissue macrophages. The Schwann cells now begin to proliferate rapidly and become arranged in parallel cords within the persistent basement membrane. The endoneurial sheath and the contained cords of Schwann cells are referred to as a **band fiber**. If regeneration does not occur, the axon and the Schwann cells are replaced by fibrous tissue produced by local fibroblasts.

In the central nervous system (CNS), degeneration of the axons and the myelin sheaths follows a similar course, and the debris is removed by the phagocytic activity of the microglial cells. Little is known about the role of oligodendrocytes in this process. The astrocytes now proliferate and replace the axons.

CHANGES IN THE PROXIMAL SEGMENT OF THE AXON
The changes in the proximal segment of the axon are similar to those that take place in the distal segment (see Fig. 3-44) but extend only proximally above the lesion as far as the first node of Ranvier. The proliferating cords of Schwann cells in the peripheral nerves bulge from the cut surfaces of the endoneurial tubes.

CHANGES IN THE NERVE CELL BODY
The changes that occur in the cell body following injury to its axon are referred to as **retrograde degeneration**; the changes that take place in the proximal segment of the axon commonly are included under this heading. The possible reason for these changes is that section of the axon cuts off the cell body from its supply of trophic factors derived from the target organs at the distal end of the axon.

The most characteristic change occurs in the cell body within the first 2 days following injury and reaches its maximum within 2 weeks. The Nissl material becomes fine, granular (Figs. 3-45 and 3-46), and dispersed throughout the cytoplasm, a process known as **chromatolysis**. Chromatolysis begins near the axon hillock and spreads to all

Chromatolysis

Total degeneration following severe injury

Recovery

Figure 3-46 The changes that may take place in a nerve cell body following division of one of its processes.

parts of the cell body. In addition, the nucleus moves from its central location toward the periphery of the cell, and the cell body swells and becomes rounded. The degree of chromatolysis and the degree of swelling of the cell are greatest when the injury to the axon is close to the cell body. In some neurons, very severe damage to the axon close to the cell body may lead to death of the neuron. On the other hand, damage to the most distal process may lead to little or no detectable change in the cell body. The dispersal of the Nissl material—that is, the cytoplasmic RNA—and the swelling of the cell are caused by cellular edema. The apparent loss of staining affinity of the Nissl material is due to the wide dispersal of the cytoplasmic RNA. The movement of the nucleus away from the center of the cell may be due to the cellular edema.

Synaptic terminals are seen to withdraw from the surface of the injured nerve cell body and its dendrites and are replaced by Schwann cells in the PNS and microglial cells or astrocytes in the CNS, a process called **synaptic stripping**. Its possible causes are (1) loss of plasma membrane adhesiveness following injury and (2) stimulation of the supporting cells by chemicals released from the injured neuron. If the injury is sufficiently great, the cells of the immune system—namely, monocytes and macrophages—may migrate into the area.

Neuronal Recovery

In contrast to the rapid onset of retrograde degeneration, the recovery of the nerve cell body and regeneration of its processes may take several months.

Nerve Cell Body Recovery

The nucleolus moves to the periphery of the nucleus, and polysome clusters reappear in the cytoplasm. This indicates that RNA and protein synthesis is being accelerated in preparation for the reformation of the axon. Thus, the original Nissl structure reconstitutes, cell body swelling decreases, and the nucleus returns to its characteristic central position (Fig. 3-46).

Regeneration of Peripheral Nerve Axons

Regrowth of the axons (motor, sensory, and autonomic) is possible in peripheral nerves and appears to depend on the presence of endoneurial tubes and the special qualities possessed by Schwann cells. Sprouts from the axons grow from the proximal stump and into the distal stump toward the nerve's end organs. The following mechanisms are thought to be involved: (1) the axons are attracted by chemotropic factors secreted by the Schwann cells in the distal stump, (2) growth-stimulating factors exist within the distal stump, and (3) inhibitory factors are present in the perineurium to inhibit the axons from leaving the nerve.

The satisfactory regeneration of axons and the return of normal function depend on the following factors:

1. In crush nerve injuries, in which the axon is divided or its blood supply has been interfered with but the endoneurial sheaths remain intact, regeneration is likely.
2. In nerves that have been completely severed, the chance of recovery is much less because the regenerating fibers from the proximal stump may be directed to an incorrect destination in the distal stump—that is, cutaneous fibers entering incorrect nerve endings or motor nerves supplying incorrect muscles.

3. If the distance between the proximal and distal stumps of the completely severed nerve is greater than a few millimeters or the gap becomes filled with proliferating fibrous tissue or is simply filled by adjacent muscles that bulge into the gap, then the chances of recovery are very poor. The outgrowing axonal sprouts escape into the surrounding connective tissue and form a tangled mass or **neuroma**. In these cases, early close surgical approximation of the severed ends, if possible, greatly facilitates the chances of recovery.
4. When mixed nerves (those containing sensory, motor, and autonomic fibers) are completely severed, the chances of a good recovery are very much less than when the nerve is purely sensory or purely motor. The reason for this is that the regenerating fibers from the proximal stump may be guided to an incorrect destination in the distal stump; for example, cutaneous fibers may enter motor endoneurial tubes and vice versa.
5. Inadequate physiotherapy to the paralyzed muscles will result in their degeneration before the regenerating motor axons have reached them.
6. The presence of infection at the site of the wound will seriously interfere with the process of regeneration.

If the proximal and distal stumps of the severed nerve are in close apposition, the following regenerative processes take place (see Fig. 3-44). The Schwann cells, having undergone mitotic division, now fill the space within the basal lamina of the endoneurial tubes of the proximal stump as far proximally as the next node of Ranvier and in the distal stump as far distally as the end organs. Where a small gap exists between the proximal and distal stumps, the multiplying Schwann cells form a number of cords to bridge the gap.

Each proximal axon end now gives rise to multiple fine sprouts or filaments with bulbous tips. These filaments, as they grow, advance along the clefts between the Schwann cells and thus cross the interval between the proximal and distal nerve stumps. Many such filaments now enter the proximal end of each endoneurial tube and grow distally in contact with the Schwann cells (Fig. 3-47). Although the filaments from many different axons may enter a single endoneurial tube, only one filament persists, the remainder degenerate, and that one filament grows distally to reinnervate a motor or sensory end organ. While crossing the gap between the severed nerve ends, many filaments fail to enter an endoneurial tube and grow out into the surrounding connective tissue. Note that the formation of multiple sprouts or filaments from a single proximal axon greatly increases the chances that a neuron will become connected to a sensory or motor ending. Why one filament within a single endoneurial tube should be selected to persist while the remainder degenerate remains unknown.

Once the axon has reached the end organ, the adjacent Schwann cells start to lay down a myelin sheath. This process begins at the site of the original lesion and extends in a distal direction. By this means, the nodes of Ranvier and the Schmidt–Lanterman incisures are formed.

Many months may elapse before the axon reaches its appropriate end organ, depending on the site of the nerve injury. The rate of growth has been estimated to be approximately 2 to 4 mm per day. However, in light of the almost certain delay incurred by the axons as they cross the site of the injury, an overall regeneration rate of 1.5 mm per

Fragmentation of axons and myelin

Axons growing along endoneural tubes

Figure 3-47 Photomicrograph of a longitudinal section of the distal stump of the sciatic nerve showing evidence of degeneration and axon regeneration following injury. (Courtesy Dr. M. J. T. Fitzgerald.)

day is a useful figure to remember clinically. Even if all the difficulties outlined above are overcome and a given neuron reaches the original end organ, the enlarging axonal filament within the endoneurial tube reaches only about 80% of its original diameter. For this reason, the conduction velocity will not be as great as that of the original axon. Moreover, a given motor axon tends to innervate more muscle fibers than formerly; thus, the control of muscle is less precise.

Regeneration of Central Nervous System Axons

In the CNS, axons attempt to regenerate, as evidenced by sprouting of the axons, but the process ceases after about 2 weeks. Long-distance regeneration is rare, and the injured axons make few new synapses. Evidence that restoration of function takes place does not exist. The regeneration process is aborted by the absence of endoneurial tubes (which are necessary to guide the regenerating axons), the failure of oligodendrocytes to serve in the same manner as Schwann cells, and the laying down of scar tissue by the active astrocytes. Absence of nerve growth factors in the CNS or that the neuroglial cells may produce nerve growth-inhibiting factors is also possible.

Research has shown that the Schwann cell basal laminae contain laminin and cell-adhesion molecules of the immunoglobulin family, both of which stimulate axon growth. The CNS contains only low concentrations of these molecules. In the embryo, when axon growth actively takes place in both the CNS and PNS, growth-promoting factors are present in both systems. Later in development, these factors disappear in the CNS. Myelin in the CNS inhibits axonal growth, and myelination in the CNS occurs late in the development process when growth of the main nervous pathways is complete.

Central axons may not be as good at regeneration as peripheral axons. In tissue culture, peripheral axons are more successful at growth than central axons. Moreover, the ability of central axons to grow decreases with age.

NEUROBIOLOGIC RESEARCH INTO CENTRAL NERVOUS SYSTEM REGENERATION

Because traumatic injury to the CNS produces such devastating disabilities that are largely irreversible, neurobiologists are now enthusiastically pressing forward with research in this area. Differences are known to exist between the environment in the CNS and PNS. Moreover, the ability of central axons in lower vertebrates, such as frogs, to regenerate provides an enormous stimulus for future work.

Research has taken the following directions:

1. Molecules present in the PNS, such as laminins and neurotrophins, have been introduced into the CNS at the site of injury to promote axon growth.
2. Schwann cells have been grafted into the CNS, and central axons will grow into the graft.
3. Attempts have been made to reduce the inhibitory factors present in the CNS. Infusion of antibodies at the site of injury has been carried out with some success.
4. The introduction of anti-inflammatory agents to suppress the neuroglial and monocyte response has been used with success. **Methylprednisolone** is now commonly used as soon as possible after the incident in all patients with spinal cord injuries.

Although a vast amount of research still needs to be done, a combination of treatments may provide the return of some function to these patients with CNS injuries.

Transneuronal Degeneration

The responses of a single neuron to injury were considered in the previous section. In the CNS, if one group of neurons is injured, then a second group farther along the pathway, serving the same function, may also show degenerative changes. This phenomenon is referred to as **anterograde transneuronal degeneration**. For example, if the axons of the ganglion cells of the retina are severed, not only do the distal ends of the axons that go to the lateral geniculate bodies undergo degeneration but also the neurons in the lateral geniculate bodies with which these axons form synapses undergo degeneration. In fact, a further set of neurons may be involved in the degenerative process in the visual cortex.

In situations in the CNS in which multiple neurons synapse with a single distal neuron, injury to one of the proximal neurons is not followed by degeneration of the distal neuron.

Experimentation on animals with artificial lesions of the CNS has shown that **retrograde transneuronal degeneration** may occur in certain situations.

Neuronal Degeneration Associated with Senescence

Many neurons degenerate and disappear during fetal development. This process is believed to be due to their failure to establish adequate functional connections. During postnatal life, further gradual neuronal degeneration continues to occur. In old age, an individual may have lost up to 20% of the original number of neurons. This may account to some extent for the loss of efficiency of the nervous system that is associated with senescence.

Atrophy of Voluntary Muscle and Other End Organs Following Peripheral Nerve Degeneration

Voluntary muscle undergoes degenerative changes following motor nerve section. First, the response to acetylcholine (ACh) is altered, followed by gradual wasting of the sarcoplasm, and finally loss of the fibrils and striations. Eventually, the muscle completely atrophies and is replaced by fibrous tissue. Reinnervation of the muscle halts its degeneration and, if the muscle atrophy is not too advanced, normal structure and function return.

Furthermore, if the motor nerve that supplies fast white voluntary muscle fibers is exchanged for a motor nerve that supplies slow red voluntary muscle fibers, the muscle fibers change their structural and functional properties to comply with the new type of innervation. This experimental result strongly suggests not only that voluntary muscle cells are dependent on the presence of intact motor nerves but also that the nerve has some trophic influence on the muscle and even determines the type of muscle that it innervates.

Another end organ, the taste bud, also depends on the integrity of the sensory nerve. If the nerve is sectioned, the taste bud quickly atrophies. Once the sensory nerve regenerates into the mucous membrane, new taste buds develop.

Traumatic Lesions of Peripheral Nerves

Seddon (1944) described three clinical types of nerve injury:

- **Neuropraxia** is a transient block. The paralysis is incomplete, recovery is rapid and complete, and microscopic evidence of nerve degeneration does not exist. Pressure is the most common cause. It is essentially a temporary interference in function.
- **Axonotmesis** is a nerve lesion in which the axons are damaged but the surrounding connective tissue sheaths remain more or less intact. Wallerian degeneration occurs peripherally. Functional recovery is more rapid and more complete than after complete section of the nerve trunk because the nerve fibers, although severely damaged, for the most part retain their normal anatomical relationships to one another, owing to the preservation of the connective tissue sheaths. Crush injuries, traction, and compression are the most common causes.
- **Neurotmesis** is complete section of the nerve trunk.

Symptoms and Signs of Neurotmesis

Completely dividing a peripheral nerve can be seen in the clinic as paralysis or anesthesia, or both. The magnitude of injury is assessed by reflexive response, muscle strength, and distribution of cutaneous sensation loss.

MOTOR CHANGES

The muscles that are innervated show flaccid paralysis and rapidly waste. The reflexes in which the muscles participate are lost. The paralyzed muscle ceases to respond to faradic stimulation after 4 to 7 days. After 10 days, the muscle responds only sluggishly to galvanic stimulation, and the strength of the current must be greater than that required for a normal innervated muscle. This altered response of muscle to electrical stimulation is known as the **reaction of degeneration**.

SENSORY CHANGES

Cutaneous sensibility is completely lost over the area exclusively supplied by the nerve. This area is surrounded by a zone of partial sensory loss where adjacent sensory nerves overlap. The skin area in which the sensation of light touch is lost is much greater than the area lost to pinprick.

VASOMOTOR, SUDOMOTOR, AND TROPHIC CHANGES

Section of a peripheral nerve results in the interruption of postganglionic sympathetic fibers traveling in the nerve. As a result of the loss of vascular control, the skin area at first becomes red and hot. Later, the affected area becomes blue and colder than normal, especially in cold weather. Because of the loss of sudomotor control, the sweat glands cease to produce sweat, and the skin becomes dry and scaly. Nail growth becomes retarded as the direct result of poor peripheral circulation. If a large area of the body is denervated, as in cases in which the sciatic nerve is sectioned, the bones undergo decalcification as a result of disuse and loss of circulatory control.

RECOVERY FROM NEUROTMESIS

Assuming that the divided peripheral nerve has been carefully sutured together, a clinician must be aware of the symptoms and signs of recovery and their sequence.

MOTOR RECOVERY

Regenerating motor axons grow at an average rate of about 1.5 mm per day. The proximal muscles will recover first, and the distal muscles will recover later. The muscles may respond to faradic stimulation before voluntary control returns.

SENSORY RECOVERY

Sensory recovery occurs before voluntary movement returns. The part of the nerve distal to the section becomes very sensitive to mechanical stimulation once the regenerating sensory axons have entered the distal segment. Simple tapping of the distal nerve trunk gives rise to a tingling sensation in the area of cutaneous distribution of the nerve. This sign is referred to as the **Tinel sign**. Recovery of deep cutaneous sensibility—that is, pain caused by deep pressure—is the first sign of recovery. This is followed by the return of poorly localized, superficial cutaneous pain. Vasomotor control also returns at about this time. Later, the sensations of heat and cold are recovered. Light touch and tactile discrimination are the last sensations to return; these sensations return many months later and are often incomplete.

Specific Spinal Nerve Injuries

Table 3-3 summarizes the important features found in cervical and lumbosacral root syndromes (a detailed description of the neurologic deficits following the many spinal nerve injuries seen in clinical practice is beyond the scope of this book). Tables that summarize the branches of the brachial

Table 3-3   Important Features Found in Cervical and Lumbosacral Root Syndromes

Root Injury	Dermatome Pain	Muscles Supplied	Movement Weakness	Reflex Involved
C5	Lateral side of upper part of arm	Deltoid and biceps brachii	Shoulder abduction, elbow flexion	Biceps
C6	Lateral side of forearm	Extensor carpi radialis longus and brevis	Wrist extensors	Brachioradialis
C7	Middle finger	Triceps and flexor carpi radialis	Extension of elbow and flexion of wrist	Triceps
C8	Medial side of forearm	Flexor digitorum superficialis and profundus	Finger flexion	None
L1	Groin	Iliopsoas	Hip flexion	Cremaster
L2	Anterior part of thigh	Iliopsoas, sartorius, hip adductors	Hip flexion, hip adduction	Cremaster
L3	Medial side of knee	Iliopsoas, sartorius, quadriceps, hip adductors	Hip flexion, knee extension, hip adduction	Patellar
L4	Medial side of calf	Tibialis anterior, quadriceps	Foot inversion, knee extension	Patellar
L5	Lateral side of lower leg and dorsum of foot	Extensor hallucis longus, extensor digitorum longus	Toe extension, ankle dorsiflexion	None
S1	Lateral edge of foot	Gastrocnemius, soleus	Ankle plantar flexion	Ankle jerk
S2	Posterior part of thigh	Flexor digitorum longus, flexor hallucis longus	Ankle plantar flexion, toe flexion	None

(Table 3-4) and lumbar and sacral (Table 3-5) plexuses and their distribution are also included. These tables can assist the reader in determining the specific nerve lesion associated with a particular motor or sensory deficit in the upper or lower limbs.

Cranial nerve injuries are considered in Chapter 11.

Basic Clinical Principles Underlying Peripheral Nerve Injuries

- In open, dirty wounds, which carry a high risk of infection, the sectioned nerve should be ignored, and the wound infection should be treated. Later, when the wound has healed satisfactorily, the nerve should be explored, and the cut ends of the nerve should be sutured together.
- For a patient with a healed wound and no evidence of nerve recovery, the treatment should be conservative. Sufficient time should be allowed to elapse to enable the regenerating nerve fibers to reach the proximal muscles. If recovery fails to occur, the nerve should be explored surgically.
- In cases in which connective tissue, bone fragments, or muscles come to lie between the cut ends of a severed nerve, the nerve should be explored; if possible, the cut ends of the nerve should be brought together and sutured.
- The nutrition of the paralyzed muscles must be maintained with adequate physiotherapy. Warm baths, massage, and warm clothing help to maintain adequate circulation.
- The paralyzed muscles must not be allowed to be stretched by antagonist muscles or by gravity. Moreover, excessive shortening of the paralyzed muscles leads to contracture of these muscles.

- Mobility must be preserved by daily passive movements of all joints in the affected area. Failure to do this results in the formation of adhesions and consequent limitation of movement.

Once voluntary movement returns in the most proximal muscles, the physiotherapist can assist the patient in performing active exercises. This not only aids in the return of a normal circulation to the affected part but also helps the patient to learn once again the complicated muscular performance of skilled movements.

Nerve Transplantation

Nerve grafts have been used with some success to restore muscle tone in facial nerve palsy. In mixed nerve injuries, nerve grafts have succeeded only in restoring some sensory function and slight muscle activity. The presence of two suture lines and the increased possibility of mixing the nerve fibers is probably the reason for the lack of success with nerve grafts. In most nerve injuries, even when the gap between the proximal and distal ends is as great as 10 cm, mobilizing the nerve or altering its position in relation to joints so that the proximal and distal ends may be brought together without undue tension is usually possible; the ends are then sutured together.

Peripheral Nerve Tumors

A peripheral nerve consists essentially of nerve fibers (axons), each of which is associated with Schwann cells; the fibers are either myelinated or nonmyelinated. The nerve

Table 3-4   Branches of the Brachial Plexus and Their Distribution

Branches	Distribution
Roots	
Dorsal scapular nerve (C5)	Rhomboid minor, rhomboid major, levator scapulae muscles
Long thoracic nerve (C5–C7)	Serratus anterior muscle
Upper Trunk	
Suprascapular nerve (C5–C6)	Supraspinatus and infraspinatus muscles
Nerve to subclavius (C5–C6)	Subclavius
Lateral Cord	
Lateral pectoral nerve (C5–C7)	Pectoralis major muscle
Musculocutaneous nerve (C5–C7)	Coracobrachialis, biceps brachii, brachialis muscles; supplies skin along lateral border of forearm when it becomes the lateral cutaneous nerve of forearm
Lateral root of median nerve (C5–C7)	See medial root of median nerve
Posterior Cord	
Upper subscapular nerve (C5–C6)	Subscapularis muscle
Thoracodorsal nerve (C6–C8)	Latissimus dorsi muscle
Lower subscapular nerve (C5–C6)	Subscapularis and teres major muscles
Axillary nerve (C5–C6)	Deltoid and teres minor muscles; upper lateral cutaneous nerve of arm supplies skin over lower half of deltoid muscle
Radial nerve (C5–C8, T1)	Triceps, anconeus, part of brachialis, brachioradialis, extensor carpi radialis longus; via deep radial nerve branch supplies extensor muscles of forearm: supinator, extensor carpi radialis brevis, extensor carpi ulnaris, extensor digitorum, extensor digiti minimi, extensor indicis, abductor pollicis longus, extensor pollicis longus, extensor pollicis brevis; skin, lower lateral cutaneous nerve of arm, posterior cutaneous nerve of arm, and posterior cutaneous nerve of forearm; skin on lateral side of dorsum of hand and dorsal surface of lateral 3½ fingers; articular branches to elbow, wrist, and hand
Medial Cord	
Medial pectoral nerve (C8, T1)	Pectoralis major and minor muscles
Medial cutaneous nerve of arm joined by intercostal brachial nerve from second intercostal nerve (C8, T1–T2)	Skin of medial side of arm
Medial cutaneous nerve of forearm (C8, T1)	Skin of medial side of forearm
Ulnar nerve (C8, T1)	Flexor carpi ulnaris and medial half of flexor digitorum profundus, flexor digiti minimi, opponens digiti minimi, abductor digiti minimi, adductor pollicis, third and fourth lumbricals, interossei, palmaris brevis, skin of medial half of dorsum of hand and palm, skin of palmar and dorsal surfaces of medial 1½ fingers
Medial root of median nerve (with lateral root) forms median nerve (C5–C8, T1)	Pronator teres, flexor carpi radialis, palmaris longus, flexor digitorum superficialis, abductor pollicis brevis, flexor pollicis brevis, opponens pollicis, first two lumbricals (by way of anterior interosseous branch), flexor pollicis longus, flexor digitorum profundus (lateral half), pronator quadratus, palmar cutaneous branch to lateral half of palm and digital branches to palmar surface of lateral 3½ fingers; articular branches to elbow, wrist, and carpal joints

Table 3-5 Branches of the Lumbar and Sacral Plexuses and Their Distribution

Branches	Distribution
Femoral nerve (L2–L4)	Iliacus, pectineus, sartorius, quadriceps femoris muscles; skin, medial cutaneous and intermediate cutaneous nerves of thigh, saphenous nerve to medial side of leg, medial side of foot as far as ball of big toe; articular branches to hip and knee joints
Obturator nerve (L2–L4)	Pectineus, adductor longus, adductor brevis, adductor magnus (adductor portion), gracilis muscles; skin, medial side of thigh; articular branches to hip and knee joints
Sciatic nerve (L4–L5, S1–S3)	
Common peroneal nerve	Biceps femoris muscle (short head); skin, lateral cutaneous nerve of calf, sural communicating branch to lateral side of leg, lateral side of foot, and little toe
Superficial peroneal nerve	Peroneus longus and brevis muscles; skin, lower leg, and dorsum of foot
Deep peroneal nerve	Tibialis anterior, extensor hallucis longus, extensor digitorum longus, peroneus tertius, extensor digitorum brevis muscles; skin, cleft between the first and second toes; articular branches to tibiofibular, ankle, and foot joints
Tibial nerve	Semitendinosus, biceps femoris (long head), semimembranosus, adductor magnus (hamstring part), gastrocnemius, soleus, plantaris, popliteus, tibialis posterior, flexor digitorum longus, flexor hallucis longus muscles; skin, medial side of ankle; articular branches to hip, knee, and ankle joints
Medial plantar nerve	Abductor hallucis, flexor digitorum brevis, flexor hallucis brevis, first lumbrical muscles; skin, medial side of sole of foot; articular branches to foot joints
Lateral plantar nerve	Flexor accessorius, abductor digiti minimi, flexor digiti minimi brevis, second, third, and fourth lumbricals, adductor hallucis, all interossei muscles; skin of lateral side of sole of foot

fibers are arranged in parallel bundles and are surrounded by connective tissue sheaths.

A **benign fibroma** or a **malignant sarcoma** may arise in the connective tissue of the nerve and does not differ from similar tumors elsewhere. **Neurilemmomas** are believed to arise from Schwann cells. They arise from any nerve trunk, cranial or spinal, and in any part of its course. Primary tumors of the axons are very rare.

Blood Vessels, Lymphatics, and Endoneurial Spaces within Peripheral Nerves

Peripheral nerves receive branches from arteries in the regions they pass through. The anastomotic network that exists within a nerve is considerable, and local ischemia does not occur if a single artery is obstructed.

A plexus of lymph vessels lies within the epineurial connective tissues, and this drains to regional lymph nodes.

As demonstrated by the results of experiments in which dyes have been injected into peripheral nerves, spaces exist between individual nerve fibers. These endoneurial spaces evidently provide a potential route for the ascent of **tetanus toxin** to the spinal cord.

Local Anesthetic Action on Nerve Conduction

Local anesthetics are drugs that block nerve conduction when applied locally to a nerve fiber in suitable concentrations. Their site of action is the axolemma (plasma membrane), and they interfere with the transient increase in permeability of the axolemma to Na^+, K^+, and other ions. The sensitivity of nerve fibers to local anesthetics is related to the size of the nerve fibers (see Table 2-3). Small nerve

fibers are more susceptible than large fibers; small fibers are also slower to recover.

Cocaine has been used clinically to block nerve conduction. Unfortunately, it is a strong stimulant of the cerebral cortex and readily causes addiction. **Procaine** is a synthetic compound that is widely used as a local anesthetic agent.

Apparent Recovery of Central Nervous System Function

Axon regeneration in the brain and spinal cord is minimal following a lesion, yet considerable functional recovery often occurs. Several explanations exist, and more than one mechanism may be involved.

1. Nerve fiber function may be impaired from compression by edema fluid. Once the edema subsides, a substantial recovery may take place.
2. The damaged nerve fiber proximal to the lesion may form new synapses with neighboring normal neurons.
3. Following a lesion to branches of a nerve, all the neurotransmitters may pass down the remaining branches, producing a greater effect.
4. Following a lesion of an afferent neuron, an increased number of receptor sites may develop on a postsynaptic membrane. This may result in the second neuron responding to neurotransmitter substances from neighboring neurons.
5. Nonfunctioning neurons may take over the function of damaged neurons.
6. The damaged nerve fiber proximal to the lesion may form new synapses with neighboring normal neurons.

7. The normal neighboring nerve fibers may give off branches distal to the lesion, which then follow the pathway previously occupied by the damaged fibers.
8. If a particular function, such as the contraction of voluntary muscle, is served by two neural pathways in the CNS and one pathway is damaged, the remaining undamaged pathway may take over the entire function. Thus, conceivably, if the corticospinal tract is injured, the corticoreticulospinal tract may take over the major role of controlling the muscle movement.
9. With intensive physiotherapy, patients may be trained to use other muscles to compensate for the loss of paralyzed muscles.

Herpes Zoster

Herpes zoster, or shingles, is a relatively common condition caused by the reactivation of the latent varicella zoster virus in a patient who has previously had chickenpox. The infection is found in the first sensory neuron in a cranial or spinal nerve. The lesion is seen as an inflammation and degeneration of the sensory neuron with the formation of vesicles with inflammation of the skin. The first symptom is pain in the distribution of the sensory neuron, followed in a few days by a skin eruption. The condition occurs most frequently in patients over age 50 years.

Polyneuropathy

Polyneuropathy is an impairment of function of many peripheral nerves simultaneously. The many causes include infection (endotoxin of diphtheria, Guillain–Barré syndrome [see Clinical Example at beginning of chapter]), metabolic disorders (vitamins B_1 and B_{12} deficiency, poisoning by heavy metals, drugs), and endocrine disorders (diabetes). Axon degeneration and/or segmental demyelination may take place, and the neuron cell body may be involved. In mild cases, the condition is reversible, but in severe cases, it may be permanent. Both sensory and motor symptoms and signs may be evident.

Receptors

Sensory endings are found throughout the body in both somatic and visceral areas. Their wide distribution is fortunate, because they enable us to react to changes in the external and internal environment.

To make a diagnosis or study the effect of treatment on a disease process, a clinician relies almost entirely on the patient's ability to describe changes in subjective sensations or to respond to specific stimuli during a physical examination. Such descriptions, such as "knifelike pain," "dull and aching pain," "colicky pain," "pins and needles," and "cannot feel anything" are very familiar to the practicing clinician. Each main type of sensation that can be experienced, such as pain, temperature, and touch and pressure, is called a **modality** of sensation. The type of modality felt by a patient from a particular part of the body is determined by the specific area of the CNS to which the afferent nerve fiber passes. However, remembering that axons carrying specific modalities are associated with one or more anatomically distinct receptors is clinically useful (Table 3-6).

Sensory Receptors and Age

With life expectancy increasing, many patients now reach the age when sensory receptor degeneration can cause

Table 3-6	Receptors and Associated Functions
Receptor	**Associated Function**
Free nerve endings	Pain, touch, pressure, tickle sensations, possibly cold and heat
Merkel discs	Touch and pressure
Hair follicle receptor	Touch
Meissner corpuscles	Touch (two-point tactile discrimination)
Pacinian corpuscles	Pressure and vibration
Ruffini corpuscles	Stretch
Neuromuscular spindles	Elongation of muscle (stretch)
Neurotendinous spindles	Tension

disequilibrium. This critical age varies in different individuals, but once it starts, the sensory systems progressively deteriorate, involving not only visual and auditory systems but also proprioception and the ability to integrate the afferent information entering the CNS.

Sensory Modality Examination

An accurate physical examination may enable the neurologist to make a precise diagnosis. He or she may be able to determine whether a particular sensation can or cannot be appreciated or whether it is less than normal. The clinician will be able to determine the precise area over the surface of the body where impairment of sensation is found. The following sensations are usually tested:

1. **Light touch.** This is tested by gently touching the skin with a wisp of cotton; the patient has the eyes closed and responds "yes" whenever the stimulus is felt. Recognize that different areas of the skin normally exhibit different thresholds for touch. The back and buttocks are less sensitive than the face or fingertips. On hairy surfaces, the slightest movement of a hair usually can be felt.
2. **Localization of touch.** After detecting the light touch with the eyes closed, the patient is asked to place a finger on the exact site touched. Failure to accomplish this may be due to damage to the cerebral cortex.
3. **Two-point tactile discrimination.** Two blunt points are applied to the skin surface while the patient's eyes are closed. Gradually, the points are brought closer together until the patient is unable to distinguish two definite points. A normal person is able to distinguish two separate points on the tip of the index finger when they are separated by a distance greater than about 3 mm. On the back, however, they have to be separated by as much as 3 to 4 cm.
4. **Pain.** The skin may be touched with the sharp end of a pin. First, the pain threshold is established and then the areas of diminished or lost pain sensation are mapped out. Apply the stimulus in an irregular manner, first using the sharp end of the pin and then the dull head, with the patient responding "sharp" or "dull." Certain diseases, such as tabes dorsalis or polyneuropathy

(polyneuritis), may produce a delay of up to 3 seconds before the patient recognizes the sharp pain.

5. **Pressure pain.** This poorly localized pain is perceived by deep pressure on a muscle or by squeezing a tendon.

6. **Temperature testing.** Test tubes filled with hot or cold water may be used. When the test tubes are applied to the skin, the patient responds with either "warm" or "cold." First, the temperature threshold is established and then the areas of diminished or lost temperature sensation are mapped out.

7. **Vibration.** When the handle of a vibrating tuning fork is applied to the skin over bone (e.g., the medial malleolus of the tibia or the olecranon process of the ulna), a tingling sensation is felt. This is due to the stimulation of superficial and deep pressure receptors. The patient is asked to respond when the first vibration is felt as well as when the vibration can no longer be detected. The perception of vibration in the legs is usually diminished after age 60 years.

8. **Appreciation of form (stereognosis).** With the patient's eyes closed, the examiner places common objects, such as coins or keys, in the patient's hands. The patient normally should be able to identify objects by moving them around in the hand and feeling them with the fingers.

9. **Passive movements of joints.** This test may be carried out on the fingers or toes. With the patient completely relaxed and in the supine position with eyes closed, the digit is flexed or extended irregularly. After each movement, the patient is asked, "Is the digit 'up' or 'down'?" A normal individual not only can determine that passive movement is taking place but also is aware of the direction of the movement.

10. **Postural sensibility.** This is the ability to describe the position of a limb when it is placed in that position while the patient's eyes are closed. Another way to perform the test is to ask the patient, with eyes closed, to place the limb on the opposite side in the same position as the other limb. The application and interpretation of the results of these tests will be understood more fully when the afferent or sensory pathways have been discussed (see Chapter 4).

Phantom Limb

Wherever a particular sensory pathway is stimulated along its course from the receptor to the sensory cortex of the brain, the sensation experienced by the individual is referred to the site of the receptor. For example, if the pain fibers from the receptors in the little finger are stimulated in the ulnar nerve at the elbow, the individual will experience pain in the little finger and not at the elbow.

Following the amputation of a limb, the patient may experience severe pain in the absent limb due to pressure on the nerve fibers at the end of the stump. This phenomenon is referred to clinically as **phantom limb**.

Action of Drugs and Other Agents on Skeletal Neuromuscular Junctions

Table 3-7 gives some examples of drugs and diseases affecting the motor endplates in skeletal muscle.

Neuromuscular Blocking Agents

***d*-Tubocurarine** produces flaccid paralysis of skeletal muscle, first affecting the extrinsic muscles of the eyes and then those of the face, the extremities, and finally the diaphragm.

Table 3-7 Drugs and Diseases Affecting the Motor Endplates in Skeletal Muscle

Drug or Disease	Increasing ACh Release	Decreasing ACh Release	Acting on ACh Receptors		AChE Inhibition
			Depolarizing Blockade	ACh Receptor Blockade	
Drug					
4-Aminopyridines	Yes				
Guanidine hydrochloride	Yes				
Succinylcholine			Yes		
d-Tubocurarine				Yes	
Dimethyltubocurarine				Yes	
Gallamine				Yes	
Benzoquinonium				Yes	
Physostigmine					Yes
Neostigmine					Yes
Disease					
Botulinum toxin		Yes			
Myasthenia gravis			Destruction of receptors		

ACh, acetylcholine; AChE, acetylcholinesterase.

Dimethyltubocurarine, **gallamine**, and **benzoquinonium** have similar effects.

These drugs combine with the receptor sites at the postsynaptic membrane normally used by ACh and thus block the neurotransmitter action of ACh. Therefore, they are referred to as competitive blocking agents, as they are competing for the same receptor site as ACh. As these drugs are slowly metabolized, the paralysis passes off.

Decamethonium and **succinylcholine** also paralyze skeletal muscle, but their action differs from that of competitive blocking agents because they produce their effect by causing depolarization of the motor endplate. Acting like ACh, they depolarize the postsynaptic membrane, and the muscle contracts once. This is followed by flaccid paralysis and blockage of neuromuscular activity. Although the blocking action endures for some time, the drugs are metabolized, and the paralysis passes off. The actual paralysis is produced by the continued depolarization of the postsynaptic membrane. Remember that continuous depolarization does not produce continuous skeletal muscle contraction. Repolarization has to take place before further depolarization can occur.

Neuromuscular blocking agents are commonly used with general anesthetics to produce the desired degree of muscle relaxation without using larger doses of general anesthetics. Because the respiratory muscles are paralyzed, facilities for artificial respiration are essential.

Anticholinesterases

Physostigmine and **neostigmine** have the capacity to combine with acetylcholinesterase (AChE) and prevent the esterase from inactivating ACh. In addition, neostigmine has a direct stimulating action on skeletal muscle. The actions of both drugs are reversible, and they have been used with success in the treatment of myasthenia gravis.

Bacterial Toxins

Clostridium botulinum, the causative organism in certain cases of food poisoning, produces a toxin that inhibits the release of ACh at the neuromuscular junction. Death results from paralysis of the respiratory muscles. The course of the disease can be improved by the administration of calcium gluconate or guanidine, which promotes the release of ACh from the nerve terminals.

Motor Nerve and Skeletal Muscle

Not only does the motor nerve control the activity of the muscle it supplies but also its integrity is essential for the muscle's normal maintenance. Following section of a motor nerve, the muscle fibers rapidly atrophy and are replaced by connective tissue. The total bulk of the muscle may be 75% reduced in as little as 3 months. This degree of atrophy does not occur if the muscle simply is immobilized; that is, it is not just disuse atrophy. Apparently, the maintenance of normal muscle is dependent on the continued reception of ACh at the postsynaptic membrane at the neuromuscular junction.

Denervation Supersensitivity of Skeletal Muscle

After approximately 2 weeks of denervation, skeletal muscle fibers respond to externally applied ACh at sites other than the neuromuscular junctions. This supersensitivity could be explained on the basis that many new ACh receptors have developed along the length of the muscle fibers following denervation.

Myasthenia Gravis

Myasthenia gravis is a common disease characterized by drooping of the upper eyelids (ptosis), double vision (diplopia), difficulty in swallowing (dysphagia), difficulty in talking (dysarthria), and general muscle weakness and fatigue. Initially, the disease most often involves the muscles of the eye and the pharynx, and the symptoms can be relieved with rest. In the progressive form of the disease, the weakness becomes steadily worse, and ultimately death occurs.

The condition is an autoimmune disorder in which antibodies are produced against the nicotinic ACh receptors on the postsynaptic membrane. The cause of the autoimmune disorder is unknown. The antibodies interfere with the synaptic transmission by reducing the number of receptors or by blocking the interaction of ACh with its receptors. The size of the junctional folds is also reduced, and the width of the synaptic cleft is increased. Together, these changes result in reduced amplitude in endplate potentials. The condition can be temporarily relieved by AChE drugs such as **neostigmine,** which potentiates ACh's action.

In adults with myasthenia gravis, about 70% show evidence of hyperplasia of their thymus glands. In the thymus, T cells, which mediate immune protection, undergo maturation. Excessive synthesis of thymic hormones that stimulate the development of T cells may contribute to the autoimmune response.

A rare congenital form of myasthenia gravis may exist from birth, with no abnormal antibody present. The causes of the congenital disease include AChE deficiency at the motor endplates, impaired release of ACh, impaired capacity of the receptors to interact with ACh, and a reduced number of ACh receptors.

Hypokalemic Periodic Paralysis and Hyperkalemic Paralysis

Hypokalemic periodic paralysis and hyperkalemic paralysis are diseases due to decreased or increased blood potassium levels. The ability of ACh to initiate electrical changes in the postsynaptic membrane of the neuromuscular junction can be greatly influenced by the level of blood potassium, and this blood change is responsible for the paralysis in these patients.

Action of Drugs on Neuromuscular Junctions in Smooth and Cardiac Muscle and Nerve Endings on Secretory Cells

In normal body physiology, ACh released from postganglionic parasympathetic fibers can bring about depolarization and resulting contraction of smooth muscle fibers. ACh, however, is a useless drug to be administered by the clinician, because it is rapidly destroyed by the **cholinesterases**. Also, its actions are so widespread that it cannot be used selectively. By slightly changing the structure, as in the case of **methacholine chloride** or **carbachol**, the drugs are less susceptible to destruction by the cholinesterases but still possess the ability to react with the receptors.

Atropine and **scopolamine** are drugs that compete with ACh for the same receptors. These drugs are competitive antagonists of ACh at receptor sites of smooth muscle, cardiac muscle, and various secretory cells.

Norepinephrine is released from postganglionic sympathetic fibers and can bring about depolarization of smooth muscle in the walls of arteries, for example, resulting in their contraction. At other sites, such as the bronchi, it causes smooth muscle relaxation. Sympathetic receptors have been classified as α and β. The functions associated with α-receptors are vasoconstriction, mydriasis (dilatation of the pupil), and relaxation of the smooth muscle of the intestine. β-Receptors are associated with vasodilatation, cardioacceleration, bronchial relaxation, and intestinal relaxation.

Phenoxybenzamine has been found to block α-receptors, whereas **propranolol** blocks β-receptors. The structure of these receptors is not known.

Sensory Perception Abnormalities

Abnormalities in sensory perception should be looked for on the face, trunk, and limbs. Areas of diminished pain sensation (**hypalgesia**) or touch sensation (**hypesthesia**) or heightened sensation (**hyperesthesia**) should be identified. Abnormal sensations (**paresthesia**), such as pins and needles, may be experienced by a patient who has a lesion located anywhere along the sensory pathway from the peripheral nerve to the cerebral cortex. The areas of sensory abnormality should be precisely defined and recorded, with each modality being recorded separately.

Testing sensory function requires practice and experience. Many patients have difficulty in responding to a clinician's examination of the sensory system. Some individuals try to assist the examiner by wrongfully anticipating the correct response. This problem can largely be overcome by testing for cutaneous sensibility with the patient's eyes closed. In this way, the patient cannot see which areas of skin are being tested. Other patients find it difficult to understand exactly what information is required of them. Some intelligent patients respond more to differences in intensity of stimulation rather than giving a simple "yes" or "no" answer to the question "Can you feel anything?" The clinician must always be aware of the possibility of hysteria, which occurs when a patient complains of sensory loss that has no neuroanatomical explanation. For example, a total loss of skin sensation on one side of the face, including the angle of the jaw, would infer that the patient has a lesion involving the fifth cranial nerve in the pons and the greater auricular nerve (C2–C3), which is anatomically very unlikely. Patience and objectivity are required, and if doubt exists as to the accuracy of the assessment, the patient should be reexamined on another occasion.

Segmental Innervation of the Skin

Because large nerve plexuses are present at the roots of the upper and lower limbs, a single spinal nerve may send both motor and sensory fibers to several peripheral nerves, and conversely, a single peripheral nerve may receive nerve fibers from many spinal nerves. Moreover, a lesion of a segment of the spinal cord, or posterior root, or spinal nerve will result in a sensory loss that is different from that occurring after a lesion of a peripheral nerve.

The area of skin supplied by a single spinal nerve and, therefore, a single segment of the spinal cord is called a **dermatome**. A clinician should remember that dermatomes overlap and that, in the trunk, at least three contiguous spinal nerves have to be sectioned to produce a region of complete anesthesia. Remember also that the degree of overlap for painful and thermal sensations is much greater than that for tactile sensation. A clinician should have a working knowledge of the segmental (dermatomal) innervation of skin, because with a pin or a piece of cotton, he or she can determine whether the sensory function of a particular spinal nerve or segment of the spinal cord is normal. When examining the dermatomal charts, note that because of the development of the upper limbs, the anterior rami of the lower cervical and first thoracic spinal nerves have lost their cutaneous innervation of the trunk anteriorly, and at the level of the second costal cartilage, the fourth cervical dermatome is contiguous with the second thoracic dermatome. In the sensory innervation of the head, the trigeminal (fifth cranial) nerve supplies a large area of the face and scalp, and its cutaneous area is contiguous with that of the second cervical segment.

Because the dermatomes run longitudinally along the long axis of the upper limbs, sensation should be tested by dragging a wisp of cotton or a pin along the long axis of the medial and lateral borders of the limbs. On the trunk, the dermatomes run almost horizontally, so the stimulus should be applied by moving in a vertical direction.

Segmental Innervation of the Muscles

Remember that most skeletal muscles are innervated by more than one spinal nerve and, therefore, by the same number of segments of the spinal cord. Complete destruction of one segment of the spinal cord as the result of trauma or pressure from a tumor will cause weakness of all the muscles that are innervated from that segment. To paralyze a muscle completely, several adjacent segments of the spinal cord have to be destroyed.

Because of the presence of the cervical, brachial, and lumbosacral plexuses, the axons of motor anterior gray column cells are redistributed into a number of peripheral nerves. Knowing this, the clinician, is able to distinguish between a lesion of a segment of the spinal cord, an anterior root, or a spinal nerve on the one hand and a lesion of a peripheral nerve on the other hand. For example, the musculocutaneous nerve of the arm, which receives nerve fibers from the fifth, sixth, and seventh cervical segments of the spinal cord, supplies a finite number of muscles—namely, the biceps brachii, the brachialis, and the coracobrachialis muscles—and section of that nerve would result in total paralysis of these muscles; a lesion of the fifth, sixth, and seventh cervical spinal segments, or their anterior roots or their spinal nerves, would result in paralysis of these muscles and also partial paralysis of many other muscles, including the deltoid, supraspinatus, teres minor, and infraspinatus.

The segmental innervation of the biceps brachii, triceps, brachioradialis, muscles of the anterior abdominal wall, quadriceps femoris, gastrocnemius, and soleus should be memorized, as testing them is possible by eliciting their reflex contraction (see p. 110).

Muscle Tone

Skeletal muscle tone is due to the presence of a few muscle fibers within a muscle being in a state of full contraction all the time. Muscle tone is controlled reflexly from afferent nerve endings situated in the muscle itself. Therefore, any disease process that interferes with any part of the reflex arc will abolish the muscle tone. Some examples are syphilitic infection of the posterior root (tabes dorsalis); destruction of the motor anterior gray column cells, as in poliomyelitis or syringomyelia; destruction of a segment of the spinal cord by trauma or pressure from a tumor; section of an anterior root; pressure on a spinal nerve by a prolapsed intervertebral disc; and section of a peripheral nerve, as in a stab wound. All these clinical conditions will result in loss of muscle tone.

Although the basic mechanism underlying muscle tone is the integrity of the spinal segmental reflex, this reflex activity is influenced by nervous impulses received by the anterior horn cells from all levels of the brain and spinal cord. Spinal shock, which follows injury to the spinal cord and is caused by loss of functional activity of neurons, will result in diminished muscle tone. Cerebellar disease also results in diminished muscle tone because the cerebellum facilitates the stretch reflex. The reticular formation normally tends to increase muscle tone, but its activity is inhibited by higher cerebral centers. Therefore, if the higher cerebral control is interfered with by trauma or disease, the inhibition is lost and the muscle tone is exaggerated (decerebrate rigidity). Primary degeneration of the muscles themselves (myopathies) can also cause loss of muscle tone.

Posture

The posture of an individual depends on the degree and distribution of muscle tone and, therefore, on the activity of the motor neurons that supply the muscles. The motor neurons in the anterior gray columns of the spinal cord are the points where the nervous impulses converge from many posterior nerve roots and the descending fibers from many different levels of the brain and spinal cord. The successful coordination of all these nervous influences results in a normal posture.

When someone is in the standing posture, remarkably little muscular activity is taking place in the muscles of the limbs and trunk. This is because the center of gravity of any part of the body is mainly above the joints on which its weight is directed. Moreover, in many joints, such as the hip and the knee, the ligaments are very strong and support the body in the erect posture. However, a person cannot remain standing if all muscles are paralyzed. Once a person starts to fall, either forward, backward, or laterally, the muscle spindles and other stretch receptors immediately increase their activity, and the reflex arcs come into play; thus, reflex compensatory muscle contractions take place to restore the state of balance. The eyes and the receptors in the membranous labyrinth also play a vital part in the maintenance of balance. The importance of the eyes in maintaining the erect position can easily be tested in a normal person. Once the eyes are closed, the person shows a tendency to sway slightly because he or she now must rely exclusively on muscle and labyrinthine receptors to preserve his or her balance.

Pathologic alteration in muscle tone will therefore affect posture. For example, in hemiplegia or in Parkinson disease, in which hypertonicity exists, posture will be changed. As with cerebellar disease, hypotonicity will cause drooping of the shoulder on the affected side. Lesions involving peripheral nerves that innervate antigravity muscles will produce wristdrop (radial nerve) and footdrop (common peroneal nerve).

Clinical Observation of Muscular Activity

Magnitude of muscle injury is evaluated through observation of size, tone, and the presence of involuntary movements.

Muscular Power

Ask the patient to perform movements for which the muscle under examination is primarily responsible. Next, ask the patient to perform each movement against resistance and compare the strengths of the muscles on the two sides of the body. Section of the peripheral nerve that supplies the muscle or disease affecting the anterior gray column cells (e.g., poliomyelitis) will clearly reduce the power of or paralyze the muscles involved.

Muscle Wasting

Muscle wasting occurs within 2 to 3 weeks after section of the motor nerve. In the limbs, it is easily tested by measuring the diameter of the limbs at a given point over the involved muscle and comparing the measurement obtained with that at the same site on the opposite limb.

Muscular Fasciculation

Twitching of groups of muscle fibers is seen most often in patients with chronic disease that affects the anterior horn cells (e.g., progressive muscular atrophy).

Muscular Contracture

Muscular contracture occurs most commonly in the muscles that normally oppose paralyzed muscles. The muscles contract and undergo permanent shortening.

Muscle Tone

A muscle without tone—that is, one in which the simple spinal reflex arcs are not functioning—is noncontractile and doughlike on palpation. Degrees of loss of tone may be tested by passively moving the joints and comparing the resistance to the movements by the muscles on the two sides of the body. Increase in muscle tone can occur following the removal of the cerebral inhibition on the reticular formation.

Muscular Coordination

To determine muscular coordination, ask the patient to touch, with the eyes open, the tip of the nose with the tip of the forefinger and then ask to repeat the process with the eyes closed. A similar test of the lower limbs may be carried out with the patient lying down. Ask the patient to place one heel on the opposite knee, with the eyes open and then ask to repeat the process with the eyes closed.

Another test is to ask the patient to quickly supinate and pronate both forearms simultaneously. Disease of the cerebellum, for example, which coordinates muscular activity, would result in impaired ability to perform these rapid repetitive movements.

Involuntary Movement of Muscles

Tic is a coordinated, repetitive movement involving one or more muscles.

Choreiform movements are quick, jerky, irregular movements that are nonrepetitive. Swift grimaces and sudden movements of the head or limbs are examples of this condition.

Athetosis consists of slow, sinuous, writhing movements that most commonly involve the distal segments of the limbs.

Tremor is the alternating contraction of the agonists and antagonists of a joint.

Myoclonus consists of shocklike muscular contractions of a portion of a muscle, an entire muscle, or a group of muscles.

Tonic spasm refers to a sustained contraction of a muscle or group of muscles, as in the tonic phase of an epileptic seizure.

Neurologic Sensory and Motor Symptoms—Are They Always of Primary Neurologic Origin?

A neurologic diagnosis depends on determining the site of the lesion and the nature of the pathology causing the disease. The clinician cannot consider the nervous system in isolation, because the neurologic symptoms and signs may depend on disorders mainly involving another system. For example, a cerebral embolism may follow the formation of a blood clot on the ventricular wall of a patient with coronary thrombosis. A cerebral abscess may follow the formation of a lung abscess. Therefore, neurologic examination in many patients should be accompanied by a more general physical examination involving other systems.

Key Concepts

Nerve Fibers

- Myelinated nerve fibers are surrounded by segmented, discontinuous myelin sheaths from supporting neuroglia cells.
- In the PNS, multiple Schwann cells wrap around a single axon in a tight spiral.
- In the CNS, a single oligodendrocyte will extend multiple myelin processes that cover portions of multiple nerve fibers.
- Some smaller axons do not require myelination, such as fine sensory or postganglionic autonomic nerves.

Peripheral Nerves

- The 31 pairs of spinal nerves and 12 pairs of cranial nerves each carry sensory and/or motor nerve fibers.
- Spinal nerves carrying sensory information have a dorsal root ganglion, formed by the collection of unipolar cell bodies. Cranial nerves carrying sensory fibers also have sensory ganglia.
- Sympathetic and parasympathetic nerves have autonomic ganglia, formed by the collection of postsynaptic autonomic cell bodies, located away from the brain and spinal cord.
- Peripheral nerve bundles may divide into branches that join neighboring peripheral nerves, forming a nerve plexus. This allows nerve fibers from different spinal cord segments to be distributed efficiently in different nerve trunks to various parts of the body.

Conduction in Peripheral Nerves

- Reversing the negative resting potential by diffusion of sodium (Na^+) and potassium (K^+) across the plasma membrane, resulting in propagation of electrical depolarization down the fiber, is called an action potential.
- For a short time after the action potential, the nerve is unable to be excited because the sodium channels are inactivated. This is called the absolute refractory period.

- Conduction velocity is positively affected by factors such as fiber diameter and myelination.

Receptor Endings

- Sensory receptors are classified by functional type (mechanoreceptors, thermoreceptors, nociceptors, electromagnetic receptors, and chemoreceptors) and anatomical type (encapsulated or nonencapsulated).
- Free nerve endings are nonencapsulated and typically detect pain, crude touch, pressure, and tickle sensations.
- Merkel discs are nonencapsulated endings found in hairless skin and are considered to be slowly adapting touch receptors.
- Hair follicle receptors are nonencapsulated endings that surround the hair follicle and respond to bending the hair.
- Meissner corpuscles are encapsulated ending found in the dermal papillae of the skin and function as rapidly adapting fine touch detectors.
- Pacinian corpuscles are encapsulated endings in the skin that respond to vibration sensations.
- Ruffini corpuscles are encapsulated stretch receptors in the skin.
- Neuromuscular and neurotendinous spindles are found in muscles and tendons to detect muscle stretch and muscle tension, respectively.

Effector Endings

- Skeletal muscle is innervated by large myelinated nerve fibers derived from motor neurons in the anterior gray horns of the spinal cord.
- A single nerve fiber terminates on multiple muscle fibers at a site referred to as a neuromuscular junction or motor endplate.
- Smooth muscle and cardiac muscle fibers are innervated by sympathetic and parasympathetic parts of the autonomic system.

Clinical Problem Solving

1. A 20-year-old man is seen in the emergency department following an automobile accident. A diagnosis of fracture dislocation of the fourth thoracic vertebra is made, with injury to the spinal cord as a complication. A laminectomy is performed to decompress the spinal cord in order to avoid permanent injury to the tracts of the cord. What is a nerve tract in the spinal cord? How does this differ in structure from a peripheral nerve?

2. Multiple sclerosis is an example of a demyelinating disease of the nervous system. Many other diseases of the nervous system also have the common pathologic feature of destruction of the myelin sheaths of nerve fibers. How does myelination normally take place in peripheral nerves and central nervous system tracts? When does myelination of nerves normally take place?

3. The myelin sheath is said to be formed in the peripheral nervous system (PNS) by the rotation of Schwann cells on the axon so that the plasma membrane becomes wrapped around the axon in a spiral. In the central nervous system (CNS), do the oligodendrocytes rotate on the axons in a similar manner to form myelin?

4. A 26-year-old man is involved in a street brawl and receives a knife wound to the right arm at about the midhumeral level. Physical examination reveals that the median nerve has been sectioned. Motor loss consists of paralysis of the pronator muscles of the forearm and the long flexor muscles of the wrist and fingers, with the exception of the flexor carpi ulnaris and the medial half of the flexor digitorum profundus. As a result, the right forearm is kept in the supine position; wrist flexion is weak and accompanied by adduction. The latter deviation is due to the paralysis of the flexor carpi radialis and the strength of both the flexor carpi ulnaris and the medial half of the flexor digitorum profundus. No flexion is possible at the interphalangeal joints of the index and middle fingers, although weak flexion of the metacarpophalangeal joints of these fingers was attempted by the interossei. When the patient is asked to make a fist of his right hand, the index and, to a lesser extent, the middle fingers tends to remain straight, while the ring and little fingers flex. The latter two fingers are weakened by the loss of the flexor digitorum superficialis. Flexion of the terminal phalanx of the thumb is lost due to paralysis of the flexor pollicis longus. The muscles of the thenar eminence are paralyzed, and the right thumb is laterally rotated and adducted.

Sensory loss of the skin of the right hand involves the lateral half of the palm and the palmar aspect of the lateral three and a half fingers. There is also sensory loss of the skin of the distal parts of the dorsal surfaces of the lateral three and a half fingers.

The skin areas involved in sensory loss become warmer and drier than normal, evidencing vasomotor changes. This is due to arteriolar dilatation and absence of sweating resulting from loss of sympathetic nervous control.

(a) Describe the changes that would take place in the median nerve proximal and distal to the site of section. (b) How would you treat this case? (c) What will be the first signs and symptoms to indicate that the nerve is regenerating adequately? (d) Which function will return first—sensory or muscular? (e) About how long will it take for the nerve to regenerate and reach its end organs?

5. A 45-year-old woman with a right-sided facial palsy is examined. When questioned, she says that 3 years previously she had experienced a weakness of the right side of the face and some degree of loss of taste sensation following a ride in an open car on a cold day. A diagnosis of Bell palsy was made. What is Bell palsy? How would you treat this patient?

6. A family with five small children move into an old house. Six months later, the mother notices that her 1-year-old son is becoming somnolent and quiet. Whereas previously he was very active and crawled around the house, he now tends to lie about the floor, uninterested in his toys. He has also stopped eating well and is very constipated. The mother decides to take him to a pediatrician when, as she puts it, the child suddenly "threw a fit." Examination reveals no positive physical signs except for a dark line between the gums and teeth. When questioned further, the mother admits that the child liked sucking the peeling paint on the railings outside the house. A diagnosis of chronic lead poisoning is made. This is confirmed by finding that the blood lead level was in excess of 50 μg per 100 mL. What effect does lead have on the nervous system?

7. A 54-year-old man suddenly develops severe pain down both legs in the distribution of the sciatic nerve. He also notices numbness in the buttocks and perineum and recently notes that he cannot feel the passage of urine or feces. A diagnosis is made of central protrusion posteriorly of the intervertebral disc between the third and fourth lumbar vertebrae. The symptoms indicate that the cauda equina is being pressed on. Can regeneration occur in the cauda equina?

8. By what anatomical route is tetanus toxin believed to pass from a wound to the central nervous system?

9. Following an automobile accident, a 35-year-old man is seen in the emergency department with fractures of the fifth and sixth ribs on the right side. In order to relieve the pain and discomfort experienced by the patient when breathing, the clinician decides to block the right fifth and sixth intercostal nerves by

injecting a local anesthetic, lidocaine (Xylocaine), around the nerve trunks. What is the effect of the local anesthetic agent on the nerve fibers? Are the large-diameter or the small-diameter nerve fibers more susceptible to the action of the drug?

10. A 65-year-old man, on returning home from a party, finds that he cannot climb the stairs. He has consumed a large amount of whiskey and seems to have lost control of his legs. He sits down on a chair in the hallway and is soon in a deep, stuporous sleep, with his right arm suspended over the back of the chair. The next morning, he wakes with a severe headache and loss of the use of his right arm and hand. During examination in the emergency department, the patient is found to have severe paralysis involving branches of the medial cord of the brachial plexus and the radial nerve. The diagnosis is neuropraxia, which occurred as the result of the pressure of the back of the chair on the involved nerves. What is neuropraxia? How does this differ from axonotmesis and neurotmesis? What is the prognosis in this patient? How would you treat this case?

11. A well-known politician is attending a rally when a youth suddenly steps forward and shoots him in the back. Examination in the emergency department shows that the bullet has entered the back obliquely and is lodged in the vertebral canal at the level of the eighth thoracic vertebra. The patient cannot feel anything below this level and is paralyzed from the waist downward. At the operation, a laminectomy is performed, and the bullet is removed. Considerable damage to the spinal cord is noted. What changes take place in the spinal cord when the nerve fibers are damaged? Does regeneration take place in the central nervous system?

12. An 18-year-old woman visits her physician because she has burns, which she cannot feel, on the tips of the fingers of the right hand. She also mentions that she has weakness of her right hand. On physical examination, severe scarring of the fingers of the right hand is noted. Obvious atrophy of the small muscles of the right hand is also found. Testing the sensory modalities of the skin of the entire patient shows total loss of pain and temperature sensation of the distal part of the right upper limb. The left hand has diminished sensibility to pain and temperature. Definite muscular weakness is demonstrated in the small muscles of the right hand, and a small amount of weakness also is found in the muscles of the left hand. A diagnosis of syringomyelia was made. (a) Using your neuroanatomical knowledge, describe the type of sensory nerve endings that are sensitive to pain and temperature. (b) How would you examine a patient to determine cutaneous pain and temperature sensory loss?

13. A 35-year-old man, while walking past some workmen who are digging a hole in the road, suddenly becomes aware of a foreign body in his left eye. Because the cornea is extremely sensitive, he suffers considerable discomfort. What sensory endings are present in the cornea? Is the cornea sensitive to stimuli other than pain?

14. A 60-year-old man visits his physician because for the past 3 months he has been experiencing an agonizing stabbing pain over the middle part of the right side of his face. The stabs last a few seconds but might be repeated several times. "The pain is the worst I have ever experienced," he tells his clinician. He has noticed particularly that a draft of cold air on his face or the touching of a few scalp hairs in the temporal region can trigger the pain. Physical examination reveals no sensory or motor loss of the trigeminal nerve. A diagnosis of trigeminal neuralgia is made. Using your knowledge of neuroanatomy, explain why hairs are so sensitive to touch.

15. A 50-year-old man is diagnosed as suffering from tabes dorsalis. On physical examination, many signs of the syphilitic disease are present, including a total lack of deep sensation to pain. Intense squeezing of the calcaneus tendon or the testicles produces no response. Using your knowledge of neuroanatomy, explain how deep pain sensation is normally experienced.

16. While carrying out a physical examination of a patient, the clinician asks the patient to cross his knees and relax his leg muscles. The left ligamentum patellae are then struck smartly with a reflex hammer, which immediately produces an involuntary partial extension of the left knee joint (the knee-jerk test is positive). How does the central nervous system receive nervous information from the quadriceps femoris muscle in order that it may respond reflexly by extending the knee?

17. A 55-year-old man suffering from syphilis of the spinal cord presents characteristic symptoms and signs of tabes dorsalis. He has experienced severe stabbing pains in the abdomen and legs for the last 6 months. When asked to walk, the patient is seen to do so with a broad base, slapping the feet on the ground. How would you test the patient's ability to perceive the position of his lower extremities and his vibratory sense? Using your knowledge of neuroanatomy, explain how a normal individual is able to perceive the position of the extremities and detect vibrations.

18. Using your knowledge of pharmacology, name two drugs that act as competitive blocking agents on skeletal neuromuscular junctions. Name the chemical substance against which these agents are competing. Name the sites at which the blocking agents are believed to act.

19. Name a drug that will bring about flaccid paralysis of skeletal muscle by causing depolarization of the postsynaptic membrane.

20. In cases of severe food poisoning, the organism *Clostridium botulinum* may be found to be responsible. How does this organism cause paralysis of the respiratory muscles?

21. During a ward round, an orthopedic surgeon states that the degree of muscular atrophy that occurs in a limb immobilized in a cast is totally different from

the degree of muscular atrophy that follows section of the motor nerve supply to muscles. The surgeon asks a medical student to explain this difference. How would you account for this difference in the degree of muscular atrophy?

22. A 57-year-old man visits his physician because of pain in the right buttock that extends down the right leg, the back of the thigh, the outer side and back of the calf, and the outer border of the foot. The patient gives no history of previous injury but states that the pain started about 3 months ago as a dull, low backache. Since that time, the pain has increased in intensity and has spread down the right leg. When asked if the pain has ever disappeared, he replied that on two separate occasions the pain has diminished in intensity, but his back remains "stiff" all the time. He says the pain is aggravated by stooping or by coughing and sneezing. Sometimes, he experiences a "pins and needles" sensation along the outer border of his right foot. After a complete physical examination, a diagnosis is made of herniation of a lumbar intervertebral disc. Using your knowledge of anatomy, state which intervertebral disc is most likely to have been herniated.

23. A 61-year-old woman is seen by her physician because she is experiencing a shooting, burning pain in the left side of her chest. Three days later, a group of localized papules appears on the skin covering the left fifth intercostal space. One day later, the papules become vesicular; a few days later, the vesicles dry up into crusts. The crusts later separate, leaving small permanent scars. The patient also notices some loss of sensibility over the left side of the chest. A diagnosis of herpes zoster is made. Using your knowledge of anatomy, state the segment of the spinal cord involved with the disease.

24. While examining the sensory innervation of the skin of the head and neck in a patient, a medical student has difficulty remembering the dermatomal pattern at the junction of the head with the neck and at the junction of the neck with the thorax. Are the dermatomes arranged in a special manner in these areas? If so, what is the underlying reason for this?

25. On physical examination, a 30-year-old man is found to have weakness and diminished tone of the rhomboid muscles, deltoids, and biceps brachii on both sides of the body. The degree of weakness is greater on the right side. The biceps tendon jerk is absent on the right side and diminished on the left side. The triceps jerks are normal on both sides of the body. The muscles of the trunk and lower limb show increased tone and exhibit spastic paralysis. Radiology of the vertebral column reveals the presence of vertebral destruction due to a tumor arising within the vertebral canal. Using your knowledge of anatomy, answer the following questions: (a) Which vertebra is likely to have the tumor within the vertebral canal? (b) Name the segments of the spinal cord that are being pressed on by the tumor. (c) Which segments of the spinal cord participate in the reflex arcs responsible for the biceps brachii tendon jerk?

(d) Why do the rhomboid and deltoid muscles exhibit diminished muscle tone, whereas the muscles of the lower limb exhibit increased tone?

26. Name three clinical conditions that could result in a loss of tone of skeletal muscle.

27. A 69-year-old man with advanced tabes dorsalis is asked to stand with his toes and heels together and his eyes closed. He immediately starts to sway violently, and if the nurse had not held on to his arm, he would have fallen to the ground (positive Romberg test). Why was it vital for this patient to keep his eyes open in order to remain upright?

28. A 63-year-old man with moderately advanced Parkinson disease is disrobed and asked to walk in a straight line in the examining room. The physician observes that the patient has his head and shoulders stooped forward, the arms slightly abducted, the elbow joints partly flexed, and the wrists slightly extended with the fingers flexed at the metacarpophalangeal joints and extended at the interphalangeal joints. On starting to walk, the patient leaned forward and slowly shuffles his feet. The farther he leans forward, the more quickly he moves his legs, so that by the time he has crossed the room, he is almost running. The patient's face is masklike and exhibits few emotional movements. The hands show a coarse tremor, and the muscles of the upper and lower limbs show increased tone in the opposing muscle groups when the joints are passively moved. Parkinson disease, or the parkinsonian syndrome, can be caused by a number of pathologic conditions, but they usually interfere in the normal function of the corpus striatum or the substantia nigra or both. Using your knowledge of the anatomy and physiology of muscle action, explain the different signs seen in this important syndrome.

29. A 10-year-old girl is taken to a neurologist because of a 6-month history of epileptic attacks. The parents describe the attacks as starting with sudden involuntary movements of the trunk, arms, or legs. Sometimes, the muscle movements are slight, but at other times, they are so violent that she has been known to throw an object in her hand across the room. At yet other times, the patient just falls to the ground as the result of a sudden loss of muscle tone. Having hit the ground, the patient will immediately rise to her feet. On one occasion, she severely bruised her head and shoulder by striking a chair and a table. One month ago, the parents notice that their daughter appears to lose consciousness briefly. On that occasion, she is carrying on a normal conversation when she suddenly stops and her gaze becomes fixed. After a few seconds, she becomes alert and continues her conversation. This patient is suffering from a form of epilepsy known as petit mal. What is the correct term for the sudden involuntary contraction of the muscles of the trunk or extremities? Name the condition of a patient who suddenly loses all muscle tone and falls to the ground.

30. A 45-year-old man suffering from amyotrophic lateral sclerosis is examined by a third-year medical student. The student found that the flexor and extensor muscles of the knee and ankle joints of the right leg are weaker than those of the left leg. However, she is of the opinion that the muscles of the left leg also are somewhat weaker than normal. On palpation of the extensor muscles of the right thigh, twitching of the muscle fibers in the quadriceps muscle is detected. Marked atrophy of the muscles of both legs also is noted. Cutaneous sensory loss in either limb is not evident. Amyotrophic lateral sclerosis is a condition in which the motor anterior horn cells of the spinal cord and brainstem degenerate with secondary degeneration of the nervous tracts in the lateral and anterior portions of the spinal cord. Why do you think this patient had weakness and atrophy of the muscles of the lower limbs? What is the correct clinical term for the twitching of the muscle fibers in the extensor muscles of the right knee?

31. A 12-year-old girl is diagnosed as suffering from a medulloblastoma of the cerebellum. Clinical and radiologic examinations reveal that the tumor is predominantly invading the right cerebellar hemisphere. Knowing that the cerebellum is concerned with the coordination of motor activity so that complex voluntary movements involving antagonistic muscle groups can take place in a precise manner, what should you test for to demonstrate loss of cerebellar function? Describe the test for each parameter.

 Answers and Explanations to Clinical Problem Solving

1. Nervous tracts are bundles of nerve fibers found in the brain and spinal cord, most of which are myelinated. Some of the main structural differences between a myelinated nerve tract and a myelinated peripheral nerve fiber are as follows:

   Nerve Tract
   Oligodendrocyte
   Mesaxon absent
   Schmidt–Lanterman incisures present
   Nerve fibers supported by neuroglia
   Peripheral Nerve Fiber
   Schwann cell
   Mesaxon present
   Schmidt–Lanterman incisures present
   Nerve fibers supported by connective tissue sheaths, endoneurium, perineurium, and epineurium

2. Myelination is fully described on page 72. Myelin sheaths begin to form during fetal development and during the first year postnatally.

3. No. In the CNS, a single oligodendrocyte may be responsible for the formation of myelin for as many as 60 nerve fibers. Clearly, it would not be possible for an oligodendrocyte to rotate on each axon as does the Schwann cell in the PNS. In the CNS, the process of the oligodendrocyte is believed to grow in length and wrap itself around the axon.

4. (a) The microscopic changes that occur in the proximal and distal segments of a divided peripheral nerve are fully described on page 105. Remember that in the proximal segment, the changes occur only as far proximally as the next node of Ranvier, whereas the changes spread distally from the site of the lesion and include its terminations. (b) If one bears in mind the considerations outlined on page 109 and that the surgeon has the experience to perform nerve suture, the following treatment should be instituted. If the knife was clean, the nerve should be immediately sutured, and any arterial damage should be repaired. On the other hand, if the knife was contaminated or the wound was more than 6 hours old, the wound should be treated, and the nerve should be ignored. In the latter case, when the wound has healed and there is no sign of residual infection, the nerve ends should be explored and sutured together without tension. In either case, the paralyzed muscles are protected with a suitable splint, and the joints are gently exercised daily. (c) Once the regenerating axons have entered the distal segment, the nerve distal to the section becomes very sensitive to mechanical stimulation (Tinel sign). (d) Sensory recovery occurs first. Deep pressure sensation is the first sign of recovery. This is followed by the return of superficial cutaneous pain and vasomotor control of blood vessels. Later, the sensations of heat and cold return. Later still, light touch and tactile discrimination reappear. Sensory recovery occurs before there is return of voluntary movement. (e) For clinical purposes, a figure of 1.5 mm per day is the average rate of regeneration. Use this figure to determine approximately how long it will take for a regenerating nerve to reach its end organs.

5. Bell palsy is produced by swelling of the seventh cranial nerve (facial nerve) in the facial nerve canal of the skull. Its cause is unknown, although it often follows exposure to cold. Since the facial canal is bony, the nerve cannot expand and consequently becomes compressed and ischemic. In severe cases, the muscles of facial expression are paralyzed on one side of the face, and there is loss of taste sensation in the anterior part of the tongue on the same side. Massage of the paralyzed muscles should be undertaken to preserve their integrity until nerve function returns. The majority of patients recover completely. In this patient, a serious residual palsy existed after 3 years. A treatment that has been successful in many cases is to section the hypoglossal nerve below and behind the angle of the mandible and to anastomose its proximal end to the distal

end of the facial nerve. Although the right half of the tongue would be paralyzed, this causes little disability. A reasonable return of facial movement can be expected. The patient learns to move the face instead of the tongue by practicing in front of a mirror. Note that both the hypoglossal and facial nerves are peripheral nerves; therefore, regeneration is possible. The prognosis is especially good since the hypoglossal nerve is purely a motor nerve.

6. Lead causes neuronal degeneration in the central nervous system and demyelination in the tracts of the spinal cord and peripheral nerves. The treatment is to remove the child from the source of the lead and to aid rapid excretion by administering calcium disodium versenate—a chelating agent. Nontoxic lead versenate is excreted in the urine.

7. Yes. The cauda equina consists of the anterior and posterior roots of the spinal nerves below the level of the first lumbar segment of the spinal cord. These are peripheral nerves with endoneurial sheaths and Schwann cells. Therefore, if adequate treatment is promptly instituted, regeneration will take place.

8. As the result of experiments in which dyes have been injected into peripheral nerves, spaces have been demonstrated between individual nerve fibers in the endoneurium. These spaces are believed to provide the route for the ascent of the tetanus toxin to the spinal cord.

9. Lidocaine is a local anesthetic that blocks nerve conduction when applied to a nerve fiber. The anesthetic acts on the axolemma and interferes with the transient increase in permeability of the axolemma to Na^+ ions and, in the resting axon, reduces the permeability of the axolemma to Na^+, K^+, and other ions. The small-diameter pain fibers are more susceptible to the action of this drug.

10. *Neuropraxia* is the term applied to a transient nerve block. Pressure is the most common cause, and this case was due to the pressure of the upper edge of the chair back on the brachial plexus in the axilla. The loss of function is probably caused by ischemia of the nerve fibers. Microscopic evidence of degeneration does not exist. *Axonotmesis* is the term applied to a nerve lesion in which the axons are damaged but the surrounding connective tissue sheaths remain intact. *Neurotmesis* is the term applied to complete section of the nerve trunk.

The prognosis in this patient is excellent for rapid, complete recovery. The paralyzed muscles must not be stretched by antagonist muscles or by gravity. Therefore, suitable splints should be applied, and gentle passive movement of the joints should be performed once daily.

11. Degeneration in the CNS occurs in a manner similar to that found in the peripheral nervous system. The axon breaks up into small fragments, and the debris is digested by the neighboring microglial cells. The myelin sheath is broken down into lipid droplets, which are also phagocytosed by the microglial cells.

The axons attempt to regenerate, as evidenced by sprouting of the axons, but no evidence shows that restoration of function ever occurs. The reasons for the failure of regeneration are fully described on page 107.

12. Syringomyelia is a chronic disease of the spinal cord that is due to a developmental abnormality in the formation of the central canal. It is characterized by the appearance of a fluid-filled cavity within the spinal cord that gradually enlarges, causing destruction of surrounding nervous tissue. In this patient, the cavity or syrinx was located in the lower cervical and upper thoracic segments of the cord, causing destruction of the ascending tracts that serve pain and temperature from the upper limbs. The cavity was encroaching on the motor anterior horn cells of both sides as well, causing weakness of the small muscles of the hands.

(a) As is now generally accepted, the type of sensation felt is determined not by a specific receptor but by the specific area of the central nervous system to which the afferent nerve fiber passes. Free nerve endings are commonly associated with axons serving pain and temperature. (b) The examination of a patient to test different sensory modalities is discussed on page 113.

13. The only sensory receptors present in the cornea are free nerve endings. The cornea is sensitive to touch and temperature changes in addition to pain.

14. All hair follicles are richly innervated. Free nerve endings are found as a branching network that winds around the follicle below the entrance of the sebaceous duct. Merkel discs also are found in the epidermis of the follicle. The hair shaft acts as a lever, so the slightest movement of the hair readily stimulates the nerve endings in the hair follicle. In this patient suffering from trigeminal neuralgia, the temporal region of the scalp was the trigger area, which, on stimulation, initiated the intense stabs of pain in the distribution of the maxillary division of the trigeminal nerve.

15. Numerous free nerve endings are found in the connective tissue of tendons and the testes. Normally, squeezing these structures elicits an aching type of pain. In tabes dorsalis, the disease process affects the sensory neurons in the posterior roots of the spinal nerves.

16. Striking the ligamentum patellae with a reflex hammer causes elongation of the intrafusal fibers of the muscle spindles of the quadriceps muscle and stimulation of the annulospiral and flower-spray endings. The nerve impulses reach the spinal cord in the afferent neurons within the femoral nerve and enter the cord at the level of L2–L4. The afferent neurons synapse with the large α motor neurons in the anterior gray horns of the spinal cord. Nerve impulses now pass via the efferent motor neurons in the femoral nerve and stimulate the extrafusal muscle fibers of the quadriceps muscle, which then contracts. The muscle spindle afferent impulses

inhibit the motor neurons of the antagonist muscles (see reciprocal inhibition, p. 92).

17. To test position sense, the patient is placed in the supine position and is asked to close the eyes. The big toe is grasped at the sides between the thumb and index finger and extended and flexed. The patient is asked, on completion of each movement, "Is the toe pointing up or down?" Another simple test is to ask the patient, again with the eyes closed, to place the right heel on the left shin and run it down the shin to the dorsum of the left foot. The patient is then asked to repeat the performance with the left heel on the right shin.

    Vibratory sense can be tested by placing the handle of a vibrating tuning fork on the tibial tuberosity, the anterior border of the tibia, and the medial or lateral malleoli. The patient is asked to indicate when the vibration is first felt and when it ceases. Symmetrical points on the two limbs may be compared, and the clinician can use his or her own limbs as a control. In the normal individual, the sense of position depends on the central nervous system receiving adequate information from the pressure receptors (Pacinian corpuscles) in the joint capsules and ligaments, touch receptors (free nerve endings) in the tissues in and around joints, and the stretch receptors in the muscles and tendons (especially the neurotendinous spindles).

    Vibration sense is normally believed to be due to the stimulation of superficial and deep pressure receptors (Pacinian corpuscles).

    Appreciation of the passive movements of joints, postural sensibility, and vibration sense is often lost in tabes dorsalis due to syphilitic destruction of the posterior columns of the spinal cord and degeneration of the posterior roots.

18. *d*-Tubocurarine, dimethyltubocurarine, gallamine, and benzoquinonium are examples of competitive blocking agents. These drugs compete with the neurotransmitter acetylcholine (ACh). The competitive blocking agents are believed to combine with the same sites at the postsynaptic membrane (sarcolemma) of the motor endplate normally used by ACh.

19. Decamethonium and succinylcholine paralyze skeletal muscle by depolarizing the motor endplate.

20. *C. botulinum* produces a toxin that inhibits the release of acetylcholine at the motor endplate. Death results from paralysis of the respiratory muscles.

21. Skeletal muscles that are not used, such as in a limb fitted with a splint immobilizing a fracture, undergo disuse atrophy. The longer the muscles are not used, the greater the degree of atrophy. In severe cases, the atrophy may amount to as much as 25% of the muscle mass. The muscle fibers rapidly atrophy following section of a motor nerve, so the total mass of the muscle may be reduced by as much as 75% in as little as 3 months. The precise reason for this severe atrophy is not understood. Apparently, the maintenance of normal muscle depends on the continued reception of acetylcholine and trophic substances from the nerve terminals at the postsynaptic membrane at the neuromuscular junction. The latter mechanism would be impossible if the motor nerve was sectioned and the distal end had degenerated.

22. Your knowledge of the dermatomes of the lower limb will enable you to ascertain that the patient's pain was felt in the area of distribution of the fifth lumbar and first sacral nerve roots. The involvement of these roots is usually due to herniation of the fourth or fifth lumbar intervertebral disc.

23. Herpes zoster is a viral infection of the posterior root ganglia (or sensory ganglia of the cranial nerves), the posterior root, or the posterior gray horn of the spinal cord. This patient experienced pain and had a skin eruption in the area of distribution of the fifth left intercostal nerve. The virus was producing an acute inflammation at some point along the course of the sensory neurons of the fifth segment of the spinal cord on the left side.

24. The trigeminal (5th cranial) nerve innervates the skin of the greater part of the face. The next dermatome that occurs inferior to this is that of the 2nd cervical nerve. The 6th to the 12th cranial nerves do not innervate the skin of the face. At the junction of the neck with the thorax, the 4th cervical dermatome is contiguous with the 2nd thoracic dermatome; the anterior rami of the lower cervical and 1st thoracic spinal nerves lose their cutaneous distribution on the neck and trunk during the development of the upper limb.

25. (a) The physical examination revealed weakness of the rhomboid, deltoid, and biceps brachii muscles, which are innervated by the fifth and sixth cervical segments of the spinal cord. These spinal cord segments lie within the vertebral foramina of the sixth and seventh cervical vertebrae, respectively. (b) The fifth and sixth cervical segments of the spinal cord are being pressed on. (c) The biceps brachii reflex arc involves the fifth and sixth segments of the spinal cord. (d) The rhomboid and deltoid muscles show diminished muscle tone because the reflex arcs on which their tone depends travel through the compressed segments of the spinal cord; that is, the reflex arcs were no longer functioning normally. Because of the pressure of the tumor on the cervical region of the spinal cord, the nervous pathways passing down to lower segments of the spinal cord were interrupted. This resulted in the motor anterior gray column cells of the segments of the cord below the level of compression receiving diminished information from the higher centers, with a consequent increase in muscle tone.

26. Any disease process that can interrupt the normal functioning of the basic spinal reflex arc on which skeletal muscle tone is dependent will cause loss of muscle tone. Some examples are spinal shock following trauma to the spinal cord; section of or pressure on a spinal nerve, a posterior root, or an anterior root; syringomyelia; and poliomyelitis.

27. Tabes dorsalis, which is a syphilitic infection of the brain and spinal cord, produces degeneration of the central processes of the posterior root ganglion cells and also, usually, the ganglion cells themselves. The lower thoracic and lumbar sacral segments of the cord are involved first, and the interruption of the proprioceptive fibers results in impairment of appreciation of posture and the tendency to fall down if one closes the eyes while standing. Eyesight in this patient compensated for lack of proprioception.

28. In a normal individual, standing and walking are largely automatic, but as you have read in this chapter, these activities are highly complex and require the proper integration of neural mechanisms at all levels of the spinal cord and brain. The basic mechanism underlying muscle tone is the spinal segmental reflex. In order to maintain normal posture, these reflex arcs must receive adequate nervous input from higher levels of the nervous system. Diseases involving the corpus striatum (caudate and lentiform nuclei) or the substantia nigra result in an alteration in the pattern of nervous impulses impinging on the anterior horn cells of the spinal cord, hence the abnormal muscle tone. The increased tone is equal in extent in opposing muscle groups. The tremor of the parkinsonian syndrome is produced by the alternating movements of the agonist and antagonist muscles of a joint. The tremor is most prominent when the limb is at rest, ceases temporarily when voluntary movement is performed, and then starts again when the movement is completed. The tremor ceases when the patient is asleep. In Parkinson disease, neuronal degeneration is seen in the substantia nigra, resulting in the loss of inhibitory control of the substantia nigra over the lentiform nucleus, putamen, and caudate nucleus.

29. The syndrome of petit mal commonly has three sets of symptoms: (a) myoclonic jerks, in which the patient experiences sudden involuntary contraction of the muscles of the trunk and extremities; (b) akinetic seizures, in which all muscles of the body suddenly lose tone; and (c) brief losses of consciousness, in which the patient loses contact with the environment for a few seconds.

30. Destruction of the anterior gray column cells in the lumbar and sacral regions of the spinal cord resulted in paralysis and atrophy of the muscles of both legs. The twitching of groups of muscle fibers is referred to as *muscular fasciculation* and is commonly seen in patients with chronic disease affecting the anterior horn cells.

31. (a) Muscular hypotonia, which is present on the same side of the body as the lesion. Passively move the joints on the right side of the body and then on the left side, and compare the resistance to these movements by the muscles on the two sides of the body. (b) Posture. The shoulder girdle on the affected side drops because of loss of muscle tone. With the patient disrobed, ask her to stand up straight with her back toward you. With a unilateral cerebellar lesion, the shoulder on the affected side may be lower than that on the opposite, normal side. (c) Disorders of voluntary movement (ataxia) due to loss of muscle coordination. (d) Nystagmus. This is an involuntary to-and-fro movement of the eyes. It is commonly demonstrated in cerebellar disease and is due to lack of muscle coordination. When the eyes are turned horizontally, quick, rhythmic jerks occur in the direction of gaze. In unilateral cerebellar lesions, the amplitude of nystagmus is greater and its rate is slower when the eyes are rotated toward the side of the lesion than when they are displaced to the opposite side.

❓ Review Questions

Directions: Each of the numbered items in this section is followed by answers. Select the ONE lettered answer that is CORRECT.

1. The following statements concern nerves:
   (a) *Nerve tract* is the name given to a nerve fiber in the peripheral and central nervous systems (PNS and CNS).
   (b) The supporting cell of a myelinated nerve fiber in the CNS is called an oligodendrocyte.
   (c) A node of Ranvier in peripheral nerves is where two Schwann cells come together and cover the exposed part of the plasma membrane of the axon.
   (d) Nodes of Ranvier are absent from myelinated nerve fibers in the CNS.
   (e) The major dense line of myelin consists of two inner lipid layers of the plasma membrane that are fused together.

2. The following statements concern nerves:
   (a) The minor dense line of myelin is made up of protein.
   (b) Incisures of Schmidt–Lanterman are caused by the mesaxons of the Schwann cells.
   (c) Only five or six unmyelinated axons may share a single Schwann cell in the peripheral nervous system (PNS).
   (d) The node of Ranvier is the site of nerve activity.
   (e) *Chromatolysis* is the term used to describe the changes in the arrangement of Nissl material within the axon following injury.

3. The following statements concern an oligodendro-cyte:
   (a) A single oligodendrocyte may be associated with one segment of myelin on a single axon.
   (b) Incisures of Schmidt–Lanterman are not present in the myelinated fibers of the central nervous system (CNS).
   (c) Myelination in the CNS occurs by the rotation of the axon within the oligodendrocytic process and the wrapping of it around the axon.
   (d) A nonmyelinated axon in the CNS has a special relationship with the oligodendrocyte.
   (e) A single oligodendrocyte may be associated with the myelin sheaths of as many as 60 axons.

4. The following statements concern spinal nerves:
   (a) There are 26 pairs.
   (b) They are formed by the union of anterior and posterior nerve roots.
   (c) The posterior ramus contains only sensory axons.
   (d) The anterior root contains only sensory axons.
   (e) The posterior root ganglion contains bipolar neurons enveloped in capsular cells.

5. The following statements concern peripheral nerve plexuses:
   (a) They are formed by a network of connective tissue fibers.
   (b) Bundles of nerve fibers do not branch, and, in most instances, the individual nerve fibers do not branch.
   (c) Plexuses at the roots of the limbs are formed from posterior rami of spinal nerves.
   (d) The plexuses of the autonomic nervous system possess a network of efferent nerve fibers and no nerve cells.
   (e) A plexus situated at the root of a limb permits nerve fibers from different segments of the spinal cord to become rearranged so that they more easily travel to different parts of the limb.

6. The following statements concern nerve conduction:
   (a) Adequate stimulus decreases the permeability of the axolemma to Na^+ ions at the point of stimulation.
   (b) During the absolute refractory period, a very strong stimulus will excite the nerve fiber.
   (c) As the action potential moves along the axon, the entry of Na^+ ions into the axon increases and the permeability to K^+ ions decreases.
   (d) A typical action potential is about +40 mV.
   (e) In the resting unstimulated nerve fiber, the interior of the axolemma is positive to the exterior.

7. The following statements concern the propagation of a nerve impulse:
   (a) Conduction velocity is smallest in nerve fibers having a large cross-sectional diameter.
   (b) In nonmyelinated nerve fibers, the action potential occurs along the length of the fiber.
   (c) A myelinated nerve fiber can be stimulated only between the nodes of Ranvier.

(d) Saltatory conduction occurs only in the central nervous system.
(e) At the node of Ranvier, the action potential has no effect on the surrounding tissue fluid.

8. The following statements concern Wallerian degeneration:
   (a) Myelin breaks down into droplets that are phagocytosed by the Schwann cells.
   (b) The axon rapidly disappears.
   (c) Schwann cells round off and do not multiply.
   (d) In the central nervous system (CNS), debris is removed by the astrocyte cells.
   (e) In the peripheral nervous system (PNS), tissue macrophages play no part in the digestion of the nerve fragments.

9. The following statements concern the failure of regeneration of nerve fibers in the central nervous system (CNS):
   (a) Endoneurial tubes are present.
   (b) Oligodendrocytes have a basement membrane.
   (c) Oligodendrocytes fail to multiply and form a band fiber, as do Schwann cells in the peripheral nervous system (PNS).
   (d) Blood supply is not usually adequate.
   (e) Nerve growth factors are not present.

10. The following factor may explain the partial return of function following injury to the spinal cord:
    (a) Edema fluid persists at the site of injury.
    (b) Nonfunctional neurons never take over the function of damaged neurons.
    (c) Reduction in the number of receptor sites may occur on the postsynaptic membranes.
    (d) Some of the axons completely regenerate.
    (e) With training, the patient may use other muscles to compensate for the loss of paralyzed muscles.

11. The following statements concern receptor endings:
    (a) Rods and cones of the eyes are chemoreceptors.
    (b) Taste and smell endings are electromagnetic receptors.
    (c) Free nerve endings have no Schwann cells covering their tips.
    (d) Merkel discs are fast-adapting touch receptors.
    (e) Meissner corpuscles are absent from the skin of the palm of the hand and the sole of the foot.

12. The following statements concern receptor endings:
    (a) Pacinian corpuscles are slowly adapting mechanoreceptors.
    (b) Ruffini corpuscles are fast-adapting stretch receptors found in the dermis of hairy skin.
    (c) Each Pacinian corpuscle has no capsule but has a central core containing the nerve ending.
    (d) Annulospiral endings in skeletal muscle do not possess intrafusal muscle fibers.
    (e) The number of Meissner corpuscles considerably diminishes between birth and old age.

13. The following statements concern cutaneous receptors:
    (a) Different histologic types of receptors transmit different types of nerve impulses.

(b) The type of sensation felt is determined by the specific area of the central nervous system (CNS) to which the sensory nerve fiber passes.

(c) Transduction at the receptor is the process by which the stimulus is changed into the mechanical energy of the nerve impulse.

(d) When applied to the receptor, the stimulus brings about a change in the potential of the plasma membranes of the capsule cells and not the nerve ending.

(e) If small enough, the receptor potential will generate an action potential in the afferent sensory nerve fiber.

14. The following statements concern the function of a neuromuscular spindle:

(a) It gives rise to intermittent afferent nerve impulses.

(b) Only active muscle movement causes an increase in the rate of passage of nerve impulses in the afferent nerve fiber.

(c) The neuromuscular spindle keeps the central nervous system (CNS) informed about muscle activity.

(d) The neuromuscular spindle directly influences the control of voluntary movement.

(e) Flower-spray endings are situated mainly on the nuclear bag fibers close to the equatorial region.

15. The following statements concern the neurotendinous spindles:

(a) They are situated in tendons some distance away from the musculotendinous junction.

(b) The nerve terminates in a single club-shaped ending.

(c) Each has a fibrous capsule, loosely arranged collagen fibers, and tendon cells.

(d) Neurotendinous spindles are found only in slow-acting muscles.

(e) The neurotendinous spindle is activated by changes in muscle tension and stimulates muscle contraction.

16. The following statements concern the neuromuscular junctions in skeletal muscle:

(a) Each terminal branch of the motor nerve ends as an axon covered with fine connective tissue.

(b) Each axon lies in a groove on the surface of the muscle fiber formed by the infolding of the muscle plasma membrane (sarcolemma).

(c) Having caused depolarization of the postsynaptic membrane, acetylcholine (ACh) is reabsorbed into the axon terminal.

(d) ACh is released from the axon terminal when the nerve impulse leaves the initial segment of the axon.

(e) Schwann cells form the floor for the groove on the surface of the muscle fiber.

17. The following statements concern the neuromuscular junctions on smooth and cardiac muscle:

(a) In smooth muscle, the autonomic nerve fiber exerts control over a single muscle fiber.

(b) In smooth muscle, the wave of contraction does not pass from one muscle fiber to another.

(c) In cardiac muscle, the wave of contraction spreads slowly from one muscle fiber to another by way of desmosomes and gap junctions.

(d) Autonomic nerve fibers terminate on smooth muscle as unmyelinated fibers.

(e) At the site of the neuromuscular junction, the axon is completely surrounded by Schwann cells.

18. The following statements concern skin sensations and dermatomes:

(a) To produce a region of complete anesthesia on the trunk, at least three segments of the spinal cord have to be damaged.

(b) When contiguous spinal nerves are sectioned, the area of tactile loss is always smaller than the area of loss of painful and thermal sensations.

(c) The dermatome present on the medial side of the wrist is C5.

(d) The dermatome present on the point of the shoulder is C2.

(e) The dermatomes for the limbs run almost horizontally.

19. The following statements concern muscle reflexes:

(a) The biceps brachii tendon reflex involves the C5–C6 segments of the spinal cord.

(b) The triceps tendon reflex involves the T1 segment of the spinal cord.

(c) The patellar tendon reflex (knee jerk) involves L5–S1 segments of the spinal cord.

(d) A tumor pressing on the second, third, and fourth lumbar segments of the spinal cord is likely to interfere with the ankle jerk.

(e) The abdominal superficial reflexes involve T3–T5 segments of the spinal cord.

20. The following statements concern the dermatomes of the trunk and lower limbs:

(a) The T8 dermatome includes the skin of the umbilicus.

(b) The L5 dermatome lies over the lateral side of the knee joint.

(c) The L2 dermatome lies over the medial side of the knee joint.

(d) The S2 dermatome runs along the lateral side of the foot.

(e) The L1 dermatome lies over the inguinal ligament.

21. The following statements concern muscle innervation:

(a) A motor unit consists of the posterior root ganglion and all the neuromuscular spindles to which it is connected.

(b) In the small muscles of the hand, one nerve fiber supplies large numbers of muscle fibers.

(c) Neurotendinous spindles are innervated by nonmyelinated nerve fibers.

(d) Muscle tone is dependent on the integrity of a simple monosynaptic reflex arc.

(e) The γ motor efferent fibers innervate the extrafusal fibers of a muscle spindle.

22. The following statements concern skeletal muscle action:
    (a) When a muscle begins to contract, the larger motor units are stimulated first.
    (b) Muscle fatigue is caused by an exhaustion of the presynaptic vesicles at the neuromuscular junction.
    (c) When a prime mover contracts, the antagonistic muscles are inhibited.
    (d) When a muscle is paralyzed, it does not immediately lose its normal tone.
    (e) To paralyze a muscle completely, destroying several adjacent segments of the spinal cord or their nerve roots is not necessary.
23. The following statements concern posture:
    (a) In the standing position, the line of gravity passes through the odontoid process of the axis, behind the centers of the hip joints, and in front of the knee and ankle joints.
    (b) Posture depends on the strength of the joint ligaments and not on the degree and distribution of muscle tone.
    (c) A particular posture can often be maintained for long periods by groups of muscle fibers in a muscle contracting together continuously.
    (d) The cerebral cortex has no role in the maintenance of normal posture.
    (e) Nerve impulses arising in the eyes and ears cannot influence posture.
24. The following clinical observation on muscle activity can be made:
    (a) Muscle contracture is a condition in which the muscle contracts for a long period of time.
    (b) Muscle fasciculation is seen with chronic disease that affects sensory nerves supplying muscles.
    (c) Muscle atrophy does not take place when a limb is immobilized in a splint.
    (d) Muscle wasting can occur if only the efferent motor nerve fibers to a muscle are sectioned.
    (e) Wasting does not occur in the muscles acting on the shoulder joint in patients with painful pericapsulitis involving that joint.

 Answers and Explanations to Review Questions

1. B is correct. The supporting cell of a myelinated nerve fiber in the CNS is called an oligodendrocyte. A. *Nerve tract* is the name given to a nerve fiber in the CNS. C. A node of Ranvier in peripheral nerves is where two Schwann cells terminate and the plasma membrane of the axon is exposed (see p. 72). D. Nodes of Ranvier are present in myelinated nerve fibers in the CNS. E. The major dense line of myelin consists of two inner protein layers of the plasma membrane that are fused together.
2. D is correct. The node of Ranvier is the site of nerve activity. A. The minor dense line of myelin is made up of lipid. B. Incisures of Schmidt–Lanterman represent where the dark major dense line is not formed as a result of the localized persistence of Schwann cell cytoplasm (Fig. 3-7). C. As many as 15 or more unmyelinated axons may share a single Schwann cell in the PNS. E. *Chromatolysis* is the term used to describe the changes in the arrangement of Nissl material within the cytoplasm of the nerve cell body following injury (see p. 106).
3. E is correct. A single oligodendrocyte may be associated with the myelin sheaths of as many as 60 axons (see p. 72). A. A single oligodendrocyte may be associated with several segments of myelin on a single axon. B. Incisures of Schmidt–Lanterman are present in the myelinated fibers of the CNS. C. Myelination in the CNS occurs by the growth in length of the oligodendrocytic process and the wrapping of it around the axon. D. A nonmyelinated axon in the CNS has no special relationship with the oligodendrocyte (see p.79).
4. B is correct. Spinal nerves are formed by the union of anterior and posterior nerve roots (Fig. 3-1). A. There are 31 pairs of spinal nerves. C. The posterior ramus of a spinal nerve contains both motor and sensory axons. D. The anterior root of a spinal nerve contains only motor axons. E. The posterior root ganglion of a spinal nerve contains unipolar neurons enveloped in capsular cells.
5. E is correct. A peripheral nerve plexus situated at the root of a limb permits nerve fibers from different segments of the spinal cord to become rearranged so that they more easily travel to different parts of the limb (see p. 81). A. Peripheral nerve plexuses are formed by a network of nerve fibers. B. In peripheral nerve plexuses, bundles of nerve fibers branch, but in most instances, the individual nerve fibers do not branch. C. The peripheral nerve plexuses at the roots of the limbs are formed from the anterior rami of the spinal nerves. D. The nerve plexuses of the autonomic nervous system possess a network of nerve fibers and nerve cells.
6. D is correct. In nerve conduction, a typical action potential is about +40 mV (see pp. 44–45). A. In nerve conduction, an adequate stimulus increases the permeability of the axolemma to Na^+ ions at the point of stimulation. B. During the absolute refractory period of nerve conduction, no stimulus, no matter how strong, will excite the nerve fiber. C. During nerve conduction, the action potential moves along the axon; the entry of Na^+ ions into the axon ceases, and the permeability of the plasma membrane of the axon to K^+ ions increases (see p. 44). E. In the resting unstimulated nerve fiber, the interior of the plasma membrane (axolemma) is negative to the exterior.
7. B is correct. In nonmyelinated nerve fibers, the action potential occurs along the length of the fiber.

A. Conduction velocity is greatest in nerve fibers having a large cross-sectional diameter. C. A myelinated nerve fiber can be stimulated only at the nodes of Ranvier. D. Saltatory conduction occurs in both the peripheral and central nervous systems. E. At the node of Ranvier, the action potential sets up an electrical current in the surrounding tissue fluid (see p. 72).

8. A is correct. In Wallerian degeneration, the myelin breaks down into droplets that are phagocytosed by the Schwann cells. B. In Wallerian degeneration, the axon first breaks up into fragments before it is phagocytosed by the surrounding Schwann cells (see p. 105). C. In Wallerian degeneration, the Schwann cells proliferate rapidly and become arranged in parallel cords within the persistent basement membrane. D. In Wallerian degeneration in the CNS, the debris is removed by the microglial cells. E. In Wallerian degeneration in the PNS, the tissue macrophages are very active in removing the nerve fragments.

9. C is correct. Following injury to the CNS, the oligodendrocytes fail to multiply and form a band fiber as do Schwann cells in the damaged PNS (see p. 106). A. The absence of endoneurial tubes may be important in the failure in the regeneration of injured CNS tissue (see p. 106). B. Oligodendrocytes have no basement membrane. D. Blood supply to the central nervous tissue is usually adequate. E. In the CNS, no nerve growth factors are present.

10. E is correct. The partial return of function seen in spinal cord injuries may be due in part to the patient using other muscles to compensate for the loss of the paralyzed muscles. A. Following injury to the central nervous system, the edema fluid usually subsides at the site of injury and will result in some clinical improvement (see p. 107). B. Nonfunctional neurons may take over the function of damaged neurons. C. The receptor sites on the postsynaptic membrane may increase in number and be responsible for some posttraumatic improvement. D. Evidence does not show that destroyed axons in the central nervous system completely regenerate after injury.

11. C is correct. Free nerve endings have no Schwann cells covering their tips (see p. 84). A. The rods and cones of the eyes are examples of electromagnetic receptors. B. Taste and smell receptors are chemoreceptors. D. Merkel discs are slow-adapting touch receptors. E. Meissner corpuscles are present in the skin of the palm of the hand and the sole of the foot.

12. E is correct. The number of Meissner corpuscles is considerably reduced between birth and old age. A. Pacinian corpuscles are fast-adapting mechanoreceptors. B. Ruffini corpuscles are slow-adapting stretch receptors found in the dermis of hairy skin. C. Each Pacinian corpuscle has a lamellated capsule and a central core containing the nerve ending (Figs. 3-23 and 3-24). D. Annulospiral endings in skeletal muscle do possess intrafusal muscle fibers.

13. B is correct. The type of sensation felt is determined by the specific area of the CNS to which the sensory nerve fiber passes (see p. 89). A. Although a variety of histologic types of receptors exist, their nerves only transmit the same nerve impulses. C. Transduction at the receptor is the process by which the energy of the stimulus is changed into electrochemical energy of the nerve impulse. D. When applied to the receptor, the stimulus brings about a change in the potential of the plasma membrane of the nerve ending (see p. 89). E. If large enough, the receptor potential will generate an action potential in the afferent sensory nerve fiber.

14. C is correct. The neuromuscular spindle keeps the CNS informed about muscle activity (see p. 89). A. The neuromuscular spindle gives rise to afferent nerve impulses all the time. B. When active or passive muscle movement occurs, the rate of passage of nerve impulses in the afferent nerve fibers of the neuromuscular spindles increases. D. The neuromuscular spindle indirectly influences the control of voluntary movement (see p. 90). E. Flower-spray endings are situated mainly on the nuclear chain fibers some distance from the equatorial region (Fig. 3-25).

15. C is correct. Each neurotendinous spindle has a fibrous capsule, loosely arranged collagen fibers, and tendon cells (see p. 92). A. Neurotendinous spindles are situated in tendons close to the musculotendinous junction. B. The nerve ends within the spindle by branching and terminating in club-shaped endings. D. Neurotendinous spindles are found in fast- and slow-acting muscles. E. The neurotendinous spindle is activated by changes in muscle tension and inhibits muscle contraction.

16. B is correct. At a neuromuscular junction, each axon lies in a groove on the surface of the muscle fiber formed by the infolding of the muscle plasma membrane (sarcolemma) (Fig. 3-30). A. At a neuromuscular junction, each terminal branch of the motor nerve ends as a naked axon. C. Having caused depolarization of the postsynaptic membrane, ACh is immediately hydrolyzed in the synaptic cleft by acetylcholinesterase (see p. 96). D. ACh is released from the axon terminal when the nerve impulse reaches the neuromuscular junction. E. At the neuromuscular junction, the Schwann cells form a cap or roof for the groove on the surface of the muscle fiber.

17. D is correct. Autonomic nerve fibers terminate on smooth muscle fibers as unmyelinated fibers (see p. 98). A. In neuromuscular junctions of smooth muscle, the autonomic nerve fiber exerts control over several muscle fibers (see p. 98). B. In smooth muscle, the wave of contraction passes from one muscle fiber to another by means of gap junctions. C. In cardiac muscle, the wave of contraction spreads rapidly from one muscle fiber to another by way of desmosomes and gap junctions. E. At the site of a neuromuscular junction involving smooth muscle, the axon lies in a shallow groove on the muscle surface, and the Schwann cell is retracted to expose the axolemma (Fig. 3-34).

18. A is correct. To produce a region of complete anesthesia on the trunk, at least three segments of the spinal cord have to be damaged (see p. 98). B. When contiguous spinal nerves are sectioned, the area of tactile loss is always greater than the area of loss of painful and thermal sensations. C. The dermatome present on the medial side of the wrist is C8. D. The dermatomes present on the point of the shoulder are C3–C4. E. Limb dermatomes run almost vertically (see Figs. 3-36 and 3-37).

19. A is correct. The biceps brachii tendon reflex involves C5–C6 segments of the spinal cord (see p. 100). B. The triceps tendon reflex involves the C6–C7 and C8 segments of the spinal cord. C. The patellar tendon reflex (knee jerk) involves the L2–L4 segments of the spinal cord. D. A tumor pressing on the S1–S2 segments of the spinal cord is likely to interfere with the ankle jerk. E. The abdominal superficial reflexes involve T6–T12 segments of the spinal cord.

20. E is correct. The L1 dermatome lies over the inguinal ligament (see Fig. 3-36). A. The T10 dermatome includes the skin of the umbilicus; the T8 dermatome involves the skin between the xiphoid process and the umbilicus. B. The L5 dermatome lies over the anterior and lateral surfaces of the leg below the knee. C. The L2 dermatome lies over the anterior and lateral surfaces of the thigh. D. The S2 dermatome extends down the middle of the posterior surface of the thigh and leg (see Fig. 3-37).

21. D is correct. Muscle tone is dependent on the integrity of a simple reflex arc (see p. 101). A. A motor unit consists of a motor neuron in the anterior gray column (horn) of the spinal cord and all the muscle fibers it supplies (Fig. 3-39). B. In the small muscles of the hand, one nerve fiber supplies only a few muscle fibers. C. Neurotendinous spindles are innervated by myelinated nerve fibers. E. The γ motor efferent fibers innervate the intrafusal fibers of a muscle spindle.

22. C is correct. In voluntary muscle movement, when a prime mover contracts, the antagonistic muscles are inhibited (see p. 92). A. When a muscle begins to contract, the smaller motor units are stimulated first. B. Muscle fatigue is caused by reduced adenosine triphosphate within the muscle fibers. D. When a muscle is paralyzed, it immediately loses its normal tone (see p. 101). E. To paralyze a muscle completely, destroying several adjacent segments of the spinal cord or their nerve roots is usually necessary.

23. A is correct. In the standing position, the line of gravity passes through the odontoid process of the axis, behind the centers of the hip joints, and in front of the knee and ankle joints (see p. 102). B. Posture depends on the degree and distribution of muscle tone. C. A particular posture can often be maintained for long periods by different groups of muscle fibers in a muscle contracting in relays. D. The cerebral cortex makes an important contribution to the maintenance of normal posture (see p. 102). E. Nerve impulses arising in the eyes and the ears can greatly influence posture.

24. D is correct. Muscle wasting can occur if only the efferent motor nerve fibers to a muscle are sectioned (see p. 109). A. Muscle contracture is a condition in which the muscle contracts and undergoes permanent shortening; it occurs frequently in muscles that normally oppose paralyzed muscles. B. Muscle fasciculation is seen with chronic disease that affects anterior horn cells or the motor nuclei of cranial nerves. C. Muscle atrophy takes place when a limb is immobilized in a splint. E. Wasting occurs in the muscles acting on the shoulder joint in patients with painful pericapsulitis involving that joint.

4

Spinal Cord and Ascending, Descending, and Intersegmental Tracts

CHAPTER OBJECTIVES

- To learn how injuries to the spinal cord can occur

- To understand the position of the main nervous pathways and nerve cell groups in the spinal cord as well as be able to correlate radiologic evidence of bone injury with segmental levels of the spinal cord and neurologic deficits

- To review the basic structure of the delicate spinal cord and the positions and functions of the various ascending and descending tracts that lie within it

- To make simple line drawings of each of the ascending and descending tracts, showing their cells of origin, their course through the central nervous system, and their destination

A 35-year-old man is galloping his horse when he attempts to jump over a farm gate. The horse refuses to jump, and he is thrown to the ground. His head strikes a log, and his head and neck are excessively flexed. On initial evaluation in the emergency department after he regains consciousness, he is found to have signs and symptoms of severe neurologic deficits in the upper and lower extremities. A lateral radiograph of the cervical region of the spine shows fragmentation of the body of the fourth cervical vertebra with backward displacement of a large bony fragment on the left side.

After stabilization of the vertebral column by using skeletal traction to prevent further neurologic damage, a complete examination reveals that the patient has signs and symptoms indicating incomplete hemisection of the spinal cord on the left side.

Any medical personnel involved in the evaluation and treatment of a patient with spinal cord injuries must know the structure of the spinal cord and the arrangement and functions of the various nerve tracts passing up and down this vital conduit in the central nervous system.

Because of the devastating nature of spinal cord injuries and the prolonged disability that results, all concerned with the care of such patients must be trained to prevent any additional cord injury and provide the best chance for recovery. All medical personnel must have a clear picture of the extent of the cord lesion and the possible expectations for the return of function.

Spinal cord injuries are common and can occur as a result of automobile and motorcycle accidents, falls, sports injuries, and gunshot wounds. Spinal cord and spinal nerve damage may also be associated with vertebral fractures; vertebral infections; vertebral tumors, both primary and secondary; and herniated intervertebral discs. The student must learn the course and connections of the various tracts within the spinal cord in order to be able to diagnose and understand the treatment of cord injuries. Particular attention should be paid as to whether a specific tract crosses the midline to the opposite side of the central nervous system (CNS) or remains on the same side. If the tract does cross the midline, the level of the crossover is important.

The assessment of neurologic damage requires not only an understanding of the main nervous pathways within the spinal cord but an ability to correlate radiologic evidence of bone injury with segmental levels of the spinal cord. The close relationship of the spinal cord to the bony vertebral column necessitates a brief review of the vertebral column before the spinal cord is considered.

BRIEF REVIEW OF THE VERTEBRAL COLUMN

The vertebral column is the central bony pillar of the body. It supports the skull, pectoral girdle, upper limbs, and thoracic cage and, by way of the pelvic girdle, transmits body weight to the lower limbs. Within its cavity lie the spinal cord, spinal nerve roots, and the covering meninges, to which the vertebral column gives great protection.

Vertebral Column Composition

The vertebral column (Figs. 4-1 and 4-2) is composed of 33 vertebrae—7 cervical, 12 thoracic, 5 lumbar, 5 sacral (fused to form the sacrum), and 4 coccygeal (the lower 3 are commonly fused). Because it is segmented and made up of vertebrae, joints, and pads of fibrocartilage called **intervertebral discs**, it is a flexible structure. The intervertebral discs form about a quarter of the length of the column.

Vertebra General Characteristics

Although vertebrae show regional differences, they all possess a common pattern (Fig. 4-2B). A **typical vertebra** consists of a rounded **body** anteriorly and a **vertebral arch** posteriorly. These enclose a space called the **vertebral foramen**, through which run the spinal cord and its coverings. The vertebral arch consists of a pair of cylindrical **pedicles**, which form the sides of the arch, and a pair of flattened **laminae**, which complete the arch posteriorly.

The vertebral arch gives rise to seven processes: one spinous, two transverse, and four articular.

The **spinous process**, or **spine**, is directed posteriorly from the junction of the two laminae. The transverse processes are directed laterally from the junction of the laminae and the pedicles. Both the spinous and transverse processes serve as levers and receive attachments of muscles and ligaments.

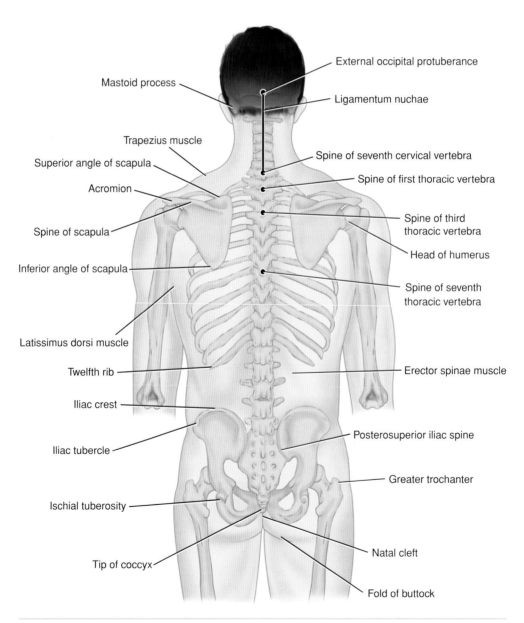

Figure 4-1   Posterior view of the skeleton showing the vertebral column. The surface marking of the external occipital protuberance of the skull, the ligamentum nuchae (*solid black line*) and some important palpable spines (*solid dots*) are also shown.

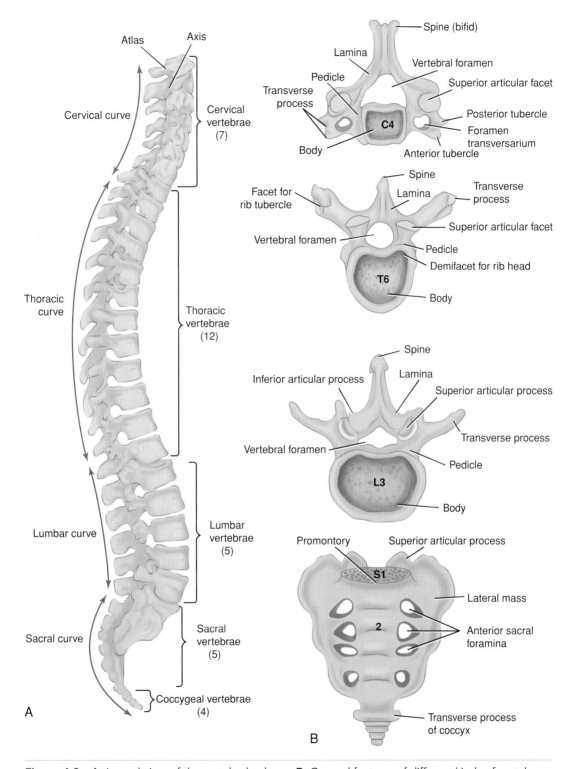

Figure 4-2 A: Lateral view of the vertebral column. **B:** General features of different kinds of vertebrae.

The **articular processes** are vertically arranged and consist of two superior and two inferior processes. They arise from the junction of the laminae and the pedicles. The two superior articular processes of one vertebral arch articulate with the two inferior articular processes of the arch above, forming two synovial joints.

The pedicles are notched on their upper and lower borders, forming the **superior** and **inferior vertebral notches**. On each side, the superior notch of one vertebra and the inferior notch of an adjacent vertebra together form an **intervertebral foramen**. These foramina, in an articulated skeleton, serve to transmit

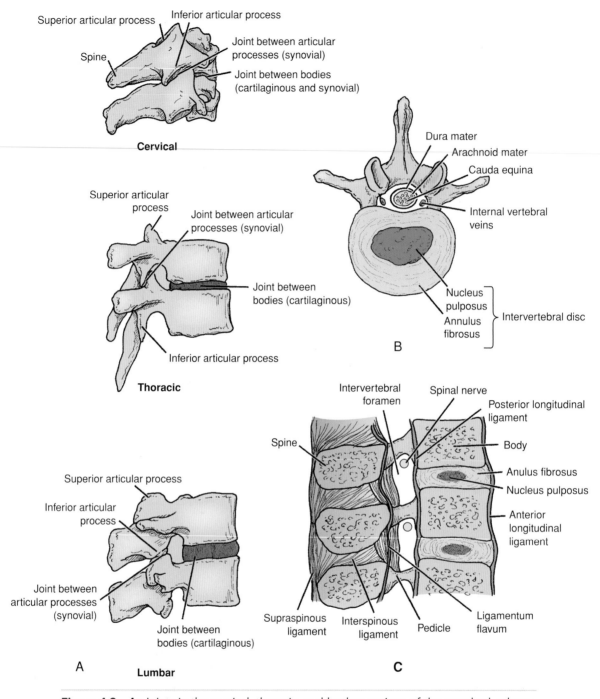

Figure 4-3   A: Joints in the cervical, thoracic, and lumbar regions of the vertebral column. **B:** Third lumbar vertebra seen from above showing the relationship between intervertebral disc and cauda equina. **C:** Lumbar vertebrae in sagittal section showing vertebral ligament relationships.

the spinal nerves and blood vessels. The anterior and posterior nerve roots of a spinal nerve unite within these foramina with their coverings of dura to form the segmental spinal nerves.

Vertebral Column Joints

Below the axis, the vertebrae articulate with each other by means of cartilaginous joints between their bodies and by synovial joints between their articular processes.

Joints Between Two Vertebral Bodies

Sandwiched between the vertebral bodies is an intervertebral disc of fibrocartilage (Fig. 4-3).

Intervertebral Discs

The intervertebral discs are thickest in the cervical and lumbar regions, where the movements of the vertebral column are greatest. They serve as shock absorbers when the load on the vertebral column is suddenly increased. Unfortunately, their resilience is gradually lost with advancing age.

Each disc consists of a peripheral part, the annulus fibrosus, and a central part, the nucleus pulposus (Fig. 4-3B,C). The **annulus fibrosus** is composed of fibrocartilage, which is strongly attached to the vertebral bodies and the anterior and posterior longitudinal ligaments of the vertebral column.

The **nucleus pulposus** in the young is an ovoid mass of gelatinous material. It is normally under pressure and situated slightly nearer to the posterior than to the anterior margin of the disc. The upper and lower surfaces of the bodies of adjacent vertebrae that abut onto the disc are covered with thin plates of hyaline cartilage.

The semifluid nature of the nucleus pulposus allows it to change shape and permits one vertebra to rock forward or backward on another. A sudden increase in the compression load on the vertebral column flattens the nucleus pulposus, which is accommodated by the resilience of the surrounding annulus fibrosus. Sometimes, the outward thrust is too great for the annulus fibrosus and it ruptures, allowing the nucleus pulposus to herniate and protrude into the vertebral canal, where it may press on the spinal nerve roots, the spinal nerve, or even the spinal cord.

With advancing age, the nucleus pulposus becomes smaller and is replaced by fibrocartilage. The collagen fibers of the annulus degenerate, and, as a result, the annulus cannot always contain the nucleus pulposus under stress. In old age, the discs are thin and less elastic, and distinguishing the nucleus from the annulus is no longer possible.

Ligaments

The **anterior** and **posterior longitudinal ligaments** run as continuous bands down the anterior and posterior surfaces of the vertebral column from the skull to the sacrum (Fig. 4-3C). The anterior ligament is wide and is strongly attached to the front and sides of the vertebral bodies and to the intervertebral discs. The posterior ligament is weak and narrow and is attached to the posterior borders of the discs.

Joints Between Two Vertebral Arches

The joints between two vertebral arches consist of synovial joints between the superior and inferior articular processes of adjacent vertebrae (Fig. 4-3A).

Ligaments

Refer to Figure 4-3C.

- The **supraspinous ligament** runs between the tips of adjacent spines.
- The **interspinous ligament** connects adjacent spines.
- The **intertransverse ligaments** run between adjacent transverse processes.
- The **ligamentum flavum** connects the laminae of adjacent vertebrae.

In the cervical region, the supraspinous and interspinous ligaments are greatly thickened to form the strong **ligamentum nuchae**.

Vertebral Joint Nerve Supply

The joints between the vertebral bodies are innervated by the small meningeal branches of each spinal nerve (Fig. 4-4). The joints between the articular processes are innervated by branches from the posterior rami of the spinal nerves; the joints of any particular level receive nerve fibers from two adjacent spinal nerves.

The atlanto-occipital joints and the atlanto-axial joints should be reviewed in a textbook of gross anatomy.

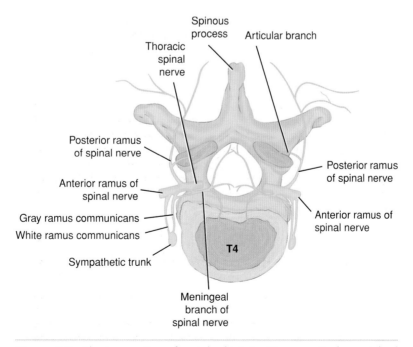

Figure 4-4 The innervation of vertebral joints. At any particular vertebral level, the joints receive nerve fibers from two adjacent spinal nerves.

SPINAL CORD

The spinal cord is roughly cylindrical in shape. It begins superiorly at the foramen magnum in the skull, where it is continuous with the **medulla oblongata** of the brain, and it terminates inferiorly in the adult at the level of the **lower border of the first lumbar vertebra**. In the young child, it is relatively longer and usually ends at the upper border of the third lumbar vertebra. Thus, it occupies the upper two thirds of the **vertebral canal** of the vertebral column and is surrounded by the three meninges, the **dura mater**, the arachnoid mater, and the **pia mater**. Further protection is provided by the **cerebrospinal fluid** (**CSF**), which surrounds the spinal cord in the **subarachnoid space**.

In the cervical region, where it gives origin to the brachial plexus, and in the lower thoracic and lumbar regions, where it gives origin to the lumbosacral plexus, the spinal cord is fusiformly enlarged; the enlargements are referred to as the **cervical** and **lumbar enlargements** (Fig. 4-5). Inferiorly, the spinal cord tapers off into the **conus medullaris**, from the apex of which a prolongation of the pia mater, the **filum terminale**, descends to attach to the posterior

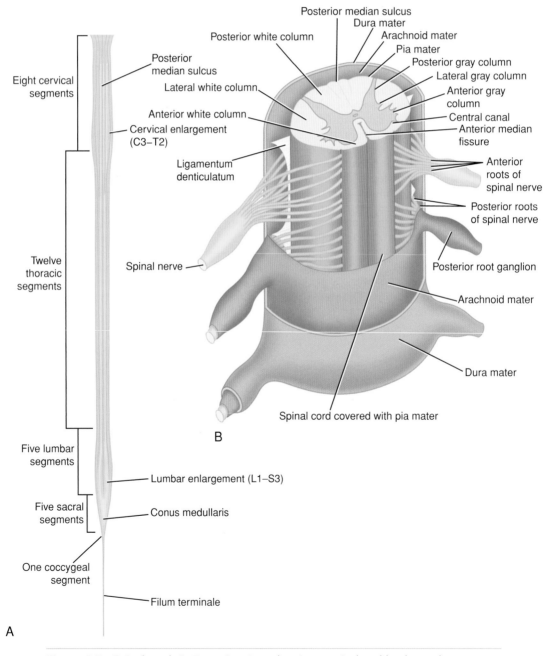

Figure 4-5   Spinal cord. **A:** Posterior view, showing cervical and lumbar enlargements. **B:** Three segments of the spinal cord showing the coverings of dura mater, arachnoid mater, and pia mater.

surface of the coccyx. The cord possesses a deep longitudinal fissure called the **anterior median fissure** in the midline anteriorly and a shallow furrow called the **posterior median sulcus** on the posterior surface (Fig. 4-5B).

Along the entire length of the spinal cord, 31 pairs of spinal nerves are attached by the **anterior** or **motor roots** and the **posterior** or **sensory roots** (Fig. 4-5B). Each root is attached to the cord by a series of rootlets, which extend the whole length of the corresponding

segment of the cord. Each posterior nerve root possesses a **posterior root ganglion**, the cells of which give rise to peripheral and central nerve fibers.

Spinal Cord Structure

The spinal cord is composed of an inner core of gray matter, which is surrounded by an outer covering of white matter (Fig. 4-6); there is no indication that the cord is segmented.

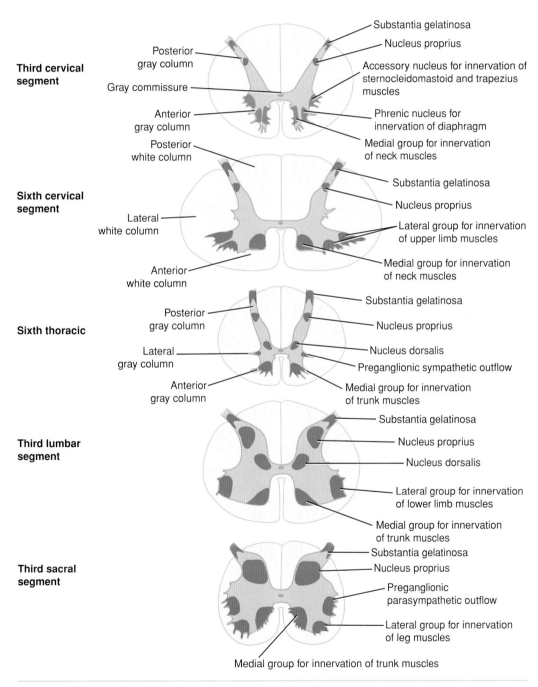

Figure 4-6 Transverse sections of the spinal cord at different levels showing the arrangement of the gray matter and white matter.

Table 4-1   Comparison of Structural Details in Different Regions of the Spinal Cord[a]

Region	Shape	White Matter	Anterior Gray Column	Posterior Gray Column	Lateral Gray Column
				Gray Matter	
Cervical	Oval	Fasciculus cuneatus and fasciculus gracilis present	Medial group of cells for neck muscles; central group of cells for accessory nucleus (C1–C5) and phrenic nucleus (C3–C5); lateral group of cells for upper limb muscles	Substantia gelatinosa present, continuous with Sp.N. of cranial nerve V at level C2; nucleus proprius present; nucleus dorsalis (Clarke column) absent	Absent
Thoracic	Round	Fasciculus cuneatus (T1–T6) and fasciculus gracilis present	Medial group of cells for trunk muscles	Substantia gelatinosa, nucleus proprius, and visceral afferent nucleus present.	Present; gives rise to preganglionic sympathetic fibers
Lumbar	Round to oval	Fasciculus cuneatus absent; fasciculus gracilis present	Medial group of cells for lower limb muscles; central group of cells for lumbosacral nerve	Substantia gelatinosa, nucleus proprius, nucleus dorsalis (Clarke column) at L1–L4, and visceral afferent nucleus present	Present (L1–L2 [3]); gives rise to preganglionic sympathetic fibers
Sacral	Round	Small amount; fasciculus cuneatus absent; fasciculus gracilis present	Medial group of cells for lower limb and perineal muscles	Substantia gelatinosa and nucleus proprius present	Absent; group of cells present at S2–S4, for parasympathetic outflow

[a]The information in this table is useful for identifying the specific level of the spinal cord from which a section has been taken.

For a comparison of the structural details in different regions of the spinal cord, see Table 4-1.

Gray Matter

On cross section, the gray matter is seen as an H-shaped pillar with **anterior** and **posterior gray columns**, or **horns**, united by a thin **gray commissure** containing the small **central canal**. A small **lateral gray column** or **horn** is present in the thoracic and upper lumbar segments of the cord. The amount of gray matter present at any given level of the spinal cord is related to the amount of muscle innervated at that level. Thus, its size is greatest within the cervical and lumbosacral enlargements of the cord, which innervate the muscles of the upper and lower limbs, respectively (Figs. 4-7 to 4-10; also see Fig. 4-6).

Structure

As in other CNS regions, spinal cord gray matter consists of a mixture of nerve cells and their processes, neuroglia, and blood vessels. The nerve cells are multipolar, and the neuroglia forms an intricate network around the nerve cell bodies and their neurites.

ANTERIOR GRAY COLUMN NERVE CELL GROUPS

Most nerve cells are large and multipolar, and their axons pass out in the anterior roots of the spinal nerves as α **efferents,** which innervate skeletal muscles. The smaller nerve cells are also multipolar, and the axons of many of these pass out in the anterior roots of the spinal nerves as γ **efferents**, which innervate the intrafusal muscle fibers of neuromuscular spindles.

For practical purposes, the nerve cells of the anterior gray column can be divided into three basic groups or columns: medial, central, and lateral (Fig. 4-6).

The medial group is present in most segments of the spinal cord and is responsible for innervating the skeletal muscles of the neck and trunk, including the intercostal and abdominal musculature.

The central group is the smallest and is present in some cervical and lumbosacral segments. In the cervical part of the cord, some of these nerve cells (segments C3–C5) specifically innervate the diaphragm and are collectively referred to as the phrenic nucleus (Fig. 4-7). In the upper five or six cervical segments, some of the nerve cells innervate the sternocleidomastoid and trapezius muscles and are referred to as the **accessory nucleus**. The axons of these cells form the spinal part of the accessory nerve. The **lumbosacral nucleus** present in the second lumbar down to the first sacral segment of the cord is made up of nerve cells whose axons have an unknown distribution.

The lateral group is present in the cervical and lumbosacral segments of the cord and is responsible for

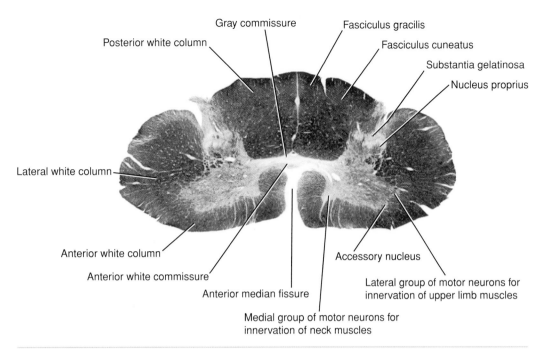

Figure 4-7 Transverse section of the spinal cord at the level of the fifth cervical segment. (Weigert stain.)

innervating the skeletal muscles of the limbs (Figs. 4-6, 4-7, 4-9, and 4-10).

POSTERIOR GRAY COLUMN NERVE CELL GROUPS
Two of the four nerve cell groups of the posterior gray column extend throughout the length of the cord; the other two are restricted to the thoracic and lumbar segments.

The **substantia gelatinosa group** is situated at the apex of the posterior gray column throughout the length of the spinal cord (Figs. 4-6 to 4-10). It is largely

composed of Golgi type II neurons and receives afferent fibers concerned with pain, temperature, and touch from the posterior root. Furthermore, it receives input from descending fibers from supraspinal levels. Pain and temperature inputs are thought to be modified by excitatory or inhibitory information from other sensory inputs and by information from the cerebral cortex.

The **nucleus proprius** is a group of large nerve cells situated anterior to the substantia gelatinosa throughout the spinal cord (Figs. 4-6 to 4-10). This nucleus constitutes the main bulk of cells present in the posterior

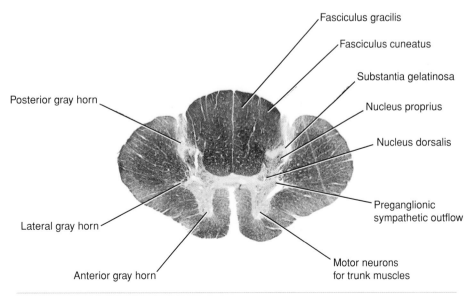

Figure 4-8 Transverse section of the spinal cord at the level of the second thoracic segment. (Weigert stain.)

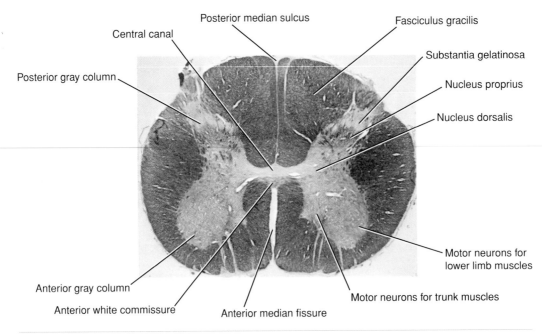

Figure 4-9 Transverse section of the spinal cord at the level of the fourth lumbar segment. (Weigert stain.)

gray column and receives fibers from the posterior white column that are associated with the senses of position and movement (proprioception), two-point discrimination, and vibration.

The **nucleus dorsalis (Clarke column)** is a group of nerve cells situated at the base of the posterior gray column and extending from the eighth cervical segment

caudally to the third or fourth lumbar segment (Figs. 4-6 to 4-9). Most of the cells are comparatively large and are associated with proprioceptive endings (neuromuscular spindles and tendon spindles).

The **visceral afferent nucleus** is a group of nerve cells of medium size situated lateral to the nucleus dorsalis; it extends from the first thoracic to

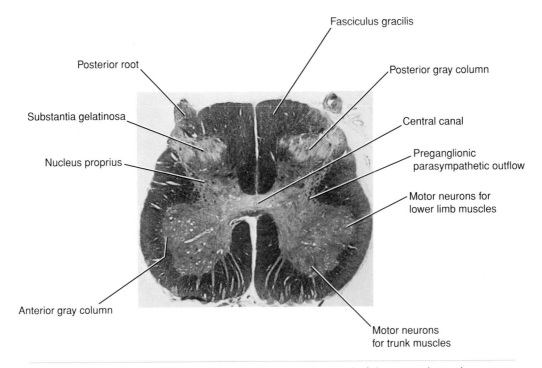

Figure 4-10 Transverse section of the spinal cord at the level of the second sacral segment. (Weigert stain.)

the third lumbar segment of the spinal cord. It is believed to be associated with receiving visceral afferent information.

LATERAL GRAY COLUMN NERVE CELL GROUPS

The intermediolateral group of cells form the small lateral gray column, which extends from the first thoracic to the second or third lumbar segment of the spinal cord (Figs. 4-6 and 4-8). The cells are relatively small and give rise to preganglionic sympathetic fibers.

A similar group of cells found in the second, third, and fourth sacral segments of the spinal cord give rise to preganglionic parasympathetic fibers (Figs. 4-6 and 4-10).

GRAY COMMISSURE AND CENTRAL CANAL

In transverse sections of the spinal cord, the anterior and posterior gray columns on each side are connected by a transverse **gray commissure**; the gray matter resembles the letter H (Figs. 4-6 to 4-10). The **central canal** is situated in the center of the gray commissure. The part of the gray commissure that is situated posterior to the central canal is the **posterior gray commissure**; the anterior part is the **anterior gray commissure**.

The central canal is present throughout the spinal cord. Superiorly, it is continuous with the central canal of the caudal half of the medulla oblongata; above this, it opens into the cavity of the fourth ventricle. Inferiorly in the conus medullaris, it expands into the fusiform **terminal ventricle** and terminates below within the root of the filum terminale. It is filled with CSF and is lined with ciliated columnar epithelium, the **ependyma**.

Thus, the central canal is closed inferiorly and opens superiorly into the fourth ventricle.

White Matter

The white matter, for purposes of description, may be divided into **anterior**, **lateral**, and **posterior white columns** or **funiculi** (Figs. 4-5 to 4-10). The anterior column on each side lies between the midline and the point of emergence of the anterior nerve roots; the lateral column lies between the emergence of the anterior nerve roots and the entry of the posterior nerve roots; the posterior column lies between the entry of the posterior nerve roots and the midline.

Structure

As in other CNS regions, the spinal cord white matter consists of a mixture of nerve fibers, neuroglia, and blood vessels. It surrounds the gray matter, and its white color is due to the high proportion of myelinated nerve fibers.

NERVE FIBER TRACT ARRANGEMENT

The arrangement of the nerve fiber tracts within the spinal cord has been deduced as the result of animal experimentation and study of the human spinal cord for degenerative nerve fibers resulting from injury or disease. Although some nerve tracts are concentrated in certain areas of the white matter, considerable overlap is present. For purposes of description, the spinal tracts are divided into ascending, descending, and intersegmental tracts, and their relative positions in the white matter are described below. A simplified diagram, showing the general arrangement of the major tracts, is shown in Figure 4-11.

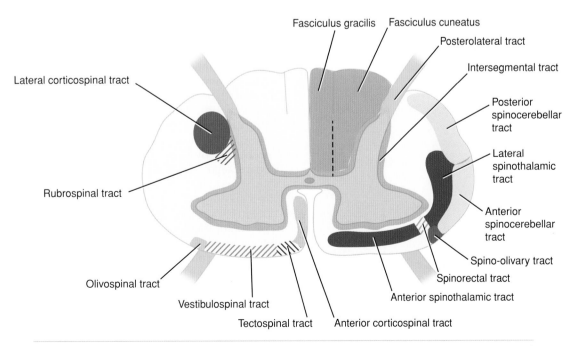

Figure 4-11 Transverse section of the spinal cord at the midcervical level showing the general arrangement of the ascending tracts on the right and the descending tracts on the left.

ASCENDING TRACTS

On entering the spinal cord, the sensory nerve fibers of different sizes and functions are sorted out and segregated into nerve bundles or **tracts** in the white matter (Fig. 4-12; also see Fig. 4-11). Some of the nerve fibers serve to link different segments of the spinal cord, while others ascend from the spinal cord to higher centers and thus connect the spinal cord with the brain. These bundles of the ascending fibers are referred to as the **ascending tracts**.

The ascending tracts conduct two types of afferent information, which may or may not reach consciousness. **Exteroceptive** information originates from outside the body, such as pain, temperature, and touch. **Proprioceptive** information originates from inside the body, for example, from muscles and joints.

Anatomical Organization

General information from the peripheral sensory endings is conducted through the nervous system by a series of neurons. In its simplest form, the ascending pathway to consciousness consists of three neurons (Fig. 4-12). The first neuron, the **first-order neuron**, has its cell body in the **posterior root ganglion** of the spinal nerve. A peripheral process connects with a sensory receptor ending, whereas a central process enters the spinal cord through the posterior root to synapse on the second-order neuron. The **second-order neuron** gives rise to an axon that decussates (crosses to the opposite side) and ascends to a higher level of the CNS, where it synapses with the **third-order neuron**. The third-order neuron is usually in the thalamus and gives rise to a projection fiber that passes to a sensory region of the cerebral cortex. This three-neuron chain is the most common arrangement, but some afferent pathways use more or fewer neurons. Many of the neurons in the ascending pathways branch and give a major input into the reticular formation, which, in turn, activates the cerebral cortex, maintaining wakefulness. Other branches pass to motor neurons and participate in reflex muscular activity.

Functions

Painful and thermal sensations ascend in the lateral spinothalamic tract; light (crude) touch and pressure ascend in the anterior spinothalamic tract (Fig. 4-13). Discriminative touch—that is, the ability to localize accurately the area of the body touched and also to be aware that two points are touched simultaneously, even though they are close together (two-point discrimination)—ascends in the posterior white columns. Also ascending in the posterior white columns is information from muscles and joints pertaining to movement and position of different parts of the body. In addition, vibratory sensations ascend in the posterior white column. Unconscious information from muscles, joints, the skin, and subcutaneous tissue reaches the cerebellum by way of the anterior and posterior spinocerebellar tracts and by the cuneocerebellar tract. Pain, thermal, and tactile information are passed to the superior colliculus of the midbrain through the spinotectal tract for the purpose of spinovisual reflexes. The spinoreticular tract provides a pathway from the muscles, joints, and skin to the reticular formation, while the spino-olivary tract provides an indirect pathway for further afferent information to reach the cerebellum.

Pain and Temperature Pathways

The pain and thermal receptors in the skin and other tissues are free nerve endings. The pain impulses are transmitted to the spinal cord in fast-conducting

Cerebral cortex

Thalamus

3

2

Sensory ending

1

Figure 4-12   Simplest form of the ascending sensory pathway from the sensory nerve ending to the cerebral cortex. Note the three neurons involved.

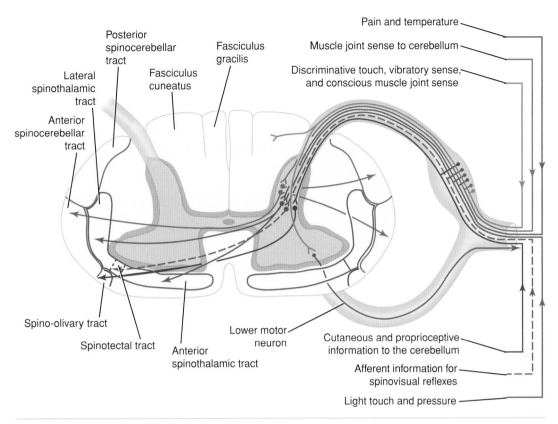

Figure 4-13 Transverse section of the spinal cord showing the origin of the main ascending sensory tracts. Note that the sensations of pain and temperature ascend in the lateral spinothalamic tract, and light touch and pressure ascend in the anterior spinothalamic tract.

δ A-type fibers and slow-conducting C-type fibers. The fast-conducting fibers alert the individual to initial sharp pain, and the slow-conducting fibers are responsible for prolonged burning, aching pain. The sensations of heat and cold also travel by δ A and C fibers.

The main somatosensory pathways are summarized in Table 4-2.

Table 4-2 Main Somatosensory Pathways to Consciousness[a]

Sensation	Receptor	First-Order Neuron	Second-Order Neuron	Third-Order Neuron	Pathways	Destination
Pain and temperature	Free nerve endings	Posterior root ganglion	Substantia gelatinosa	Ventral posterolateral nucleus of thalamus	Lateral spinothalamic, spinal lemniscus	Posterior central gyrus
Light touch and pressure	Free nerve endings	Posterior root ganglion	Substantia gelatinosa	Ventral posterolateral nucleus of thalamus	Anterior spinothalamic, spinal lemniscus	Posterior central gyrus
Discriminative touch, vibratory sense, conscious muscle joint sense	Meissner corpuscles, pacinian corpuscles, muscle spindles, tendon organs	Posterior root ganglion	Nuclei gracilis and cuneatus	Ventral posterolateral nucleus of thalamus	Fasciculi gracilis and cuneatus, medial lemniscus	Posterior central gyrus

[a]Note that all ascending pathways send branches to the reticular activating system.

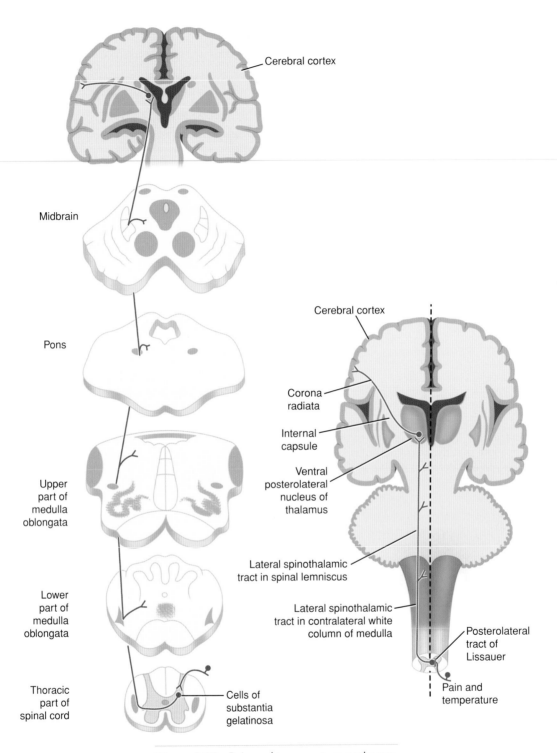

Figure 4-14 Pain and temperature pathways.

Lateral Spinothalamic Tract

Axons entering the spinal cord from the posterior root ganglion proceed to the tip of the posterior gray column and divide into ascending and descending branches (Fig. 4-14). These branches travel for a distance of one or two segments of the spinal cord and form the **posterolateral tract of Lissauer**. These fibers of the

first-order neuron terminate by synapsing with cells in the posterior gray column, including cells in the substantia gelatinosa. Substance P, a peptide, is thought to be the neurotransmitter at these synapses.

Axons of the second-order neurons now **cross obliquely to the opposite side in the anterior gray and white commissures within one spinal segment of** the cord, ascending in the contralateral white column as the lateral spinothalamic tract. The lateral spinothalamic tract lies medial to the anterior spinocerebellar tract. As the lateral spinothalamic tract ascends through the spinal cord, new fibers are added to the anteromedial aspect of the tract. Thus, in the upper cervical segments of the cord, the sacral fibers are lateral and the cervical segments are medial. The fibers carrying pain are situated slightly anterior to those conducting temperature.

As the lateral spinothalamic tract ascends through the medulla oblongata, it lies near the lateral surface and between the inferior olivary nucleus and the nucleus of the spinal tract of the trigeminal nerve. It is now accompanied by the anterior spinothalamic tract and the spinotectal tract; together they form the **spinal lemniscus**.

The spinal lemniscus continues to ascend through the posterior part of the pons. In the midbrain, it lies in the tegmentum lateral to the medial lemniscus. Many of the fibers of the lateral spinothalamic tract end by synapsing with the third-order neuron in the ventral posterolateral nucleus of the thalamus. Crude pain and temperature sensations are probably appreciated and emotional reactions initiated here.

Axons of the third-order neurons in the ventral posterolateral nucleus of the thalamus now pass through the posterior limb of the internal capsule and the corona radiata to reach the somesthetic area in the postcentral gyrus of the cerebral cortex. The contralateral half of the body is represented as inverted, with the hand and mouth situated inferiorly and the leg situated superiorly, and with the foot and anogenital region on the medial surface of the hemisphere. (For details, see Chapter 7.) From here, the information is transmitted to other regions of the cerebral cortex to be used by motor areas and the parietal association area. The role of the cerebral cortex is interpreting the quality of the sensory information at the level of consciousness.

Pain Reception

The perception of pain is a complex phenomenon that is influenced by the emotional state and past experiences of the individual. Pain is a sensation that warns of potential injury and alerts the person to avoid or treat it.

Pain can be divided into two main types: **fast pain** and **slow pain**. Fast pain is experienced within about 0.1 second after the pain stimulus is applied; slow pain is felt 1.0 second or later after the stimulation. Fast pain is described by the patient as sharp pain, acute pain, or pricking pain and is the type of pain felt after pricking the finger with a needle. Fast pain is almost confined to the skin.

Slow pain is described as burning pain, aching pain, and throbbing pain and is produced on tissue destruction, as for example, in the development of an abscess or in severe arthritis. Slow pain can occur in any tissue of the body.

All types of pain reception take place in free nerve endings. Fast pain is experienced by mechanical or thermal types of stimuli, and slow pain may be elicited by mechanical, thermal, and chemical stimuli.

Many chemical substances have been found in extracts from dam**aged tissue that will excite free nerve endings. These include serotonin; histamine; bradykinin; acids**, such as **lactic acid**; and **K$^+$ ions.** The threshold for pain endings can be lowered by prostaglandins and substance P, but they cannot stimulate the endings directly by themselves.

The individual should be aware of the existence of stimuli that, if allowed to persist, will cause tissue destruction; pain receptors have little or no adaptation.

Pain Conduction to the Central Nervous System

Fast pain travels in peripheral nerves in large diameter A δ axons at velocities between 6 and 30 msec. Slow pain travels in the small-diameter C fibers at velocities between 0.5 and 2.0 msec. The fast pain impulses reach consciousness first to alert the individual to danger so that a suitable protective response may take place. Slow pain is appreciated later and lasts much longer.

Pain Conduction in the Central Nervous System

Afferent pain fibers enter the spinal cord, for example, in the posterior roots of a spinal nerve and terminate predominantly in the superficial layers of the posterior gray horn. The main excitatory neurotransmitter released by A δ fibers and C fibers is the amino acid **glutamate**. Substance P, a neuropeptide, is also released from C fibers. Whereas glutamate is a fast-acting localized neurotransmitter, substance P has a slow release and diffuses widely in the posterior horn and can influence many neurons.

The initial sharp, pricking, fast-acting pain fibers stimulate the second-order neurons of the lateral spinothalamic tract. The axons immediately cross to the opposite side of the spinal cord and ascend to the thalamus where they are relayed to the sensory postcentral gyrus. The burning, aching, slow-acting pain fibers also stimulate the second-order neurons of the lateral spinal thalamic tract in the posterior gray horn and ascend with the axons of the fast-acting pain fibers. However, most of the incoming slow fibers to the spinal cord probably take part in additional relays involving several neurons in the posterior horn before ascending in the spinal cord. The repeated arrival of noxious stimuli through C fibers in the posterior gray horn during severe injury results in an increased response of the second-order neurons. This **winding up** phenomenon is attributed to the release of the neurotransmitter glutamate from C fibers.

The fast type of pain is precisely localized. For example, if someone hits a thumb with a hammer, where the injury has occurred is clear. The slow type of pain is only poorly localized. For example, in a patient with osteoarthritis of the hip joint, the individual can only vaguely localize the pain to the hip area and not to the specific site of the disease. This may be explained by the fact that fast pain fibers directly ascend the spinal cord in the lateral spinothalamic tract, whereas the slow pain fibers take part in multiple relays in the posterior gray horn before ascending to higher centers.

Other Terminations of the Lateral Spinothalamic Tract

As is now generally agreed, fast pain impulses travel directly up to the ventral posterolateral nucleus of the thalamus and are then relayed to the cerebral cortex.

The majority of the slow pain fibers in the lateral spinothalamic tract terminate in the reticular formation, which then activates the entire nervous system. In the lower areas of the brain, the individual becomes aware of the chronic, nauseous, suffering type of pain.

As the result of research using the positron emission tomography scan, the postcentral gyrus, the cingulate gyrus of the limbic system, and the insular gyrus are sites concerned with the reception and interpretation of nociceptor information. The postcentral gyrus is responsible for the interpretation of pain in relation to past experiences. The cingulate gyrus is involved with the interpretation of the emotional aspect of pain, whereas the insular gyrus is concerned with the interpretation of pain stimuli from the internal organs of the body and brings about an autonomic response.

Reception of pain information by the CNS is modulated first in the posterior gray horns of the spinal cord and at other sites at higher levels.

Pain Control in the Central Nervous System

Massage and the application of liniments to painful areas in the body can relieve pain. The technique of acupuncture, which was discovered several thousand years ago in China, is also beneficial in relieving pain. Low-frequency electrical stimulation of the skin also relieves pain in certain cases.

Gating Theory

Although the precise mechanism for the phenomena described above is not understood, the gating theory suggested that, at the site where the pain fiber enters the CNS, inhibition could occur by means of connector neurons excited by large, myelinated afferent fibers carrying information of nonpainful touch and pressure. The excess tactile stimulation produced by massage, for example, "closed the gate" for pain. Once the nonpainful tactile stimulation ceased, however, "the gate was opened," and information on the painful stimuli ascended the lateral spinothalamic tract. Although the gate theory may partially explain the phenomena, the analgesia system is probably involved with the liberation of enkephalins and endorphins in the posterior gray columns.

Analgesia System

Stimulation of certain areas of the brainstem can reduce or block sensations of pain. These areas include the periventricular area of the diencephalon, the periaqueductal gray matter of the midbrain, and midline nuclei of the brainstem. Fibers of the reticulospinal tract are believed to pass down to the spinal cord and synapse on cells concerned with pain sensation in the posterior gray column. The analgesic system can suppress both sharp pricking pain and burning pain sensations.

Recently, two compounds with morphinelike actions, **enkephalins** and **endorphins**, have been isolated in the CNS. These compounds and **serotonin** serve as neurotransmitter substances in the analgesic system of the brain, and they may inhibit the release of substance P in the posterior gray column.

Light (Crude) Touch and Pressure Pathways

These pathways are summarized in Table 4-2.

Anterior Spinothalamic Tract

Axons enter the spinal cord from the posterior root ganglion and proceed to the tip of the posterior gray column, where they divide into ascending and descending branches (Fig. 4-15). These branches travel for a distance of one or two segments of the spinal cord, contributing to the posterolateral tract of Lissauer. These fibers of the first-order neuron are believed to terminate by synapsing with cells in the substantia gelatinosa group in the posterior gray column.

Axons of the second-order neuron now **cross very obliquely to the opposite side in the anterior gray and white commissures within several spinal segments** and ascend in the opposite anterolateral white column as the anterior spinothalamic tract. As the anterior spinothalamic tract ascends through the spinal cord, new fibers are added to the medial aspect of the tract. Thus, in the upper cervical segments of the cord, the sacral fibers are mostly lateral and the cervical segments are mostly medial.

As the anterior spinothalamic tract ascends through the medulla oblongata, it accompanies the lateral spinothalamic tract and the spinotectal tract, all of which form the **spinal lemniscus**.

The spinal lemniscus continues to ascend through the posterior part of the pons, and the tegmentum of the midbrain and the fibers of the anterior spinothalamic tract terminate by synapsing with the third-order neuron in the ventral posterolateral nucleus of the thalamus. Crude awareness of touch and pressure is believed to be appreciated here.

Axons of the third-order neurons in the ventral posterolateral nucleus of the thalamus pass through the posterior limb of the **internal capsule** and the **corona radiata** to reach the somesthetic area in the postcentral gyrus of the cerebral cortex. The contralateral half of the body is represented inverted, with the hand and mouth situated inferiorly, as described previously. (For details, see Chapter 7.) The conscious appreciation of touch and pressure depends on the activity of the cerebral cortex. The sensations can be only crudely

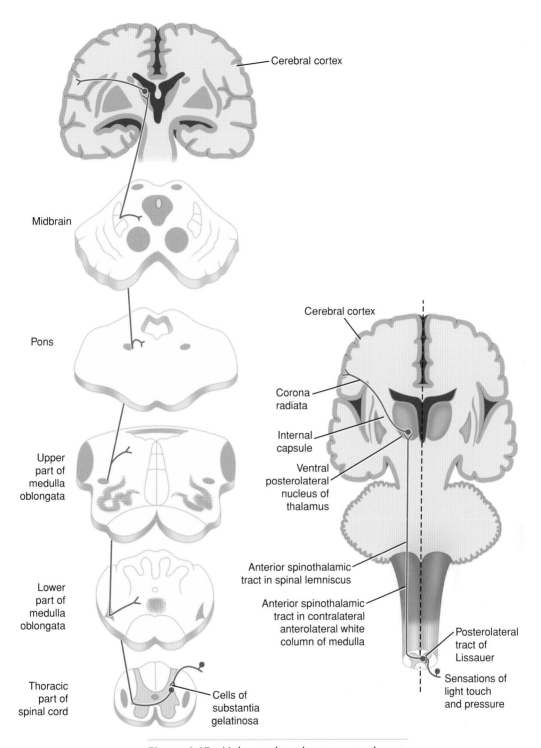

Figure 4-15   Light touch and pressure pathways.

localized, and very little discrimination of intensity is possible.

Discriminative Touch, Vibratory Sense, and Conscious Muscle Joint Sense

These pathways are summarized in Table 4-2.

Posterior White Column: Fasciculus Gracilis and Fasciculus Cuneatus

Axons enter the spinal cord from the posterior root ganglion and pass directly to the posterior white column of the same side (Fig. 4-16). Here, the fibers divide into long ascending and short descending branches. The

Figure 4-16 Discriminative touch, vibratory sense, and conscious muscle joint sense pathways.

descending branches pass down a variable number of segments, giving off collateral branches that synapse with cells in the posterior gray horn, with internuncial neurons, and with anterior horn cells. These short descending fibers are clearly involved with intersegmental reflexes.

Long ascending fibers may also end by synapsing with cells in the posterior gray horn, with internuncial neurons, and with anterior horn cells. This distribution may extend over numerous segments of the spinal cord. As in the case of the short descending fibers, they are involved with intersegmental reflexes.

Many of the long ascending fibers travel upward in the posterior white column as the **fasciculus gracilis** and **fasciculus cuneatus**. The fasciculus gracilis is present throughout the length of the spinal cord and contains the long ascending fibers from the sacral, lumbar, and lower six thoracic spinal nerves. The fasciculus cuneatus is situated laterally in the upper thoracic and cervical segments of the spinal cord and is separated from the fasciculus gracilis by a septum. The fasciculus cuneatus contains the long ascending fibers from the upper six thoracic and all the cervical spinal nerves.

Fibers of the fasciculus gracilis and fasciculus cuneatus ascend **ipsilaterally** and terminate by synapsing on the second-order neurons in the **nuclei gracilis** and **cuneatus** of the medulla oblongata. The axons of the second-order neurons, called the **internal arcuate fibers**, sweep anteromedially around the central gray matter and **cross the median plane,** decussating with the corresponding fibers of the opposite side in the **sensory decussation**. The fibers then ascend as a single compact bundle, the **medial lemniscus**, through the medulla oblongata, the pons, and the midbrain. The fibers terminate by synapsing on the third-order neurons in the ventral posterolateral nucleus of the thalamus.

Axons of the third-order neuron leave and pass through the posterior limb of the **internal capsule** and **corona radiata** to reach the somesthetic area in the postcentral gyrus of the cerebral cortex. The contralateral half of the body is represented inverted, with the hand and mouth situated inferiorly, as described previously. (For details, see Chapter 7.) In this manner, the impressions of touch with fine gradations of intensity, exact localization, and two-point discrimination can be appreciated. Vibratory sense and the position of the different parts of the body can be consciously recognized.

Many fibers in the fasciculus cuneatus from the cervical and upper thoracic segments, having terminated on the second-order neuron of the nucleus cuneatus, are relayed and travel as the axons of the second-order neurons to enter the cerebellum through the inferior cerebellar peduncle of the same side. This pathway is the **cuneocerebellar tract**, and the fibers are known as the **posterior external arcuate fibers**. The function of these fibers is to convey information of muscle joint sense to the cerebellum.

Muscle Joint Sense Pathways to the Cerebellum

Muscle joint sense pathways to the cerebellum are summarized in Table 4-3.

Posterior Spinocerebellar Tract

Axons entering the spinal cord from the posterior root ganglion enter the posterior gray column and terminate by synapsing on the second-order neurons at the base of the posterior gray column (Fig. 4-17). These neurons are known collectively as the **nucleus dorsalis (Clarke column)**. Axons of the second-order neurons enter the posterolateral part of the lateral white column on the **same side** and ascend as the posterior spinocerebellar tract to the medulla oblongata. Here, the tract joins the inferior cerebellar peduncle and terminates in the cerebellar cortex. Note that it does not ascend to the cerebral cortex. Because the nucleus dorsalis (Clarke column) extends only from the eighth cervical segment caudally to the third or fourth lumbar segment, axons entering the spinal cord from the posterior roots of the lower lumbar and sacral segments ascend in the posterior white column until they reach the third or fourth lumbar segment, where they enter the nucleus dorsalis.

The posterior spinocerebellar fibers receive muscle joint information from the muscle spindles, tendon organs, and joint receptors of the trunk and lower limbs. This information concerning tension of muscle tendons and the movements of muscles and joints is used by the cerebellum in the coordination of limb movements and the maintenance of posture.

Anterior Spinocerebellar Tract

Axons entering the spinal cord from the posterior root ganglion terminate by synapsing with the second-order neurons in the **nucleus dorsalis** at the base of the posterior gray column (Fig. 4-17). Most axons of the second-order neurons **cross** to the opposite side and ascend as the anterior spinocerebellar tract in the contralateral white column; a minority ascend as the anterior spinocerebellar tract in the lateral white column of the **same side**. The fibers, having ascended through the medulla oblongata and pons, enter the cerebellum through the superior cerebellar peduncle and terminate in the cerebellar cortex. Those fibers that crossed over to the opposite side in the spinal cord are believed to **cross back** within the cerebellum. The anterior spinocerebellar tract conveys muscle joint information from the muscle spindles, tendon organs, and joint receptors of the trunk and the upper and lower limbs. It is also believed that the cerebellum receives information from the skin and superficial fascia by this tract.

Table 4-3	Muscle Joint Sense Pathways to the Cerebellum				
Sensation	**Receptor**	**First-Order Neuron**	**Second-Order Neuron**	**Pathways**	**Destination**
Unconscious muscle joint sense	Muscle spindles, tendon organs, joint receptors	Posterior root ganglion	Nucleus dorsalis	Anterior and posterior spinocerebellar	Cerebellar cortex

Figure 4-17 Unconscious muscle joint sense pathways to the cerebellum.

Cuneocerebellar Tract

These fibers are described on page 142. They originate in the nucleus cuneatus and enter the cerebellum through the inferior cerebellar peduncle of the **same side** (Fig. 4-16). They are known as the **posterior external arcuate fibers**, and their function is to convey information of muscle joint sense to the cerebellum.

Other Ascending Pathways

The spinotectal, spinoreticular, and spino-olivary tracts are shown in Figure 4-18.

Spinotectal Tract

Axons enter the spinal cord from the posterior root ganglion and travel to the gray matter where they synapse on unknown second-order neurons. Axons of the second-order neurons **cross the median plane** and ascend as the spinotectal tract in the anterolateral white column lying close to the lateral spinothalamic tract. After passing through the medulla oblongata and pons, they terminate by synapsing with neurons in the superior colliculus of the midbrain. This pathway provides afferent information for spinovisual reflexes and brings about movements of the eyes and head toward the source of the stimulation.

Spinoreticular Tract

Axons enter the spinal cord from the posterior root ganglion and terminate on unknown second-order neurons in the gray matter. Axons from these second-order neurons ascend the spinal cord as the spinoreticular tract in the lateral white column mixed with the lateral spinothalamic tract. Most of the fibers are **uncrossed** and terminate by synapsing with neurons of the reticular formation in the medulla oblongata, pons, and midbrain. The spinoreticular tract provides an afferent

Superior colliculus

Midbrain

Pons

Spinoreticular tract passing to reticular formation

Inferior cerebellar peduncle

Inferior olivary nucleus

Medulla oblongata

Spinoreticular tract in lateral white column of medulla

Spinotectal tract in anterolateral white column of medulla

Spino-olivary tract in anterolateral white column of medulla

Afferent information for spinovisual reflexes

From cutaneous and proprioceptive organs

Afferent information that influences consciousness

Figure 4-18   Spinotectal, spinoreticular, and spino-olivary tracts.

pathway for the reticular formation, which plays an important role in influencing levels of consciousness. (For details, see p. 204.)

Spino-olivary Tract

Axons enter the spinal cord from the posterior root ganglion and terminate on unknown second-order neurons in the posterior gray column. Axons from the second-order neurons **cross the midline** and ascend as the spino-olivary tract in the white matter at the junction of the anterior and lateral columns. The axons end by synapsing on third-order neurons in the inferior olivary nuclei in the medulla oblongata. Axons of the third-order neurons cross the midline and

enter the cerebellum through the inferior cerebellar peduncle. The spino-olivary tract conveys information to the cerebellum from cutaneous and proprioceptive organs.

Visceral Sensory Tracts

Sensations that arise in viscera located in the thorax and abdomen enter the spinal cord through the posterior roots. The cell bodies of the first-order neuron are situated in the posterior root ganglia. The peripheral processes of these cells receive nerve impulses from pain and stretch receptor endings in the viscera. The causes of visceral pain include ischemia, chemical damage, spasm of smooth muscle, and distention. The central processes, having entered the spinal cord, synapse with second-order neurons in the gray matter, probably in the posterior or lateral gray columns.

Axons of the second-order neurons are believed to join the spinothalamic tracts and ascend and terminate on third-order neurons in the ventral posterolateral nucleus of the thalamus. The final destination of these axons is probably in the postcentral gyrus of the cerebral cortex.

Many of the visceral afferent fibers that enter the spinal cord branch participate in reflex activity.

DESCENDING TRACTS

Motor neurons situated in the anterior gray columns of the spinal cord send axons to innervate skeletal muscle through the anterior roots of the spinal nerves. These motor neurons are referred to as the **lower motor neurons** and constitute the final common pathway to the muscles (Fig. 4-19).

Lower motor neurons are constantly bombarded by nervous impulses that descend from the medulla, pons, midbrain, and cerebral cortex as well as those that enter along sensory fibers from the posterior

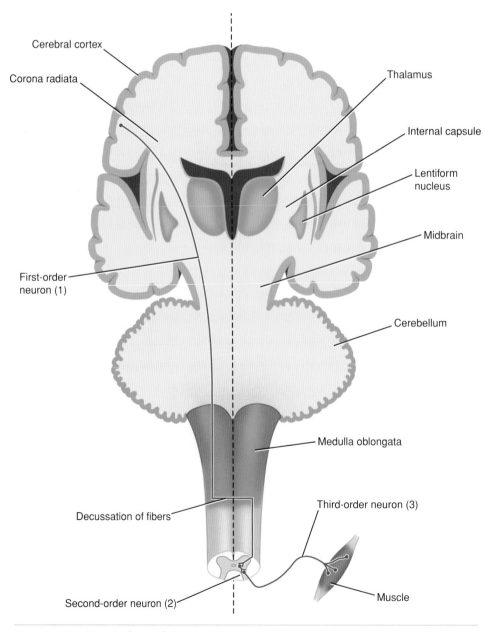

Figure 4-19   Simple form of the descending motor pathway from the cerebral cortex to the skeletal muscle. Note the three neurons involved.

Table 4-4   Main Descending Pathways to the Spinal Cord[a]

Pathway	Function	Origin	Site of Crossover	Destination	Branches to
Corticospinal tracts	Rapid, skilled, voluntary movements, especially distal ends of limbs	Primary motor cortex (area 4), secondary motor cortex (area 6), parietal lobe (areas 3, 1, and 2)	Most cross at decussation of pyramids and descend as lateral corticospinal tracts; some continue as anterior corticospinal tracts and cross over at level of destination	Internuncial neurons or α motor neurons	Cerebral cortex, basal nuclei, red nucleus, olivary nuclei, reticular formation
Reticulospinal tracts	Inhibit or facilitate voluntary movement; hypothalamus controls sympathetic, para-sympathetic outflows	Reticular formation	Some cross at various levels	α and γ motor neurons	Multiple branches as they descend
Tectospinal tract	Reflex postural movements concerning sight	Superior colliculus	Soon after origin	α and γ motor neurons	?
Rubrospinal tract	Facilitates activity of flexor muscles and inhibits activity of extensor muscles	Red nucleus	Immediately	α and γ motor neurons	?
Vestibulospinal tract	Facilitates activity of extensor inhibits flexor muscles	Vestibular nuclei	Uncrossed	α and γ motor neurons	?
Olivospinal tract	??	Inferior olivary nuclei	Cross in brainstem	? α and γ motor neurons	—
Descending autonomic fibers	Control sympathetic and parasympathetic systems	Cerebral cortex, hypothalamus, amygdaloid complex, reticular formation		Sympathetic and parasympathetic outflows	—

[a]Note that the corticospinal tracts are believed to control the prime mover muscles (especially the highly skilled movements), whereas the other descending tracts are important in controlling the simple basic movements. For simplicity, the internuncial neurons are omitted from this table.

roots. Nerve fibers that descend in the white matter from different supraspinal nerve centers are segregated into nerve bundles called the **descending tracts**. These supraspinal neurons and their tracts are referred to as the **upper motor neurons**, and they provide numerous separate pathways that can influence motor activity.

A summary of the main descending pathways in the spinal cord is shown in Table 4-4.

Anatomical Organization

Control of skeletal muscle activity from the cerebral cortex and other higher centers is conducted through the nervous system by a series of neurons (Fig. 4-19). The descending pathway from the cerebral cortex is often made up of three neurons. The first neuron, the **first-order neuron**, has its cell body in the cerebral cortex. Its axon descends to synapse on the **second-order neuron**, an internuncial neuron, situated in the anterior gray column of the spinal cord. The axon of the second-order neuron is short and synapses with the **third-order neuron**, the lower motor neuron, in the anterior gray column. The axon of the third-order neuron innervates the skeletal muscle through the anterior root and spinal nerve. In some instances, the axon of the first-order neuron terminates directly on the third-order neuron (as in reflex arcs).

Functions

Corticospinal tracts (Fig. 4-20) are the pathways concerned with voluntary, discrete, skilled movements, especially those of the distal parts of the limbs. **Reticulospinal tracts** may facilitate or inhibit the activity of the α and γ motor neurons in the anterior gray columns and may, therefore, facilitate or inhibit voluntary

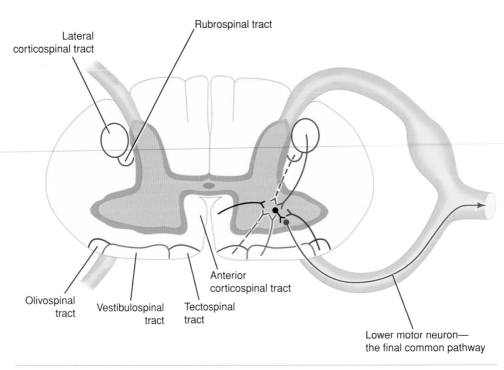

Figure 4-20 Transverse section of the spinal cord showing the termination of the descending motor tracts. Note that the existence of the olivospinal tract as a separate pathway is now in considerably doubt.

movement or reflex activity. The **tectospinal tract** is concerned with reflex postural movements in response to visual stimuli. Those fibers that are associated with the sympathetic neurons in the lateral gray column are concerned with the pupillodilation reflex in response to darkness. The **rubrospinal tract** acts on both the α and γ motor neurons in the anterior gray columns and facilitates the activity of flexor muscles and inhibits the activity of extensor or antigravity muscles. The **vestibulospinal tract**, by acting on the motor neurons in the anterior gray columns, facilitates the activity of the extensor muscles, inhibits the activity of the flexor muscles, and is concerned with the postural activity associated with balance. The **olivospinal tract** may play a role in muscular activity, but some doubt its existence. The **descending autonomic fibers** are concerned with the control of visceral activity.

Corticospinal Tracts

Fibers of the corticospinal tract arise as axons of pyramidal cells situated in the fifth layer of the cerebral cortex (Fig. 4-21). About a third of the fibers originate from the primary motor cortex (area 4), another third from the secondary motor cortex (area 6), and the final third from the parietal lobe (areas 3, 1, and 2); thus, two thirds of the fibers arise from the precentral gyrus, and one third of the fibers arise from the postcentral gyrus. These fibers do not control motor activity but influence sensory input to the nervous system. Because electrical stimulation of different parts of the precentral gyrus produces movements of different parts of the opposite side of the body, we can represent the parts of the body in this area of the cortex. Such a homunculus is shown in Figure 4-21. Note that the region controlling the face is situated inferiorly, and the region controlling the lower limb is situated superiorly and on the medial surface of the hemisphere. The homunculus is a distorted picture of the body, with the various parts having a size proportional to the area of the cerebral cortex devoted to their control. Interestingly, most corticospinal fibers are myelinated and are relatively slow-conducting, small fibers.

The descending fibers converge in the **corona radiata** and then pass through the posterior limb of the **internal capsule**. Here, the fibers are organized so that those closest to the genu are concerned with cervical portions of the body, while those situated more posteriorly are concerned with the lower extremity. The tract then continues through the middle three fifths of the **basis pedunculi of the midbrain**. Here, the fibers concerned with cervical portions of the body are situated medially, while those concerned with the leg are placed laterally.

On entering the pons, the tract is broken into many bundles by the **transverse pontocerebellar fibers** (see Figs. 5-19 to 5-22). In the medulla oblongata, the bundles become grouped together along the anterior border to form a swelling known as the **pyramid** (hence the alternative name, **pyramidal tract**) (see Figs. 5-11 and 5-12). At the junction of the medulla oblongata and the spinal cord, most of the fibers **cross** the midline at the **decussation of the pyramids** (Fig. 4-21) and enter the lateral white column of the

Figure 4-21 Corticospinal tracts.

spinal cord to form the **lateral corticospinal tract** (Fig. 4-20). The remaining fibers do not cross in the decussation but descend in the anterior white column of the spinal cord as the **anterior corticospinal tract** (Figs. 4-20 and 4-21). These fibers eventually **cross** the midline and terminate in the anterior gray column of the spinal cord segments in the cervical and upper thoracic regions.

The lateral corticospinal tract descends the length of the spinal cord; its fibers terminate in the anterior gray column of all the spinal cord segments.

Most corticospinal fibers synapse with internuncial neurons, which, in turn, synapse with α motor neurons and some γ motor neurons. Only the largest corticospinal fibers synapse directly with the motor neurons.

The corticospinal tracts are not the sole pathway for serving voluntary movement. Rather, they form the pathway that confers speed and agility to voluntary movements and is thus used in performing rapid skilled movements. Many of the simple, basic voluntary movements are mediated by other descending tracts.

Branches

1. Branches are given off early in their descent and return to the cerebral cortex to inhibit activity in adjacent regions of the cortex.
2. Branches pass to the caudate and lentiform nuclei, the red nuclei, and the olivary nuclei and the reticular formation. These branches keep the subcortical regions informed about the cortical motor activity. Once alerted, the subcortical regions may react and send their own nervous impulses to the α and γ motor neurons by other descending pathways.

Reticulospinal Tracts

Throughout the midbrain, pons, and medulla oblongata, groups of scattered nerve cells and nerve fibers exist that are collectively known as the **reticular formation**. From the pons, these neurons send axons, which are mostly **uncrossed**, down into the spinal cord and form the **pontine reticulospinal tract** (Fig. 4-22). From the medulla, similar neurons send axons, which are crossed and uncrossed, to the spinal cord and form the **medullary reticulospinal tract**.

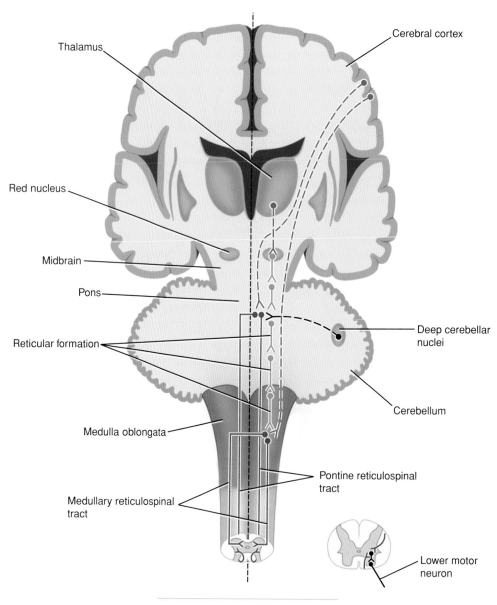

Figure 4-22 Reticulospinal tracts.

Reticulospinal fibers from the pons descend through the anterior white column, while those from the medulla oblongata descend in the lateral white column. Both sets of fibers enter the anterior gray columns of the spinal cord and may facilitate or inhibit α and γ motor neuron activity. By these means, the reticulospinal tracts influence voluntary movements and reflex activity. The reticulospinal fibers are also now thought to include the descending autonomic fibers. The reticulospinal tracts thus provide a pathway by which the hypothalamus can control the sympathetic outflow and the sacral parasympathetic outflow.

Tectospinal Tract

Fibers of this tract arise from nerve cells in the **superior colliculus** of the midbrain (Fig. 4-23). Most

of the fibers **cross** the midline soon after their origin and descend through the brainstem close to the **medial longitudinal fasciculus**. The tectospinal tract descends through the anterior white column of the spinal cord close to the anterior median fissure (Fig. 4-20). The majority of the fibers terminate in the anterior gray column in the upper cervical segments of the spinal cord by synapsing with internuncial neurons. These fibers are believed to be concerned with reflex postural movements in response to visual stimuli.

Rubrospinal Tract

The **red nucleus** is situated in the tegmentum of the midbrain at the level of the superior colliculus (Fig. 4-24). The axons of neurons in this nucleus cross

Figure 4-23 Tectospinal tract.

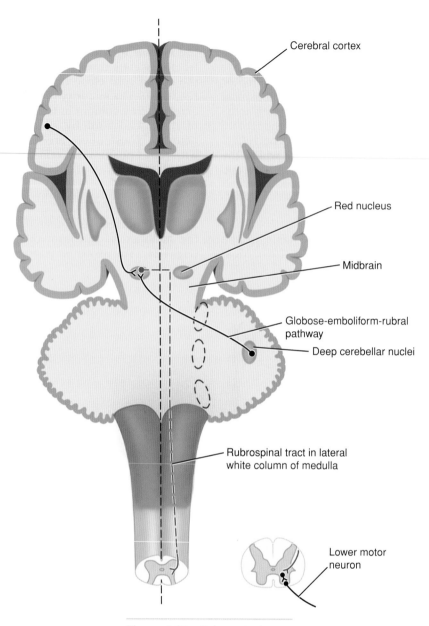

Figure 4-24 Rubrospinal tract.

the midline at the level of the nucleus and descend as the rubrospinal tract through the pons and medulla oblongata to enter the lateral white column of the spinal cord (Fig. 4-20). The fibers terminate by synapsing with internuncial neurons in the anterior gray column of the cord.

Neurons of the red nucleus receive afferent impulses through connections with the cerebral cortex and the cerebellum. This is believed to be an important indirect pathway by which the cerebral cortex and the cerebellum can influence α and γ motor neuron activity. The tract facilitates the activity of the flexor muscles and inhibits the activity of the extensor or antigravity muscles.

Vestibulospinal Tract

Vestibular nuclei are situated in the pons and medulla oblongata beneath the floor of the fourth ventricle (Fig. 4-25). The vestibular nuclei receive afferent fibers from the inner ear through the vestibular nerve and from the cerebellum. Neurons of the lateral vestibular nucleus give rise to the axons that form the vestibulospinal tract. The tract descends **uncrossed** through the medulla and through the length of the spinal cord in the anterior white column (Fig. 4-20). The fibers terminate by synapsing with internuncial neurons of the anterior gray column of the spinal cord.

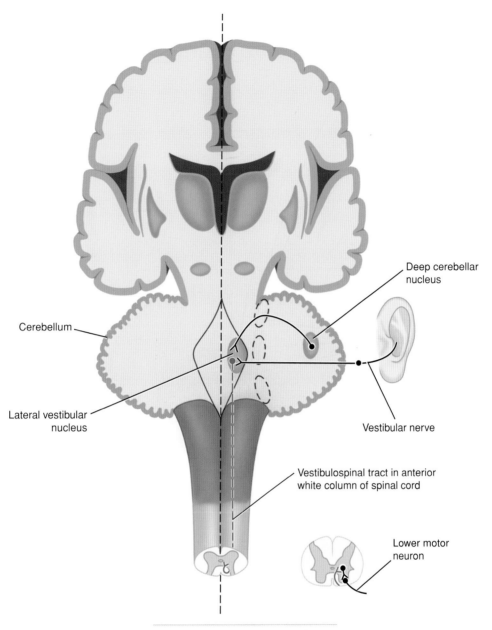

Figure 4-25 Vestibulospinal tract.

The inner ear and the cerebellum, by means of this tract, facilitate the activity of the extensor muscles and inhibit the activity of the flexor muscles in association with the maintenance of balance.

Olivospinal Tract

The olivospinal tract was thought to arise from the inferior olivary nucleus and to descend in the lateral white column of the spinal cord (Fig. 4-26), to influence the activity of the motor neurons in the anterior gray column. Many now doubt that it exists.

Descending Autonomic Fibers

The higher centers of the CNS associated with the control of autonomic activity are situated in the cerebral cortex, hypothalamus, amygdaloid complex, and reticular formation. Although distinct tracts have not been recognized, investigation of spinal cord lesions has demonstrated that descending autonomic tracts do exist and probably form part of the reticulospinal tract.

The fibers arise from neurons in the higher centers and cross the midline in the brainstem. They are

Cerebral cortex

Globus pallidus

Red nucleus

Descending tracts
from higher centers

Inferior olivary nucleus

Ascending spino-olivary
tract

Olivospinal tract in anterior
white column of medulla

Lower motor
neuron

Figure 4-26 Olivospinal tract. The existence of this tract as a separate pathway is doubtful.

believed to descend in the lateral white column of the spinal cord and to terminate by synapsing on the autonomic motor cells in the lateral gray columns in the thoracic and upper lumbar (sympathetic outflow) and midsacral (parasympathetic) levels of the spinal cord.

INTERSEGMENTAL TRACTS

Short ascending and descending tracts that originate and end within the spinal cord exist in the anterior, lateral, and posterior white columns. The function of these pathways is to interconnect the neurons of different segmental levels, and the pathways are particularly important in intersegmental spinal reflexes.

Reflex Arc

A **reflex** may be defined as an involuntary response to a stimulus. It depends on the integrity of the reflex arc (Fig. 4-27). In its simplest form, a reflex arc consists of the following anatomical structures: (1) a receptor organ, (2) an afferent neuron, (3) an effector neuron, and (4) an effector organ. A reflex arc involving only one synapse is referred to as a **monosynaptic reflex arc**. Interruption of the reflex arc at any point along its course would abolish the response.

In the spinal cord, reflex arcs play an important role in maintaining muscle tone, which is the basis for body posture. The receptor organ is situated in the skin, muscle, or tendon. The cell body of the afferent neuron is

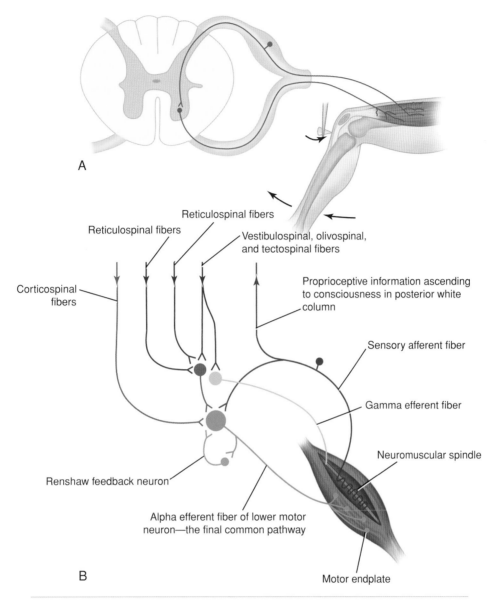

A

Reticulospinal fibers

Reticulospinal fibers

Vestibulospinal, olivospinal, and tectospinal fibers

Corticospinal fibers

Proprioceptive information ascending to consciousness in posterior white column

Sensory afferent fiber

Gamma efferent fiber

Neuromuscular spindle

Renshaw feedback neuron

Alpha efferent fiber of lower motor neuron—the final common pathway

B

Motor endplate

Figure 4-27 A: A monosynaptic reflex arc. **B:** Multiple neurons synapsing with the lower motor neuron. Note the presence of the Renshaw feedback neuron.

located in the posterior root ganglion, and the central axon of this first-order neuron terminates by synapsing on the effector neuron. Since the afferent fibers are of large diameter and are rapidly conducting and because of the presence of only one synapse, a very quick response is possible.

Physiologic study of the electrical activity of the effector neuron shows that a prolonged asynchronous discharge follows the very quick monosynaptic discharge. The reason for this later discharge is that the afferent fibers entering the spinal cord frequently branch, and the branches synapse with many internuncial neurons, which ultimately synapse with the effector neuron (Fig. 4-28). These additional neuronal circuits prolong the bombardment of the effector neurons after the initial stimulation by the afferent neuron has ceased. The presence of internuncial neurons also results in the spread of the afferent stimulus to neurons at different segmental levels of the spinal cord.

The **law of reciprocal innervation** is important to understand in considering reflex skeletal muscle activity. Simply stated, it means that the flexor and extensor reflexes of the same limb cannot be made to contract simultaneously. For this law to work, the afferent nerve fibers responsible for flexor reflex muscle action must have branches that synapse with the extensor motor neurons of the same limb, causing them to be inhibited.

Another interesting property of spinal reflexes is that the evocation of a reflex on one side of the body causes opposite effects on the limb of the other side of the body. This **crossed extensor reflex** is demonstrated when afferent stimulation of the reflex arc that causes the ipsilateral limb to flex results in the contralateral limb being extended.

Posterior root ganglion

Spinal nerve

A

Anterior root

B

Figure 4-28 **A:** Multiple branching of afferent fibers entering the spinal cord and the presence of many internuncial neurons that synapse with the effector neuron. **B:** Law of reciprocal innervation and the crossed extensor reflex.

Influence of Higher Neuronal Centers on Spinal Reflex Activity

The spinal segmental reflex arc involving motor activity is greatly influenced by higher centers in the brain. These influences are mediated through the corticospinal, reticulospinal, tectospinal, rubrospinal, and vestibulospinal tracts. In the clinical condition known as spinal shock (see p. 167), which follows the sudden removal of these influences by spinal cord severance, the segmental spinal reflexes are depressed. When the spinal shock disappears in a few weeks, the segmental spinal reflexes return, and the muscle tone is increased. This **decerebrate rigidity** is due to the overactivity of the γ efferent nerve fibers to the muscle spindles, which results from the release of these neurons from the higher centers. The next stage may be **paraplegia in extension** with domination of the increased tone of the extensor muscles over the flexor muscles. Some neurologists believe that this condition is due to incomplete severance of all the descending tracts with persistence of the vestibulospinal tract. Should all the descending tracts be severed, the condition of **paraplegia in flexion** occurs. In this condition, the reflex responses are flexor in nature, and the tone of the extensor muscles is diminished.

RENSHAW CELLS AND LOWER MOTOR NEURON INHIBITION

Lower motor neuron axons give off collateral branches as they pass through the white matter to reach the anterior roots of the spinal nerve. These collaterals synapse on neurons described by Renshaw, which, in turn, synapse on the lower motor neurons (Fig. 4-27). These internuncial neurons are believed to provide feedback on the lower motor neurons, inhibiting their activity.

Clinical Notes

General Anatomical Features of Clinical Importance

The spinal cord may be described, for practical purposes, as consisting of columns of motor and sensory nerve cells (gray matter) surrounded by ascending and descending tracts (white matter). It lies within the vertebral canal and is protected by three surrounding fibrous membranes, the meninges. It is cushioned against trauma by cerebrospinal fluid (CSF) and is held in position by the denticulate ligaments on each side and the filum terminale inferiorly. The spinal cord is segmented, and paired posterior (sensory) and anterior (motor) roots corresponding to each segment of the cord leave the vertebral canal through the intervertebral foramina.

The spinal cord is shorter than the vertebral column and terminates inferiorly in the adult at the level of the lower border of the first lumbar vertebra. The subarachnoid space extends inferiorly beyond the end of the cord and ends at the level of the lower border of the second sacral vertebra.

Because of the shortness of the spinal cord relative to the length of the vertebral column, the nerve roots of the lumbar and sacral segments have to take an oblique course downward to reach their respective intervertebral foramina; the resulting leash of nerve roots forms the cauda equina.

A spinal tap needle may be inserted into the subarachnoid space below the level of the second lumbar vertebra without damaging the spinal cord. (For details, see p. 19.)

Anterior and Posterior Nerve Root Lesions

Each nerve root has a covering of pia, arachnoid, and dura mater. The anterior and posterior roots unite in the intervertebral foramina to form the spinal nerves. Here, the meninges fuse with the epineurium of the spinal nerves. Either or both spinal nerve roots may be involved in syphilitic spinal meningitis or pyogenic meningitis. The posterior roots may be involved in tabes dorsalis and herpes zoster. Their anatomical location, both in the vertebral canal and in the intervertebral foramina, exposes them to compression from tumors of the vertebral column and to irritation from abnormal constituents of CSF, such as blood following a subarachnoid hemorrhage. A herniated intervertebral disc, a primary or secondary vertebral tumor, vertebral destruction by tumor or infection, or a fracture dislocation can press on the spinal nerve roots in the intervertebral foramina. Even severe scoliosis can compress the nerve roots.

A lesion of one posterior spinal nerve root will produce pain in the area of skin innervated by that root and in the muscles that receive their sensory nerve supply from that root. Movements of the vertebral column in the region of the lesion will heighten the pain, and coughing and sneezing will also make it worse by raising the pressure within the vertebral canal. Before loss of sensation in the dermatome occurs, the patient might experience hyperalgesia and hyperesthesia.

A lesion of an anterior root will result in paralysis of any muscle that is supplied exclusively by that root and a partial paralysis of any muscle that is supplied partially by that root. In both cases, fasciculation and muscle atrophy occur.

Clinical Significance of Ascending Tract Lamination

Within the anterolateral white column of the spinal cord, the axons of the spinothalamic tracts from the sacral and lumbar segments of the body are deflected laterally by axons crossing the midline at successively higher levels. Within the posterior white column, the axons from the sacral and lumbar segments of the body are pushed medially by the axons from higher segments of the body. This deflection of the tracts produces lamination; thus, in the spinothalamic tracts (anterolateral system), the cervical to sacral segments are located from medial to lateral, whereas in the posterior white column (medial lemniscus system), the sacral to cervical segments are located from medial to lateral. This is shown diagrammatically in Figure 4-29.

Ascending Tract Injury

The detailed information described above is of practical value in patients experiencing external pressure exerted on the spinal cord in the region of the spinothalamic tracts. It explains, for example, why patients will experience a loss of pain and temperature sensations first in the sacral dermatomes of the body and, if the pressure increases, in the other higher segmental dermatomes of the body.

Lateral Spinothalamic Tract

Destruction of this tract produces contralateral loss of pain and thermal sensibilities below the level of the lesion. Therefore, the patient will not respond to pinprick or recognize hot and cold objects placed in contact with the skin.

Anterior Spinothalamic Tract

Destruction of this tract produces contralateral loss of light touch and pressure sensibilities below the level of the lesion. Remember that discriminative touch will still be present, because this information is conducted through the fasciculus gracilis and fasciculus cuneatus. The patient will not feel the light touch of a piece of cotton placed against the skin or feel pressure from a blunt object placed against the skin.

Fasciculus Gracilis and Fasciculus Cuneatus

Destruction of these tracts cuts off the supply of information from the muscles and joints to consciousness; thus, the individual does not know about the position and movements of the ipsilateral limbs below the level of the lesion. With the patient's eyes closed, he or she is unable to tell where the limb or part of the limb is in space. For example, if you passively dorsiflex the patient's big toe, he or she is unable to tell you whether the toe is pointing upward or downward. The patient has impaired muscular control, and the movements are jerky or ataxic.

The patient also has loss of vibration sense below the level of the lesion on the same side. This is easily tested by applying a vibrating tuning fork to a bony prominence, such as the lateral malleolus of the fibula or the styloid process of the radius.

Tactile discrimination will also be lost on the side of the lesion. This is tested most easily by gradually separating the two points of a compass until the patient can appreciate them as two separate points, not as one, when they are applied to the skin surface. Tactile discrimination

Figure 4-29 Segmental organization of the tracts in the posterior, lateral, and anterior white columns of the spinal cord.

varies from one part of the body to another. In a normal individual, the points have to be separated by about 3 to 4 mm before they are recognized as separate points on the tips of the fingers. On the back, however, the points have to be separated by 65 mm or more before they can be recognized as separate points.

The sense of general light touch would be unaffected, as these impulses ascend in the anterior spinothalamic tracts.

Note that a spinal cord lesion so localized that it affects one sensory tract only is extremely rare; usually, several ascending and descending tracts are involved.

Somatic and Visceral Pain

Somatic pain has been considered extensively in this chapter. The sense organs for somatic pain are the naked nerve endings. The initial sharp pain is transmitted by fast-conducting fibers, and the more prolonged burning pain travels in the slow-conducting nerve fibers (see p. 143).

In the viscera, special receptors, chemoreceptors, baroreceptors, osmoreceptors, and stretch receptors are sensitive to a variety of stimuli, including ischemia, stretching, and chemical damage. Afferent fibers from the visceral receptors reach the central nervous system (CNS) via the sympathetic and parasympathetic parts of the autonomic nervous system. Once within the CNS, the pain impulses travel by the same ascending tracts as the somatic pain and ultimately reach the postcentral gyrus.

Visceral pain is poorly localized and often associated with salivation, nausea, vomiting, tachycardia, and sweating. Visceral pain may be referred from the organ involved to a distant area of the body (**referred pain**).

Treatment of Acute Pain

Drugs such as salicylates can be used to reduce the synthesis of prostaglandin, a substance that sensitizes free nerve endings to painful stimuli. Local anesthetics, such as procaine, can be used to block nerve conduction in peripheral nerves.

Narcotic analgesics, such as morphine and codeine, reduce the affective reaction to pain and act on the opiate receptor sites in the cells in the posterior gray column of the spinal cord as well as other cells in the analgesic system in the brain likely by inhibiting the release of glutamate, substance P, and other transmitters from the sensory nerve endings. To minimize the side effects of morphine given by systemic injection, the narcotic can be given by local injection directly into the posterior gray horn of the spinal cord or by injection indirectly into the CSF in the subarachnoid space. Long-term cancer pain has been treated successfully by the continuous infusion of morphine into the spinal cord.

Treatment of Chronic Pain

New techniques, such as acupuncture and electrical stimulation of the skin, are now being used with success. Relief of pain can be achieved by the use of placebos in a few patients. The anticipation of the relief of pain is thought to stimulate the release of endorphins, which inhibit the normal pain pathway.

Relief of Pain by Rhizotomy or Cordotomy

Surgical relief of pain has been used extensively in patients with terminal cancer. Posterior rhizotomy or division of the posterior root of a spinal nerve effectively severs the conduction of pain into the CNS. It is a relatively simple procedure, but, unfortunately, the operation deprives the patient of other sensations besides pain. Moreover, if the pain sensation is entering the spinal cord through more than one spinal nerve, it may be necessary to divide several posterior roots.

Thoracic cordotomy has been performed with success in patients with severe pain originating from the lower abdomen or pelvis. Essentially, the operation consists of dividing the lateral spinothalamic tracts by inserting a knife into the anterolateral quadrant of the

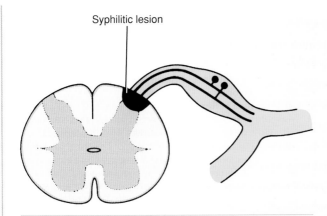

Syphilitic lesion

Figure 4-30 Site of a syphilitic lesion on the spinal cord.

spinal cord. Remember that the lateral spinothalamic fibers have originated in cells of the substantia gelatinosa in the opposite posterior gray column and that they cross the spinal cord obliquely and reach their tract in the white column three or four segments higher than their posterior root of entry. Cervical cordotomy has been performed successfully in patients with intractable pain in the neck or thorax.

Tabes Dorsalis

Tabes dorsalis is caused by syphilis. The organism causes a selective destruction of nerve fibers at the point of entrance of the posterior root into the spinal cord, especially in the lower thoracic and lumbosacral regions (Fig. 4-30). The following symptoms and signs may be present: (1) stabbing pains in the lower limbs, which may be very severe; (2) paresthesia, with numbness in the lower limbs; (3) hypersensitivity of skin to touch, heat, and cold; (4) loss of sensation in the skin of parts of the trunk and lower limbs and loss of awareness that the urinary bladder is full; (5) loss of appreciation of posture or passive movements of the limbs, especially the legs; (6) loss of deep pain sensation, such as when the muscles are forcibly compressed or when the Achilles tendon is compressed between the finger and thumb; (7) loss of pain sensation in the skin in certain areas of the body, such as the side of the nose or the medial border of the forearm, the thoracic wall between the nipples, or the lateral border of the leg; (8) ataxia of the lower limbs as the result of loss of proprioceptive sensibility (the unsteadiness in gait is compensated to some extent by vision; however, in the dark or if the eyes are closed, the ataxia becomes worse and the person may fall); (9) hypotonia as the result of loss of proprioceptive information that arises from the muscles and joints; and (10) loss of tendon reflexes, owing to degeneration of the afferent fiber component of the reflex arc (the knee and ankle tendon jerks are lost early in the disease).

Muscle Activity

Muscle tone is a state of continuous partial contraction of a muscle and is dependent on the integrity of a monosynaptic reflex arc (see description on p. 160). The receptor organs are the muscle spindles. The afferent neuron enters the spinal cord through the posterior root and synapses with the effector neuron or lower motor neuron in the anterior gray column. The lower motor neuron supplies the muscle fibers by traveling through the anterior roots, the spinal nerves, and peripheral nerves.

Muscle Tone

Muscle tone is abolished if any part of that simple reflex arc is destroyed. An atonic muscle feels soft and flabby and atrophies rapidly. Normal muscle tone exhibits a certain resilience or elasticity, and, when a muscle is passively stretched by moving a joint, a certain degree of resistance is felt. Normal muscle tone depends on the integrity of the monosynaptic reflex arc described above and the control superimposed on it by impulses received through the descending tracts from supraspinal levels. Note that muscle spindles are excitatory to muscle tone, whereas neurotendinous receptors are inhibitory to muscle tone.

Voluntary Movement

Voluntary movement is initiated by the individual. A series of different muscles are made to contract for the purpose of reaching a goal. This would suggest that the descending tracts that influence the activity of the lower motor neurons are driven by information received by the sensory systems, the eyes, the ears, and the muscles themselves and are affected further by past afferent information that has been stored in the memory. Moreover, the whole process may be colored by past and present emotional input. The limbic structures appear to play a role in emotion, motivation, and memory and may influence the initiation process of voluntary movement by their projections to the cerebral cortex.

The descending pathways from the cerebral cortex and brainstem, that is, the upper motor neurons, influence the activity of the lower motor neurons either directly or through internuncial neurons. Most of the tracts originating in the brainstem that descend to the spinal cord also are receiving input from the cerebral cortex.

The corticospinal tracts are believed to control the prime mover muscles, especially those responsible for the highly skilled movements of the distal parts of the limbs. The other supraspinal descending tracts play a major role in the simple basic voluntary movements and, in addition, adjust muscle tone so that easy and rapid movements of the joints can take place.

Interestingly, the basal ganglia and cerebellum do not give rise directly to descending tracts that influence the activities of the lower motor neuron, yet these parts of the nervous system greatly influence voluntary movements. This influence is accomplished indirectly by fibers that project to the cerebral cortex and brainstem nuclei, which are the sites of origin of the descending tracts.

Pyramidal and Extrapyramidal Tracts

The term **pyramidal tract** is used commonly by clinicians and refers specifically to the corticospinal tracts. The term came into common usage when it was learned that the corticospinal fibers become concentrated on the anterior part of the medulla oblongata in an area referred to as the **pyramids**.

The term **extrapyramidal tracts** refers to all the descending tracts other than the corticospinal tracts.

Upper Motor Neuron Lesions

Damage to descending tracts produces a variety of clinical signs, depending on the specific location.

Corticospinal Tract (Pyramidal Tract) Lesions

Lesions restricted to the corticospinal tracts produce the following clinical signs:

1. The **Babinski sign** is present. The great toe becomes dorsally flexed, and the other toes fan outward in response to scratching the skin along the lateral aspect of the sole of the foot. The normal response is plantar flexion of all the toes. Remember that the Babinski sign is normally present during the first year of life because the corticospinal tract is not myelinated until the end of the first year of life.
2. The explanation for the Babinski sign is thought to be that, normally, the corticospinal tracts produce plantar flexion of the toes in response to sensory stimulation of the skin of the sole. When the corticospinal tracts are nonfunctional, the influence of the other descending tracts on the toes becomes apparent, and a kind of withdrawal reflex takes place in response to stimulation of the sole, with the great toe being dorsally flexed and the other toes fanning out.
3. The **superficial abdominal reflexes** are absent. The abdominal muscles fail to contract when the skin of the abdomen is scratched. This reflex is dependent on the integrity of the corticospinal tracts, which exert a tonic excitatory influence on the internuncial neurons.
4. The **cremasteric reflex** is absent. The cremaster muscle fails to contract when the skin on the medial side of the thigh is stroked. This reflex arc passes through the first lumbar segment of the spinal cord. This reflex is dependent on the integrity of the corticospinal tracts, which exert a tonic excitatory influence on the internuncial neurons.
5. **Fine-skilled voluntary movements are lost.** This occurs especially at the distal end of the limbs.

Lesions of Other Descending Tracts (Extrapyramidal Tracts)

The following clinical signs are present in lesions restricted to the other descending tracts:

1. **Severe paralysis** with little or no muscle atrophy (except secondary to disuse).
2. **Spasticity** or **hypertonicity** of the muscles. The lower limb is maintained in extension, and the upper limb is maintained in flexion.
3. **Exaggerated deep muscle reflexes** and clonus may be present in the flexors of the fingers, the quadriceps femoris, and the calf muscles.
4. **Clasp-knife reaction.** When passive movement of a joint is attempted, muscle spasticity produces resistance. The muscles, on stretching, suddenly give way due to neurotendinous organ-mediated inhibition.

In clinical practice, organic lesions restricted only to the pyramidal tracts or only to the extrapyramidal tracts are rare. Usually, both sets of tracts are affected to a variable extent, producing both groups of clinical signs. As the pyramidal tracts normally tend to increase muscle tone and the extrapyramidal tracts inhibit muscle tone, the balance between these opposing effects will be altered, producing different degrees of muscle tone.

Lower Motor Neuron Lesions

Trauma, infection (poliomyelitis), vascular disorders, degenerative diseases, and neoplasms may all produce a lesion of the lower motor neuron by destroying the cell body in the anterior gray column or its axon in the anterior root or spinal nerve. The following clinical signs are present with lower motor neuron lesions:

1. Muscles exhibit **flaccid paralysis**.
2. Muscles **atrophy**.
3. Muscles **lose reflexes**.
4. **Muscular fasciculation** (muscle twitching) is seen only with slow destruction of the lower motor neuron cell.
5. **Muscular contracture** (shortening of the paralyzed muscles) occurs more often in the antagonist muscles whose action is no longer opposed by the paralyzed muscles.
6. Normally innervated muscles respond to stimulation by the application of faradic (interrupted) current, and the contraction continues as long as the current is passing. Galvanic or direct current causes contraction only when the current is turned on or turned off. When the lower motor neuron is cut, a muscle will no longer respond to interrupted electrical stimulation 7 days after nerve section, although it still will respond to direct current. After 10 days, the response to direct current also ceases. This change in muscle response to electrical stimulation is known as the **reaction of degeneration**.

Types of Paralysis

Hemiplegia is a paralysis of one side of the body and includes the upper limb, one side of the trunk, and the lower limb.

Monoplegia is paralysis of one limb only.

Diplegia is paralysis of two corresponding limbs (i.e., arms or legs).

Paraplegia is paralysis of the two lower limbs.

Quadriplegia is paralysis of all four limbs.

Relationship of Muscular Signs and Symptoms to Nervous System Lesions

The type of abnormal muscle tone resulting from nervous system damage will depend on the location of the lesion.

Hypotonia

Hypotonia exists when the muscle tone is diminished or absent. It occurs when any part of the monosynaptic stretch reflex arc is interrupted. It also occurs in cerebellar disease as the result of diminished influence on the γ motor neurons from the cerebellum.

Hypertonia

Hypertonia (spasticity, rigidity) exists when the muscle tone is increased. It occurs when lesions exist that involve supraspinal centers or their descending tracts but *not* the corticospinal tract. It also may occur at the local spinal segmental level and be produced by local excitation of the stretch reflex by sensory irritation (e.g., spasm of back muscles secondary to prolapsed intervertebral disc, spasm of abdominal muscles secondary to peritonitis).

Tremors

Tremors are rhythmic involuntary movements that result from the contraction of opposing muscle groups. These may be slow, as in **parkinsonism,** or fast, as in toxic tremors from thyrotoxicosis. They may occur at rest, as in parkinsonism, or with action, the so-called intention tremor, as seen in cerebellar disease.

Spasms

Spasms are sudden, involuntary contractions of large groups of muscles. Examples of spasms are seen in paraplegia and are due to lesions involving the descending tracts but not the corticospinal tract.

Athetosis

Athetosis are continuous, slow, involuntary, dysrhythmic movements that are always the same in the same patient and disappear during sleep. They impede voluntary movement. Athetosis occurs with lesions of the corpus striatum.

Chorea

Chorea consists of a series of continuous, rapid, involuntary, jerky, coarse, purposeless movements, which may occur during sleep. Chorea occurs with lesions of the corpus striatum.

Dystonia

Dystonia consists of frequent, maintained contractions of hypertonic muscles, leading to bizarre postures. It occurs with lesions of the lentiform nucleus.

Myoclonus

Myoclonus is a sudden contraction of an isolated muscle or part of a muscle. It occurs irregularly and commonly involves a muscle of a limb. It may be present with diseases that involve the reticular formation and the cerebellum. Normal myoclonic jerks sometimes occur in individuals as they are falling asleep and are believed to be due to a sudden temporary reactivation of the reticular formation.

Hemiballismus

Hemiballismus is a rare form of involuntary movement confined to one side of the body. It usually involves the proximal extremity musculature, and the limb involved is made to fly about in all directions. The lesion responsible occurs in the opposite subthalamic nucleus.

Acute Spinal Cord Injury

The incidence of acute spinal cord injuries in the United States is about 10,000 per year. The injury is catastrophic, because little or no regeneration of the severed nerve tracts takes place (see p. 71) and the individual is permanently disabled. Treatment has been restricted to anatomical realignment and stabilization of the vertebral column or decompression of the spinal cord. During the recovery process, the patient goes through intensive rehabilitation to optimize remaining neurologic function. Apart from improved management of medical complications, very little new therapy has been successful despite an enormous amount of research into the problem of neuronal regeneration in the spinal cord. Recently, the use of certain drugs (GM$_1$ ganglioside and methylprednisolone) administered to the patient soon after injury has resulted in some improvement in the neurologic deficit. Animal experiments appear to indicate that these drugs enhance the functional recovery of damaged neurons.

Chronic Compression of the Spinal Cord

If acute spinal cord injury is excluded, the causes of compression may be divided into extradural and intradural, which is further divided into those that arise outside the spinal cord (extramedullary) and those that arise within the cord (intramedullary).

Extradural causes include herniation of an intervertebral disc, infection of the vertebrae with tuberculosis, and primary and secondary tumors of the vertebra; leukemic deposits and extradural abscesses may also compress the spinal cord. The two common extramedullary tumors are meningiomas and nerve fibromas. Intramedullary causes include primary tumors of the spinal cord, such as gliomas.

The clinical signs and symptoms are produced by an interference with the normal anatomical and physiologic functions of the spinal cord. Pressure on the spinal arteries causes ischemia of the spinal cord with degeneration of nerve cells and their fibers. Pressure on the spinal veins causes edema of the spinal cord with interference in the function of the neurons. Finally, direct pressure on the white and gray matter of the spinal cord and the spinal nerve roots interferes with nerve conduction. At the same time, CSF circulation is obstructed, and the composition of the fluid changes below the level of obstruction.

Clinical Signs

One of the earliest signs is pain, which may be local pain in the vertebra involved or pain radiating along the distribution of one or more spinal nerve roots. The pain is made worse by coughing or sneezing and is usually worse at night, when the patient is recumbent.

Interference with motor function occurs early. Involvement of the anterior gray column motor cells at the level of the lesion results in partial or complete paralysis of muscles, with loss of tone and muscle wasting. The early involvement of the corticospinal and other descending tracts produces muscular weakness, increased muscle tone (spasticity), increased tendon reflexes below the level of the lesion, and an extensor plantar response. The degree of sensory loss will depend on the nerve tracts involved. A lesion of the posterior white columns of the spinal cord will cause loss of muscle joint sense (proprioception), vibration sense, and tactile discrimination below the level of the lesion on the same side. Involvement of the lateral spinal thalamic tracts will cause loss of pain and heat and cold sensations on the opposite side of the body below the level of the lesion. A more detailed discussion of the symptoms and signs following injury to the ascending and descending tracts in the spinal cord is given on pages 163 and 166.

Because many spinal tumors are benign and can be successfully removed (provided that irreversible damage to the spinal cord has not occurred as a result of compression of the blood supply), an early accurate diagnosis is essential. The following investigations should be performed: (1) radiography of the vertebral column, including computed tomography (CT) and magnetic resonance imaging (MRI); (2) spinal tap; and (3) myelography when determining the diagnosis is difficult.

Clinical Syndromes Affecting the Spinal Cord

Myelopathy stems from a number of causes, including trauma, developmental abnormality, infection, autoimmune destruction, and genetic disease.

Spinal Shock Syndrome

Spinal shock syndrome is a clinical condition that follows acute severe damage to the spinal cord. All cord functions below the level of the lesion become depressed or lost, and sensory impairment and flaccid paralysis occur. The segmental spinal reflexes are depressed due to the removal of influences from the higher centers that are mediated through the corticospinal, reticulospinal, tectospinal, rubrospinal, and vestibulospinal tracts. Spinal shock, especially when the lesion is at a high level of the cord, may also cause severe hypotension from loss of sympathetic vasomotor tone.

In most patients, the shock persists for less than 24 hours, whereas in others, it may persist for as long as 1 to 4 weeks. As the shock diminishes, the neurons regain their excitability, and the effects of the upper motor neuron loss on the segments of the cord below the lesion, for example, spasticity and exaggerated reflexes, appear.

The presence of spinal shock can be determined by testing for anal sphincter reflex activity. The reflex can be initiated by placing a gloved finger in the anal canal and stimulating the anal sphincter to contract by squeezing the glans penis or clitoris or gently tugging on an inserted Foley catheter. An absent anal reflex indicates spinal shock. A cord lesion involving the sacral segments of the cord would nullify this test, insofar as the neurons giving rise to the inferior hemorrhoidal nerve to the anal sphincter (S2–S4) would be nonfunctioning.

Destructive Spinal Cord Syndromes

When neurologic impairment is identified following the disappearance of spinal shock, it can often be categorized into one of the following syndromes: (1) complete cord transection syndrome, (2) anterior cord syndrome, (3) central cord syndrome, or (4) Brown-Séquard syndrome or hemisection of the cord. Clinical findings often indicate a combination of lower motor neuron injury (at the level of destruction of the cord) and upper motor neuron injury (for those segments below the level of destruction).

COMPLETE CORD TRANSECTION SYNDROME

Complete cord transection syndrome (Fig. 4-31) results in complete loss of all sensibility and voluntary movement below the level of the lesion. It can be caused by fracture dislocation of the vertebral column, by a bullet or stab wound, or by an expanding tumor. The following characteristic clinical features will be seen *after* the period of spinal shock has ended:

1. Bilateral lower motor neuron paralysis and muscular atrophy in the segment of the lesion results from damage to the neurons in the anterior gray columns (i.e., lower motor neuron) and possibly from damage to the nerve roots of the same segment.
2. In bilateral spastic paralysis below the level of the lesion, bilateral Babinski sign is present, and, depending on the level of the segment of the spinal cord damaged, bilateral loss of the superficial abdominal and cremaster reflexes occurs. All these signs are caused by an interruption of the corticospinal tracts on both sides of the cord. The bilateral spastic paralysis is produced by the cutting of the descending tracts other than the corticospinal tracts.
3. In bilateral loss of all sensations below the level of the lesion, loss of tactile discrimination and vibratory and proprioceptive sensations is due to bilateral destruction of the ascending tracts in the posterior white columns. The loss of pain, temperature, and light touch sensations is caused by section of the lateral and anterior spinothalamic tracts on both sides. Because these tracts cross obliquely, the loss of thermal and light touch sensations occurs two or three segments below the lesion distally.

4. Bladder and bowel functions are no longer under voluntary control, because all the descending autonomic fibers have been destroyed.

With a complete fracture dislocation at the L2–L3 vertebral level (i.e., a level below the lower end of the cord in the adult), no cord injury occurs. Neural damage is confined to the cauda equina, and lower motor neuron, autonomic, and sensory fibers are involved.

ANTERIOR CORD SYNDROME

Anterior cord syndrome (Fig. 4-31) can be caused by cord contusion during vertebral fracture or dislocation, from injury to the anterior spinal artery or its feeder arteries with resultant ischemia of the cord, or by a herniated intervertebral disc. The following characteristic clinical features are seen *after* the period of spinal shock has ended:

1. Bilateral lower motor neuron paralysis in the segment of the lesion and muscular atrophy is caused by damage to the neurons in the anterior gray columns (i.e., lower motor neuron) and possibly by damage to the anterior nerve roots of the same segment.
2. In bilateral spastic paralysis below the level of the lesion, the extent depends on the size of the injured area of the cord. The bilateral paralysis is caused by the interruption of the anterior corticospinal tracts on both sides of the cord. The spasticity is produced by the interruption of tracts other than the corticospinal tracts.
3. Bilateral loss of pain, temperature, and light touch sensations below the level of the lesion are caused by interruption of the anterior and lateral spinothalamic tracts on both sides.
4. Tactile discrimination and vibratory and proprioceptive sensations are preserved because the posterior white columns on both sides are undamaged.

CENTRAL CORD SYNDROME

Central cord syndrome is most often caused by hyperextension of the cervical region of the spine (Fig. 4-31). The cord is pressed on anteriorly by the vertebral bodies and posteriorly by the bulging of the ligamentum flavum, causing damage to the central region of the spinal cord. Radiographs of these injuries often appear normal because no fracture or dislocation has occurred. The following characteristic clinical features are seen *after* the period of spinal shock has ended:

1. Bilateral lower motor neuron paralysis in the segment of the lesion and muscular atrophy is caused by damage to the neurons in the anterior gray columns (i.e., lower motor neuron) and possibly by damage to the nerve roots of the same segment.
2. In bilateral spastic paralysis below the level of the lesion with characteristic sacral "sparing," lower limb fibers are affected less than upper limb fibers because the descending fibers in the lateral corticospinal tracts are laminated, with the upper limb fibers located medially and the lower limb fibers located laterally (Fig. 4-29).
3. In bilateral loss of pain, temperature, light touch, and pressure sensations below the level of the lesion with characteristic sacral "sparing," because the ascending fibers in the lateral and anterior spinothalamic tracts are also laminated, with the upper limb fibers located medially and the lower limb fibers located laterally, the upper limb fibers are more susceptible to damage than the lower limb fibers.

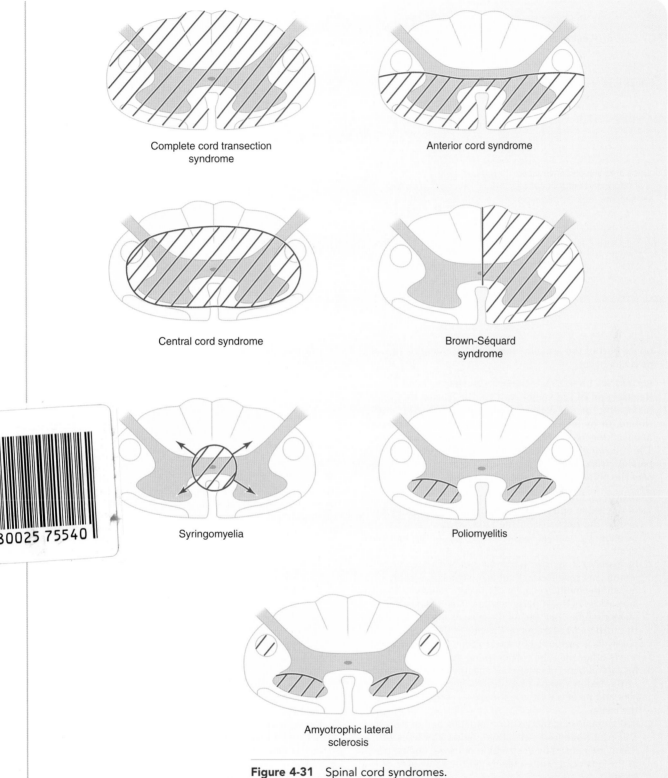

Complete cord transection
syndrome

Anterior cord syndrome

Central cord syndrome

Brown-Séquard
syndrome

Syringomyelia

Poliomyelitis

Amyotrophic lateral
sclerosis

Figure 4-31 Spinal cord syndromes.

Thus, the clinical picture of a patient with a history of a hyperextension injury of the neck, presenting with motor and sensory tract injuries involving principally the upper limb, would strongly suggest central cord syndrome. The sparing of the lower part of the body may be evidenced

by (1) the presence of perianal sensation, (2) good anal sphincter tone, and (3) the ability to move the toes slightly. In patients whose damage is caused by edema of the spinal cord alone, the prognosis is often very good. Mild central cord syndrome that consists only of paresthesias of the

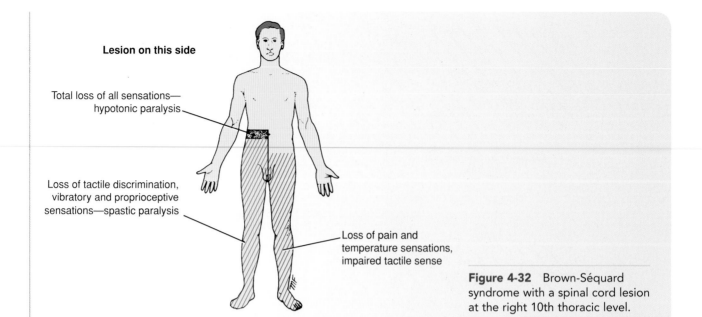

Lesion on this side

Total loss of all sensations—
hypotonic paralysis

Loss of tactile discrimination,
vibratory and proprioceptive
sensations—spastic paralysis

Loss of pain and
temperature sensations,
impaired tactile sense

Figure 4-32 Brown-Séquard syndrome with a spinal cord lesion at the right 10th thoracic level.

upper part of the arm and some mild arm and hand weakness can occur.

BROWN-SÉQUARD SYNDROME (CORD HEMISECTION)

Hemisection of the spinal cord can be caused by fracture dislocation of the vertebral column, by a bullet or stab wound, or by an expanding tumor (Fig. 4-31). Incomplete hemisection is common; complete hemisection is rare. The following characteristic clinical features are seen in patients with complete hemisection of the cord (Fig. 4-32) *after* the period of spinal shock has ended:

1. Ipsilateral lower motor neuron paralysis in the segment of the lesion and muscular atrophy are caused by damage to the neurons on the anterior gray column and possibly by damage to the nerve roots of the same segment.
2. In ipsilateral spastic paralysis below the level of the lesion, an ipsilateral Babinski sign is present, and, depending on the segment of the cord damaged, an ipsilateral loss of the superficial abdominal reflexes and cremasteric reflex occurs. All these signs are due to loss of the corticospinal tracts on the side of the lesion. Spastic paralysis is produced by interruption of the descending tracts other than the corticospinal tracts.
3. Ipsilateral band of cutaneous anesthesia in the segment of the lesion results from destruction of the posterior root and its entrance into the spinal cord at the level of the lesion.
4. Ipsilateral loss of tactile discrimination and of vibratory and proprioceptive sensations below the level of the lesion are caused by destruction of the ascending tracts in the posterior white column on the same side of the lesion.
5. Contralateral loss of pain and temperature sensations below the level of the lesion is due to destruction of the crossed lateral spinothalamic tracts on the same side of the lesion. Because the tracts cross obliquely, the sensory loss occurs two or three segments below the lesion distally.
6. Contralateral but not complete loss of tactile sensation below the level of the lesion condition is caused

by destruction of the crossed anterior spinothalamic tracts on the side of the lesion. Here, again, because the tracts cross obliquely, the sensory impairment occurs two or three segments below the level of the lesion distally. The contralateral loss of tactile sense is incomplete because discriminative touch traveling in the ascending tracts in the contralateral posterior white column remains intact.

Syringomyelia

Syringomyelia, which is due to a developmental abnormality in the formation of the central canal, most often affects the brainstem and cervical region of the spinal cord. At the site of the lesion, cavitation and gliosis in the central region of the neuroaxis occurs (Fig. 4-33). The following characteristic signs and symptoms are found:

1. Pain and temperature sensations are lost in dermatomes on both sides of the body related to the affected segments of the cord. This loss commonly has a shawllike distribution caused by the interruption of the lateral spinothalamic tracts as they cross the midline in the anterior gray and white commissures. The patient commonly complains of accidental burning injuries to the fingers.
2. Tactile discrimination, vibratory sense, and proprioceptive sense are normal because the ascending tracts in the posterior white column are unaffected.
3. Lower motor neuron weakness is present in the small muscles of the hand. It may be bilateral, or one hand may suffer before the other. As the lesion expands in the lower cervical and upper thoracic region, it destroys the anterior horn cells of these segments. Later, the other muscles of the arm and shoulder girdles undergo atrophy.
4. Bilateral spastic paralysis of both legs may occur, with exaggerated deep tendon reflexes and the presence of a positive Babinski response. These signs are produced by the further expansion of the lesion laterally into the white column to involve the descending tracts.

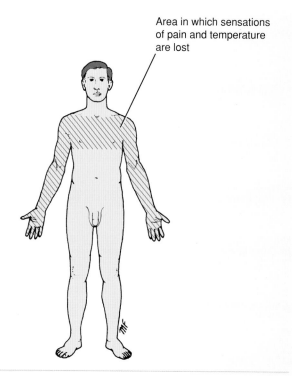

Area in which sensations of pain and temperature are lost

Figure 4-33 Skin area in which the sensations of pain and temperature are lost in syringomyelia.

5. Horner syndrome may be present. This is caused by the interruption of the descending autonomic fibers in the reticulospinal tracts in the lateral white column by the expanding lesion.

Poliomyelitis

Poliomyelitis is an acute viral infection of the neurons of the anterior gray columns of the spinal cord (Fig. 4-31) and cranial nerve motor nuclei. Immunization has greatly reduced the incidence of poliomyelitis, which was once a feared disease. Paralysis and muscle wasting follow motor nerve cell death. Lower limb muscles are more often affected than those of the upper limb. In severe poliomyelitis, respiration may be threatened due to the paralysis spreading to the intercostal muscles and diaphragm. Muscles of the face, pharynx, larynx, and tongue may also be paralyzed. Improvement usually begins at the end of the first week as the edema in the affected area subsides, and function returns to the neurons that have not been destroyed.

Multiple Sclerosis

Multiple sclerosis is a common disease confined to the CNS, causing demyelination of the ascending and descending tracts. It is a disease of young adults, and the cause is unknown. Autoimmunity, infection, and heredity, alone or in combination, may play a role in its etiology. A breach in the integrity of the blood–brain barrier in an individual who is genetically predisposed to the disease may be responsible. This could result in the invasion of the brain and spinal cord by some infection allowing leukocytes to enter the normally immunologically protected CNS. Inflammation

and demyelination with loss of the myelin sheath results in the breakdown of the insulation around the axons, and the velocity of the action potentials is reduced and ultimately becomes blocked. Although myelin is relatively rich in lipid (70% to 80%), it also contains proteins that play a role in myelin compaction. Many of these proteins in the myelin of the CNS differ from those in the peripheral nervous system. Experimentally, basic myelin proteins injected into animals have been shown to produce a strong immune response, and CNS demyelination occurs. Mutations in the structure of myelin protein can possibly occur and be responsible for some inherited forms of demyelination. Also possible is that autoantigens develop in multiple sclerosis.

The course of multiple sclerosis is chronic with exacerbations and remissions. Because of the widespread involvement of different tracts at different levels of the neuroaxis, the signs and symptoms are multiple, but remissions do occur. Weakness of the limbs is the most common sign of the disease. Ataxia due to involvement of the tracts of the cerebellum may occur, but spastic paralysis may also be present.

Recent research has suggested that the remissions in multiple sclerosis may in part be explained by the remodeling of the demyelinated axonal plasma membrane so that it acquires a higher than normal number of sodium channels, which permit conduction of action potentials despite the loss of myelin.

Patients who have the progressive form of the disease without remissions have substantial damage to the axons as well as the myelin. This would suggest that multiple sclerosis is not just a demyelinating disease but one with axonal pathology also.

Amyotrophic Lateral Sclerosis

Amyotrophic lateral sclerosis (Lou Gehrig disease) is a disease confined to the corticospinal tracts and the motor neurons of the anterior gray columns of the spinal cord (Fig. 4-31). It is rarely familial and is inherited in about 10% of patients. Amyotrophic lateral sclerosis is a chronic progressive disease of unknown etiology. Typically, it occurs in late middle age and is inevitably fatal in 2 to 6 years. The lower motor neuron signs of progressive muscular atrophy, paresis, and fasciculations are superimposed on the signs and symptoms of upper motor neuron disease with paresis, spasticity, and Babinski response. The motor nuclei of some cranial nerves may also be involved.

Parkinson Disease

Parkinson disease is associated with neuronal degeneration in the substantia nigra and, to a lesser extent, in the globus pallidus, putamen, and caudate nucleus. The degeneration of the inhibitory nigrostriate fibers results in a reduction in the release of the neurotransmitter dopamine within the corpus striatum. This leads to hypersensitivity of the dopamine receptors in the postsynaptic neurons in the corpus striatum, which become overactive. The characteristic signs of the disease include tremor and cogwheel rigidity (hyperkinetic activity) and difficulty initiating voluntary movements, which are slow (hypokinetic activity).

Pernicious Anemia

Pernicious anemia, a form of megaloblastic anemia, is caused by vitamin B$_{12}$ deficiency. The disease may produce extensive damage to the tracts in the posterior and lateral white columns of the spinal cord as well as peripheral nerve degeneration. Widespread sensory and motor losses may be present due to involvement of the ascending and descending tracts of the spinal cord.

Vertebral Column Radiography

The views commonly used in radiography are anteroposterior, lateral, and oblique. Vertebral destruction due to tuberculosis or primary or secondary tumors of the vertebrae or fractures due to trauma usually can be revealed by radiographic examination. Erosion of the pedicles by a tumor within the intervertebral foramina may be seen. Narrowing of the space between the vertebral bodies with bony spurs because of osteoarthritic changes in adjacent vertebral bodies can also be seen.

Computed Tomography and Magnetic Resonance Imaging

CT scans of the vertebrae and joints can be obtained (Fig. 4-34). A protrusion of an intervertebral disc can be identified, and the presence of narrowing of the vertebral canal (**spinal stenosis**) can be diagnosed.

Sagittal MRI is increasingly being used to replace CT and myelography. The parts of a vertebra, the intervertebral disc, the posterior longitudinal ligament, and meningeal sac (**thecal sac**) can easily be identified (Fig. 4-35).

Myelography

The subarachnoid space can be studied radiographically by the injection of a contrast medium into the subarachnoid space by spinal tap. Iodized oil has been used with success. This technique is referred to as **myelography** (Figs. 4-36 and 4-37).

If the patient is sitting in the upright position, the oil sinks to the lower limit of the subarachnoid space at the level of the lower border of the second sacral vertebra. By placing the patient on a tilting table, the oil can be made to gravitate gradually to higher levels of the vertebral column.

A normal myelogram will show pointed lateral projections at regular intervals at the intervertebral space levels because the opaque medium fills the lateral extensions of the subarachnoid space around each spinal nerve. The presence of a tumor or a prolapsed intervertebral disc may obstruct the movement of the oil from one region to another when the patient is tilted.

With the recent technologic advances in CT scans and MRIs, intrusive procedures such as myelography are usually not required to make a diagnosis.

Figure 4-34 Horizontal (axial) CT scan of the fourth lumbar vertebra.

Spinal cord contained within the meninges

Epidural fat

Body of fourth lumbar vertebra

Spinous process of fourth lumbar vertebra

Prolapsed intervertebral discs

Posterior longitudinal ligament

L5-S1 intervertebral disc

First sacral vertebra

Figure 4-35 Sagittal MRI of the lumbosacral part of the vertebral column showing several prolapsed intervertebral discs. (*Courtesy Dr. Pait.*)

Figure 4-36 Posteroanterior myelogram of the cervical region of a 22-year-old woman.

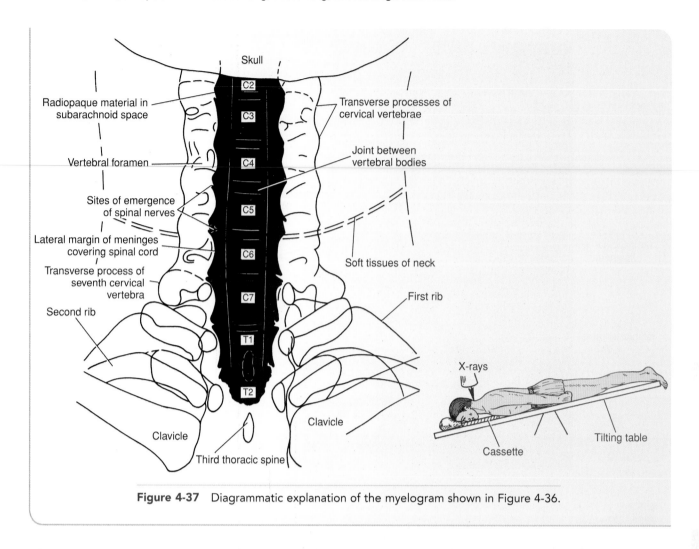

Figure 4-37 Diagrammatic explanation of the myelogram shown in Figure 4-36.

Key Concepts

Vertebral Column

- The vertebral column is composed of 33 vertebrae—7 cervical, 12 thoracic, 5 lumbar, 5 sacral (fused), and 4 coccygeal (fused).
- Because it is segmented and made up of vertebrae, joints, and intervertebral discs, it is a flexible structure.
- The vertebral arch encloses a space called the vertebral foramen. The collective vertebral foramina form the vertebral canal—the housing of the spinal cord.

Spinal Cord

- Roughly cylindrical, the spinal cord extends from the rostral end of the medulla oblongata to the eventual tapering of the cord, called the conus medullaris.

- Within the vertebral canal, the spinal cord is covered by three layers of meninges, the dura mater, arachnoid mater, and pia mater. Between the latter two, is the subarachnoid space, which is filled with CSF.
- The spinal cord is composed of an inner core of gray matter surrounded by an outer covering of white matter.
- On cross section, the gray matter is seen as an H-shaped pillar with anterior and posterior columns or horns. A lateral gray column is present in thoracic and upper lumbar segments.
- Most nerve cells in the anterior columns are large, alpha and multipolar, and their axons pass out in the anterior roots of the spinal nerves.
- The substantia gelatinosa of the posterior gray column is largely composed of neurons receiving

afferent fibers concerned with pain, temperature, and touch from the posterior root.

- The nucleus proprius is situated anterior to the substantia gelatinosa throughout the spinal cord and communicates information regarding the senses of proprioception, two-point discrimination, and vibration with the posterior white columns.
- The lateral gray column extends from T1 to L2(3) segments and contains cells that give rise to preganglionic sympathetic fibers.
- The white matter of the spinal cord can be described as anterior, lateral, and posterior columns formed from multiple myelinated nerve bundles, or tracts.

Ascending Tracts

- Pain and temperature sensations ascend in the lateral spinothalamic tract; light touch and pressure ascend in the anterior spinothalamic tract. Together, these are also referred to as the anterolateral system.
- First-order axons entering the spinal cord with pain and temperature information, synapse on second-order neurons of the substantia gelatinosa, cross obliquely to the opposite side through the anterior gray and white commissure, and ascend in the contralateral white column as the lateral spinothalamic tract. The anterior spinothalamic ascends in the contralateral anterior white column.
- As the anterolateral system tracts ascend through the medulla oblongata and pons, they form the spinal lemniscus and eventually synapse on third-order neurons in the ventral posterolateral nucleus of the thalamus.
- First-order axons carrying discriminative touch and vibration sensations enter the dorsal horn and continue traveling upward in the posterior white column as the fasciculus gracilis (sacral, lumbar, and lower thoracic spinal nerves) and

fasciculus cuneatus (thoracic and cervical spinal nerves). Fibers of these fasciculi synapse on the second-order neurons of the ipsilateral nuclei gracilis and cuneatus in the medulla oblongata, respectively.

- The axons of the second-order neurons cross anteromedially as the internal arcuate fibers and ascend a compact bundle, called the medial lemniscus, until synapsing with third-order neurons in the ventral posterolateral nucleus of the thalamus.

Descending Tracts

- Motor neurons situated in the anterior gray columns of the spinal cord send axons through the anterior roots to the spinal nerves and are often referred to as lower motor neurons. This is the final pathway to the muscles.
- Corticospinal tracts are pathways concerned with voluntary movement of muscles. Axons of pyramidal cells in the motor cortex descend through the internal capsule, form the cerebral peduncles of the midbrain, then separates into smaller bundles throughout the pons. As the axons approach the medulla, they coalesce, forming the pyramid of the rostral medulla oblongata and cross caudal medulla as the decussation of the pyramids. The axons continue as the lateral corticospinal tract of the spinal cord until they synapse on the lower motor neurons of the anterior horns.
- Reticulospinal tracts may facilitate or inhibit voluntary movements or reflex activity.
- Tectospinal tracts are concerned with reflex postural movements in response to visual stimuli while vestibulospinal tracts are concerned with postural activity associated with balance.
- The rubrospinal tract facilitates the activity of flexor muscles and inhibits the activity of extensor muscles.

❓ Clinical Problem Solving

1. A 53-year-old widower is admitted to the hospital complaining of a burning pain over his right shoulder region and the upper part of his right arm. The pain started 3 weeks previously and, since that time, has progressively worsened. The pain is accentuated when the patient moves his neck or coughs. Two years previously, he had been treated for osteoarthritis of his vertebral column. The patient states that he had been a football player at college and continued to take an active part in the game until he was 42 years old. Physical examination reveals weakness, wasting, and fasciculation of the right deltoid and biceps brachii muscles. The right biceps tendon reflex is absent. Radiologic examination reveals extensive spur formation on the bodies of the fourth, fifth,

and sixth cervical vertebrae. The patient demonstrates hyperesthesia and partial analgesia in the skin over the lower part of the right deltoid and down the lateral side of the arm. Using your knowledge of neuroanatomy, make the diagnosis. How is the pain produced? Why is the pain made worse by coughing?

2. A 66-year-old woman is admitted to the hospital because of her increasing difficulty with walking. Two weeks before admission, she had been able to walk with the help of a stick. Since that time, walking has become increasingly difficult, and for the past 2 days, she cannot walk at all. She has complete control of micturition and defecation. On examination, the handgrip is weak on both sides, but power is normal in the proximal segments of the upper extremities. The tendon reflexes of the upper limbs and the sensory functions are normal. Both lower limbs show muscular weakness with increased muscle tone, especially on the left side. The knee jerks and ankle jerks (tendon reflexes) in both lower limbs are grossly exaggerated, and extensor plantar responses are seen bilaterally. The patient has a loss of sensation of pain below the fifth thoracic dermatome on both sides of the body. Postural sense is impaired in both great toes, and vibration sense is absent below the fifth thoracic segmental level. Radiologic examination, including an MRI, of the vertebral column shows nothing abnormal. A myelogram in the lumbar region reveals a complete block at the lower border of the fourth thoracic vertebra. Using your knowledge of neuroanatomy, suggest a possible diagnosis. How would you treat this patient? Name the tracts in the spinal cord that are responsible for pain sensation conduction. What is the position of these tracts in the spinal cord? Name the tracts responsible for the conduction of postural sense and vibration sense from the spinal cord to the brain. Why did the patient have increasing difficulty in walking? Why were the tendon reflexes in the lower limbs exaggerated, and why did the patient exhibit bilateral extensor plantar responses?

3. A 20-year-old male student celebrates the passing of an examination by drinking several beers at a party. On the way home, he drives his car head-on into a bridge abutment. On examination in the emergency department, he is found to have a fracture dislocation of the ninth thoracic vertebra with signs and symptoms of severe damage to the spinal cord. On physical examination, he has an upper motor neuron paralysis of the left leg. He also has loss of muscle joint sense of the left leg. On testing of cutaneous sensibility, he has a band of cutaneous hyperesthesia extending around the abdominal wall on the left side at the level of the umbilicus. Just below this, he has a narrow band of anesthesia and analgesia. On the right side, total analgesia, thermoanesthesia, and partial loss of tactile sense of the skin of the abdominal wall below the level of the umbilicus and involving the whole of the right leg are present. Using your knowledge of neuroanatomy, state the level at which the spinal cord was damaged. Was the spinal cord completely sectioned? If not, on which side did the hemisection occur? Explain the sensory losses found on examination in this patient.

4. A 35-year-old woman is admitted to the hospital for investigation. She has symptoms of analgesia and thermoanesthesia on the medial side of the left hand that persist for 6 months. Three weeks prior to her admittance, she had severely burned the little finger of her left hand on a hot stove and was unaware that the burn had occurred until she smelled the burning skin. On physical examination, she is found to have considerably reduced pain and temperature sense involving the eighth cervical and first thoracic dermatomes of the left hand. However, her sense of tactile discrimination is perfectly normal in these areas. Examination of the right arm shows a similar but much less severe dissociated sensory loss involving the same areas. No further abnormal signs are discovered. Using your knowledge of neuroanatomy, state which tract or tracts were involved in this pathologic process. Name this disease.

5. A 60-year-old man walks into the neurology clinic, and the clinician pays particular attention to his gait. The patient raises his feet unnecessarily high and brings them to the ground in a stamping manner. While he is waiting for the clinician, he is seen to stand with his feet wide apart. On questioning, the patient says that he is finding it increasingly difficult to walk and is starting to use a stick, especially when he goes out for walks in the dark. The clinician asks the patient to stand with his toes and heels together and to close his eyes. The patient immediately starts to sway, and the nurse has to steady him to prevent him from falling. On further examination, the patient is found to have loss of muscle joint sense of both legs and is unable to detect any feeling of vibration when a vibrating tuning fork was placed on the medial malleolus of either leg. No other sensory losses are noted. Using your knowledge of neuroanatomy, name the ascending pathways that are involved, by disease, in this patient. Name a disease that could be responsible for these findings.

6. A 68-year-old man has an advanced inoperable carcinoma of the prostate with multiple metastases in the lumbar vertebrae and hip bones. Apart from the severe intractable pain, the patient is still able to enjoy life among his family. After a full discussion of the prognosis with the patient and his wife, the wife turned to the clinician and says, "Can't you do something to stop this terrible pain so that my husband can die happy?" What can a

clinician do to help a patient under these circumstances?

7. A third-year medical student attends a lecture on the effects of vertebral column trauma. The orthopedic surgeon describes very superficially the different neurologic deficits that may follow injury to the spinal cord. At the end of the lecture, the student says he does not understand what was meant by the term *spinal shock*. He cannot understand what the underlying mechanism for this condition is. He also asks the surgeon to explain what was meant by paraplegia in extension and paraplegia in flexion. Can the surgeon explain why one condition sometimes passes into the other? These are good questions. Can you answer them?

8. While examining a patient with right-sided hemiplegia caused by a cerebrovascular accident, the neurologist asks the student which clinical signs can be attributed to an interruption of the corticospinal tracts and which signs can be attributed to damage to other descending tracts. Using your knowledge of neuroanatomy, answer this question.

9. A large civilian aircraft is forced to abort its take-off because three tires have burst as the plane speeds along the runway. The pilot miraculously manages to halt the plane as it veers off the runway and comes to an abrupt halt in a ditch. All the passengers escape injury, but one of the flight attendants is admitted to the emergency department with suspected spinal cord injury. On questioning, the 25-year-old patient says that although she had her seatbelt fastened, she was thrown violently forward on impact. She says she cannot feel anything in either leg and cannot move her legs. On examination, complete motor and sensory loss is noted in both legs below the inguinal ligament as well as absence of all deep tendon reflexes of both legs. Twelve hours later, she is able to move the toes and ankle of her left lower limb, and she has a return of sensations to her right leg except for loss of tactile discrimination, vibratory sense, and proprioceptive sense. She has a band of complete anesthesia over her right inguinal ligament. Her left leg shows total analgesia, thermoanesthesia, and partial loss of tactile sense. Her right leg is totally paralyzed, and the muscles are spastic. A right-sided Babinski response is seen as well as right-sided ankle clonus. The right knee jerk is exaggerated.

Using your knowledge of neuroanatomy, explain the symptoms and signs found in this patient. Which vertebra was damaged?

10. Why is moving a patient with suspected vertebral column fracture or dislocation so dangerous?

11. An 18-year-old man is admitted to the hospital following a severe automobile accident. After a complete neurologic investigation, his family is told that he will be paralyzed from the waist down for the rest of his life. The neurologist outlines to the medical personnel the importance of preventing complications in these cases. The common complications are the following: (a) urinary infection, (b) bedsores, (c) nutritional deficiency, (d) muscular spasms, and (e) pain. Using your knowledge of neuroanatomy, explain the underlying reasons for these complications. How long after the accident would giving an accurate prognosis in this patient be possible?

12. A 67-year-old man is brought to the neurology clinic by his daughter because she notices that his right arm has a tremor. Apparently, this had started about 6 months previously and is becoming steadily worse. When questioned, the patient says he notices that the muscles of his limbs sometimes felt stiff, but he has attributed this to old age. While talking, the patient rarely smiles and then only with difficulty. He infrequently blinks his eyes. The patient tends to speak in a low, faint voice. When asked to walk, the patient has normal posture and gait, although he tends to hold his right arm flexed at the elbow joint. When he is sitting, the fingers of the right hand are alternately contracting and relaxing, and a fine tremor involving the wrist and elbow on the right side is seen. The tremor is worse when the arm is at rest. When he is asked to hold a book in his right hand, the tremor stops momentarily, but it starts again immediately after the book is placed on the table. The daughter says that when her father falls asleep, the tremor stops immediately. On examination, passive movements of the right elbow and wrist show increased tone, and cogwheel rigidity is noted. The patient has neither cutaneous or deep sensibility sensory loss, and the reflexes are normal. Using your knowledge of neuroanatomy, make a diagnosis. Which regions of the brain are diseased?

13. Name a center in the central nervous system that may be responsible for the following clinical signs: (a) intention tremor, (b) athetosis, (c) chorea, (d) dystonia, and (e) hemiballismus.

 Answers and Explanations to Clinical Problem Solving

1. This patient was suffering from spondylosis, which is a general term used for degenerative changes in the vertebral column caused by osteoarthritis. In the cervical region, the growth of osteophytes was exerting pressure on the anterior and posterior roots of the fifth and sixth spinal nerves. As the result of repeated trauma and aging, degenerative changes occurred at the articulating

surfaces of the fourth, fifth, and sixth cervical vertebrae. Extensive spur formation resulted in narrowing of the intervertebral foramina with pressure on the nerve roots. The burning pain, hyperesthesia, and partial analgesia were due to pressure on the posterior roots, and weakness, wasting, and fasciculation of the deltoid and biceps brachii muscles were due to pressure on the anterior roots. Movements of the neck presumably intensified the symptoms by exerting further traction or pressure on the nerve roots. Coughing or sneezing raised the pressure within the vertebral canal and resulted in further pressure on the nerve roots.

2. The patient was operated on and laminectomy of the third, fourth, and fifth thoracic vertebrae was carried out. At the level of the fourth thoracic vertebra, a small swelling was seen on the posterior surface of the spinal cord; it was attached to the dura mater. Histologic examination showed that it was a meningioma. The tumor was easily removed, and the patient successfully recovered from the operation. Power of the lower limbs progressively returned, with the patient walking without a stick. This patient emphasizes the importance of making an early, accurate diagnosis because benign extramedullary spinal tumors are readily treatable. The lateral spinal thalamic tracts are responsible for the conduction of pain impulses up the spinal cord. These tracts are situated in the lateral white columns of the spinal cord (see p. 141). Postural sense and vibration sense are conducted up the spinal cord in the posterior white column through the fasciculus cuneatus from the upper limbs and the upper part of the thorax and in the fasciculus gracilis from the lower part of the trunk and the leg. The difficulty in walking was due to pressure on the corticospinal tracts in the lateral white column. The exaggeration in the tendon reflexes of the lower limbs and the bilateral extensor plantar responses were due to the pressure on the descending tracts in the spinal cord at the level of the tumor. This also resulted in spastic paralysis of the muscles of the lower limbs.

3. A fracture dislocation of the 9th thoracic vertebra would result in severe damage to the 10th thoracic segment of the spinal cord. The unequal sensory and motor losses on the two sides indicate a left hemisection of the cord. The narrow band of hyperesthesia on the left side was due to the irritation of the cord immediately above the site of the lesion. The band of anesthesia and analgesia was due to the destruction of the cord on the left side at the level of the 10th thoracic segment; that is, all afferent fibers entering the cord at that point were interrupted. The loss of pain and thermal sensibilities and the loss of light touch below the level of the umbilicus on the right side were caused by the interruption of the lateral

and anterior spinothalamic tracts on the left side of the cord.

4. This patient has the early signs and symptoms of syringomyelia. The gliosis and cavitation had resulted in interruption of the lateral and anterior spinothalamic tracts as they decussated in the anterior gray and white commissures of the spinal cord at the level of the eighth cervical and first thoracic segments of the spinal cord. Because of uneven growth of the cavitation, the condition was worse on the left side than the right. Because tactile discrimination was normal in both upper limbs, the fasciculus cuneatus in both posterior white columns was unaffected. This dissociated sensory loss is characteristic of this disease.

5. The peculiar stamping gait and the swaying posture on closing the eyes are the characteristic signs of loss of appreciation of proprioceptive sensation from the lower limbs. These, together with the inability to detect the vibrations of a tuning fork placed on the medial malleoli of both legs, indicated that the patient had a lesion involving the fasciculus gracilis in both posterior white columns. Further questioning of this patient indicated that he had been treated for syphilis. The diagnosis was tabes dorsalis.

6. The treatment of intractable pain in terminal cancer is a difficult problem. Narcotic drugs with their strong analgesic action are generally used. The likelihood that these drugs will be habit-forming is accepted in a dying patient. Alternative treatments include the continuous infusion of morphine directly into the spinal cord (see p. 164) or the surgical section of the nerve fibers carrying the sensations of pain into the nervous system. The techniques of posterior rhizotomy and cordotomy are described on page 164.

7. Spinal shock is a temporary interruption of physiologic function of the spinal cord following injury. It may in part be a vascular phenomenon involving the gray matter of the spinal cord; on the other hand, some authorities believe it is due to the sudden interruption of the influence of the higher centers on the local segmental reflexes. Whatever the cause, it usually disappears after 1 to 4 weeks. The condition is characterized by flaccid paralysis and loss of sensation and reflex activity below the level of the lesion; this includes paralysis of the bladder and rectum.

Paraplegia in extension and paraplegia in flexion follow severe injury to the spinal cord. Paraplegia in extension indicates an increase in the extensor muscle tone owing to the overactivity of the γ efferent nerve fibers to the muscle spindles as the result of the release of these neurons from the higher centers. However, some neurologists believe that the vestibulospinal tracts are intact in these cases. Should all the descending tracts be severed, the condition of paraplegia in flexion occurs where the reflex responses are flexor in nature when a noxious stimulus is applied. Recall that paraplegia in extension and paraplegia in flexion occur only after spinal shock has ceased. Paraplegia in extension may change to paraplegia in flexion if the damage to the spinal cord becomes more extensive and the vestibulospinal tracts are destroyed.

8. If this patient is assumed to have a lesion in the left internal capsule following a cerebral hemorrhage, the corticospinal fibers would have been interrupted as they descended through the posterior limb of the internal capsule. Because most of these fibers crossed to the right side at the decussation of the pyramids or lower down at the segmental level of the spinal cord, the muscles of the opposite side would have been affected. Interruption of these corticospinal fibers would have produced the following clinical signs: (a) a positive Babinski sign; (b) loss of superficial abdominal and cremasteric reflexes; and (c) loss of performance of fine, skilled voluntary movements, especially at the distal ends of the limbs.

In patients with severe hemorrhage into the internal capsule, subcortical connections between the cerebral cortex and the caudate nucleus and the globus pallidus and other subcortical nuclei may be damaged. Moreover, some of the nuclei themselves may be destroyed. The interruption of other descending tracts from these subcortical centers would produce the following clinical signs: (a) severe paralysis on the opposite side of the body; (b) spasticity of the paralyzed muscles; (c) exaggerated deep muscle reflexes on the opposite side of the body to the lesion (clonus may be demonstrated); and (d) clasp-knife reaction, which may be felt in the paralyzed muscles.

9. A lateral radiograph of the thoracic part of the vertebral column showed a fracture dislocation involving the 10th vertebra. The first lumbar segment of the spinal cord is related to this vertebra. The first lumbar dermatome overlies the inguinal ligament, and total anesthesia over the right ligament would suggest a partial lesion of the spinal cord involving the total sensory input at that level. Loss of tactile discrimination and vibratory and proprioceptive senses in the right leg was caused by interruption of the ascending tracts in the posterior white column on the right side of the spinal cord. Loss of pain and temperature senses in the skin of the left leg was due to destruction of the crossed lateral spinothalamic tracts on the right side at the level of the lesion. Loss of tactile sense in the skin of the left leg was caused by the destruction of the crossed anterior spinothalamic tracts on the right side. Spastic paralysis of the right leg and the right-sided ankle clonus were due to the interruption of the right-sided descending tracts other than the corticospinal tracts. The

right-sided Babinski response was brought about by the interruption of the corticospinal fibers on the right side.

The complete motor and sensory loss of both legs and the absence of all deep tendon reflexes of both legs during the first 12 hours were due to spinal shock.

10. The spinal cord occupies the vertebral canal of the vertebral column, and therefore, under normal circumstances, it is well protected. Unfortunately, once the integrity of the bony protection is destroyed by a fracture dislocation, especially in the thoracic region, where the canal is of small diameter, the bone can damage the cord and sever it just as a knife cuts through butter. All patients suspected of having an injury to the spine must be handled with great care to prevent the bones undergoing further dislocation and causing further injury to the cord. The patient should be carefully lifted by multiple supports under the feet, knees, pelvis, back, shoulders, and head and placed on a rigid stretcher or board for transportation to the nearest medical center.

11. Urinary infection secondary to bladder dysfunction is extremely common in paraplegic patients. The patient has not only lost control of the bladder but also does not know when it is full. An indwelling Foley catheter is placed in the bladder immediately for continuous drainage, and antibiotic therapy is instituted.

Bedsores are very common in patients who have lost all sensory perception over their bony points, such as the ischial tuberosities and the sacrum. Bedsores are best prevented by (a) keeping the skin scrupulously clean, (b) frequently changing the position of the patient, and (c) keeping soft padding beneath the bony points.

Nutritional deficiency is common in active individuals who are suddenly confined to their beds and who are paralyzed. Loss of appetite must be combated by giving the patients a high-calorie diet that has all the required ingredients, especially vitamins.

Muscle spasms occur in paraplegia in extension or paraplegia in flexion and may follow only minor stimuli. The cause is unknown, but neuronal irritation at the site of injury may be responsible. Warm baths are helpful, but, occasionally, in extreme cases, nerve section may be necessary.

Pain occurs in the anesthetic areas in about 25% of patients who have a complete section of the spinal cord. The pain may be burning or shooting and superficial, or deep visceral. Here again, neuronal irritation at the site of injury may be responsible. Analgesics should be tried, but in some individuals, rhizotomy or even chordotomy may be necessary.

An accurate prognosis is not possible until the stage of spinal shock has ended, and this may last as long as 4 weeks.

12. The characteristic coarse tremor of the right hand (pill rolling) and right arm, the unsmiling masklike face with unblinking eyes, and the cogwheel rigidity of the involved muscles make the diagnosis of early Parkinson disease (paralysis agitans) certain. Degenerative lesions occur in the substantia nigra and other subcortical nuclei, including the lentiform nucleus. The loss of normal function of these subcortical areas and the absence of their influence on the lower motor neurons are responsible for the increased tone and tremor.

13. (a) Intention tremor occurs in cerebellar disease. (b) Athetosis occurs in lesions of the corpus striatum. (c) Chorea occurs in lesions of the corpus striatum. (d) Dystonia occurs in disease of the lentiform nucleus. (e) Hemiballismus occurs in disease of the opposite subthalamic nucleus.

Review Questions

Directions: Each of the numbered items in this section is followed by answers. Select the ONE lettered answer that is CORRECT.

1. The following statements concern the spinal cord:
   (a) The anterior and posterior gray columns on the two sides are united by a white commissure.
   (b) The terminal ventricle is the expanded lower end of the fourth ventricle.
   (c) The larger nerve cell bodies in the anterior gray horns give rise to α efferent nerve fibers in the anterior roots.
   (d) The substantia gelatinosa groups of cells are located at the base of each posterior gray column.
   (e) The nucleus dorsalis (Clarke column) is a group of nerve cells found in the posterior gray column and restricted to the lumbar segments of the cord.
2. The following statements concern the white columns of the spinal cord:
   (a) The posterior spinocerebellar tract is situated in the posterior white column.
   (b) The anterior spinothalamic tract is found in the anterior white column.
   (c) The lateral spinothalamic tract is found in the anterior white column.
   (d) The fasciculus gracilis is found in the lateral white column.
   (e) The rubrospinal tract is found in the anterior white column.
3. The following statements concern the spinal cord:
   (a) The spinal cord has a cervical enlargement for the brachial plexus.
   (b) The spinal cord possesses spinal nerves that are attached to the cord by anterior and posterior rami.
   (c) In the adult, the spinal cord usually ends inferiorly at the lower border of the fourth lumbar vertebra.
   (d) The ligamentum denticulatum anchors the spinal cord to the pedicles of the vertebra along each side.
   (e) The central canal does not communicate with the fourth ventricle of the brain.

Directions: Matching Questions. Questions 4 through 9 apply to the following figure. Match the numbers listed on the left with the appropriate lettered structure listed on the right. Each lettered option may be selected once, more than once, or not at all.

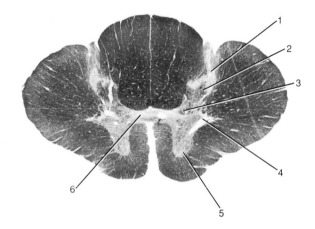

4. Number 1   (a) Nucleus proprius
5. Number 2   (b) Preganglionic sympathetic outflow
6. Number 3   (c) Nucleus dorsalis
7. Number 4   (d) Substantia gelatinosa
8. Number 5   (e) None of the above
9. Number 6

Directions: Each of the numbered items in this section is followed by answers. Select the ONE lettered answer that is CORRECT.

10. The following statements concern the cell of origin of the tracts listed below:
    (a) The fasciculus cuneatus arises from cells in the substantia gelatinosa.
    (b) The anterior spinothalamic arises from cells in the posterior root ganglion.
    (c) The fasciculus gracilis arises from cells in the nucleus dorsalis (Clarke column).
    (d) The anterior spinocerebellar arises from cells in the posterior root ganglion.
    (e) The lateral spinothalamic arises from cells in the substantia gelatinosa.

11. The following statements concern the courses taken by the tracts listed below:
    (a) The fasciculus gracilis does not cross to the opposite side of the neural axis.
    (b) The spinotectal tract does not cross to the opposite side of the spinal cord.
    (c) The lateral spinothalamic tract does not cross to the opposite side of the spinal cord.
    (d) The posterior spinocerebellar tract crosses to the opposite side of the neural axis.
    (e) The anterior spinothalamic tract immediately crosses to the opposite side of the spinal cord.

12. The following statements concern the nucleus of termination of the tracts listed below:
    (a) The posterior white column tracts terminate in the inferior colliculus.
    (b) The spinoreticular tract terminates on the neurons of the hippocampus.
    (c) The spinotectal tract terminates in the inferior colliculus.
    (d) The anterior spinothalamic tract terminates in the ventral posterolateral nucleus of the thalamus.
    (e) The anterior spinocerebellar tract terminates in the dentate nucleus of the cerebellum.

13. The following statements relate sensations with the appropriate nervous pathways:
    (a) Two-point tactile discrimination travels in the lateral spinothalamic tract.
    (b) Pain travels in the anterior spinothalamic tract.
    (c) Unconscious muscle joint sense travels in the anterior spinocerebellar tract.
    (d) Pressure travels in the posterior spinothalamic tract.
    (e) Vibration travels in the posterior spinocerebellar tract.

14. The following statements concern the gating theory of pain:
    (a) Stimulation of small non–pain-conducting fibers in a peripheral nerve may reduce pain sensitivity.
    (b) Massage applied to the skin over a painful joint may reduce pain sensitivity.
    (c) Stimulation of δ A- and C-type fibers in a spinal nerve posterior root may decrease pain sensitivity.
    (d) Degeneration of large non–pain-conducting fibers in a peripheral nerve decreases pain sensitivity.
    (e) Inhibition of pain conduction in the spinal cord does not involve connector neurons.

15. The following statements concern the reception of pain:
    (a) Serotonin is not a transmitter substance in the analgesic system.
    (b) Substance P is thought to be the neurotransmitter at the synapses where the first-order neuron terminates on the cells in the posterior gray column of the spinal cord.
    (c) Enkephalins and endorphins may stimulate substance P release in the posterior gray column of the spinal cord.

    (d) Many of the tracts conducting the initial, sharp, pricking pain terminate in the dorsal anterolateral nucleus of the thalamus.
    (e) The slow-conducting C-type fibers are responsible for prolonged, burning pain.

16. The following statements concern the corticospinal tracts:
    (a) They occupy the posterior limb of the internal capsule.
    (b) They are mainly responsible for controlling the voluntary movements in proximal limb muscles.
    (c) They arise as axons of the pyramidal cells in the fourth layer of the cerebral cortex.
    (d) Those that control the movements of the upper limb originate in the precentral gyrus on the medial side of the cerebral hemisphere.
    (e) Those that are concerned with the movements of the lower limb are located in the medial area of the middle three fifths of the basis pedunculi.

17. The following statements concern the course taken by the tracts listed below:
    (a) The rubrospinal tract crosses the midline of the neuroaxis in the medulla oblongata.
    (b) The tectospinal tract (most of the nerve fibers) crosses the midline in the posterior commissure.
    (c) The vestibulospinal tract crosses the midline in the midbrain.
    (d) The lateral corticospinal tract crosses the midline in the medulla oblongata.
    (e) The anterior corticospinal tract crosses the midline in the midbrain.

18. The following statements concern the nerve cells of origin for the tracts listed below:
    (a) The vestibulospinal tract originates from cells of the medial vestibular nucleus situated in the pons.
    (b) The tectospinal tract originates from cells in the inferior colliculus.
    (c) The lateral corticospinal tract originates from cells in area 4 of the cerebral cortex.
    (d) The rubrospinal tract originates from cells in the reticular nucleus.
    (e) The reticulospinal tract originates from cells in the reticular formation that is confined to the midbrain.

19. The following statements concern muscle movement:
    (a) Muscular fasciculation is seen only with rapid destruction of lower motor neurons.
    (b) Muscle spindle afferent nerve fibers send information only to the spinal cord.
    (c) In Parkinson disease, dopamine-secreting neurons that originate in the vestibular nucleus degenerate.
    (d) Brain neuronal activity preceding a voluntary movement is limited to the precentral gyrus (area 4).
    (e) Hyperactive ankle-jerk reflexes and ankle clonus indicate release of lower motor neuron supraspinal inhibition.

20. After a hemorrhage into the left internal capsule in a right-handed person, the following sign or symptom might be present:
    (a) Left homonymous hemianopia
    (b) Right astereognosis
    (c) Left hemiplegia
    (d) Normal speech
    (e) Left-sided positive Babinski response
21. A patient with a traumatic lesion of the left half of the spinal cord at the level of the eighth cervical segment might present the following sign(s) and symptom(s):
    (a) Loss of pain and temperature sensations on the left side below the level of the lesion
    (b) Loss of position sense of the right leg
    (c) Right hemiplegia
    (d) Left positive Babinski sign
    (e) Right-sided lower motor paralysis in the segment of the lesion and muscular atrophy

Directions: Each of the numbered items in this section is followed by answers. Select the ONE lettered answer that is BEST in each case.

22. Which of the signs and symptoms listed below indicate a cerebellar lesion?
    (a) Cogwheel rigidity
    (b) Hemiballismus
    (c) Chorea
    (d) Intention tremor
    (e) Athetosis
23. Which of the following regions of white matter would not contain corticospinal fibers?
    (a) Pyramid of medulla oblongata
    (b) Lateral white column of the spinal cord
    (c) Cerebral peduncle of the midbrain
    (d) Anterior limb of the internal capsule
    (e) Corona radiata

Directions: Each case history is followed by questions. Read the case history, then select the ONE BEST lettered answer.

A 59-year-old woman was experiencing pain in the back and showed evidence of loss of pain and temperature sensations down the back of her left leg. Three years previously, she underwent a radical mastectomy followed by radiation and chemotherapy for advanced carcinoma of her right breast.

Examination showed that she was experiencing pain over the lower part of the back, with loss of the skin sensations of pain and temperature down the back of her left leg in the area of the S1–S3 dermatomes. No other neurologic deficits were identified. Radiographic examination of the vertebral column showed evidence of metastases in the bodies of the 9th and 10th thoracic vertebrae. An MRI revealed an extension of one of the metastases into the vertebral canal, with slight indentation of the spinal cord on the right side.

24. The pain in the back could be explained in this patient by the following facts **except**:
    (a) Osteoarthritis of the joints of the vertebral column
    (b) Metastases in the bodies of the 9th and 10th thoracic vertebrae
    (c) Tumor pressure on the spinal nerve posterior roots
    (d) A prolapsed intervertebral disc pressing on the spinal nerves
    (e) Spasm of the postvertebral muscles following tumor pressure on the posterior white columns of the spinal cord
25. Loss of pain and temperature sensations down the back of the patient's left leg in the area of the S1–S3 dermatomes could be explained by the following factual statements **except**:
    (a) Lateral spinothalamic tracts in the spinal cord conduct the sensations of pain.
    (b) Lateral spinothalamic tracts are laminated, with the sacral segments of the body located most laterally.
    (c) The sacral segments of the tracts are the most exposed to external cord pressure from a metastasizing tumor.
    (d) Loss of temperature sensations in the leg could be explained by tumor pressure on the anterior spinothalamic tract.
26. The severe intractable pain in the back in this patient could be treated by the following methods **except**:
    (a) Prescription of salicylates in large doses
    (b) Intramuscular injection of morphine or even the direct injection of the opiate into the spinal cord
    (c) Posterior rhizotomy
    (d) Cordotomy
    (e) Injection of opiates into the subarachnoid space

 Answers and Explanations to Review Questions

1. C is correct. The larger nerve cell bodies in the anterior gray horns give rise to α efferent nerve fibers in the anterior roots. A. The anterior and posterior gray columns on the two sides of the spinal cord are united by a gray commissure formed of gray matter. B. The terminal ventricle is the expanded lower end of the central canal. D. The substantia gelatinosa group of cells is located at the apex of each posterior gray column throughout the length of the spinal cord. E. The nucleus dorsalis (Clarke column) is a group of nerve cells found in the posterior gray column and extending from the eighth cervical segment of the cord to the third or fourth lumbar segment.
2. B is correct. In the spinal cord, the anterior spinothalamic tract is found in the anterior white column. A. The posterior spinocerebellar tract is situated in the lateral white column. C. The lateral spinothalamic tract is found in the lateral white

column. D. The fasciculus gracilis is found in the posterior white column. E. The rubrospinal tract is found in the lateral white column.

3. A is correct. The spinal cord has a cervical enlargement for the brachial plexus (Fig. 4-5). B. The spinal cord possesses spinal nerves that are attached to the cord by anterior and posterior nerve roots. C. In the adult, the spinal cord usually ends inferiorly at the lower border of the first lumbar vertebra. D. The ligamentum denticulatum anchors the spinal cord to the dura mater along each side. E. The central canal, which contains cerebrospinal fluid, communicates with the fourth ventricle of the brain.

4. D is correct.

5. A is correct.

6. C is correct.

7. B is correct.

8. E is correct. The structure is the anterior gray horn.

9. E is correct. The structure is the gray commissure.

10. E is correct. In the spinal cord, the lateral spinothalamic tract arises from cells in the substantia gelatinosa. A. The fasciculus cuneatus arises from cells in the posterior root ganglion. B. The anterior spinal thalamic arises from cells in the substantia gelatinosa. C. The fasciculus gracilis arises from cells in the posterior root ganglion. D. The anterior spinocerebellar arises from cells in Clarke column.

11. A is correct. The fasciculus gracilis does not cross to the opposite side of the neural axis. B. The spinotectal tract crosses to the opposite side of the spinal cord. C. The lateral spinothalamic tract crosses to the opposite side of the spinal cord. D. The posterior spinocerebellar tract does not cross to the opposite side of the spinal cord. E. The anterior spinothalamic tract crosses very obliquely to the opposite side of the spinal cord.

12. D is correct. The anterior spinothalamic tract terminates in the ventral posterolateral nucleus of the thalamus. A. The posterior white column tracts terminate in the nucleus gracilis and cuneatus. B. The spinoreticular tract terminates on the neurons of the reticular formation in the medulla, pons, and midbrain. C. The spinotectal tract terminates in the superior colliculus. E. The anterior spinocerebellar tract terminates in the cerebellar cortex.

13. C is correct. Unconscious muscle joint sense travels in the anterior spinocerebellar tract. A. Two-point tactile discrimination travels in the fasciculus cuneatus. B. Pain travels in the lateral spinothalamic tract. D. Pressure travels in the anterior spinothalamic tract. E. Vibration travels in the fasciculus gracilis.

14. B is correct concerning the gating theory of pain. Massage applied to the skin over a painful joint may reduce pain sensitivity. A. Stimulation of large non–pain-conducting fibers in a peripheral nerve may reduce pain sensitivity. C. Stimulation of δ A- and C-type fibers in a spinal nerve posterior root may increase pain sensitivity. D. Degeneration of large non–pain-conducting fibers in a peripheral nerve increases pain sensitivity. E. Inhibition of pain conduction in the spinal cord could be brought about by means of connector neurons.

15. E is correct. The slow-conducting C-type fibers are responsible for prolonged, burning pain. A. Serotonin is a transmitter substance in the analgesic system. B. Substance P is a peptide and is thought to be the neurotransmitter at the synapses where the first-order neuron terminates on the cells in the posterior gray column of the spinal cord. C. Enkephalins and endorphins may inhibit the release of substance P in the posterior gray column of the spinal cord. D. Many of the tracts conducting the initial, sharp, pricking pain terminate in the ventral posterolateral nucleus of the thalamus.

16. A is correct. The corticospinal tracts occupy the posterior limb of the internal capsule (Fig. 4-11). B. The corticospinal tracts are mainly responsible for controlling the voluntary movements in the distal muscles of the limbs. C. They arise as axons of the pyramidal cells in the fifth layer of the cerebral cortex. D. Those that control the movements of the upper limb originate in the precentral gyrus on the lateral side of the cerebral hemisphere. E. Those that are concerned with the movements of the lower limb are located in the lateral area of the middle three fifths of the basis pedunculi.

17. D is correct. The lateral corticospinal tract crosses the midline in the medulla oblongata (Fig. 4-21). A. The rubrospinal tract crosses the midline of the neuroaxis in the midbrain. B. The tectospinal tract (most of the nerve fibers) crosses the midline in the midbrain. C. The vestibulospinal tract does not cross the midline and descends through the medulla oblongata and spinal cord in the anterior white column (Figs. 4-20 and 4-25). E. The anterior corticospinal tract crosses the midline in the spinal cord.

18. C is correct. The lateral corticospinal tract originates from cells in area 4 of the cerebral cortex. A. The vestibulospinal tract originates from cells of the lateral vestibular nucleus situated in the pons. B. The tectospinal tract originates from cells in the superior colliculus. D. The rubrospinal tract originates from cells in the red nucleus. E. The reticulospinal tract originates from cells in the reticular formation in the midbrain, pons, and medulla oblongata.

19. E is correct. Hyperactive ankle-jerk reflexes and ankle clonus indicate lower motor neuron release from supraspinal inhibition. A. Muscular fasciculation is seen only with slow destruction of the lower motor neurons. B. Muscle spindle afferent nerve fibers send information to the brain as well as to the spinal cord. C. In Parkinson disease, dopamine-secreting neurons decrease in the substantia nigra. D. Brain neuronal activity preceding a voluntary movement is not limited to the precentral gyrus (area 4).

20. B is correct. Right astereognosis. A. Right homonymous hemianopia is seen. C. Right hemiplegia is present. D. Aphasia is present. E. A right-sided positive Babinski response is seen.

21. D is correct. Left positive Babinski sign is present. A. Pain and temperature sensations are lost on the right side below the level of the lesion. B. Position sense of the left leg is lost. C. Left hemiplegia is present. E. Left-sided lower motor paralysis is seen in the segment of the lesion and muscular atrophy.

22. D is correct. Intention tremor is present. A. Cogwheel rigidity occurs in Parkinson disease when the muscle resistance is overcome as a series of jerks. B. Hemiballismus is a rare form of involuntary movement confined to one side of the body; it occurs in disease of the subthalamic nuclei. C. Chorea consists of a series of continuous, rapid, involuntary, jerky, coarse, purposeless movements, which may take place during sleep; it occurs with lesions of the corpus striatum. E. Athetosis consists of continuous, slow, involuntary, dysrhythmic movements that are always the same in the same individual, and they disappear during sleep; it occurs with lesions of the corpus striatum.

23. D is correct. The anterior limb of the internal capsule does not contain corticospinal fibers.

24. E is correct. Spasm of the postvertebral muscles would not be produced by pressure on the posterior white columns of the spinal cord.

25. D is correct. The sensation of temperature travels in the lateral spinothalamic tract along with the pain impulses.

26. A is correct. Salicylates, such as aspirin, sodium salicylate, and diflunisal, are used clinically only for the relief of mild to moderate pain, as found in patients suffering from headache and dysmenorrhea.

5 Brainstem

CHAPTER OBJECTIVES

- To review the anatomy of the brainstem
- To develop a three-dimensional picture of the interior of the brainstem
- To know the positions of several of the cranial nerve nuclei, the olivary nuclear complex, and the paths

taken by the various ascending and descending nerve tracts as they ascend to the higher brain centers or descend to the spinal cord

- To assess the signs and symptoms presented by a patient and identify the exact location of a structural lesion

A 58-year-old woman is referred to a neurologist because of recent onset of difficulty with walking. The neurologist notes that she stands and walks with her left arm flexed at the elbow and the left leg extended (left hemiparesis). While walking, she has difficulty flexing the left hip and knee and dorsiflexing the ankle; the forward motion is possible by swinging the left leg outward at the hip to avoid dragging the foot on the ground. Her left arm remains motionless.

Neurologic examination shows no signs of facial paralysis, but tongue weakness is evident. On protrusion, the tongue deviates toward the right side (right hypoglossal nerve palsy). Cutaneous sensations are found to be normal, but muscle joint sense, tactile discrimination, and vibratory sense on the left side of the body are impaired.

Based on the neurologic findings, a diagnosis of right-sided medial medullary syndrome is made. The medial part

of the right side of the medulla oblongata receives its arterial supply from the right vertebral artery. Occlusion of this artery or its branch to the medulla results in destruction of the right pyramid (left hemiparesis), destruction of the right hypoglossal nucleus and nerve (right hypoglossal palsy), and destruction of the medial lemniscus on the right side (left-sided loss of muscle joint sense, vibratory sense, and tactile discrimination). The absence of facial palsy showed that the facial nerve nuclei, the facial nerves, and the corticobulbar fibers to the facial nuclei were intact. The sparing of the sensations of touch, pain, and temperature showed that the spinal lemniscus was intact.

This diagnosis is possible as the result of carefully sorting out the neurologic findings. A clear knowledge of the position and function of the various nerve tracts and nuclei in the medulla oblongata is essential before a clinician can reach a diagnosis in this case.

SKULL ANATOMY

Head injuries from blunt trauma and penetrating missiles are associated with a high mortality and disabling morbidity. Because of the close relationship that exists between the skull and the underlying brain and cranial nerves (CNs), as well as their common involvement in many diseases, a brief review of the anatomy of the skull will first be considered.

Adult Skull

The skull is composed of several separate bones united at immobile joints called **sutures**. The connective tissue

between the bones is called a **sutural ligament**. The mandible is an exception, united to the skull by the mobile temporomandibular joint.

The bones of the skull can be divided into those of the **cranium** and those of the face. The **vault** is the upper part of the cranium, and the **base of the skull** is the lowest part of the cranium (Fig. 5-1).

The skull bones are made up of **external** and **internal tables** of compact bone separated by a layer of spongy bone called the **diploë** (Fig. 5-2). The internal table is thinner and more brittle than the external table. The bones are covered on the outer and inner surfaces with periosteum.

The **cranium** consists of the following bones, two of which are paired (Fig. 5-3; also see Fig. 5-1):

- Frontal bone 1
- Parietal bones 2
- Occipital bone 1
- Temporal bones 2
- Sphenoid bone 1
- Ethmoid bone 1

The **facial bones** consist of the following, two of which are single:

- Zygomatic bones 2
- Maxillae 2
- Nasal bones 2
- Lacrimal bones 2
- Vomer 1

- Palatine bones 2
- Inferior conchae 2
- Mandible 1

Although students do not need to know the detailed structure of each individual skull bone, they should be familiar with the skull as a whole. If possible, have a dried skull available for reference as you read the following description.

Anterior View

The **frontal bone**, or forehead bone, curves downward to make the upper margins of the orbits (see Fig. 5-1). The **superciliary arches** can be seen on either side, and the **supraorbital notch**, or **foramen**, can be recognized. Medially, the frontal bone articulates with the frontal

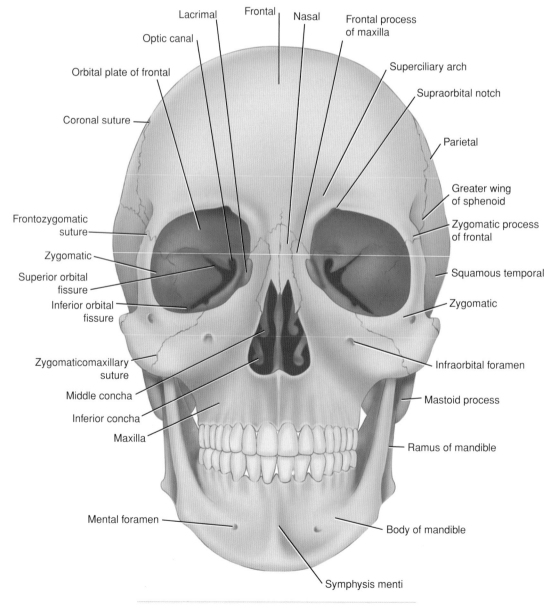

Figure 5-1   Bones of the anterior aspect of the skull.

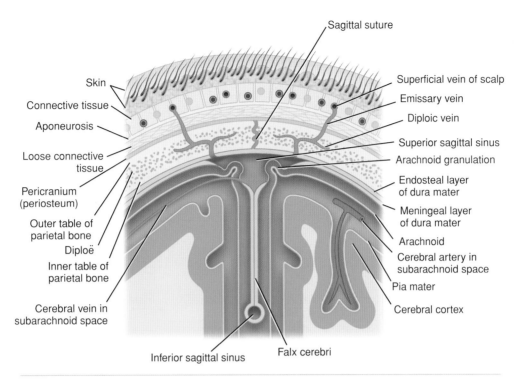

Figure 5-2   Coronal section of the upper part of the head showing the layers of the scalp, the sagittal suture of the skull, the falx cerebri, the superior and inferior sagittal venous sinuses, the arachnoid granulations, the emissary veins, and the relation of cerebral blood vessels to the subarachnoid space.

processes of the maxillae and with the nasal bones. Laterally, the frontal bone articulates with the zygomatic bone.

The **orbital margins** are bounded by the frontal bone superiorly, the zygomatic bone laterally, the maxilla inferiorly, and the processes of the maxilla and frontal bone medially.

Within the **frontal bone**, just above the orbital margins, are two hollow spaces lined with mucous membrane called the **frontal air sinuses**. These communicate with the nose and serve as voice resonators.

The two **nasal bones** form the bridge of the nose. Their lower borders, with the maxillae, make the **anterior nasal aperture**. The nasal cavity is divided into two by the bony nasal septum, which is largely formed by the **vomer**. The **superior** and **middle conchae** are shelves of bone that project into the nasal cavity from the **ethmoid** on each side; the **inferior conchae** are separate bones.

The two **maxillae** form the upper jaw, the anterior part of the hard palate, part of the lateral walls of the nasal cavities, and part of the floors of the orbital cavities. The two bones meet in the midline at the **intermaxillary** suture and form the lower margin of the nasal aperture. Below the orbit, the maxilla is perforated by the **infraorbital** foramen. The **alveolar process** projects downward and, together with the fellow of the opposite side, forms the **alveolar** arch, which carries the upper

teeth. Within each maxilla is a large, pyramid-shaped cavity lined with mucous membrane called the **maxillary** sinus. This communicates with the nasal cavity and serves as a voice resonator.

The **zygomatic bone** forms the prominence of the cheek and part of the lateral wall and floor of the orbital cavity. It articulates with the maxilla medially and with the zygomatic process of the temporal bone laterally to form the **zygomatic arch**. The zygomatic bone is perforated by two foramina for the zygomaticofacial and zygomaticotemporal nerves.

The **mandible**, or lower jaw, consists of a horizontal **body** and two vertical **rami**.

Lateral View

The **frontal bone** forms the anterior part of the side of the skull and articulates with the parietal bone at the **coronal suture** (see Fig. 5-3).

The **parietal bones** form the sides and roof of the cranium and articulate with each other in the midline at the **sagittal suture**. They articulate with the occipital bone behind, at the **lambdoid suture**.

The skull is completed at the side by the squamous part of the **occipital bone**; parts of the **temporal bone**, namely, the **squamous**, **tympanic**, **mastoid process**, **styloid process**, and **zygomatic process**; and the **greater wing of the sphenoid**. Note the position of the external

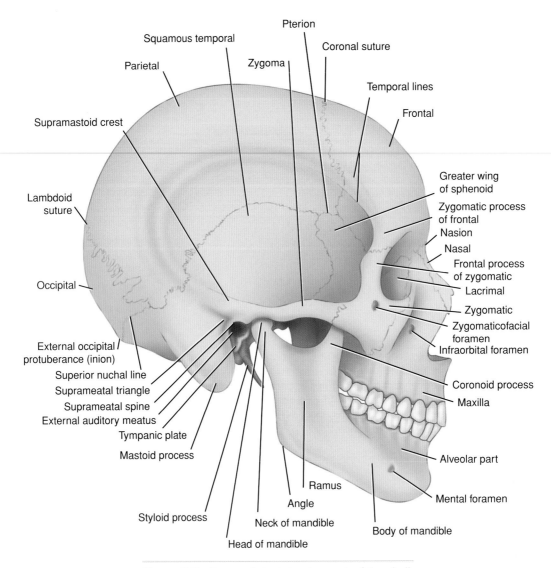

Figure 5-3 Bones of the lateral aspect of the skull.

auditory meatus. The ramus and body of the mandible lie inferiorly.

Note that the thinnest part of the lateral wall of the skull is where the anteroinferior corner of the parietal bone articulates with the greater wing of the sphenoid; this point is referred to as the **pterion**.

Clinically, the pterion is an important area because it overlies the anterior division of the **middle meningeal artery** and **vein**.

Identify the **superior** and **inferior temporal lines**, which begin as a single line from the posterior margin of the zygomatic process of the frontal bone and diverge as they arch backward. The **temporal fossa** lies below the inferior temporal line.

The **infratemporal fossa** lies below the **infratemporal crest** on the greater wing of the sphenoid. The **pterygomaxillary fissure** is a vertical fissure that lies within the fossa between the pterygoid process of the sphenoid bone and back of the maxilla. It leads medially into the **pterygopalatine fossa**.

The **inferior orbital fissure** is a horizontal fissure between the greater wing of the sphenoid bone and the maxilla. It leads forward into the orbit.

The **pterygopalatine fossa** is a small space behind and below the orbital cavity. It communicates laterally with the infratemporal fossa through the pterygomaxillary fissure, medially with the nasal cavity through the **sphenopalatine foramen**, superiorly with the skull through the **foramen rotundum**, and anteriorly with the orbit through the **inferior orbital fissure**.

Posterior View

The posterior parts of the two parietal bones (Fig. 5-4A) with the intervening **sagittal** suture are seen above. Below, the parietal bones articulate with the squamous part of the occipital bone at the **lambdoid** suture. On each side, the occipital bone articulates with the temporal bone. In the midline of the occipital bone is a roughened elevation called the **external** occipital

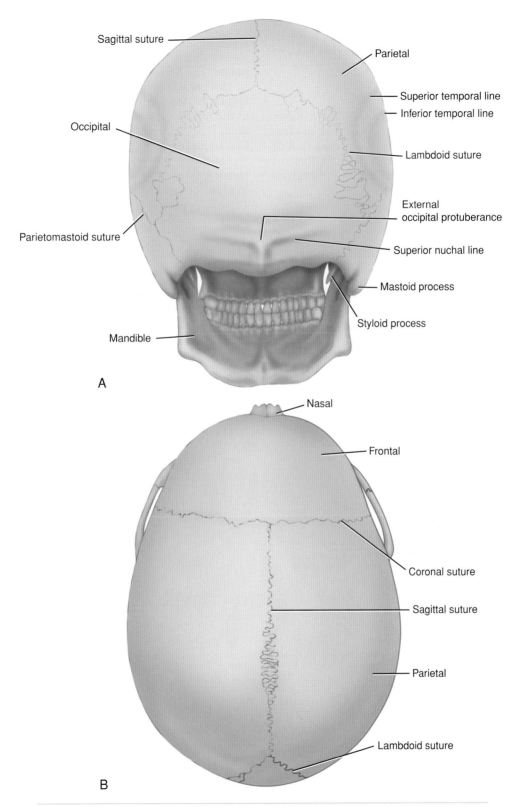

Figure 5-4 Bones of the skull viewed from the posterior (**A**) and superior (**B**) aspects.

protuberance, which gives attachment to muscles and the ligamentum nuchae. On either side of the protuberance, the **superior** nuchal lines extend laterally toward the temporal bone.

Superior View

Anteriorly, the frontal bone (see Fig. 5-4B) articulates with the two parietal bones at the **coronal suture**. Occasionally, the two halves of the frontal bone fail to fuse, leaving a midline **metopic suture**. Behind, the two parietal bones articulate in the midline at the **sagittal suture**.

Inferior View

If the mandible is discarded, the anterior part of this aspect of the skull is seen to be formed by the **hard palate** (Fig. 5-5).

The **palatal processes of the maxillae** and the **horizontal plates of the palatine bones** can be identified. In the midline anteriorly is the **incisive fossa** and **foramen**. Posterolaterally are the **greater** and **lesser palatine foramina**.

Above the posterior edge of the hard palate are the **choanae** (posterior nasal apertures). These are separated from each other by the posterior margin of the **vomer** and

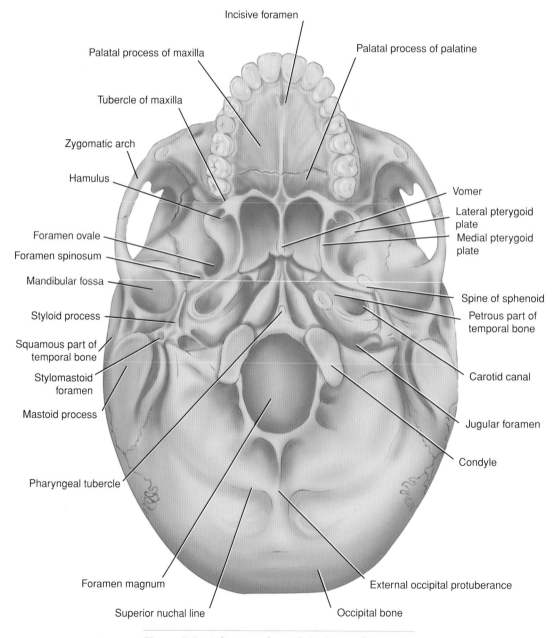

Figure 5-5 Inferior surface of the base of the skull.

are bounded laterally by the **medial pterygoid plates** of the sphenoid bone. The inferior end of the **medial pterygoid plate** is prolonged as a curved spike of bone, the **pterygoid hamulus**.

Posterolateral to the **lateral pterygoid plate**, the greater wing of the sphenoid is pierced by the large **foramen ovale** and the small **foramen spinosum**. Posterolateral to the foramen spinosum is the **spine of the sphenoid**.

Behind the spine of the sphenoid, in the interval between the greater wing of the sphenoid and the petrous part of the temporal bone, is a groove for the cartilaginous part of the **auditory tube**. The opening of the bony part of the tube can be identified.

The **mandibular fossa** of the temporal bone and the **articular tubercle** form the upper articular surfaces for the temporomandibular joint. Separating the mandibular fossa from the tympanic plate posteriorly is the **squamotympanic fissure**, through the medial end of which the chorda tympani exits from the tympanic cavity.

The **styloid process** of the temporal bone projects downward and forward from its inferior aspect. The opening of the **carotid canal** can be seen on the inferior surface of the petrous part of the temporal bone.

The medial end of the petrous part of the temporal bone is irregular and, together with the basilar part of the occipital bone and the greater wing of the sphenoid, forms the **foramen lacerum**. During life, the foramen lacerum is closed with fibrous tissue, and only a few small vessels pass through this foramen from the cavity of the skull to the exterior.

The **tympanic plate**, which forms part of the temporal bone, is C shaped on section and forms the bony part of the **external auditory meatus**. While examining this region, identify the **suprameatal crest** on the lateral surface of the squamous part of the temporal bone, the **suprameatal triangle**, and the **suprameatal spine**.

In the interval between the styloid and mastoid processes, the **stylomastoid foramen** can be seen. Medial to the styloid process, the petrous part of the temporal bone has a deep notch, which, together with a shallower notch on the occipital bone, forms the **jugular foramen**.

Behind the posterior apertures of the nose and in front of the foramen magnum are the sphenoid bone and the basilar part of the occipital bone.

The **occipital condyles** should be identified; they articulate with the superior aspect of the lateral mass of the first cervical vertebra, the atlas. Superior to the occipital condyle is the **hypoglossal canal** for transmission of the hypoglossal nerve (Fig. 5-6).

Posterior to the foramen magnum in the midline is the external occipital protuberance.

Neonatal Skull

The newborn skull (see Fig. 5-6), compared with the adult skull, has a disproportionately large cranium relative to the face. In childhood, the growth of the mandible, the maxillary sinuses, and the alveolar processes of the maxillae results in a great increase in length of the face.

The bones of the skull are smooth and unilaminar, there being no diploë present. Most of the skull bones are ossified at birth, but the process is incomplete, and the bones are mobile on each other, being connected by fibrous tissue or cartilage. The bones of the vault are not closely knit at sutures, as in the adult, but are separated by unossified membranous intervals called **fontanelles**. Clinically, the anterior and posterior fontanelles are most important and are easily examined in the midline of the vault.

The **anterior fontanelle** is diamond shaped and lies between the two halves of the frontal bone in front and the two parietal bones behind. The fibrous membrane forming the floor of the anterior fontanelle is replaced by bone and is closed by 18 months of age. The **posterior fontanelle** is triangular and lies between the two parietal bones in front and the occipital bone behind. By the end of the first year, the fontanelle is usually closed and can no longer be palpated.

The **tympanic part of the temporal bone** is merely a C-shaped ring at birth, compared with a C-shaped curved plate in the adult. The **mastoid process** is not present at birth (Fig. 5-7) and develops later in response to the pull of the sternocleidomastoid muscle when the child moves his or her head.

The mandible has right and left halves at birth, united in the midline with fibrous tissue. The two halves fuse at the **symphysis menti** by the end of the first year.

CRANIAL CAVITY

The cranial cavity contains the brain and its surrounding meninges, portions of the CNs, arteries, veins, and venous sinuses.

Vault of the Skull

The internal surface of the vault shows the coronal, sagittal, and lambdoid sutures. In the midline is a shallow sagittal groove that lodges the **superior sagittal sinus**. Several narrow grooves are present for the anterior and posterior divisions of the **middle meningeal vessels** as they pass up the side of the skull to the vault.

Base of the Skull

The interior of the base of the skull (see Fig. 5-6) is divided into three cranial fossae: anterior, middle, and posterior. The anterior cranial fossa is separated from the middle cranial fossa by the lesser wing of the sphenoid, and the middle cranial fossa is separated from the posterior cranial fossa by the petrous part of the temporal bone.

Anterior Cranial Fossa

The anterior cranial fossa lodges the frontal lobes of the cerebral hemispheres. It is bounded anteriorly by

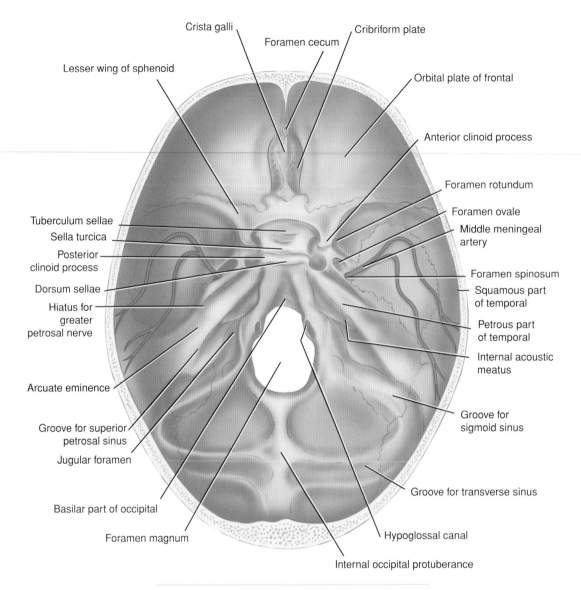

Crista galli
Foramen cecum
Cribriform plate
Lesser wing of sphenoid
Orbital plate of frontal
Anterior clinoid process
Foramen rotundum
Foramen ovale
Tuberculum sellae
Middle meningeal artery
Sella turcica
Posterior clinoid process
Foramen spinosum
Dorsum sellae
Squamous part of temporal
Hiatus for greater petrosal nerve
Petrous part of temporal
Internal acoustic meatus
Arcuate eminence
Groove for sigmoid sinus
Groove for superior petrosal sinus
Jugular foramen
Groove for transverse sinus
Basilar part of occipital
Foramen magnum
Hypoglossal canal
Internal occipital protuberance

Figure 5-6   Internal surface of the base of the skull.

the inner surface of the frontal bone, and in the midline is a crest for the attachment of the **falx cerebri**. Its posterior boundary is the sharp lesser wing of the sphenoid, which articulates laterally with the frontal bone and meets the anteroinferior angle of the parietal bone, or the pterion. The medial end of the lesser wing of the sphenoid forms the **anterior clinoid process** on each side, which gives attachment to the **tentorium cerebelli**. The median part of the anterior cranial fossa is limited posteriorly by the groove for the optic chiasma.

The floor of the fossa is formed by the ridged orbital plates of the frontal bone laterally and by the **cribriform plate** of the ethmoid medially (see Fig. 5-6). The **crista galli** is a sharp upward projection of the ethmoid bone in the midline for the attachment

of the falx cerebri. Between the crista galli and the crest of the frontal bone is a small aperture, the **foramen cecum**, for the transmission of a small vein from the nasal mucosa to the superior sagittal sinus. Alongside the crista galli is a narrow slit in the cribriform plate for the passage of the **anterior ethmoidal nerve** into the nasal cavity. The upper surface of the cribriform plate supports the **olfactory bulbs**, and the small perforations in the cribriform plate are for the **olfactory nerves**.

Middle Cranial Fossa

The middle cranial fossa consists of a small median part and expanded lateral parts (see Fig. 5-6). The median raised part is formed by the body of the sphenoid, and

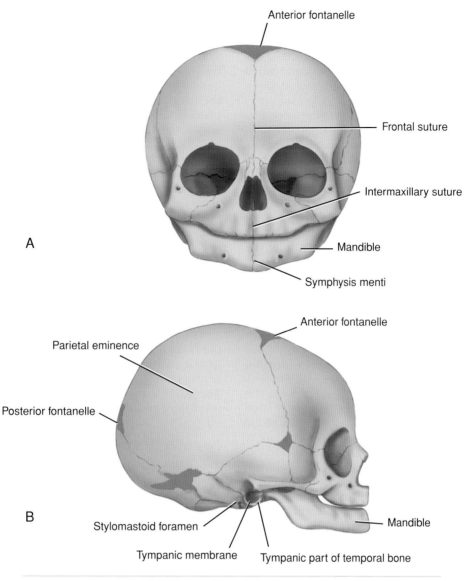

Anterior fontanelle

Frontal suture

Intermaxillary suture

Mandible

Symphysis menti

A

Anterior fontanelle

Parietal eminence

Posterior fontanelle

Stylomastoid foramen

Tympanic membrane

Tympanic part of temporal bone

Mandible

B

Figure 5-7 Neonatal skull as seen from the anterior (**A**) and lateral (**B**) aspects.

the expanded lateral parts form concavities on either side, which lodge the **temporal lobes** of the **cerebral hemispheres**.

It is bounded anteriorly by the sharp posterior edges of the lesser wings of the sphenoid and posteriorly by the superior borders of the petrous parts of the temporal bones. Laterally lie the squamous parts of the temporal bones, the greater wings of the sphenoid, and the parietal bones.

The floor of each lateral part of the middle cranial fossa is formed by the greater wing of the sphenoid and the squamous and petrous parts of the temporal bone.

The sphenoid bone resembles a bat having a centrally placed **body** with **greater** and **lesser wings** that are outstretched on each side. The body of the sphenoid contains the **sphenoid air sinuses**, which are lined

with mucous membrane and communicate with the nasal cavity; they serve as voice resonators.

Anteriorly, the **optic** canal transmits the optic nerve and the ophthalmic artery, a branch of the internal carotid artery, to the orbit. The **superior** orbital fissure, which is a slitlike opening between the lesser and greater wings of the sphenoid, transmits the lacrimal, frontal, trochlear, oculomotor, nasociliary, and abducens nerves, together with the superior ophthalmic vein. The sphenoparietal venous sinus runs medially along the posterior border of the lesser wing of the sphenoid and drains into the cavernous sinus.

The **foramen** rotundum, which is situated behind the medial end of the superior orbital fissure, perforates the greater wing of the sphenoid and transmits the maxillary nerve from the trigeminal ganglion to the pterygopalatine fossa.

The **foramen ovale** lies posterolateral to the foramen rotundum. It perforates the greater wing of the sphenoid and transmits the large sensory root and small motor root of the mandibular nerve to the infratemporal fossa.

The small **foramen spinosum** lies posterolateral to the foramen ovale and also perforates the greater wing of the sphenoid. The foramen transmits the middle meningeal artery from the infratemporal fossa into the cranial cavity. The artery then runs forward and laterally in a groove on the upper surface of the squamous part of the temporal bone and the greater wing of the sphenoid. After a short distance, the artery divides into anterior and posterior branches. The anterior branch passes forward and upward to the anteroinferior angle of the parietal bone (see Fig. 15-5). Here, the bone is deeply grooved or tunneled by the artery for a short distance before it runs backward and upward on the parietal bone. At this site, the artery may be damaged after a blow to the side of the head. The posterior branch passes backward and upward across the squamous part of the temporal bone to reach the parietal bone.

The large and irregularly shaped **foramen lacerum** lies between the apex of the petrous part of the temporal bone and the sphenoid bone (see Fig. 5-6). The inferior opening of the foramen lacerum in life is filled by cartilage and fibrous tissue, and only small blood vessels pass through this tissue from the cranial cavity to the neck.

The **carotid** canal opens into the side of the foramen lacerum above the closed inferior opening. The internal carotid artery enters the foramen through the carotid canal and immediately turns upward to reach the side of the body of the sphenoid bone. Here, the artery turns forward in the cavernous sinus to reach the region of the anterior clinoid process. At this point, the internal carotid artery turns vertically upward, medial to the anterior clinoid process, and emerges from the cavernous sinus (see Fig. 5-6).

Lateral to the foramen lacerum is an impression on the apex of the petrous part of the temporal bone for the **trigeminal ganglion**. On the anterior surface of the petrous bone are two grooves for nerves; the largest medial groove is for the **greater petrosal nerve**, a branch of the facial nerve; the smaller lateral groove is for the **lesser petrosal nerve**, a branch of the tympanic plexus. The greater petrosal nerve enters the foramen lacerum deep to the trigeminal ganglion and joins the **deep petrosal nerve** (sympathetic fibers from around the internal carotid artery), to form the **nerve of the pterygoid canal**. The lesser petrosal nerve passes forward to the foramen ovale.

The abducens nerve bends sharply forward across the apex of the petrous bone, medial to the trigeminal ganglion. Here, it leaves the posterior cranial fossa and enters the cavernous sinus.

The **arcuate eminence** is a rounded eminence found on the anterior surface of the petrous bone and is caused by the underlying **superior semicircular canal**.

The **tegmen tympani**, a thin plate of bone, is a forward extension of the petrous part of the temporal bone and adjoins the squamous part of the bone. From behind forward, it forms the roof of the mastoid antrum, the tympanic cavity, and the auditory tube. This thin plate of bone is the only major barrier that separates infection in the tympanic cavity from the temporal lobe of the cerebral hemisphere.

The median part of the middle cranial fossa is formed by the body of the sphenoid bone. In front is the **sulcus chiasmatis**, which is related to the optic chiasma and leads laterally to the **optic canal** on each side. Posterior to the sulcus is an elevation, the **tuberculum sellae**. Behind the elevation is a deep depression, the **sella turcica**, which lodges the **hypophysis cerebri**. The sella turcica is bounded posteriorly by a square plate of bone called the **dorsum sellae**. The superior angles of the dorsum sellae have two tubercles, called the **posterior clinoid processes**, which give attachment to the fixed margin of the tentorium cerebelli.

The cavernous sinus is directly related to the side of the body of the sphenoid (see Fig. 5-6). It carries in its lateral wall the third and fourth CNs and the ophthalmic and maxillary divisions of the fifth CN (see Fig. 15-6). The internal carotid artery and the sixth CN pass forward through the sinus.

Posterior Cranial Fossa

The posterior cranial fossa is deep and lodges the parts of the hindbrain, namely, the **cerebellum**, **pons**, and **medulla oblongata**. Anteriorly, the fossa is bounded by the superior border of the petrous part of the temporal bone; posteriorly, it is bounded by the internal surface of the squamous part of the occipital bone (see Fig. 5-6). The floor of the posterior fossa is formed by the basilar, condylar, and squamous parts of the occipital bone and the mastoid part of the temporal bone.

The roof of the fossa is formed by a fold of dura, the **tentorium cerebelli**, which intervenes between the cerebellum below and the occipital lobes of the cerebral hemispheres above (see Fig. 15-3).

The **foramen magnum** occupies the central area of the floor and transmits the medulla oblongata and its surrounding meninges, the ascending spinal parts of the accessory nerves, and the two vertebral arteries.

The **hypoglossal canal** is situated above the anterolateral boundary of the foramen magnum (see Fig. 5-6) and transmits the **hypoglossal nerve**.

The **jugular foramen** lies between the lower border of the petrous part of the temporal bone and the condylar part of the occipital bone. It transmits the following structures from before backward: the **inferior petrosal sinus**; the **9th, 10th, and 11th CNs**; and the large **sigmoid sinus**. The inferior petrosal sinus descends in the groove on the lower border of the petrous part of the temporal bone to reach the foramen. The sigmoid

Table 5-1   Important Openings in the Base of the Skull and the Structures That Pass Through Them

Opening in Skull	Bone of Skull	Structures Transmitted
Anterior Cranial Fossa		
Perforations in cribriform plate	Ethmoid	Olfactory nerves
Middle Cranial Fossa		
Optic canal	Lesser wing of sphenoid	Optic nerve, ophthalmic artery
Superior orbital fissure	Between lesser and greater wings of sphenoid	Lacrimal, frontal, trochlear oculomotor, nasociliary, and abducens nerves; superior ophthalmic vein
Foramen rotundum	Greater wing of sphenoid	Maxillary division of the trigeminal nerve
Foramen ovale	Greater wing of sphenoid	Mandibular division of the trigeminal nerve, lesser petrosal nerve
Foramen spinosum	Greater wing of sphenoid	Middle meningeal artery
Foramen lacerum	Between petrous part of temporal and sphenoid	Internal carotid artery
Posterior Cranial Fossa		
Foramen magnum	Occipital	Medulla oblongata, spinal part of accessory nerve, and right and left vertebral arteries
Hypoglossal canal	Occipital	Hypoglossal nerve
Jugular foramen	Between petrous part of temporal and condylar part of occipital	Glossopharyngeal, vagus, and accessory nerves; sigmoid sinus becomes internal jugular vein
Internal acoustic meatus	Petrous part of temporal	Vestibulocochlear and facial nerves

sinus turns down through the foramen to become the **internal jugular vein**.

The **internal acoustic meatus** pierces the posterior surface of the petrous part of the temporal bone. It transmits the vestibulocochlear nerve and the motor and sensory roots of the facial nerve.

The **internal occipital crest** runs upward in the midline posteriorly from the foramen magnum to the **internal occipital protuberance;** it is attached the small **falx cerebelli** over the **occipital sinus**.

On each side of the internal occipital protuberance is a wide groove for the **transverse sinus**. This groove sweeps around on either side, on the internal surface of the occipital bone, to reach the posteroinferior angle or corner of the parietal bone. The groove now passes onto the mastoid part of the temporal bone; at this point, the transverse sinus becomes the **sigmoid sinus**. The **superior petrosal sinus** runs backward along the upper border of the petrous bone in a narrow groove and drains into the sigmoid sinus. As the sigmoid sinus descends to the jugular foramen, it deeply grooves the back of the petrous bone and the mastoid part of the temporal bone. Here, it lies directly posterior to the mastoid antrum.

Table 5-1 summarizes the important openings in the base of the skull and the structures that pass through them.

Mandible

The mandible, or lower jaw, is the largest and strongest bone of the face, and it articulates with the skull at the **temporomandibular joint** (see Fig. 5-3).

The mandible consists of a horseshoe-shaped **body** and a pair of **rami** (see Fig. 5-1). The body of the mandible meets the ramus on each side at the **angle of the mandible**.

INTRODUCTION TO THE BRAINSTEM

The brainstem is made up of the medulla oblongata, the pons, and the midbrain and occupies the posterior cranial fossa of the skull (Fig. 5-8). It is stalklike in shape and connects the narrow spinal cord with the expanded forebrain (see Atlas Plates 1–8).

The brainstem has three broad functions: (1) It serves as a conduit for the ascending tracts and descending tracts connecting the spinal cord to the different parts of the higher centers in the forebrain; (2) it contains important reflex centers associated with the control of respiration and the cardiovascular system and with the control of consciousness; and (3) it contains the important nuclei of CNs III through XII.

MEDULLA OBLONGATA

The medulla oblongata connects the pons superiorly with the spinal cord inferiorly (see Fig. 5-8). The junction of the medulla and spinal cord is at the origin of the anterior and posterior roots of the first cervical spinal nerve, which corresponds approximately to the level of the foramen magnum. The medulla oblongata is conical in shape, its broad extremity being directed superiorly (Fig. 5-9). The **central** canal of the spinal cord continues upward into the lower half of the medulla; in the upper half of the medulla, it expands as the **cavity** of the fourth ventricle.

On the anterior surface of the medulla is the anterior median fissure, which is continuous inferiorly with the **anterior median fissure** of the spinal cord (see Fig. 5-9A). Swellings on each side of the median fissure are called the **pyramids**. The pyramids are composed of bundles of nerve fibers, called corticospinal fibers, which originate in large nerve cells in the precentral gyrus of the cerebral cortex. The pyramids taper inferiorly, and here the majority of the descending fibers cross over to the opposite side, forming the **decussation of the pyramids**. The **anterior external arcuate fibers** emerge from the anterior median fissure above the decussation and pass laterally over the surface of the medulla oblongata to enter the cerebellum. Posterolateral to the pyramids are the **olives**, which are oval elevations produced by the underlying **inferior olivary nuclei**. In the groove between the pyramid and the olive emerge the rootlets of the hypoglossal nerve. Posterior to the olives are the **inferior cerebellar peduncles**, which connect the medulla to the cerebellum. In the groove between the olive and the inferior cerebellar peduncle emerge the roots of the glossopharyngeal and vagus nerves and the cranial roots of the accessory nerve.

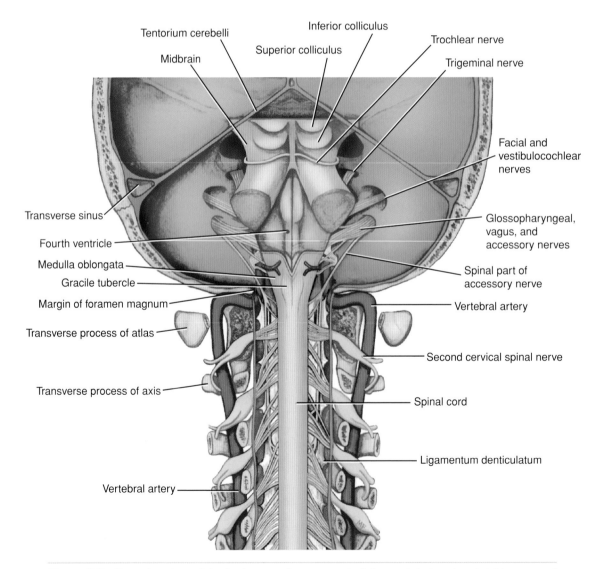

Figure 5-8 Posterior view of the brainstem after removal of the occipital and parietal bones and the cerebrum, the cerebellum, and the roof of the fourth ventricle. Laminae of the upper cervical vertebrae have also been removed.

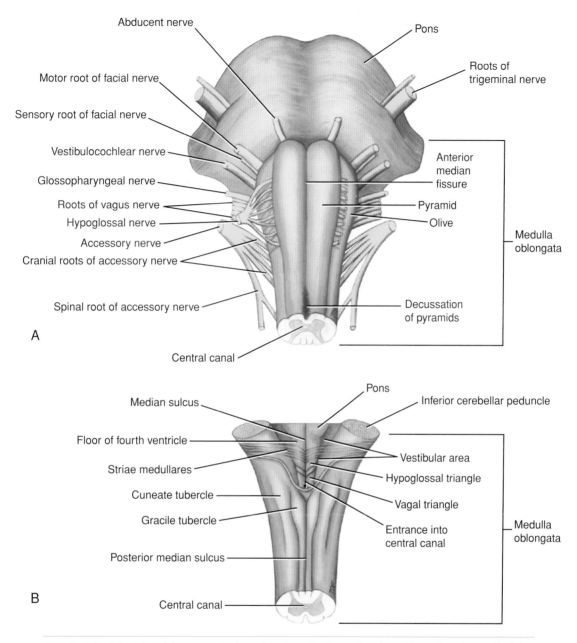

Figure 5-9   Medulla oblongata. **A:** Anterior view. **B:** Posterior view. Note that the roof of the fourth ventricle and the cerebellum have been removed.

The posterior surface of the superior half of the medulla oblongata forms the lower part of the **floor of the fourth ventricle** (see Fig. 5-9B). The posterior surface of the inferior half of the medulla is continuous with the posterior aspect of the spinal cord and possesses a **posterior median sulcus**. On each side of the median sulcus, an elongated swelling, the gracile tubercle, is produced by the underlying **gracile nucleus**. Lateral to the gracile tubercle is a similar swelling, the **cuneate tubercle**, produced by the underlying **cuneate nucleus**.

Internal Structure

As in the spinal cord, the medulla oblongata consists of white matter and gray matter, but a study of

transverse sections of this region shows that they have been extensively rearranged. This rearrangement can be explained embryologically by the expansion of the **neural tube** to form the **hindbrain vesicle**, which becomes the fourth ventricle (Fig. 5-10). The extensive lateral spread of the **fourth ventricle** results in an alteration in the position of the derivatives of the **alar** and **basal plates** of the embryo. To assist in understanding this concept, remember that, in the spinal cord, the derivatives of the alar and basal plates are situated posterior and anterior to the **sulcus limitans**, respectively; in the case of the medulla oblongata, they are situated lateral and medial to the sulcus limitans, respectively.

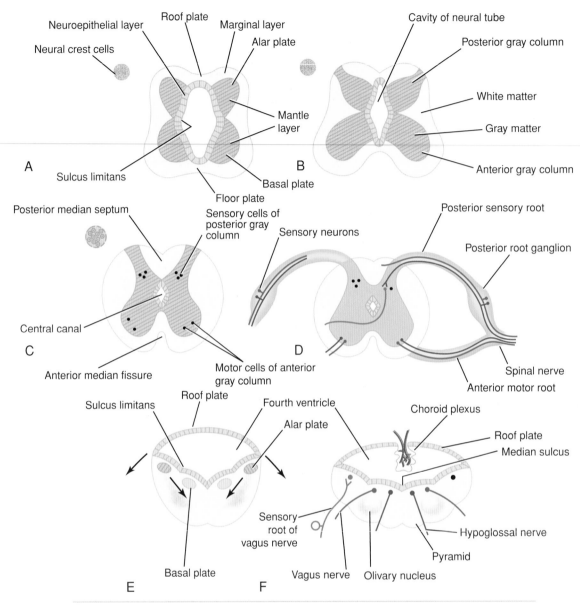

Figure 5-10 Stages in the development of the spinal cord (**A–D**) and the medulla oblongata (**E, F**). The neural crest cells will form the first afferent sensory neurons in the posterior root ganglia of the spinal nerves and the sensory ganglia of the cranial nerves.

The internal structure of the medulla oblongata is considered at four levels: (1) level of decussation of pyramids, (2) level of decussation of lemnisci, (3) level of the olives, and (4) level just inferior to the pons. Table 5-2 compares the different levels of the medulla oblongata and the major structures present at each level.

Level of Pyramid Decussation

A transverse section through the inferior half of the medulla oblongata (Figs. 5-11A and 5-12) passes through the **decussation** of the pyramids, the great motor decussation. In the superior part of the medulla, the corticospinal fibers occupy and form the pyramid, but inferiorly, about three-fourths of the fibers cross the median plane and continue down the spinal cord in the lateral white column as the **lateral** corticospinal tract. As these fibers cross the midline, they sever the continuity between the anterior column of the gray matter of the spinal cord and the gray matter that surrounds the central canal.

The **fasciculus gracilis** and the **fasciculus cuneatus** continue to ascend superiorly posterior to the central gray matter. The **nucleus gracilis** and the **nucleus cuneatus** appear as posterior extensions of the central gray matter.

Table 5-2   Levels of the Medulla Oblongata and Their Major Structures[a]

Level	Cavity	Nuclei	Motor Tracts	Sensory Tracts
Decussation of pyramids	Central canal	Nucleus gracilis, nucleus cuneatus, spinal nucleus of CN V, accessory nucleus	Decussation of corticospinal tracts, pyramids	Spinal tract of CN V, posterior spinocerebellar tract, lateral spinothalamic tract, anterior spinocerebellar tract
Decussation of medial lemnisci	Central canal	Nucleus gracilis, nucleus cuneatus, spinal nucleus of CN V, accessory nucleus, hypoglossal nucleus	Pyramids	Decussation of medial lemnisci, fasciculus gracilis, fasciculus cuneatus, spinal tract of CN V, posterior spinocerebellar tract, lateral spinothalamic tract, anterior spinocerebellar tract
Olives, inferior cerebellar peduncle	Fourth ventricle	Inferior olivary nucleus, spinal nucleus of CN V, vestibular nucleus, glossopharyngeal nucleus, vagal nucleus, hypoglossal nucleus, nucleus ambiguus, nucleus of tractus solitarius	Pyramids	Medial longitudinal fasciculus, tectospinal tract, medial lemniscus, spinal tract of CN V, lateral spinothalamic tract, anterior spinocerebellar tract
Just inferior to pons	Fourth ventricle	Lateral vestibular nucleus, cochlear nuclei		No major changes in distribution of gray and white matter

[a]Note that the reticular formation is present at all levels.
CN, cranial nerve.

The **substantia gelatinosa** in the posterior gray column of the spinal cord becomes continuous with the inferior end of the **nucleus of the spinal tract of the trigeminal nerve**. The fibers of the tract of the nucleus are situated between the nucleus and the surface of the medulla oblongata.

The lateral and anterior white columns of the spinal cord are easily identified in these sections, and their fiber arrangement is unchanged.

Level of Lemnisci Decussation

A transverse section through the inferior half of the medulla oblongata, a short distance above the level of the decussation of the pyramids, passes through the **decussation of lemnisci**, the great sensory decussation (Fig. 5-13; also see Fig. 5-11B). The decussation of the lemnisci takes place anterior to the central gray matter and posterior to the pyramids. It should be understood that the lemnisci have been formed from the **internal arcuate fibers**, which have emerged from the anterior aspects of the **nucleus gracilis** and **nucleus cuneatus**. The internal arcuate fibers first travel anteriorly and laterally around the central gray matter. They then curve medially toward the midline, where they decussate with the corresponding fibers of the opposite side.

The **nucleus of the spinal tract of the trigeminal nerve** lies lateral to the internal arcuate fibers. The **spinal tract of the trigeminal nerve** lies lateral to the nucleus.

The **lateral** and **anterior spinothalamic tracts** and the **spinotectal tracts** occupy an area lateral to the decussation of the lemnisci. They are very close to one another and collectively are known as the **spinal**

lemniscus. The **spinocerebellar, vestibulospinal,** and the **rubrospinal tracts** are situated in the anterolateral region of the medulla oblongata.

Level of the Olives

A transverse section through the olives passes across the inferior part of the fourth ventricle (Figs. 5-14 and 5-15). The amount of gray matter has increased at this level owing to the presence of the olivary nuclear complex; the nuclei of the vestibulocochlear, glossopharyngeal, vagus, accessory, and hypoglossal nerves; and the arcuate nuclei.

Olivary Nuclear Complex

The largest nucleus of this complex is the **inferior olivary nucleus**. The gray matter is shaped like a crumpled bag with its mouth directed medially; it is responsible for the elevation on the surface of the medulla called the **olive**. Smaller **dorsal** and **medial accessory olivary nuclei** also are present. The cells of the inferior olivary nucleus send fibers medially across the midline to enter the cerebellum through the inferior cerebellar peduncle. Afferent fibers reach the inferior olivary nuclei from the spinal cord (the **spino-olivary tracts**) and from the cerebellum and cerebral cortex. The function of the olivary nuclei is associated with voluntary muscle movement.

Vestibulocochlear Nuclei

The **vestibular nuclear complex** is made up of the following nuclei: (1) **medial vestibular nucleus**, (2) **inferior vestibular nucleus**, (3) **lateral vestibular nucleus**, and (4) **superior vestibular nucleus**. The details of these nuclei and their connections are discussed later.

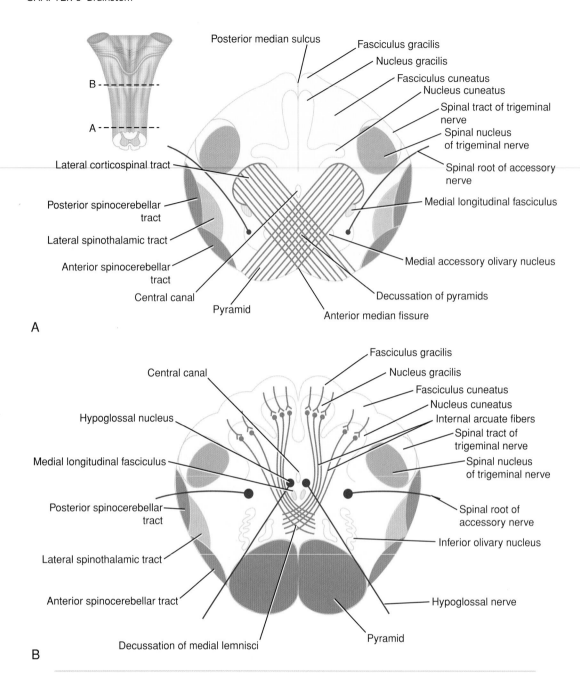

Figure 5-11 Transverse sections of the medulla oblongata. **A:** Level of decussation of the pyramids. **B:** Level of decussation of the medial lemnisci.

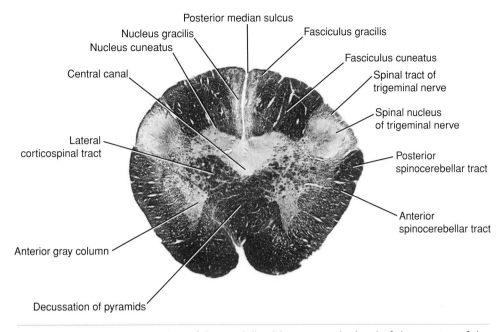

Figure 5-12 Transverse section of the medulla oblongata at the level of decussation of the pyramids. (Weigert stain.)

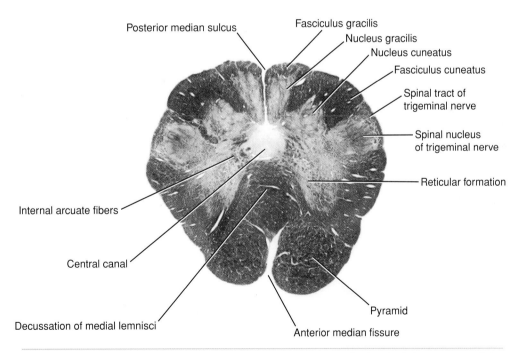

Figure 5-13 Transverse section of the medulla oblongata at the level of decussation of the medial lemnisci. (Weigert stain.)

A

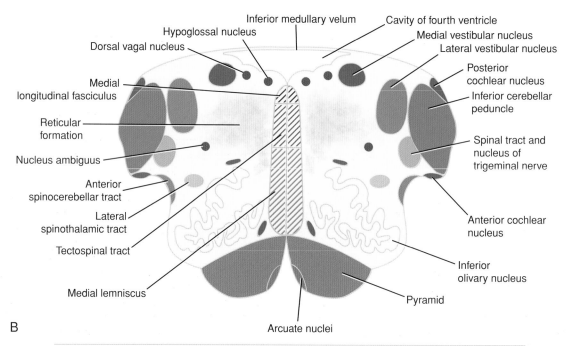

B

Figure 5-14 Transverse sections of the medulla oblongata at the level of the middle of the olivary nuclei (**A**) and the superior part of the olivary nuclei just inferior to the pons (**B**).

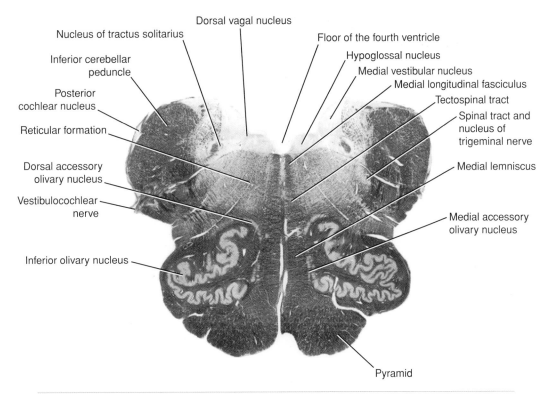

Dorsal vagal nucleus

Nucleus of tractus solitarius

Floor of the fourth ventricle

Inferior cerebellar peduncle

Hypoglossal nucleus

Posterior cochlear nucleus

Medial vestibular nucleus

Medial longitudinal fasciculus

Reticular formation

Tectospinal tract

Spinal tract and nucleus of trigeminal nerve

Dorsal accessory olivary nucleus

Medial lemniscus

Vestibulocochlear nerve

Medial accessory olivary nucleus

Inferior olivary nucleus

Pyramid

Figure 5-15 Transverse section of the medulla oblongata at the level of the middle of the olivary nuclei. (Weigert stain.)

The medial and inferior vestibular nuclei can be seen on section at this level.

The two **cochlear nuclei** are the **anterior cochlear nucleus**, situated on the anterolateral aspect of the inferior cerebellar peduncle, and the **posterior cochlear nucleus**, situated on the posterior aspect of the peduncle lateral to the floor of the fourth ventricle. The connections of these nuclei are described later (see pp. 204-207).

Nucleus Ambiguus

The nucleus ambiguus consists of large motor neurons and is situated deep within the reticular formation (Fig. 5-16; also see Fig. 5-14). The emerging nerve fibers join the glossopharyngeal, vagus, and cranial part of the accessory nerve and are distributed to voluntary skeletal muscle.

Central Gray Matter

The central gray matter lies beneath the floor of the fourth ventricle at this level (see Figs. 5-14 and 5-15). Passing from medial to lateral (see Fig. 5-16), the following important structures may be recognized: (1) the **hypoglossal nucleus**, (2) the **dorsal nucleus of the vagus**, (3) the **nucleus of the tractus solitarius**, and (4) the **medial** and **inferior vestibular nuclei**. The nucleus ambiguus has become deeply placed within the reticular formation (see Fig. 5-14). The connections and functional significance of these nuclei are described in Chapter 11.

The arcuate nuclei are thought to be inferiorly displaced **pontine nuclei** (see pp. 206-207) and are situated on the anterior surface of the pyramids. They receive nerve fibers from the cerebral cortex and send efferent fibers to the cerebellum through the **anterior external arcuate fibers**.

The **pyramids** containing the corticospinal and some corticonuclear fibers are situated in the anterior part of the medulla separated by the anterior median fissure (see Figs. 5-14 and 5-15); the corticospinal fibers descend to the spinal cord, and the corticonuclear fibers are distributed to the motor nuclei of the CNs situated within the medulla.

The **medial lemniscus** forms a flattened tract on each side of the midline posterior to the pyramid (see Figs. 5-7 and 5-15). These fibers emerge from the decussation of the lemnisci and convey sensory information to the thalamus.

The **medial longitudinal fasciculus** forms a small tract of nerve fibers situated on each side of the midline posterior to the medial lemniscus and anterior to the hypoglossal nucleus (see Figs. 5-14 and 5-15). It consists of ascending and descending fibers, the connections of which are described on page 205.

The **inferior cerebellar peduncle** is situated in the posterolateral corner of the section on the lateral side of the fourth ventricle.

The **spinal tract of the trigeminal nerve** and **its nucleus** are situated on the anteromedial aspect of the inferior cerebellar peduncle.

Figure 5-16 Position of the cranial nerve nuclei within the brainstem. The hatched area indicates the position of the vestibular nuclei.

The **anterior spinocerebellar tract** is situated near the surface in the interval between the inferior olivary nucleus and the nucleus of the spinal tract of the trigeminal nerve. The **spinal lemniscus**, consisting of the **anterior spinothalamic**, the **lateral spinothalamic**, and **spinotectal tracts**, is deeply placed.

The **reticular formation**, consisting of a diffuse mixture of nerve fibers and small groups of nerve cells, is deeply placed posterior to the olivary nucleus. The reticular formation represents, at this level, only a small part of this system, which is also present in the pons and midbrain.

The **glossopharyngeal**, **vagus**, and **cranial part of the accessory nerves** can be seen running forward and laterally through the reticular formation (see Fig. 5-14). The nerve fibers emerge between the olives and the inferior cerebellar peduncles. The **hypoglossal nerves** also run anteriorly and laterally through the reticular formation and emerge between the pyramids and the olives.

Level Just Inferior to the Pons

In comparison to the previous level, little changes in the distribution of the gray and white matter (see Figs. 5-14 and 5-16). The lateral vestibular nucleus has replaced the inferior vestibular nucleus, and the cochlear nuclei now are visible on the anterior and posterior surfaces of the inferior cerebellar peduncle.

PONS

The pons is anterior to the cerebellum (Fig. 5-17; see also Fig. 6-1) and connects the medulla oblongata to the midbrain. It is about 1 inch (2.5 cm) long and owes its name to the appearance presented on the anterior surface, which is that of a bridge connecting the right and left cerebellar hemispheres.

The anterior surface is convex from side to side and shows many transverse fibers that converge on each side to form the **middle cerebellar peduncle**. A shallow groove in the midline, the **basilar groove**, lodges the basilar artery. On the anterolateral surface of the pons, the **trigeminal nerve** emerges on each side. Each nerve consists of a smaller, medial part, known as the **motor root**, and a larger, lateral part, known as the **sensory root**. In the groove between the pons and the medulla oblongata, from medial to lateral, the **abducens**, **facial**, and **vestibulocochlear nerves** emerge.

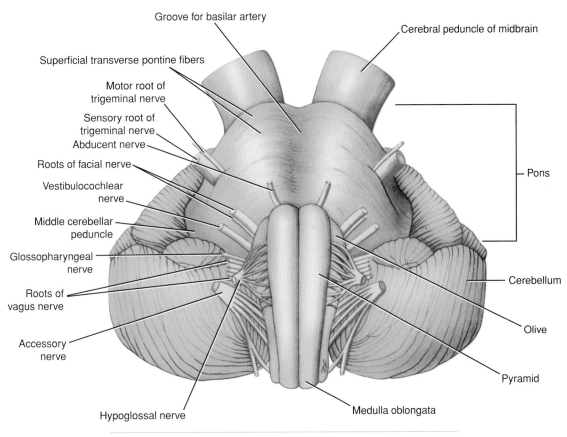

Groove for basilar artery

Cerebral peduncle of midbrain

Superficial transverse pontine fibers

Motor root of
trigeminal nerve

Sensory root of
trigeminal nerve

Abducent nerve

Roots of facial nerve

Vestibulocochlear
nerve

Middle cerebellar
peduncle

Glossopharyngeal
nerve

Roots of
vagus nerve

Accessory
nerve

Pons

Cerebellum

Olive

Pyramid

Hypoglossal nerve

Medulla oblongata

Figure 5-17 Anterior surface of the brainstem showing the pons.

The posterior surface of the pons is hidden from view by the cerebellum (Fig. 5-18). It forms the upper half of the floor of the fourth ventricle and is triangular in shape. The posterior surface is limited laterally by the **superior cerebellar peduncles** and is divided into symmetrical halves by a **median sulcus**. Lateral to this sulcus is an elongated elevation, the **medial eminence**, which is bounded laterally by a sulcus, the **sulcus limitans**. The inferior end of the medial eminence is slightly expanded to form the **facial colliculus**, which is produced by the root of the facial nerve winding around the nucleus of the abducens nerve (Fig. 5-19). The floor of the superior part of the **sulcus limitans** is bluish-gray in color and is called the **substantia ferruginea**; it owes its color to a group of deeply pigmented nerve cells. Lateral to the sulcus limitans is the **area vestibuli** produced by the underlying vestibular nuclei (see Fig. 5-18).

Internal Structure

For purposes of description, the pons is commonly divided into a posterior part, the **tegmentum**, and an anterior **basal part** by the transversely running fibers of the **trapezoid body** (see Fig. 5-19).

The structure of the pons may be studied at two levels: (1) transverse section through the caudal part, passing through the facial colliculus, and (2) transverse section through the cranial part, passing through the trigeminal nuclei. Table 5-3 compares the two levels of the pons and the major structures present at each level.

Transverse Section Through the Caudal Part

The **medial lemniscus** rotates as it passes from the medulla into the pons. It is situated in the most anterior part of the tegmentum, with its long axis running transversely. The medial lemniscus is accompanied by the spinal and lateral lemnisci.

The **facial nucleus** lies posterior to the lateral part of the medial lemniscus. The fibers of the facial nerve wind around the **nucleus of the abducens nerve**, producing the **facial colliculus**. The fibers of the facial nerve then pass anteriorly between the facial nucleus and the superior end of the nucleus of the spinal tract of the trigeminal nerve.

The **medial longitudinal fasciculus** is situated beneath the floor of the fourth ventricle on either side of the midline. The medial longitudinal fasciculus is the main pathway that connects the vestibular and cochlear nuclei with the nuclei controlling the extraocular muscles (oculomotor, trochlear, and abducens nuclei).

The **medial vestibular nucleus** is situated lateral to the abducens nucleus and is in close relationship to the inferior cerebellar peduncle. The superior part of the

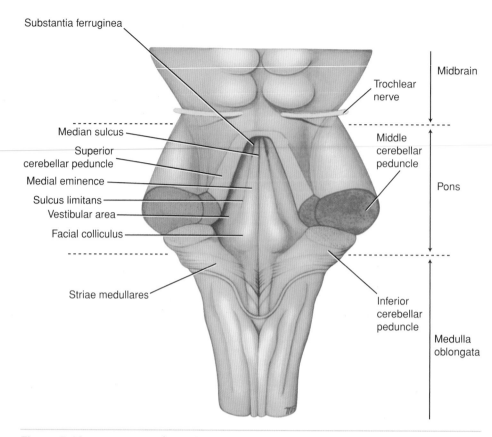

Figure 5-18   Posterior surface of the brainstem showing the pons. The cerebellum has been removed.

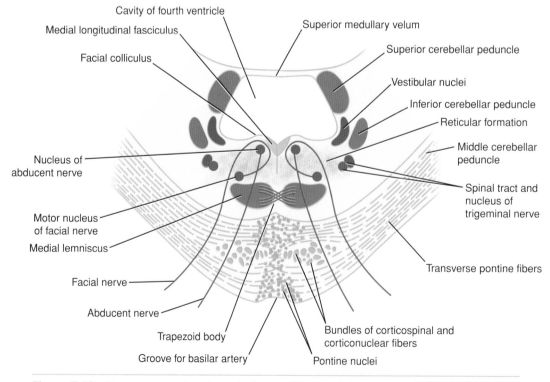

Figure 5-19   Transverse section through the caudal part of the pons at the level of the facial colliculus.

Table 5-3   Levels of the Pons and Their Major Structures[a]

Level	Cavity	Nuclei	Motor Tracts	Sensory Tracts
Facial colliculus	Fourth ventricle	Facial nucleus, abducens nucleus, medial vestibular nucleus, spinal nucleus of CN V, pontine nuclei, trapezoid nuclei	Corticospinal and corticonuclear tracts, transverse pontine fibers, medial longitudinal fasciculus	Spinal tract of CN V; lateral, spinal, and medial lemnisci
Trigeminal nuclei	Fourth ventricle	Main sensory and motor nucleus of CN V, pontine nuclei, trapezoid nuclei	Corticospinal and corticonuclear tracts, transverse pontine fibers, medial longitudinal fasciculus	Lateral, spinal, and medial lemnisci

[a]Note that the reticular formation is present at all levels.
CN, cranial nerve.

lateral and the inferior part of the superior vestibular nucleus are found at this level. The **posterior** and **anterior cochlear nuclei** are also found at this level.

The **spinal nucleus of the trigeminal nerve** and its tract lie on the anteromedial aspect of the inferior cerebellar peduncle.

The **trapezoid body** is made up of fibers derived from the cochlear nuclei and the nuclei of the trapezoid body. They run transversely in the anterior part of the tegmentum (see p. 210).

The basilar part of the pons, at this level, contains small masses of nerve cells called **pontine nuclei**. The **corticopontine fibers** of the crus cerebri of the midbrain terminate in the pontine nuclei. The axons of these cells give origin to the **transverse fibers** of the pons, which cross the midline and intersect the corticospinal

and corticonuclear tracts, breaking them up into small bundles. The transverse fibers of the pons enter the middle cerebellar peduncle and are distributed to the cerebellar hemisphere. This connection forms the main pathway linking the cerebral cortex to the cerebellum.

Transverse Section Through the Cranial Part

The internal structure of the cranial part of the pons is similar to that seen at the caudal level (Figs. 5-20 to 5-22), but it now contains the motor and principal sensory nuclei of the trigeminal nerve.

The **motor nucleus of the trigeminal nerve** is situated beneath the lateral part of the fourth ventricle within the reticular formation (see Figs. 5-20 and 5-21). The emerging motor fibers travel anteriorly through

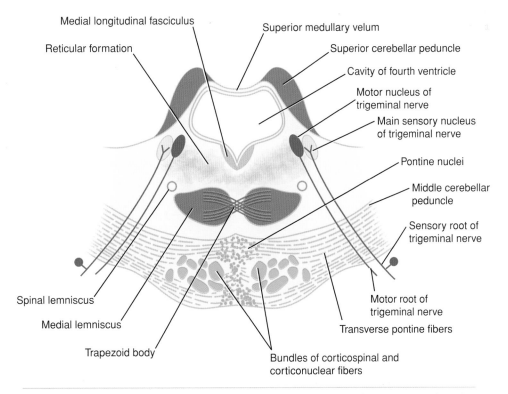

Figure 5-20   Transverse section through the pons at the level of the trigeminal nuclei.

Figure 5-21 Photomicrograph of a transverse section of the pons at the level of the trigeminal nuclei.

the substance of the pons and exit on its anterior surface.

The **principal** sensory nucleus of the trigeminal nerve is situated on the lateral side of the motor nucleus; it is continuous inferiorly with the nucleus of the spinal tract. The entering sensory fibers travel

through the substance of the pons and lie lateral to the motor fibers (see Fig. 5-20).

The **superior cerebellar peduncle** is situated posterolateral to the motor nucleus of the trigeminal nerve (see Figs. 5-20 and 5-21). It is joined by the **anterior spinocerebellar tract**.

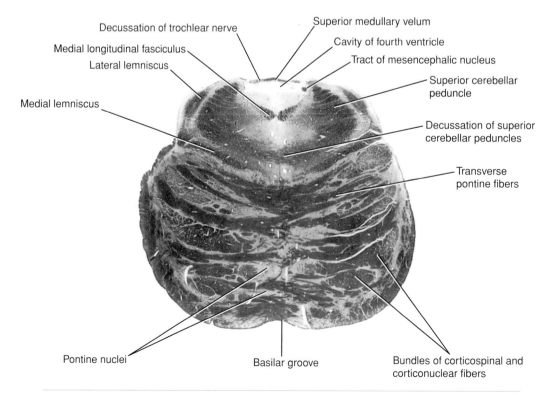

Figure 5-22 Photomicrograph of a transverse section of the most rostral part of the pons.

The **trapezoid body** and the **medial lemniscus** are situated in the same position as they were in the previous section (see Fig. 5-20). The **lateral** and **spinal lemnisci** lie at the lateral extremity of the medial lemniscus (see Figs. 5-20 and 5-22).

MIDBRAIN

The midbrain measures about 0.8 in (2 cm) in length and connects the pons and cerebellum with the forebrain (Fig. 5-23). Its long axis inclines anteriorly as it ascends through the opening in the tentorium cerebelli. The midbrain is traversed by a narrow channel, the **cerebral aqueduct**, which is filled with cerebrospinal fluid (Figs. 5-24 to 5-28).

On the posterior surface are four **colliculi** (corpora quadrigemina). These are rounded eminences that are divided into superior and inferior pairs by a vertical and a transverse groove (see Fig. 5-26). The superior colliculi are centers for visual reflexes (see p. 213), and the inferior colliculi are lower auditory centers. In the midline below the inferior colliculi, the **trochlear** nerves emerge. These are small-diameter nerves that wind around the lateral aspect of the midbrain to enter the lateral wall of the cavernous sinus.

On the lateral aspect of the midbrain, the superior and inferior brachia ascend in an anterolateral direction (see Fig. 5-23B). The **superior brachium** passes from the superior colliculus to the lateral geniculate body and the optic tract. The **inferior brachium** connects the inferior colliculus to the **medial geniculate body**.

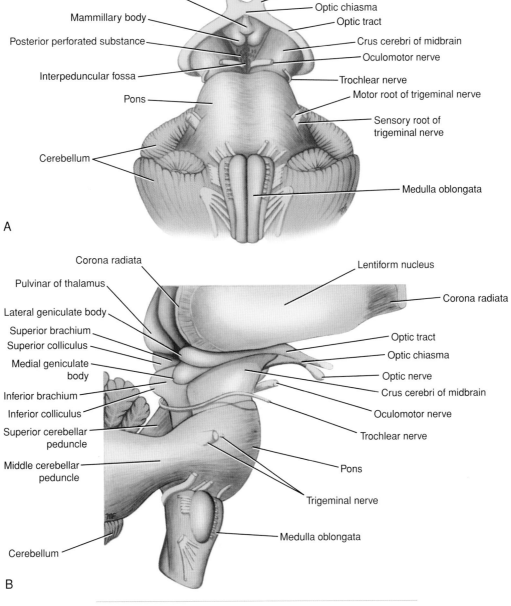

Figure 5-23   The midbrain. **A:** Anterior view. **B:** Lateral view.

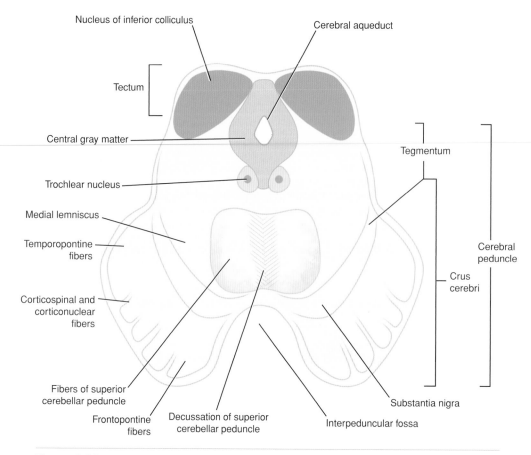

Figure 5-24 Transverse section of the midbrain through the inferior colliculi shows the division of the midbrain into the tectum and the cerebral peduncles. Note that the cerebral peduncles are subdivided by the substantia nigra into the tegmentum and the crus cerebri.

On the anterior aspect of the midbrain, a deep depression in the midline, the **interpeduncular fossa**, is bounded on either side by the **crus cerebri**. Many small blood vessels perforate the floor of the interpeduncular fossa, and this region is termed the **posterior perforated substance** (see Fig. 5-23A). The oculomotor nerve emerges from a groove on the medial side of the crus cerebri and passes forward in the lateral wall of the cavernous sinus.

Internal Structure

The midbrain comprises two lateral halves, called the **cerebral peduncles**; each of these is divided into an anterior part, the **crus cerebri**, and a posterior part, the **tegmentum**, by a pigmented band of gray matter, the **substantia nigra** (see Figs. 5-24 and 5-25). The narrow cavity of the midbrain is the **cerebral aqueduct**, which connects the third and fourth ventricles. The **tectum** is the part of the midbrain posterior to the cerebral aqueduct; it has four small surface swellings referred to previously; these are the **two superior** and **two inferior colliculi**. The cerebral aqueduct is lined by ependyma and is surrounded by the **central gray matter**. On transverse sections of the midbrain, the interpeduncular fossa can be seen to separate the crura cerebri, whereas the tegmentum is continuous across the median plane (see Fig. 5-24).

Transverse Section of the Midbrain at the Level of the Inferior Colliculi

The **inferior** colliculus, consisting of a large nucleus of gray matter, lies beneath the corresponding surface elevation and forms part of the auditory pathway (see Figs. 5-25A and 5-27). It receives many of the terminal fibers of the lateral lemniscus. The pathway then continues through the inferior brachium to the medial geniculate body.

The **trochlear nucleus** is situated in the central gray matter close to the median plane just posterior to the **medial longitudinal fasciculus**. The emerging fibers of the trochlear nucleus pass laterally and posteriorly around the central gray matter and leave the midbrain just below the inferior colliculi. The fibers of the trochlear nerve now **decussate completely** in the superior medullary velum. The **mesencephalic nuclei of the trigeminal nerve** are lateral to the cerebral aqueduct. The **decussation of the superior cerebellar peduncles** occupies the central part of the tegmentum anterior to the cerebral aqueduct. The **reticular formation** is smaller than that of the pons and is situated lateral to the decussation.

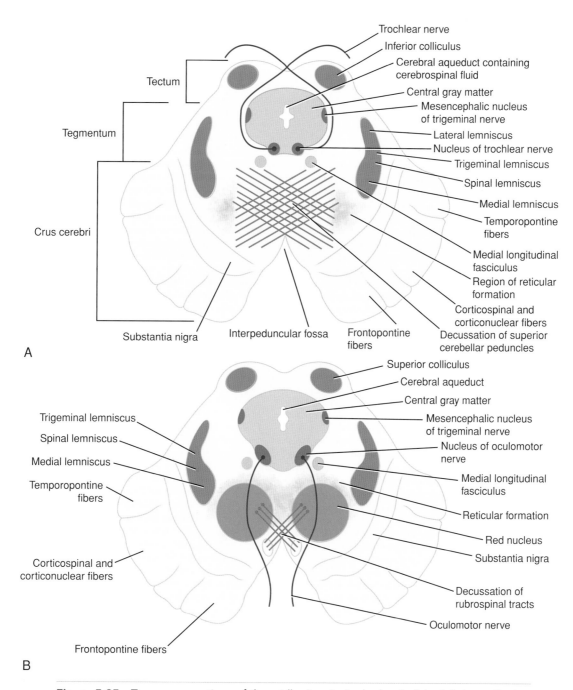

Figure 5-25 Transverse sections of the midbrain. **A:** At the level of the inferior colliculus. **B:** At the level of the superior colliculus. Note that trochlear nerves completely decussate within the superior medullary velum.

The **medial lemniscus** ascends posterior to the substantia nigra; the **spinal** and **trigeminal lemnisci** are situated lateral to the medial lemniscus (see Figs. 5-25 and 5-27). The **lateral lemniscus** is located posterior to the trigeminal lemniscus.

The **substantia nigra** is a large motor nucleus situated between the tegmentum, and the crus cerebri and is found throughout the midbrain. The nucleus is composed of medium-size multipolar neurons that

possess inclusion granules of melanin pigment within their cytoplasm. The substantia nigra is concerned with muscle tone and is connected to the cerebral cortex, spinal cord, hypothalamus, and basal nuclei.

The **crus cerebri** contains important descending tracts and is separated from the tegmentum by the substantia nigra. The corticospinal and corticonuclear fibers occupy the middle two thirds of the crus. The frontopontine fibers occupy the medial part of the crus, and

Figure 5-26 Posterior view of the brainstem showing the two superior and the two inferior colliculi of the tectum.

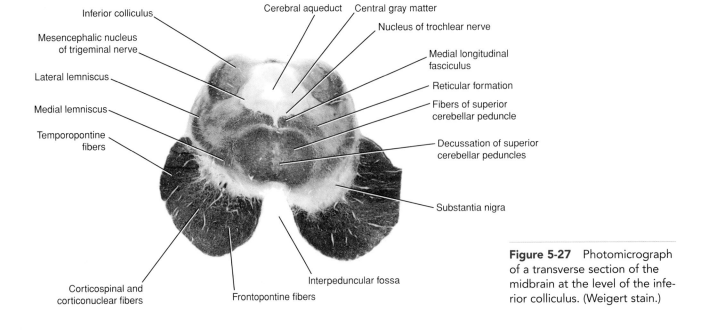

Figure 5-27 Photomicrograph of a transverse section of the midbrain at the level of the inferior colliculus. (Weigert stain.)

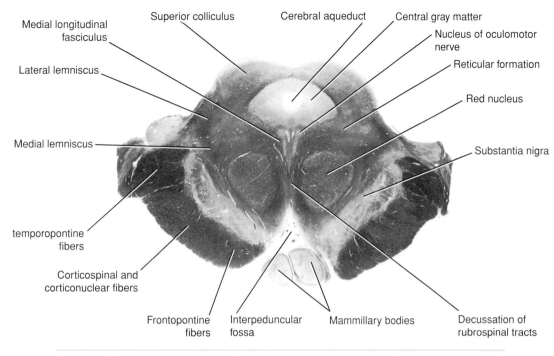

Figure 5-28 Photomicrograph of a transverse section of the midbrain at the level of the superior colliculus. (Weigert stain.)

the temporopontine fibers occupy the lateral part of the crus. These descending tracts connect the cerebral cortex to the anterior gray column cells of the spinal cord, the CN nuclei, the pons, and the cerebellum (Table 5-4).

Transverse Section of the Midbrain at the Level of the Superior Colliculi

The **superior colliculus** (see Figs. 5-25B and 5-28), a large nucleus of gray matter that lies beneath the corresponding surface elevation, forms part of the visual reflexes. It is connected to the lateral geniculate body by the superior brachium. It receives afferent fibers from the optic nerve, the visual cortex, and the spinotectal

tract. The efferent fibers form the tectospinal and tectobulbar tracts, which are probably responsible for the reflex movements of the eyes, head, and neck in response to visual stimuli. The afferent pathway for the **light reflex** ends in the **pretectal nucleus**. This is a small group of neurons situated close to the lateral part of the superior colliculus. After relaying in the pretectal nucleus, the fibers pass to the parasympathetic nucleus of the oculomotor nerve (Edinger–Westphal nucleus). The emerging fibers then pass to the oculomotor nerve. The **oculomotor nucleus** is situated in the central gray matter close to the median plane, just posterior to the **medial longitudinal fasciculus**. The fibers of the oculomotor nucleus pass anteriorly through the red nucleus

Table 5-4   Two Levels of the Midbrain and Their Major Structures[a]

Level	Cavity	Nuclei	Motor Tract	Sensory Tracts
Inferior colliculi	Cerebral aqueduct	Inferior colliculus, substantia nigra, trochlear nucleus, mesencephalic nuclei of CN V	Corticospinal and corticonuclear tracts, temporopontine, frontopontine, medial longitudinal fasciculus	Lateral, trigeminal, spinal, and medial lemnisci; decussation of superior cerebellar peduncles
Superior colliculi	Cerebral aqueduct	Superior colliculus, substantia nigra, oculomotor nucleus, Edinger–Westphal nucleus, red nucleus, mesencephalic nucleus of CN V	Corticospinal and corticonuclear tracts, temporopontine, frontopontine, medial longitudinal fasciculus, decussation of rubrospinal tract	Trigeminal, spinal, and medial lemnisci

[a]Note that the reticular formation is present at all levels.
CN, cranial nerve.

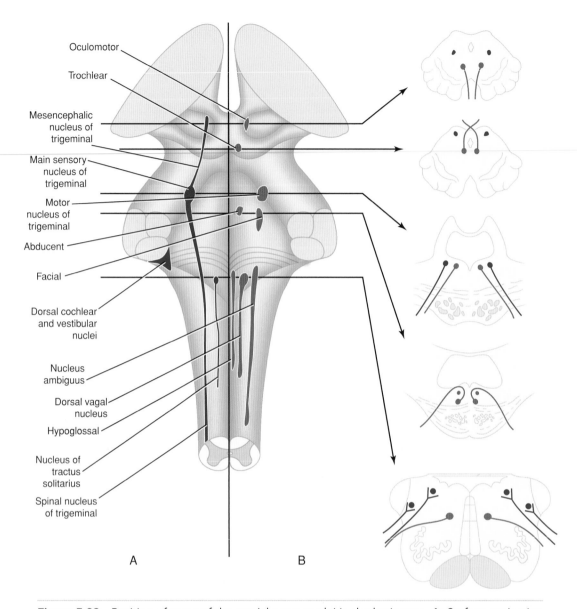

Figure 5-29 Position of some of the cranial nerve nuclei in the brainstem. **A:** Surface projection on the posterior aspect of the brainstem. **B:** Cross sections. The motor nuclei are in red and the sensory nuclei in blue.

to emerge on the medial side of the crus cerebri in the interpeduncular fossa. The nucleus of the oculomotor nerve is divisible into a number of cell groups.

The **medial**, **spinal**, and **trigeminal lemnisci** form a curved band posterior to the substantia nigra, but the **lateral lemniscus** does not extend superiorly to this level.

The **red nucleus** is a rounded mass of gray matter situated between the cerebral aqueduct and the substantia nigra. Its reddish hue, seen in fresh specimens, is due to its vascularity and the presence of an iron-containing pigment in the cytoplasm of many of its neurons. Afferent fibers reach the red nucleus from (1) the cerebral cortex through the corticospinal fibers, (2) the cerebellum through the superior cerebellar peduncle, and (3) the lentiform nucleus, subthalamic

and hypothalamic nuclei, substantia nigra, and spinal cord. Efferent fibers leave the red nucleus and pass to (1) the spinal cord through the rubrospinal tract (as this tract descends, it decussates), (2) the reticular formation through the rubroreticular tract, (3) the thalamus, and (4) the substantia nigra.

The **reticular formation** is situated in the tegmentum lateral and posterior to the red nucleus.

The **crus cerebri** contains the identical important descending tracts—the **corticospinal**, **corticonuclear**, and **corticopontine fibers**—that are present at the level of the inferior colliculus (see Table 5-4).

The continuity of the various CN nuclei through the different regions of the brainstem is shown diagrammatically in Figure 5-29.

Clinical Notes

Clinical Significance of the Medulla Oblongata

The medulla oblongata not only contains many cranial nerve (CN) nuclei that are concerned with vital functions (e.g., regulation of heart rate and respiration), but it also serves as a conduit for the passage of ascending and descending tracts connecting the spinal cord to the higher centers of the nervous system. These tracts may become involved in demyelinating diseases, neoplasms, and vascular disorders.

Raised Pressure in the Posterior Cranial Fossa

The medulla oblongata is situated in the posterior cranial fossa, lying beneath the tentorium cerebelli and above the foramen magnum. It is related anteriorly to the basal portion of the occipital bone and the upper part of the odontoid process of the axis and posteriorly to the cerebellum.

In patients with tumors of the posterior cranial fossa, the intracranial pressure is raised, and the brain—that is, the cerebellum and the medulla oblongata—tends to be pushed toward the area of least resistance; the medulla and cerebellar tonsils herniate downward through the foramen magnum. This causes headache, neck stiffness, and paralysis of the glossopharyngeal, vagus, accessory, and hypoglossal nerves owing to traction. In these circumstances, **performing a lumbar puncture is extremely dangerous** because the sudden withdrawal of cerebrospinal fluid (CSF) may precipitate further herniation of the brain through the foramen magnum and a sudden failure of vital functions, resulting from pressure and ischemia of the CN nuclei present in the medulla oblongata.

Arnold–Chiari Phenomenon

The **Arnold–Chiari malformation** is a congenital anomaly in which there is a herniation of the tonsils of the cerebellum and the medulla oblongata through the foramen magnum into the vertebral canal (Fig. 5-30). This results in the blockage of the exits in the roof of the fourth ventricle to the CSF, causing internal hydrocephalus. It is commonly associated with craniovertebral anomalies or various forms of spina bifida. Signs and symptoms related to pressure on the cerebellum and medulla oblongata and involvement of the last four CNs are associated with this condition.

Vascular Disorders

The medulla oblongata is a heterogeneous collection of nuclei and tracts, and damage to different regions will elicit the following syndromes.

LATERAL MEDULLARY SYNDROME OF WALLENBERG

The lateral part of the medulla oblongata is supplied by the posterior inferior cerebellar artery, which is usually a branch of the vertebral artery. Thrombosis of either of these arteries (Fig. 5-31) produces the following signs and symptoms: dysphagia and dysarthria due to paralysis of the ipsilateral palatal and laryngeal muscles (innervated by the nucleus ambiguus); analgesia and thermoanesthesia on the ipsilateral side of the face (nucleus and spinal tract of the trigeminal nerve); vertigo, nausea, vomiting, and nystagmus (vestibular nuclei); ipsilateral Horner syndrome (descending sympathetic fibers); ipsilateral cerebellar signs—gait and limb ataxia (cerebellum or inferior cerebellar peduncle);

Figure 5-30 Arnold–Chiari phenomenon. This coronal section of the skull shows the herniation of the cerebellar tonsil and the medulla oblongata through the foramen magnum into the vertebral canal. (From Dudek, R. W., & Louis, T. M. [2015]. *High-yield gross anatomy* (5th ed.). Baltimore, MD: Wolters Kluwer.)

and contralateral loss of sensations of pain and temperature (spinal lemniscus—spinothalamic tract).

MEDIAL MEDULLARY SYNDROME

The medial part of the medulla oblongata is supplied by the vertebral artery. Thrombosis of the medullary branch (Fig. 5-32) produces the following signs and symptoms: contralateral hemiparesis (pyramidal tract), contralateral impaired sensations of position and movement and tactile discrimination (medial lemniscus), and ipsilateral paralysis of tongue muscles with deviation to the paralyzed side when the tongue is protruded (hypoglossal nerve).

Clinical Significance of the Pons

The pons, like the medulla oblongata and the cerebellum, is situated in the posterior cranial fossa lying beneath the tentorium cerebelli. It is related anteriorly to the basilar artery, the dorsum sellae of the sphenoid bone, and the basilar part of the occipital bone. In addition to forming the upper half of the floor of the fourth ventricle, it possesses several important CN nuclei (trigeminal, abducens, facial, and vestibulocochlear) and serves as a conduit for important ascending and descending tracts (corticonuclear, corticopontine, corticospinal, medial longitudinal fasciculus and medial, spinal, and lateral lemnisci). Not surprisingly, therefore, tumors, hemorrhage, or infarcts in this area of the brain produce a variety of symptoms and signs. For example, involvement of

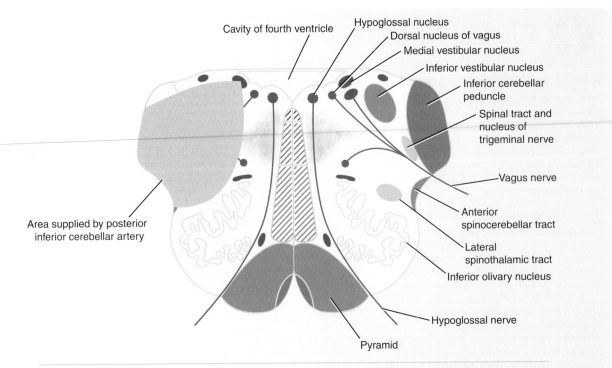

Figure 5-31 Transverse section of the medulla oblongata at the level of the inferior olivary nuclei showing the extent of the lesion producing the lateral medullary syndrome.

the corticopontocerebellar tracts will produce marked cerebellar ataxia, and voluntary movements are accompanied by a rhythmic tremor that develops and becomes further accentuated as the movements proceed (intention tumor).

Tumors

Astrocytoma of the pons occurring in childhood is the most common tumor of the brainstem. The symptoms and signs are those of ipsilateral CN paralysis and contralateral

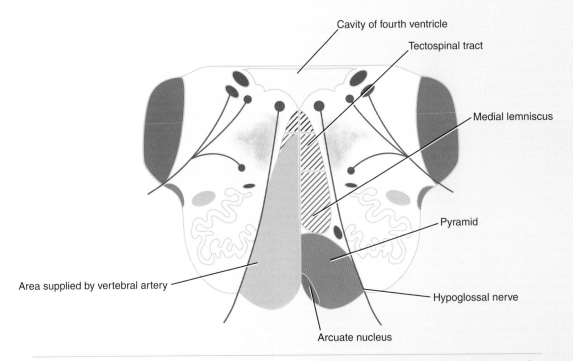

Figure 5-32 Transverse section of the medulla oblongata at the level of the inferior olivary nuclei showing the extent of the lesion producing the medial medullary syndrome.

hemiparesis: weakness of the facial muscles on the same side (facial nerve nucleus), weakness of the lateral rectus muscle on one or both sides (abducens nerve nucleus), nystagmus (vestibular nucleus), weakness of the jaw muscles (trigeminal nerve nucleus), impairment of hearing (cochlear nuclei), contralateral hemiparesis, quadriparesis (corticospinal fibers), anesthesia to light touch with the preservation of appreciation of pain over the skin of the face (principal sensory nucleus of trigeminal nerve involved, leaving spinal nucleus and tract of trigeminal intact), and contralateral sensory defects of the trunk and limbs (medial and spinal lemnisci). Involvement of the corticopontocerebellar tracts may cause ipsilateral cerebellar signs and symptoms. There may be impairment of conjugate deviation of the eyeballs due to involvement of the medial longitudinal fasciculus, which connects the oculomotor, trochlear, and abducens nerve nuclei.

Hemorrhage

The pons is supplied by the basilar artery and the anterior, inferior, and superior cerebellar arteries. If the hemorrhage occurs from one of those arteries and is unilateral, facial paralysis on the side of the lesion (involvement of the facial nerve nucleus and, therefore, a lower motor neuron palsy) and paralysis of the limbs on the opposite side (involvement of the corticospinal fibers as they pass through the pons) will result. Paralysis of conjugate ocular deviation (involvement of the abducens nerve nucleus and the medial longitudinal fasciculus) is common.

When the hemorrhage is extensive and bilateral, the pupils may be "pinpoint" (involvement of the ocular sympathetic fibers); bilateral paralysis of the face and the limbs is common. The patient may become poikilothermic because severe damage to the pons has cut off the body from the heat-regulating centers in the hypothalamus.

Infarctions

Usually, infarction of the pons is due to thrombosis or embolism of the basilar artery or its branches. If it involves the paramedian area of the pons, the corticospinal tracts, the pontine nuclei, and the fibers passing to the cerebellum through the middle cerebellar peduncle may be damaged. A laterally situated infarct will involve the trigeminal nerve, the medial lemniscus, and the middle cerebellar peduncle; the corticospinal fibers to the lower limbs also may be affected.

The clinical conditions mentioned above will be understood more clearly if the ascending and descending tracts of the brain and spinal cord are reviewed (see Chapter 4).

Clinical Significance of the Midbrain

The midbrain forms the upper end of the narrow stalk of the brain or brainstem. As it ascends out of the posterior cranial fossa through the relatively small rigid opening in the tentorium cerebelli, it is vulnerable to traumatic injury. It possesses two important CN nuclei (oculomotor and trochlear), reflex centers (the colliculi), and the red nucleus and substantia nigra, which greatly influence motor function, and the midbrain serves as a conduit for many important ascending and descending tracts. As in other parts of the brainstem, it is a site for tumors, hemorrhage, or infarcts that will produce a wide variety of symptoms and signs.

Trauma

Among the mechanisms of injuries to the midbrain, a sudden lateral movement of the head could result in the cerebral peduncles impinging against the sharp rigid free edge of the tentorium cerebelli. Sudden movements of the head resulting from trauma cause different regions of the brain to move at different velocities relative to one another. For example, the large anatomical unit, the forebrain, may move at a different velocity from the remainder of the brain, such as the cerebellum. This will result in the midbrain being bent, stretched, twisted, or torn.

Involvement of the oculomotor nucleus will produce ipsilateral paralysis of the levator palpebrae superioris; the superior, inferior, and medial rectus muscles; and the inferior oblique muscle. Malfunction of the parasympathetic nucleus of the oculomotor nerve produces a dilated pupil that is insensitive to light and does not constrict on accommodation.

Involvement of the trochlear nucleus will produce contralateral paralysis of the superior oblique muscle of the eyeball. Thus, involvement of one or both of these nuclei, or the corticonuclear fibers that converge on them, will cause impairment of ocular movements.

Cerebral Aqueduct Blockage

The cavity of the midbrain, the cerebral aqueduct, is one of the narrower parts of the ventricular system. Normally, CSF that has been produced in the lateral and third ventricles passes through this channel to enter the fourth ventricle and so escapes through the foramina in its roof to enter the subarachnoid space. In congenital hydrocephalus, the cerebral aqueduct may be blocked or replaced by numerous small tubular passages that are insufficient for normal CSF flow. A tumor of the midbrain (Fig. 5-33A) or pressure on the midbrain from a tumor arising outside the midbrain may compress the aqueduct and produce hydrocephalus. When the cerebral aqueduct is blocked, the accumulating CSF within the third and lateral ventricles produces lesions in the midbrain. The presence of the oculomotor and trochlear nerve nuclei, together with the important descending corticospinal and corticonuclear tracts, will provide symptoms and signs that are helpful in accurately localizing a lesion in the brainstem.

Vascular Lesions

The midbrain houses CN III nuclei and serves as a conduit for all ascending and descending fibers between the cerebrum and brainstem; lesions of each will result in the following syndromes.

WEBER SYNDROME

Weber syndrome (see Fig. 5-33B), which is commonly produced by occlusion of a branch of the posterior cerebral artery that supplies the midbrain, results in the necrosis of brain tissue involving the oculomotor nerve and the crus cerebri. Ipsilateral ophthalmoplegia and contralateral paralysis of the lower part of the face, the tongue, and the arm and leg also result. The eyeball is deviated laterally because of the paralysis of the medial rectus muscle; the upper lid droops (ptosis), and the pupil is dilated and fixed to light and accommodation.

BENEDIKT SYNDROME

Benedikt syndrome (see Fig. 5-33C) is similar to Weber syndrome, but the necrosis involves the medial lemniscus and red nucleus, producing contralateral hemianesthesia and involuntary movements of the limbs of the opposite side.

Figure 5-33 Pathology of the midbrain. **A:** Tumor of the midbrain blocking the cerebral aqueduct. **B:** Weber syndrome involving the oculomotor nerve and the crus cerebri following occlusion of the blood supply to the midbrain. **C:** Benedikt syndrome involving the red nucleus and the medial lemniscus following occlusion of the blood supply to the midbrain.

Key Concepts

Medulla Oblongata

- The medulla oblongata connects the pons superiorly and spinal cord inferiorly. On either side of the anterior median sulcus are the two pyramids that taper inferiorly, whereas most fibers cross at the decussation of the pyramids.

- Posterolateral to the pyramids are the olives, which are elevations produced by the underlying inferior olivary nuclei.

- The medulla oblongata contains multiple CN and cerebellar nuclei, the olivary nuclear complex, nucleus ambiguous, hypoglossal nucleus, vestibulocochlear nucleus, dorsal nucleus of the vagus, and

nucleus of the tractus solitarius, and spinal nucleus of the trigeminal nerve.

Pons

- The pons is anterior to the cerebellum and connects the medulla oblongata to the midbrain. The anterior surface is convex, and the trigeminal nerve emerges anterolaterally.

- The anterior or basal part of the pons consists of transversely running fibers, called the trapezoid body, and descending bundles of the corticospinal tract.

- The posterior part, or tegmentum, contains multiple nuclei, including facial, abducens, vestibular, pontine, trapezoid, and trigeminal (main sensory, spinal, and motor).

Midbrain

- The midbrain connects the pons and the cerebellum with the forebrain.
- The lateral halves, called the cerebral peduncles, are comprised of the crus cerebri, which contain corticospinal fibers, and the substantia nigra, a pigmented band of gray matter.

- The cerebral aqueduct, which connects the third and fourth ventricles, passes through the midbrain and divides the anterior (tegmentum) from the posterior (tectum).
- The tectum consists of four swellings, two superior and two inferior colliculi, that are associated with vision and hearing, respectively.
- The midbrain contains multiple nuclei including, inferior and superior colliculi, substantia nigra, trochlear, mesencephalic (trigeminal), oculomotor, Edinger–Westphal, and the red nucleus.

? Clinical Problem Solving

1. While carrying out a physical examination of a patient with an intracranial tumor, the neurologist turns to a medical student and asks, "What signs or symptoms would you look for that would enable you to localize the tumor to the region of the medulla oblongata?" How would you have answered that question?

2. A 6-month-old boy dies with hydrocephalus and a myelocele in the lower thoracic region. At autopsy, the hindbrain is found to be deformed. The lower part of the medulla oblongata extends inferiorly through the foramen magnum into the vertebral canal as far as the third cervical vertebra. The lower four cranial nerves are longer than normal, and the upper cervical nerve roots ascend to reach their exit from the vertebral canal. The cerebellum on the left side extends inferiorly through the foramen magnum to the third cervical vertebra, where it adheres to the spinal cord. The roof of the fourth ventricle is abnormally low. (a) What is the name of this malformation? (b) Is hydrocephalus common in this condition? (c) Is an association possible between the thoracic myelocele and the presence of part of the hindbrain in the vertebral canal?

3. A 68-year-old man is admitted to the hospital with the sudden onset of severe dizziness (vertigo), hiccups, and vomiting. He also complains of a hot, painful sensation in the skin of the right side of the face. On physical examination, the soft palate is drawn up to the left side when the patient was asked to say "ah," and the right vocal cord lacked mobility as seen on laryngoscopic examination. The patient also shows drooping of the right upper eyelid (ptosis), sunken right eye (enophthalmos), and a constricted right pupil (myosis). When asked to protrude his tongue straight out of his mouth, the patient tries to do so, but the tip of the tongue pointed to the right side. Impaired pain and temperature sensation is evident in the trunk and extremities on the left side. Using your knowledge of anatomy, make the diagnosis.

4. A pathologist, while exploring the posterior cranial fossa during an autopsy, is endeavoring to determine where the 9th, the 10th, and the cranial part of the 11th cranial nerves emerge from the hindbrain. Describe where these nerves emerge from the hindbrain.

5. A 10-year-old girl is taken to a physician because her mother has noticed that the right half of her face was weak and does not appear to react to emotional changes. Her mouth is pulled over slightly to the left, especially when she is tired. On questioning, the patient admits that food tends to stick inside her right cheek and that the right side of her face "felt funny." The mother had first noticed the facial changes 3 months previously, and the condition has progressively worsened. On examination, definite weakness of the facial muscles on the right side is noted; the facial muscles on the left side are normal. Skin sensation on stimulation of the face is normal. On testing of the ocular movements, slight weakness of the lateral rectus muscle is evident on the right side. Examination of the movements of the arm and leg shows slight weakness on the left side. Using your knowledge of neuroanatomy, relate these symptoms and signs to a lesion in the pons.

6. A 65-year-old man is admitted to the emergency department with a diagnosis of a severe pontine hemorrhage. On examination, he is found to have bilateral "pinpoint" pupils and quadriplegia. How can you explain the presence of the "pinpoint" pupils?

7. A 46-year-old man with symptoms of deafness, vertigo, and double vision (diplopia) visits his physician. On questioning, he says that he also suffers from severe headaches, which are increasing in frequency and severity. The week before, he vomited several times during one of the headache attacks.

On examination, he is found to have a slight right internal strabismus, a flattening of the skin furrows on the right side of his forehead, and a slight drooping of the right corner of his mouth. Hearing is impaired on the right side. On testing for sensory loss, sensory impairment is evident on the right side of the face in the areas supplied by the maxillary and mandibular divisions of the trigeminal nerve. Using your knowledge of anatomy, explain the symptoms and signs.

8. After a severe automobile accident that results in the death of the driver of one of the vehicles, an autopsy is performed, and the skull is opened. A massive subdural hematoma is found in the middle cranial fossa. The rapid accumulation of blood within the skull had exerted pressure on the brain above the tentorium cerebelli. The uncus of the temporal lobe has been forced inferiorly through the hiatus in the tentorium cerebelli. What effect do you think these intracranial changes had on the midbrain of this patient?

9. A 3-month-old girl is taken to a pediatrician because her mother is concerned about the large size of her head. The child is perfectly normal in every other respect. Examination of the child shows that the diameter of the head was larger than normal for the age; the fontanelles are larger than normal and are moderately tense. The scalp is shiny, and the scalp veins are dilated. The eyes are normal, and the mental and physical development of the child is within normal limits. Computed tomography and magnetic resonance imaging of the head reveal gross dilation of the third and lateral ventricles of the brain. What is your diagnosis? What possible treatment should be suggested to the mother of this child?

10. A 20-year-old man is seen by a neurologist because he has a 3-month history of double vision. On examination of the patient, both eyes at rest are turned downward and laterally. The patient is unable to move the eyes upward or medially. Both upper lids

are drooping (ptosis). Examination of both pupils shows them to be dilated, and they do not constrict when a light is shone into either eye. Facial movements and sensation are normal. Movements of the upper and lower limbs are normal. Loss of or altered skin sensations is not evident in the upper or the lower limbs. Using your knowledge of neuroanatomy, make a diagnosis and accurately locate the site of the lesion. Is the lesion unilateral or bilateral?

11. A 57-year-old man with hypertension is admitted to the hospital with a diagnosis of hemorrhage into the midbrain, possibly from a branch of the posterior cerebral artery. He is found, on physical examination, to have paralysis on the right side of the levator palpebrae superioris, the superior rectus, medial rectus, inferior rectus, and inferior oblique muscles. Furthermore, his right pupil is dilated and fails to constrict on exposure to light or on accommodation. The left eye is normal in every respect. He displays hypersensitivity to touch on the skin of the left side of his face and has loss of skin sensation on the greater part of his left arm and left leg. The left leg also displays some spontaneous slow writhing movements (athetosis). Using your knowledge of neuroanatomy, explain the signs and symptoms exhibited by this patient.

12. A 41-year-old woman is diagnosed as having a lesion in the midbrain. Physical examination reveals an oculomotor nerve palsy on the left side (paralysis of the left extraocular muscles except the lateral rectus and the superior oblique muscles) and an absence of the light and accommodation reflexes on the left side. Some weakness is evident but no atrophy of the muscles of the lower part of the face and the tongue on the right side. The right arm and leg show spastic paralysis. Sensory loss on either side of the head, trunk, or limbs is not noted. Using your knowledge of neuroanatomy, precisely place the lesion in the midbrain of this patient.

 Answers and Explanations to Clinical Problem Solving

1. Until involvement of one of the last four cranial nerves occurs, localization of a lesion to the medulla oblongata remains uncertain. For example, involvement of the main ascending sensory pathways or descending pathways may be caused by a lesion in the medulla, the pons, the midbrain, or the spinal cord. Involvement of the glossopharyngeal nerve can be detected by inadequacy of the gag reflex and loss of taste sensation on the posterior third of the tongue. Involvement of the vagus nerve can be assumed if the patient demonstrates some or all of the following symptoms: impairment of pharyngeal sensibility, difficulty in swallowing, nasal regurgitation of fluids with asymmetry of movement of the soft palate, and hoarseness of the voice with paralysis of the laryngeal muscles. The cranial part of the accessory nerve is distributed within the

vagus nerve so that testing for this nerve alone is not possible. The spinal part of the accessory nerve, which supplies the sternocleidomastoid and trapezius muscles, arises from the spinal cord and is therefore unaffected by tumors of the medulla. The hypoglossal nerve involvement may be tested by looking for wasting, fasciculation, and paralysis of half of the tongue.

2. (a) The malformation in which the cerebellum and the medulla oblongata are found in the cervical part of the vertebral canal is known as the Arnold–Chiari malformation. (b) Yes. Hydrocephalus is common in this condition. The hydrocephalus may be due to distortion or malformation of the openings in the roof of the fourth ventricle, which normally allow the cerebrospinal fluid to escape into the subarachnoid space. (c) Yes. A myelocele is commonly

associated with this malformation. The reason for this is not exactly known, although several investigators believe that the myelocele is the primary cause and that it tethers the lower part of the spinal cord to the surrounding tissues at the time when disproportionate growth of the spinal cord and the vertebral column occurs. This would serve to pull the medulla oblongata and the cerebellum inferiorly through the foramen magnum into the vertebral canal.

3. This patient is suffering from a thrombosis of the posterior inferior cerebellar artery or vertebral artery on the right side. The vertigo is caused by the involvement of the cerebellum or the vestibular nuclei or both. The hot, painful skin sensations are due to the involvement of the spinal tract and nucleus of the trigeminal nerve on the right side. The abnormal movement of the soft palate and the fixation of the right vocal cord are due to involvement of the nucleus of the vagus and accessory nerve on the right side. The ptosis, enophthalmos, and myosis (Horner syndrome) are due to involvement of the descending fibers of the sympathetic part of the autonomic nervous system. The tongue pointing to the right is caused by involvement of the right hypoglossal nucleus (the right genioglossus muscle is paralyzed). The loss of pain and temperature sensations on the opposite side of the body is due to involvement of the ascending lateral spinothalamic tracts. This characteristic clinical syndrome results from cutting off the arterial supply to a wedge-shaped area in the posterolateral part of the medulla oblongata and the inferior surface of the cerebellum.

4. The 9th, the 10th, and the cranial part of the 11th cranial nerves emerge from the medulla oblongata in a groove between the olives and the inferior cerebellar peduncles.

5. This 10-year-old girl later was found to have an astrocytoma of the pons. The right unilateral facial weakness, together with weakness of the right lateral rectus muscle of the eye, was due to involvement of the right facial and abducens nuclei by the tumor. The absence of paresthesia of the face indicated that the principal sensory nucleus of the trigeminal nerve was intact on both sides. The weakness in the movements of the left arm and left leg was due to the involvement of the corticospinal fibers in the pons. (Remember that most of these fibers cross over to the opposite side at the decussation of the pyramids in the medulla.)

6. "Pinpoint" pupils indicate that the constrictor pupillae muscles are strongly contracted and the dilator pupillae muscles are paralyzed. The dilator pupillae muscles are supplied by the sympathetic fibers, which descend through the pons (position not precisely known) to the lateral gray columns of the thoracic part of the spinal cord. Here, the fibers synapse, and the thoracolumbar sympathetic outflow occurs.

7. The deafness and vertigo were due to lesions in the cochlear and vestibular nuclei in the upper part of the pons. The double vision (diplopia) was produced by the involvement of the abducens nerve nucleus on the right side of the pons. The history of severe headaches and vomiting was due to a progressive rise in intracranial pressure caused by a tumor of the pons. The right unilateral facial palsy was due to the involvement of the right facial nerve nucleus. The sensory impairment of the skin of the middle and lower part of the right side of the face was due to the tumor involvement of the principal sensory nucleus of the right trigeminal nerve.

8. The herniated uncus and the subdural hemorrhage caused pressure of the opposite crus cerebri of the midbrain against the sharp edge of the tentorium. The distortion of the midbrain caused narrowing of the cerebral aqueduct, further raising the supratentorial pressure by blocking the passage of cerebrospinal fluid from the third to the fourth ventricle. Under these circumstances, severe hemorrhage may occur within the midbrain and affect the third and fourth cranial nerve nuclei and various important descending and ascending tracts.

9. This child had hydrocephalus. The physical examination and the special tests showed that the third and lateral ventricles of the brain were grossly dilated owing to the accumulation of cerebrospinal fluid (CSF) in these cavities. Mechanical obstruction to CSF flow from the third into the fourth ventricle through the cerebral aqueduct was present. After the possibility of the presence of cysts or resectable tumors had been excluded, it was assumed that the cause of the obstruction was a congenital atresia or malformation of the cerebral aqueduct. If the condition were progressing—that is, the block in the aqueduct was complete and the head continued to increase in size at an abnormal rate—some form of neurosurgical procedure should have been performed to shunt CSF from the third or lateral ventricles into the subarachnoid space or into the venous system of the neck.

10. Two years later, the patient died. At autopsy, a large astrocytoma that involved the central part of the tegmentum at the level of the superior colliculi was found. The patient had exhibited all signs and symptoms associated with a raised intracranial pressure. The raised pressure was due in part to the expanding tumor, but the problem was compounded by the developing hydrocephalus resulting from blockage of the cerebral aqueduct.

The symptoms and signs exhibited by the patient when he was first seen by the neurologist could be explained by the presence of the tumor in the central gray matter at the level of the superior colliculi and involving the third cranial nerve nuclei on both sides. This resulted in bilateral ptosis; bilateral ophthalmoplegia; and bilateral fixed, dilated pupils. The resting position of the eyes in a downward and lateral position was due to the action of the superior oblique muscle (trochlear nerve) and lateral rectus muscle (abducens nerve).

11. The patient had a hemorrhage in the right side of the tegmentum of the midbrain that involved the right third cranial nerve. The ascending tracts of the left trigeminal nerve also were involved. After emerging from the sensory nuclei of the left trigeminal nerve, they cross the midline and ascend through the trigeminal lemniscus on the right side. The loss of sensation seen in the left upper and lower limbs was due to involvement of the right medial and spinal lemnisci. The athetoid movements of the left leg could be explained on the basis of the involvement of the right red nucleus. The absence of spasticity of the left arm and leg would indicate that the lesion did not involve the right descending tracts. For further clarification, consult the descriptions of the various tracts (see Chapter 4).

12. Autopsy later revealed a vascular lesion involving a branch of the posterior cerebral artery. Considerable brain softening was found in the region of the substantia nigra and crus cerebri on the left side of the midbrain. The left oculomotor nerve was involved as it passed through the infarcted area. The corticonuclear fibers that pass to the facial nerve nucleus and the hypoglossal nucleus were involved as they descended through the left crus cerebri (they cross the midline at the level of the nuclei). The corticospinal fibers on the left side were also involved (they cross in the medulla oblongata), hence the spastic paralysis of the right arm and leg. The left trigeminal and left medial lemnisci were untouched, which explains the absence of sensory changes on the right side of the body. This is a good example of Weber syndrome.

 Review Questions

Directions: Each of the numbered items in this section is followed by answers. Select the ONE lettered answer that is CORRECT.

1. The following statements concern the anterior surface of the medulla oblongata:
   (a) The pyramids taper inferiorly and give rise to the decussation of the pyramids.
   (b) On each side of the midline, an ovoid swelling called the olive contains the corticospinal fibers.
   (c) The hypoglossal nerve emerges between the olive and the inferior cerebellar peduncle.
   (d) The vagus nerve emerges between the pyramid and the olive.
   (e) The abducens nerve emerges between the pons and the midbrain.

2. The following general statements concern the medulla oblongata:
   (a) The caudal half of the floor of the fourth ventricle is formed by the rostral half of the medulla.
   (b) The central canal extends throughout the length of the medulla oblongata.
   (c) The nucleus gracilis is situated beneath the gracile tubercle on the anterior surface of the medulla.
   (d) The decussation of the medial lemnisci takes place in the rostral half of the medulla.
   (e) The cerebellum lies anterior to the medulla.

3. The following statements concern the interior of the lower part of the medulla:
   (a) The decussation of the pyramids represents the crossing over from one side of the medulla to the other of a quarter of the corticospinal fibers.
   (b) The central canal of the spinal cord is not continuous upward into the medulla.
   (c) The substantia gelatinosa is not continuous with the nucleus of the spinal tract of the trigeminal nerve.

   (d) The medial lemniscus is formed by the anterior spinothalamic tract and the spinotectal tract.
   (e) The internal arcuate fibers emerge from the nucleus gracilis and nucleus cuneatus.

4. The following statements concern the interior of the upper part of the medulla:
   (a) The reticular formation consists of nerve fibers but no nerve cells.
   (b) The nucleus ambiguus constitutes the motor nucleus of the vagus, cranial part of the accessory, and hypoglossal nerves.
   (c) Beneath the floor of the fourth ventricle are located the dorsal nucleus of the vagus and the vestibular nuclei.
   (d) The medial longitudinal fasciculus is a bundle of ascending fibers on each side of the midline.
   (e) The inferior cerebellar peduncle connects the pons to the cerebellum.

5. The following statements concern the Arnold–Chiari phenomenon:
   (a) It is an acquired anomaly.
   (b) The exits in the roof of the fourth ventricle may be blocked.
   (c) The cerebellum never herniates through the foramen magnum.
   (d) It is not associated with various forms of spina bifida.
   (e) Performing a spinal tap in this condition is safe.

6. The following statements concern the medial medullary syndrome:
   (a) The tongue is paralyzed on the contralateral side.
   (b) Ipsilateral hemiplegia is evident.
   (c) Ipsilateral sensations of position and movement are impaired.
   (d) It is commonly caused by thrombosis of a branch of the vertebral artery to the medulla oblongata.
   (e) Contralateral facial paralysis is evident.

7. The following statements concern the lateral medullary syndrome:
   (a) It may be caused by a thrombosis of the anterior inferior cerebellar artery.
   (b) The nucleus ambiguus of the same side may be damaged.
   (c) Analgesia and thermoanesthesia may be evident on the contralateral side of the face.
   (d) Contralateral trunk and extremity hypalgesia and thermoanesthesia may occur.
   (e) Seizures may occur.

Directions: Matching Questions. The following questions apply to Figure 5-34. Match the numbers listed on the left with the appropriate lettered structure listed on the right. Each lettered option may be selected once, more than once, or not at all.

8. Number 1	(a) Inferior cerebellar peduncle
9. Number 2	(b) Medial lemniscus
10. Number 3	(c) Hypoglossal nucleus
11. Number 4	(d) Reticular formation
12. Number 5	(e) None of the above
13. Number 6	

Directions: Each of the numbered items in this section is followed by answers. Select the ONE lettered answer that is CORRECT.

14. The following statements concern the pons:
    (a) The trigeminal nerve emerges on the lateral aspect of the pons.
    (b) The glossopharyngeal nerve emerges on the anterior aspect of the brainstem in the groove between the pons and the medulla oblongata.
    (c) The basilar artery lies in a centrally placed groove on the anterior aspect of the pons.

(d) Many nerve fibers present on the posterior aspect of the pons converge laterally to form the middle cerebellar peduncle.
(e) The pons forms the lower half of the floor of the fourth ventricle.

15. The following important structures are located in the brainstem at the level stated:
    (a) The red nucleus lies within the midbrain.
    (b) The facial colliculus lies in the cranial part of the pons.
    (c) The motor nucleus of the trigeminal nerve lies within the caudal part of the pons.
    (d) The abducens nucleus lies within the cranial part of the pons.
    (e) The trochlear nucleus lies within the midbrain at the level of the superior colliculus.

16. The following statements concern the posterior surface of the pons:
    (a) Lateral to the median sulcus is an elongated swelling called the lateral eminence.
    (b) The facial colliculus is produced by the root of the facial nerve winding around the nucleus of the abducens nerve.
    (c) The floor of the inferior part of the sulcus limitans is pigmented and is called the substantia ferruginea.
    (d) The vestibular area lies medial to the sulcus limitans.
    (e) The cerebellum lies anterior to the pons.

17. The following statements concern a transverse section through the caudal part of the pons:
    (a) The pontine nuclei lie between the transverse pontine fibers.
    (b) The vestibular nuclei lie medial to the abducens nucleus.

Figure 5-34 Photomicrograph of transverse section of the medulla oblongata. (Weigert stain.)

(c) The trapezoid body is made up of fibers derived from the facial nerve nuclei.

(d) The tegmentum is the part of the pons lying anterior to the trapezoid body.

(e) The medial longitudinal fasciculus lies above the floor of the fourth ventricle on either side of the midline.

18. The following statements concern a transverse section through the cranial part of the pons:

(a) The motor nucleus of the trigeminal nerve lies lateral to the main sensory nucleus in the tegmentum.

(b) The medial lemniscus has rotated so that its long axis lies vertically.

(c) Bundles of corticospinal fibers lie among the transverse pontine fibers.

(d) The medial longitudinal fasciculus joins the thalamus to the spinal nucleus of the trigeminal nerve.

(e) The motor root of the trigeminal nerve is much larger than the sensory root.

19. The following statements concern the pons:

(a) It is related superiorly to the dorsum sellae of the sphenoid bone.

(b) It lies in the middle cranial fossa.

(c) Glial tumors of the pons are rare.

(d) The corticopontine fibers terminate in the pontine nuclei.

(e) The pons receives its blood supply from the internal carotid artery.

Directions: Matching Questions. The following questions apply to Figure 5-35. Match the numbers listed on the left with the appropriate lettered structure listed on the right. Each lettered option may be selected once, more than once, or not at all.

20. Number 1   (a) Basilar groove
21. Number 2   (b) Medial longitudinal fasciculus
22. Number 3   (c) Superior cerebellar peduncle
23. Number 4   (d) Superior medullary velum
24. Number 5   (e) None of the above
25. Number 6

Directions: Each of the numbered items in this section is followed by answers. Select the ONE lettered answer that is CORRECT.

26. The following statements concern the midbrain:

(a) It passes superiorly between the fixed and free borders of the tentorium cerebelli.

(b) The oculomotor nerve emerges from the posterior surface below the inferior colliculi.

(c) The superior brachium passes from the superior colliculus to the medial geniculate body.

(d) The cavity of the midbrain is called the cerebral aqueduct.

(e) The interpeduncular fossa is bounded laterally by the cerebellar peduncles.

27. The following statements concern the midbrain:

(a) The oculomotor nucleus is found within it at the level of the inferior colliculus.

(b) The trochlear nerve emerges on the anterior surface of the midbrain and decussates completely in the superior medullary velum.

(c) The trochlear nucleus is situated in the central gray matter at the level of the inferior colliculus.

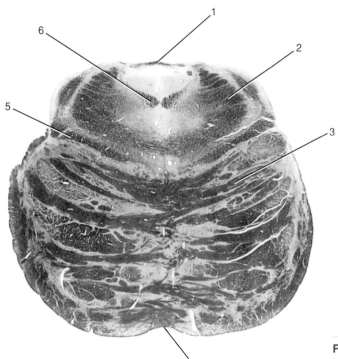

Figure 5-35 Photomicrograph of transverse section of the pons. (Weigert stain.)

(d) The lemnisci are situated medial to the central gray matter.

(e) The trigeminal lemniscus lies anterior to the medial lemniscus.

28. The following statements concern the internal structures of the midbrain:
    (a) The tectum is the part situated posterior to the cerebral aqueduct.
    (b) The crus cerebri on each side lies posterior to the substantia nigra.
    (c) The tegmentum lies anterior to the substantia nigra.
    (d) The central gray matter encircles the red nuclei.
    (e) The reticular formation is limited to the lower part of the midbrain.

29. The following statements concern the colliculi of the midbrain:
    (a) They are located in the tegmentum.
    (b) The superior colliculi are concerned with sight reflexes.
    (c) The inferior colliculi lie at the level of the oculomotor nerve nuclei.
    (d) The inferior colliculi are concerned with reflexes of smell.
    (e) The superior colliculi lie at the level of the trochlear nuclei.

30. The following statements concern the third cranial nerve nuclei:
    (a) The oculomotor nucleus is situated lateral to the central gray matter.
    (b) The sympathetic part of the oculomotor nucleus is called the Edinger–Westphal nucleus.
    (c) The oculomotor nucleus lies posterior to the cerebral aqueduct.
    (d) The nerve fibers from the oculomotor nucleus pass through the red nucleus.
    (e) The oculomotor nucleus lies close to the lateral longitudinal fasciculus.

Directions: Matching Questions. The following questions apply to Figure 5-36. Match the numbers listed on the left with the appropriate lettered structure listed on the right. Each lettered option may be selected once, more than once, or not at all.

31. Number 1	(a) Medial longitudinal fasciculus
32. Number 2	(b) Inferior colliculus
33. Number 3	(c) Medial lemniscus
34. Number 4	(d) Trochlear nucleus
35. Number 5	(e) None of the above
36. Number 6	

Directions: Each case history is followed by questions. Read the case history, then select the ONE BEST lettered answer.

A 63-year-old man complaining of difficulty in swallowing, some hoarseness of his voice, and giddiness was seen by a neurologist. All these symptoms started suddenly 4 days previously. On physical examination, he was found to have a loss of the pharyngeal gagging

Figure 5-36 Transverse section of the midbrain.

reflex on the left side, left-sided facial analgesia, and left-sided paralysis of the vocal cord.

37. Based on the clinical history and the results of the physical examination, select the **most likely** diagnosis.
    (a) Meningeal tumor in the posterior cranial fossa on the right side
    (b) Lateral medullary syndrome on the left side
    (c) Medial medullary syndrome on the left side
    (d) Lateral medullary syndrome on the right side
    (e) Medial medullary syndrome on the right side

A 7-year-old girl was seen by a neurologist because she complained to her mother that she was seeing double. Careful physical examination revealed that the double vision became worse when she looked toward the left. The patient also had evidence of a mild motor paralysis of her right lower limb without spasticity. There was also a slight facial paralysis involving the whole left side of the face.

38. Based on the clinical history and the clinical examination, the following neurologic deficits could have been present **except:**
    (a) The double vision caused by weakness of the left lateral rectus muscle.
    (b) The complete left-sided facial paralysis caused by involvement of the left seventh cranial nerve nucleus or its nerve.
    (c) The mild right hemiparesis produced by damage to the corticospinal tract on the right side.
    (d) Magnetic resonance imaging revealed the presence of a tumor of the lower part of the pons on the left side.
    (e) The left sixth cranial nerve nucleus was damaged.

A 42-year-old woman complaining of a severe, persistent headache visited her physician. At first, the headache was not continuous and tended to occur during the night. Now, the headache was present all the time and was felt over the whole head. Recently, she has begun to feel nauseous, and this has resulted in several episodes of vomiting. Last week, on looking in the mirror, she noted that her right pupil looked much larger than the left. Her right upper lid appeared to droop.

39. The physical examination revealed the following most likely findings **except:**
    (a) Weakness in raising the right eyelid upward
    (b) Severe ptosis of the right eye
    (c) Obvious dilatation of the right pupil
    (d) Ophthalmoscopic examination revealing bilateral papilledema
    (e) Evidence of paralysis of either superior oblique muscle
    (f) Examination of the lower limbs revealing mild spasticity of the left lower limb muscles

(g) Ataxia of the right upper limb
(h) Loss of taste sensation on the posterior third of the tongue on the left side

40. The combination of the clinical history and the findings in the physical examination enabled the physician to make the following **most likely** diagnosis.
    (a) Tumor involving the left cerebral hemisphere
    (b) Tumor involving the right side of the midbrain at the level of the superior colliculi
    (c) Severe migraine
    (d) Cerebral hemorrhage involving the left cerebral hemisphere
    (e) Tumor of the left side of the midbrain

 Answers and Explanations to Review Questions

1. A is correct. The pyramids of the medulla oblongata taper inferiorly and give rise to the decussation of the pyramids (see Fig. 5-9). B. On each side of the midline on the anterior surface of the medulla lateral to the pyramids, an ovoid swelling called the olive contains the olivary nucleus and does not contain the corticospinal fibers. C. The hypoglossal nerve emerges between the pyramid and the olive. D. The vagus nerve emerges between the olive and the inferior cerebellar peduncle. E. The abducens nerve emerges between the pons and the medulla oblongata (see Fig. 5-9).

2. A is correct. The caudal half of the floor of the fourth ventricle is formed by the rostral half of the medulla oblongata (see Fig. 5-9). B. The central canal in the medulla oblongata is limited to the caudal half. C. The nucleus gracilis is situated beneath the gracile tubercle on the posterior surface of the medulla. D. The decussation of the medial lemnisci takes place in the caudal half of the medulla. E. The cerebellum lies posterior to the medulla.

3. E is correct. The internal arcuate fibers emerge from the nucleus gracilis and nucleus cuneatus (see Fig. 4-16). A. The decussation of the pyramids represents the crossing over from one side of the medulla to the other of three fourths of the corticospinal fibers. B. The central canal of the spinal cord is continuous upward into the medulla. C. The substantia gelatinosa becomes continuous with the nucleus of the spinal part of the trigeminal nerve. D. The medial lemniscus is formed by the axons of cells in the nucleus gracilis and the nucleus cuneatus; the axons leave the nuclei and cross the midline as the internal arcuate fibers and then ascend to the thalamus (see Fig. 4-16).

4. C is correct. Beneath the floor of the fourth ventricle are located the dorsal nucleus of the vagus and the vestibular nuclei (see Fig. 5-14). A. The reticular formation in the upper part of the medulla oblongata consists of a mixture of nerve fibers and small nerve cells. B. The nucleus ambiguus constitutes the motor nucleus of the glossopharyngeal, vagus, and the cranial part of the accessory nerves. D. The medial longitudinal fasciculus is a bundle of ascending and descending fibers that lie posterior to the medial lemniscus on each side of the midline (see Fig. 5-14). E. The inferior cerebellar peduncle connects the medulla to the cerebellum.

5. B is correct. In the Arnold–Chiari phenomenon, the exits in the roof of the fourth ventricle may be blocked. A. It is a congenital anomaly. C. The tonsil of the cerebellum may herniate through the foramen magnum (see Fig. 5-30). D. The Arnold–Chiari phenomenon is commonly associated with various forms of spina bifida. E. Performing a spinal tap in the setting of this condition is very dangerous.

6. D is correct. The medial medullary syndrome is commonly caused by thrombosis of a branch of the vertebral artery to the medulla oblongata. A. The tongue is paralyzed on the ipsilateral side. B. Contralateral hemiplegia is evident. C. Contralateral impaired sensations of position and movement are evident. E. Facial paralysis is not evident.

7. B is correct. In the lateral medullary syndrome, the nucleus ambiguus of the same side may be damaged. A. The condition may be caused by thrombosis of the posterior inferior cerebellar artery. C. Analgesia and thermoanesthesia on the ipsilateral side of the face may occur. D. Ipsilateral trunk and extremity hypalgesia and thermoanesthesia may occur. E. Seizures usually do not occur.

8. C is correct.

9. E is correct. The structure is the medial longitudinal fasciculus.

10. B is correct.

11. E is correct. The structure is the inferior olivary nucleus.

12. D is correct.

13. A is correct.

14. C is correct. The basilar artery lies in a centrally placed groove on the anterior aspect of the pons.

A. The trigeminal nerve emerges on the anterior aspect of the pons. B. The glossopharyngeal nerve emerges on the anterior aspect of the medulla oblongata in the groove between the olive and the inferior cerebellar peduncle (see Fig. 5-9). D. The nerve fibers on the anterior aspect of the pons converge laterally to form the middle cerebellar peduncle. E. The pons forms the upper half of the floor of the fourth ventricle (see Fig. 5-18).

15. A is correct. The red nucleus lies within the midbrain (see Fig. 5-25). B. The facial colliculus lies in the caudal part of the pons (see Fig. 5-18). C. The motor nucleus of the trigeminal nerve lies within the cranial part of the pons (see Fig. 5-20). D. The abducens nucleus lies within the caudal part of the pons (see Fig. 5-19). E. The trochlear nucleus lies within the midbrain at the level of the inferior colliculus (see Fig. 5-25).

16. B is correct. On the posterior surface of the pons is the facial colliculus, which is produced by the root of the facial nerve winding around the nucleus of the abducens nerve (see Fig. 5-19). A. The medial eminence is an elongated swelling lateral to the median sulcus (see Fig. 5-26). C. The floor of the superior part of the sulcus limitans is pigmented and is called the substantia ferruginea (see Fig. 5-18). D. The vestibular area lies lateral to the sulcus limitans (see Fig. 5-18). E. The cerebellum lies posterior to the pons.

17. A is correct. The pontine nuclei lie between the transverse pontine fibers (see Fig. 5-12). B. The vestibular nuclei lie lateral to the abducens nucleus (see Fig. 5-19). C. The trapezoid body is made up of fibers derived from the cochlear nuclei and the nuclei of the trapezoid body. D. The tegmentum is the part of the pons lying posterior to the trapezoid body. E. The medial longitudinal fasciculus lies below the floor of the fourth ventricle on either side of the midline (see Fig. 5-19).

18. C is correct. In the pons, bundles of corticopontine fibers lie among the transverse pontine fibers (see Fig. 5-19). A. The motor nucleus of the trigeminal nerve lies medial to the main sensory nucleus in the tegmentum of the pons (see Fig. 5-20). B. In the cranial part of the pons, the medial lemniscus has rotated so that its long axis lies transversely (see Fig. 5-20). D. The medial longitudinal fasciculus is the main pathway that connects the vestibular and cochlear nuclei with the nuclei controlling the extraocular muscles (oculomotor, trochlear, and abducens nuclei). E. The motor root of the trigeminal nerve is much smaller than the sensory root.

19. D is correct. In the pons, the corticopontine fibers terminate in the pontine nuclei. A. The pons is related anteriorly to the dorsum sellae of the sphenoid bone. B. The pons lies in the posterior cranial fossa. C. Astrocytoma of the pons is the most common tumor of the brainstem. E. The pons receives its blood supply from the basilar artery.

20. D is correct.

21. C is correct.

22. E is correct. The structure is the transverse pontine fibers.

23. A is correct.

24. E is correct. The structure is the medial lemniscus.

25. B is correct.

26. D is correct. The cavity of the midbrain is called the cerebral aqueduct (see Fig. 5-28). A. The midbrain passes superiorly through the opening in the tentorium cerebelli posterior to the dorsum sellae. B. The oculomotor nerve emerges from the anterior surface of the midbrain at the level of the superior colliculi (see Fig. 5-25). C. The superior brachium passes from the superior colliculus to the lateral geniculate body and the optic tract and is associated with visual functions (see Fig. 5-23). E. The interpeduncular fossa is bounded laterally by the crus cerebri (see Fig. 5-25).

27. C is correct. The trochlear nucleus is situated in the central gray matter of the midbrain at the level of the inferior colliculus (see Fig. 5-25). A. In the midbrain, the oculomotor nucleus is found at the level of the superior colliculus (see Fig. 5-25). B. The trochlear nerve emerges on the posterior surface of the midbrain and decussates completely in the superior medullary velum (see Fig. 5-25). D. The lemnisci are situated lateral to the central gray matter (see Fig. 5-25). E. The trigeminal lemniscus lies posterior to the medial lemniscus (see Fig. 5-25).

28. A is correct. The tectum is the part of the midbrain situated posterior to the cerebral aqueduct (see Fig. 5-24). B. In the midbrain, the crus cerebri lies anterior to the substantia nigra (see Fig. 5-25). C. The tegmentum lies posterior to the substantia nigra (see Fig. 5-25). D. The central gray matter encircles the cerebral aqueduct (see Fig. 5-25). E. The reticular formation is present throughout the midbrain.

29. B is correct. The superior colliculi of the midbrain are concerned with site reflexes. A. The colliculi are located in the tectum (see Fig. 5-25). C. The inferior colliculi lie at the level of the trochlear nerve nuclei (see Fig. 5-25). D. The inferior colliculi are concerned with auditory reflexes. E. The superior colliculi lie at the level of the red nuclei (see Fig. 5-25).

30. D is correct. The nerve fibers from the oculomotor nucleus pass through the red nucleus (see Fig. 5-25). A. The oculomotor nucleus is situated in the central gray matter (see Fig. 5-25). B. The parasympathetic part of the oculomotor nucleus is called the Edinger–Westphal nucleus. C. The oculomotor nucleus lies anterior to the cerebral aqueduct (see Fig. 5-25). E. The oculomotor nucleus lies close to the medial longitudinal fasciculus (see Fig. 5-25).

31. E is correct. The structure is the superior colliculus.

32. E is correct. The structure is the oculomotor nucleus.

33. E is correct. The structure is decussation of the rubrospinal tract.

34. E is correct. The structures are corticospinal and corticonuclear fibers.

35. C is correct.

36. E is correct. The structure is the mesencephalic nucleus of cranial nerve V.

37. B is correct.
38. C is correct. The right-sided hemiparesis was caused by damage to the corticospinal tract on the left side of the pons. The corticospinal tract descends through the medulla and crosses to the right side of the midline at the decussation of the pyramids. The patient was later discovered to have a glioma involving the left side of the lower pons.
39. H is correct. The sensation of taste on the posterior third of the tongue is supplied by the glossopharyngeal nerve, which originates in the medulla oblongata.

40. B is correct. The combination of raised intracranial pressure (headache, vomiting, and bilateral papilledema), the involvement of the right third cranial nerve (right-sided ptosis, right pupillary dilatation, and right-sided weakness of ocular deviation upward), spasticity of the left leg (right-sided corticospinal tracts), and ataxia of the right upper limb (cerebellar connections on the right side) led the physician to make a tentative diagnosis of an intracranial tumor in the right side of the midbrain at the level of the superior colliculi. An MRI confirmed the diagnosis.

6 Cerebellum and Its Connections

CHAPTER OBJECTIVES

- To review the structure and functions of the cerebellum

- To describe the afferent and efferent connections of the cerebellum within the central nervous system

A 56-year-old woman is examined by a neurologist for a variety of complaints, including an irregular swaying gait and a tendency to drift to the right when walking. Her family recently noticed that she has difficulty in keeping her balance when standing still, and she finds that standing with her feet apart helps her keep her balance.

On examination, she has diminished tone of the muscles of her right upper limb, as seen when the elbow and wrist joints are passively flexed and extended. Similar evidence is found in the right lower limb. When asked to stretch out her arms in front of her and hold them in position, she demonstrates obvious signs of right-sided tremor. When asked to touch the tip of her nose with the left index finger, she performs the movement without any difficulty, but when she repeats the movement with her right index finger, she either misses her nose or hits it due to the irregularly contracting muscles. When she is asked to quickly pronate and supinate the forearms, the movements are normal on the left side but jerky and slow on the right side. A mild papilledema of both eyes is found. No other abnormal signs are seen.

The right-sided hypotonia, static tremor, and intention tremor associated with voluntary movements, right-sided

dysdiadochokinesia, and the history are characteristic of right-sided cerebellar disease. A computed tomography scan reveals a tumor in the right cerebellar hemisphere.

Understanding the structure and the nervous connections of the cerebellum and, in particular, knowing that the right cerebellar hemisphere influences voluntary muscle tone on the same side of the body enable the neurologist to make an accurate diagnosis and institute treatment.

The cerebellum plays a very important role in the control of posture and voluntary movements. It unconsciously influences the smooth contraction of voluntary muscles and carefully coordinates their actions, together with the relaxation of their antagonists. Students should commit the functions of the connections of the cerebellum to the remainder of the central nervous system (CNS) to memory, as this will greatly assist in the retention of the material. In this chapter, great emphasis is placed on the fact that each cerebellar hemisphere controls muscular movements on the same side of the body and that the cerebellum has no direct pathway to the lower motor neurons but exerts its control via the cerebral cortex and the brainstem.

GROSS APPEARANCE

The cerebellum is situated in the posterior cranial fossa and is covered superiorly by the tentorium cerebelli. It is the largest part of the hindbrain and lies posterior to the fourth ventricle, the pons, and the medulla oblongata (Fig. 6-1). The cerebellum is somewhat ovoid in shape and constricted in its median part. It consists of two **cerebellar hemispheres** joined by a narrow median **vermis**. The cerebellum is connected to the posterior aspect of the brainstem by three symmetrical bundles of nerve fibers called the **superior**, **middle**, and **inferior cerebellar peduncles** (see Figures 1-12 and 5-18).

The cerebellum is divided into three main lobes: the **anterior lobe**, the **middle lobe**, and the **flocculonodular lobe**. The **anterior lobe** may be seen on the superior surface of the cerebellum and is separated from the middle lobe by a wide V-shaped fissure called the **primary fissure** (Figs. 6-2 and 6-3). The **middle lobe** (sometimes called the posterior lobe), which is the largest part of the cerebellum, is situated between the primary and **uvulonodular fissures**. The **flocculonodular lobe** is situated posterior to the uvulonodular fissure (Fig. 6-3). A deep **horizontal fissure** that is found along the margin of the cerebellum separates the superior from the inferior surfaces but has

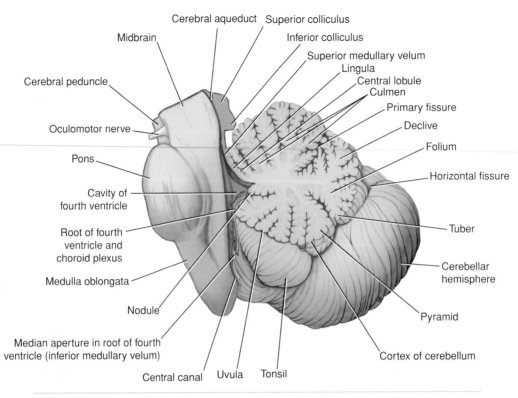

Figure 6-1 Sagittal section through the brainstem and the vermis of the cerebellum.

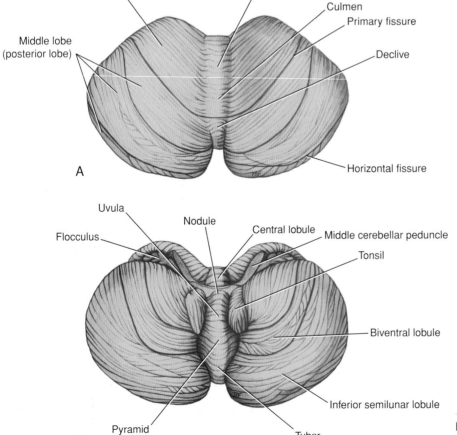

Figure 6-2 The cerebellum.
A: Superior view. **B:** Inferior view.

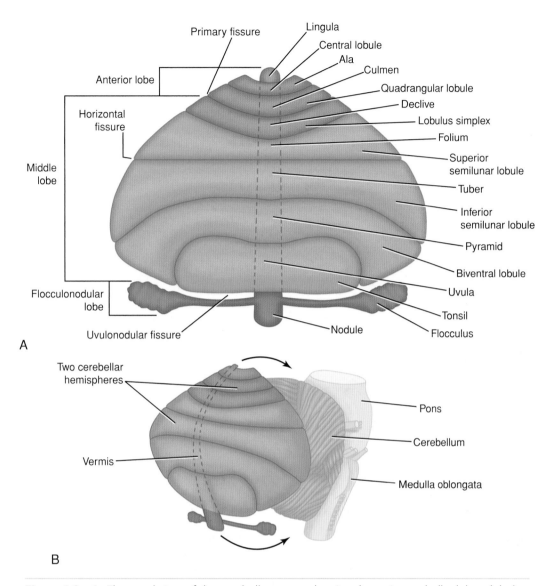

Figure 6-3 **A:** Flattened view of the cerebellar cortex showing the main cerebellar lobes, lobules, and fissures. **B:** Relationship between the diagram in (**A**) and the cerebellum.

no morphologic or functional significance (Figs. 6-2 and 6-3).

STRUCTURES

The cerebellum is composed of an outer covering of gray matter called the **cortex** and inner white matter. Embedded in the white matter of each hemisphere are three masses of gray matter forming the **intracerebellar nuclei**.

Cerebellar Cortex

The cerebellar cortex can be regarded as a large sheet with folds lying in the coronal or transverse plane. Each fold or folium contains a core of white matter covered superficially by gray matter (see Fig. 6-1).

A section made through the cerebellum parallel with the median plane divides the folia at right angles, and the cut surface has a branched appearance, called the **arbor vitae**.

The gray matter of the cortex throughout its extent has a uniform structure. It may be divided into three layers: (1) an external layer, the **molecular layer**; (2) a middle layer, the **Purkinje cell layer**; and (3) an internal layer, the **granular layer** (Figs. 6-4 and 6-5).

Molecular Layer

The molecular layer contains two types of neurons: the outer **stellate cell** and the inner **basket cell** (see Fig. 6-4). These neurons are scattered among dendritic arborizations and numerous thin axons that run parallel to the long axis of the folia. Neuroglial cells are found between these structures.

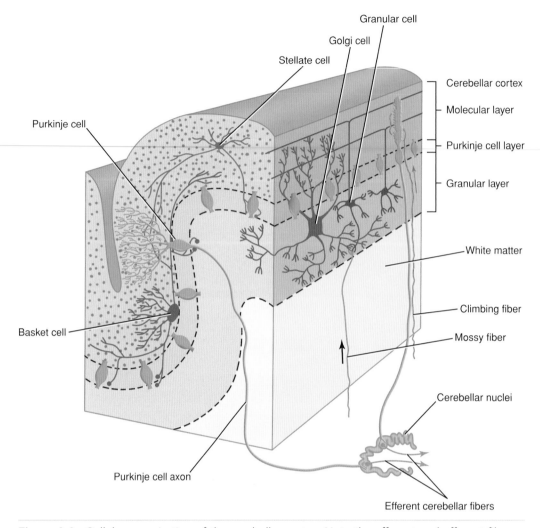

Figure 6-4 Cellular organization of the cerebellar cortex. Note the afferent and efferent fibers.

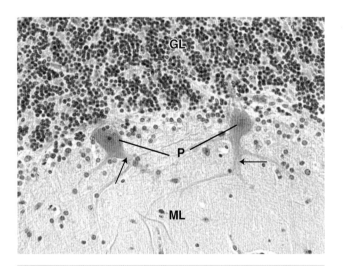

Figure 6-5 Light micrograph of the cerebellum (×132). Observe the Purkinje cells (P) with their dendritic trees (arrows) protruding into the molecular layer (ML). The heavily populated and deeply stained region is the granular layer (GL) of the cerebellum. (From Gartner, L. P. [2018]. *Color atlas and text of histology* [7th ed.]. Baltimore, MD: Wolters Kluwer.)

Purkinje Cell Layer

The Purkinje cells are large Golgi type I neurons. They are flask shaped and are arranged in a single layer (see Figs. 6-4 and 6-5). In a plane transverse to the folium, the dendrites of these cells are seen to pass into the molecular layer, where they undergo profuse branching. The primary and secondary branches are smooth, and subsequent branches are covered by short, thick **dendritic spines**. It has been shown that the spines form synaptic contacts with the parallel fibers derived from the granule cell axons.

At the base of the Purkinje cell, the axon arises and passes through the granular layer to enter the white matter. On entering the white matter, the axon acquires a myelin sheath, and it terminates by synapsing with cells of one of the intracerebellar nuclei. Collateral branches of the Purkinje axon make synaptic contacts with the dendrites of basket and stellate cells of the granular layer in the same area or in distant folia. A few of the Purkinje cell axons pass directly to end in the vestibular nuclei of the brainstem.

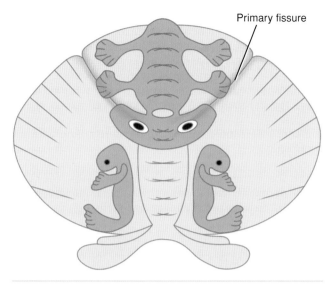

Figure 6-6 Somatosensory projection areas in the cerebellar cortex.

Granular Layer

The granular layer is packed with small cells with densely staining nuclei and scanty cytoplasm. Each cell gives rise to four or five dendrites, which make claw-like endings and have synaptic contact with mossy fiber input (see Fig. 6-4). The axon of each granule cell passes into the molecular layer, where it bifurcates at a T junction, the branches running parallel to the long axis of the cerebellar folium (see Fig. 6-4). These fibers, known as **parallel fibers**, run at right angles to the dendritic processes of the Purkinje cells. Most of the parallel fibers make synaptic contacts with the spinous processes of the dendrites of the Purkinje cells. Neuroglial

cells are found throughout this layer. Scattered throughout the granular layer are Golgi cells. Their dendrites ramify in the molecular layer, and their axons terminate by splitting up into branches that synapse with the dendrites of the granular cells (see Fig. 6-5).

Functional Areas

Clinical observations by neurologists and neurosurgeons and the experimental use of positron emission tomography have shown that the cerebellar cortex can be divided into three functional areas.

The cortex of the vermis influences the movements of the long axis of the body, namely, the neck, the shoulders, the thorax, the abdomen, and the hips (Fig. 6-6). Immediately lateral to the vermis is a so-called intermediate zone of the cerebellar hemisphere. This area has been shown to control the muscles of the distal parts of the limbs, especially the hands and feet. The lateral zone of each cerebellar hemisphere appears to be concerned with the planning of sequential movements of the entire body and is involved with the conscious assessment of movement errors.

Intracerebellar Nuclei

Four masses of gray matter are embedded in the white matter of the cerebellum on each side of the midline (Fig. 6-7). From lateral to medial, these nuclei are the **dentate**, the **emboliform**, the **globose**, and the **fastigial**.

The **dentate nucleus** is the largest of the cerebellar nuclei. It has the shape of a crumpled bag with the opening facing medially. The interior of the bag is filled with white matter made up of efferent fibers that leaves the nucleus through the opening to form a large part of the superior cerebellar peduncle.

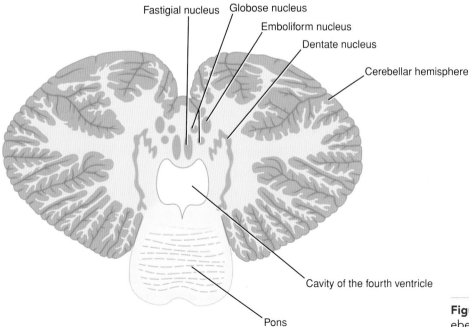

Figure 6-7 Position of the intracerebellar nuclei.

The **emboliform nucleus** is ovoid and is situated medial to the dentate nucleus, partially covering its hilus.

The **globose nucleus** consists of one or more rounded cell groups that lie medial to the emboliform nucleus.

The **fastigial nucleus** lies near the midline in the vermis and close to the roof of the fourth ventricle; it is larger than the globose nucleus.

The intracerebellar nuclei are composed of large, multipolar neurons with simple branching dendrites. The axons form the cerebellar outflow in the superior and inferior cerebellar peduncles.

White Matter

There is a small amount of white matter in the vermis; it closely resembles the trunk and branches of a tree and thus is termed the **arbor vitae** (see Fig. 6-1). There is a large amount of white matter in each cerebellar hemisphere.

The white matter is made up of three groups of fibers: (1) intrinsic, (2) afferent, and (3) efferent.

The **intrinsic fibers** do not leave the cerebellum but connect different regions of the organ. Some interconnect folia of the cerebellar cortex and vermis on the same side; others connect the two cerebellar hemispheres together.

The **afferent fibers** form the greater part of the white matter and proceed to the cerebellar cortex. They enter the cerebellum mainly through the inferior and middle cerebellar peduncles.

The **efferent fibers** constitute the output of the cerebellum and commence as the axons of the Purkinje cells of the cerebellar cortex. The great majority of the Purkinje cell axons pass to and synapse with the neurons of the cerebellar nuclei (fastigial, globose, emboliform, and dentate). The axons of the neurons then leave the cerebellum. A few Purkinje cell axons in the flocculonodular lobe and in parts of the vermis bypass the cerebellar nuclei and leave the cerebellum without synapsing.

Fibers from the dentate, emboliform, and globose nuclei leave the cerebellum through the superior cerebellar peduncle. Fibers from the fastigial nucleus leave through the inferior cerebellar peduncle.

CEREBELLAR CORTICAL MECHANISMS

As a result of extensive cytologic and physiologic research, certain basic mechanisms have been attributed to the cerebellar cortex. The climbing and the mossy fibers constitute the two main lines of input to the cortex and are **excitatory** to the Purkinje cells (Fig. 6-8).

The **climbing fibers** are the terminal fibers of the olivocerebellar tracts. They are so named because they ascend through the layers of the cortex like a

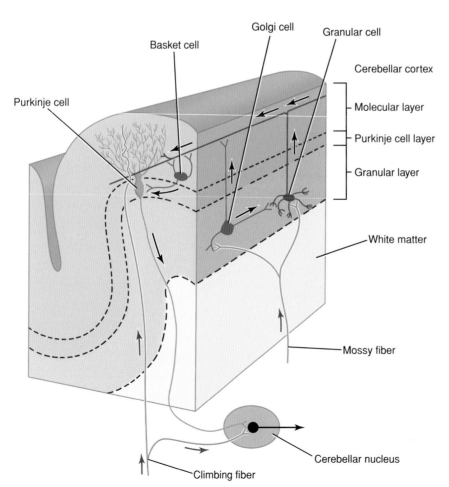

Golgi cell
Basket cell
Granular cell
Purkinje cell

Cerebellar cortex
Molecular layer
Purkinje cell layer
Granular layer
White matter
Mossy fiber
Cerebellar nucleus
Climbing fiber

Figure 6-8 Functional organization of the cerebellar cortex. The *arrows* indicate the direction taken by the nervous impulses. The red *arrows* indicate information entering the cerebellum.

vine on a tree. They pass through the granular layer of the cortex and terminate in the molecular layer by dividing repeatedly. Each climbing fiber wraps around and makes a large number of synaptic contacts with the dendrites of a Purkinje cell. A **single** Purkinje neuron makes synaptic contact with only one climbing fiber. However, one climbing fiber makes contact with 1 to 10 Purkinje neurons. A few side branches leave each climbing fiber and synapse with the stellate cells and basket cells.

The **mossy fibers** are the terminal fibers of all other cerebellar afferent tracts. They have multiple branches and exert a much more diffuse excitatory effect. A single mossy fiber may stimulate **thousands** of Purkinje cells through the granule cells. What then is the function of the remaining cells of the cerebellar cortex, namely, the stellate, basket, and Golgi cells? Neurophysiologic research, using microelectrodes, would indicate that they serve as **inhibitory** interneurons. They not only limit the area of cortex excited but also probably influence the degree of Purkinje cell excitation produced by the climbing and mossy fiber input. By this means, fluctuating **inhibitory** impulses are transmitted by the Purkinje cells to the intracerebellar nuclei, which, in turn, modify muscular activity through the motor control areas of the brainstem and cerebral cortex. Thus, the Purkinje cells form the center of a **functional unit** of the cerebellar cortex.

Intracerebellar Nuclear Mechanisms

The deep cerebellar nuclei receive afferent nervous information from two sources: (1) the inhibitory axons from the Purkinje cells of the overlying cortex and (2) the excitatory axons that are branches of the afferent climbing and mossy fibers that are passing to the overlying cortex. In this manner, a given sensory input to the cerebellum sends excitatory information to the nuclei, which a short time later receive cortical processed inhibitory information from the Purkinje cells. Efferent information from the deep cerebellar nuclei leaves the cerebellum to be distributed to the remainder of the brain and spinal cord.

Cerebellar Cortical Neurotransmitters

Pharmacologic research has suggested that the excitatory climbing and mossy afferent fibers use **glutamate** (γ-aminobutyric acid [GABA]) as the excitatory transmitter on the dendrites of the Purkinje cells. Further research has indicated that other afferent fibers entering the cortex liberate **norepinephrine** and **serotonin** at their endings that possibly modify the action of the glutamate on the Purkinje cells.

Cerebellar Peduncles

The cerebellum is linked to other parts of the central nervous system (CNS) by numerous efferent and afferent fibers that are grouped together on each side into three large bundles, or peduncles (Fig. 6-9). The superior cerebellar peduncles connect the cerebellum to the midbrain, the middle cerebellar peduncles connect the cerebellum to the pons, and the inferior cerebellar peduncles connect the cerebellum to the medulla oblongata.

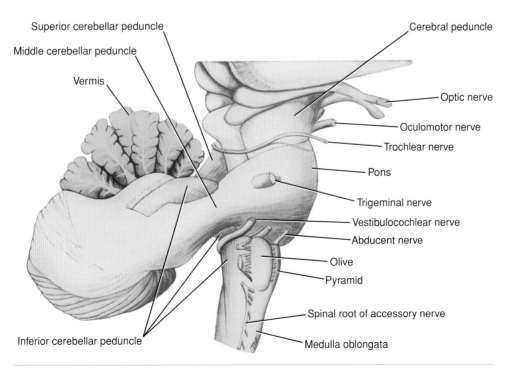

Figure 6-9 Three cerebellar peduncles connecting the cerebellum to the rest of the central nervous system.

CEREBELLAR AFFERENT FIBERS

The cerebellum receives major afferent tracts from the cerebral cortex, pons, medulla oblongata, and the spinal cord.

Cerebellar Afferent Fibers From the Cerebral Cortex

The cerebral cortex sends information to the cerebellum by three pathways: (1) the corticopontocerebellar pathway, (2) the cerebro-olivocerebellar pathway, and (3) the cerebroreticulocerebellar pathway.

Corticopontocerebellar Pathway

The corticopontine fibers arise from nerve cells in the frontal, parietal, temporal, and occipital lobes of the cerebral cortex and descend through the corona radiata and internal capsule and terminate on the pontine nuclei (Fig. 6-10). The pontine nuclei give rise to the **transverse fibers of the pons**, which cross the midline and enter the opposite cerebellar hemisphere as the middle cerebellar peduncle (see Figs. 5-18, 5-19).

Cerebro-Olivocerebellar Pathway

The cortico-olivary fibers arise from nerve cells in the frontal, parietal, temporal, and occipital lobes of the cerebral cortex and descend through the corona radiata and internal capsule to terminate bilaterally on the inferior olivary nuclei. The inferior olivary nuclei give rise to fibers that cross the midline and enter the opposite cerebellar hemisphere through the inferior cerebellar peduncle. These fibers terminate as the climbing fibers in the cerebellar cortex.

Cerebroreticulocerebellar Pathway

The corticoreticular fibers arise from nerve cells from many areas of the cerebral cortex, particularly the sensorimotor areas. They descend to terminate in the

Figure 6-10 Cerebellar afferent fibers from the cerebral cortex. The cerebellar peduncles are shown as *ovoid dotted lines*.

reticular formation on the same side and on the opposite side in the pons and medulla. The cells in the reticular formation give rise to the reticulocerebellar fibers that enter the cerebellar hemisphere on the same side through the inferior and middle cerebellar peduncles.

This connection between the cerebrum and the cerebellum is important in the control of voluntary movement. Information regarding the initiation of movement in the cerebral cortex is probably transmitted to the cerebellum so that the movement can be monitored and appropriate adjustments in the muscle activity can be made.

Cerebellar Afferent Fibers From the Spinal Cord

The spinal cord sends information to the cerebellum from somatosensory receptors by three pathways:

(1) the anterior spinocerebellar tract, (2) the posterior spinocerebellar tract, and (3) the cuneocerebellar tract.

Anterior Spinocerebellar Tract

The axons entering the spinal cord from the posterior root ganglion terminate by synapsing with the neurons in the **nucleus dorsalis** (Clarke column) at the base of the posterior gray column. Most of the axons of these neurons cross to the opposite side and ascend as the **anterior spinocerebellar tract** in the contralateral white column; some of the axons ascend as the anterior spinocerebellar tract in the lateral white column on the same side (Fig. 6-11). The fibers enter the cerebellum through the superior cerebellar peduncle and terminate as mossy fibers in the cerebellar cortex. Collateral

Figure 6-11 Cerebellar afferent fibers from the spinal cord and internal ear. The cerebellar peduncles are shown as *ovoid dotted lines.*

branches that end in the deep cerebellar nuclei are also given off. Those fibers that cross over to the opposite side in the spinal cord are thought to cross back within the cerebellum.

The anterior spinocerebellar tract is found at all segments of the spinal cord, and its fibers convey muscle joint information from the muscle spindles, tendon organs, and joint receptors of the upper and lower limbs. The cerebellum likely receives information from the skin and superficial fascia by this tract.

Posterior Spinocerebellar Tract

The axons entering the spinal cord from the posterior root ganglion enter the posterior gray column and terminate by synapsing on the neurons at the base of the posterior gray column. These neurons are known collectively as the nucleus dorsalis (Clarke column). The axons of these neurons enter the posterolateral part of the lateral white column on the same side and ascend as the **posterior spinocerebellar tract** to the medulla oblongata. Here, the tract enters the cerebellum through the inferior cerebellar peduncle and terminates as mossy fibers in the cerebellar cortex. Collateral branches that end in the deep cerebellar nuclei are also given off. The posterior spinocerebellar tract receives muscle joint information from the muscle spindles, tendon organs, and joint receptors of the trunk and lower limbs.

Cuneocerebellar Tract

These fibers originate in the nucleus cuneatus of the medulla oblongata and enter the cerebellar hemisphere on the same side through the inferior cerebellar peduncle (see Fig. 6-10). The fibers terminate as mossy fibers in the cerebellar cortex. Collateral branches that end in the deep cerebellar nuclei are also given off. The cuneocerebellar tract receives muscle joint information from the muscle spindles, tendon organs, and joint receptors of the upper limb and upper part of the thorax.

Cerebellar Afferent Fibers From the Vestibular Nerve

The vestibular nerve receives information from the inner ear concerning motion from the semicircular canals and position relative to gravity from the utricle and saccule. The vestibular nerve sends many afferent fibers directly to the cerebellum through the inferior cerebellar peduncle on the same side. Other vestibular afferent fibers pass first to the vestibular nuclei in the brainstem, where they synapse and are relayed to the cerebellum (see Fig. 6-11). They enter the cerebellum through the inferior cerebellar peduncle on the same side. All the afferent fibers from the inner ear terminate as mossy fibers in the flocculonodular lobe of the cerebellum.

Other Afferent Fibers

In addition, the cerebellum receives small bundles of afferent fibers from the red nucleus and the tectum.

The afferent cerebellar pathways are summarized in Table 6-1.

Table 6-1   Afferent Cerebellar Pathways

Pathway	Function	Origin	Destination
Corticopontocerebellar	Conveys control from cerebral cortex	Frontal, parietal, temporal, and occipital lobes	Via pontine nuclei and mossy fibers to cerebellar cortex
Cerebro-olivocerebellar	Conveys control from cerebral cortex	Frontal, parietal, temporal, and occipital lobes	Via inferior olivary nuclei and climbing fibers to cerebellar cortex
Cerebroreticulocerebellar	Conveys control from cerebral cortex	Sensorimotor areas	Via reticular formation
Anterior spinocerebellar	Conveys information from muscles and joints	Muscle spindles, tendon organs, and joint receptors	Via mossy fibers to cerebellar cortex
Posterior spinocerebellar	Conveys information from muscles and joints	Muscle spindles, tendon organs, and joint receptors	Via mossy fibers to cerebellar cortex
Cuneocerebellar	Conveys information from muscles and joints of upper limb	Muscle spindles, tendon organs, and joint receptors	Via mossy fibers to cerebellar cortex
Vestibular nerve	Conveys information of head position and movement	Utricle, saccule, and semicircular canals	Via mossy fibers to cortex of flocculonodular lobe
Other afferents	Conveys information from midbrain	Red nucleus, tectum	Cerebellar cortex

CEREBELLAR EFFERENT FIBERS

The entire output of the cerebellar cortex is through the axons of the Purkinje cells. Most of the axons of the Purkinje cells end by synapsing on the neurons of the deep cerebellar nuclei (see Fig. 6-4). The axons of the neurons that form the cerebellar nuclei constitute the efferent outflow from the cerebellum. A few Purkinje cell axons pass directly out of the cerebellum to the lateral vestibular nucleus. The efferent fibers from the cerebellum connect with the red nucleus, thalamus, vestibular complex, and reticular formation.

Globose-Emboliform-Rubral Pathway

Axons of neurons in the globose and emboliform nuclei travel through the superior cerebellar peduncle and cross the midline to the opposite side in the **decussation of the superior cerebellar peduncles** (Fig. 6-12). The fibers end by synapsing with cells of the contralateral red nucleus, which give rise to axons of the **rubrospinal tract**. Thus, this pathway crosses twice, once in the decussation of the superior cerebellar peduncle and again in the rubrospinal tract close to its origin. By this means, the globose and emboliform nuclei influence motor activity on the same side of the body.

Dentatothalamic Pathway

Axons of neurons in the dentate nucleus travel through the superior cerebellar peduncle and cross the midline to the opposite side in the **decussation of the superior cerebellar peduncle**. The fibers end by synapsing with cells in the contralateral **ventrolateral nucleus**

Figure 6-12 Cerebellar efferent fibers. The cerebellar peduncles are shown as *ovoid dotted lines.*

Table 6-2   Efferent Cerebellar Pathways[a]

Pathway	Function	Origin	Destination
Globose-emboliform-rubral	Influences ipsilateral motor activity	Globose and emboliform nuclei	To contralateral red nucleus, then via crossed rubrospinal tract to ipsilateral motor neurons in the spinal cord
Dentatothalamic	Influences ipsilateral motor activity	Dentate nucleus	To contralateral ventrolateral nucleus of the thalamus, then to contralateral motor cerebral cortex; corticospinal tract crosses midline and controls ipsilateral motor neurons in the spinal cord
Fastigial vestibular	Influences ipsilateral extensor muscle tone	Fastigial nucleus	Mainly to ipsilateral and to contralateral lateral vestibular nuclei; vestibulospinal tract to ipsilateral motor neurons in the spinal cord
Fastigial reticular	Influences ipsilateral muscle tone	Fastigial nucleus	To neurons of reticular formation; reticulospinal tract to ipsilateral motor neurons to the spinal cord

[a]Note that each cerebellar hemisphere influences the voluntary muscle tone on the same side of the body.

of the thalamus. The axons of the thalamic neurons ascend through the internal capsule and corona radiata and terminate in the primary motor area of the cerebral cortex. By this pathway, the dentate nucleus can influence motor activity by acting on the motor neurons of the opposite cerebral cortex; impulses from the motor cortex are transmitted to spinal segmental levels through the corticospinal tract. Remember that most of the fibers of the corticospinal tract cross to the opposite side in the decussation of the pyramids or later at the spinal segmental levels. Thus, the dentate nucleus is able to coordinate muscle activity on the same side of the body.

Fastigial Vestibular Pathway

The axons of neurons in the fastigial nucleus travel through the inferior cerebellar peduncle and end by projecting on the neurons of the **lateral vestibular nucleus** on both sides. Remember that some Purkinje cell axons project directly to the lateral vestibular nucleus. The neurons of the lateral vestibular nucleus form the **vestibulospinal tract**. The fastigial nucleus exerts a facilitatory influence mainly on the ipsilateral extensor muscle tone.

Fastigial Reticular Pathway

The axons of neurons in the fastigial nucleus travel through the inferior cerebellar peduncle and end by synapsing with neurons of the reticular formation. Axons of these neurons influence spinal segmental motor activity through the reticulospinal tract. The efferent cerebellar pathways are summarized in Table 6-2.

FUNCTIONS OF THE CEREBELLUM

The cerebellum receives afferent information concerning voluntary movement from the cerebral cortex and from the muscles, tendons, and joints. It also receives information concerning balance from the vestibular nerve and possibly concerning sight through the tectocerebellar tract. All this information is fed into the cerebellar cortical circuitry by the mossy fibers and the climbing fibers and converges on the Purkinje cells (see Fig. 6-8). The axons of the Purkinje cells project with few exceptions on the deep cerebellar nuclei. The output of the vermis projects to the fastigial nucleus, the intermediate regions of the cortex project to the globose and emboliform nuclei, and the output of the lateral part of the cerebellar hemisphere projects to the dentate nucleus. A few Purkinje cell axons pass directly out of the cerebellum and end on the lateral vestibular nucleus in the brainstem. Purkinje axons are generally believed to exert an inhibitory influence on the neurons of the cerebellar nuclei and the lateral vestibular nuclei.

The cerebellar output is conducted to the sites of origin of the descending pathways that influence motor activity at the segmental spinal level. In this respect, the cerebellum has no direct neuronal connections with the lower motor neurons but exerts its influence indirectly through the cerebral cortex and brainstem.

Physiologists have postulated that the cerebellum functions as a coordinator of precise movements by continually comparing the output of the motor area of the cerebral cortex with the proprioceptive information received from the site of muscle action; it is then able to bring about the necessary adjustments by influencing the activity of the lower motor neurons (Fig. 6-13). This is accomplished by controlling the timing and sequence of firing of the α and γ motor neurons. The cerebellum can possibly send back information to the motor cerebral cortex to inhibit the agonist muscles and stimulate the antagonist muscles, thus limiting the extent of voluntary movement.

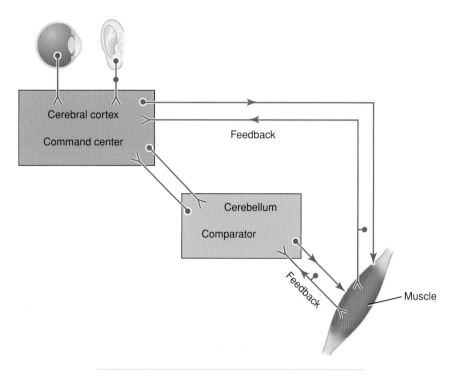

Figure 6-13 Cerebellum serving as a comparator.

Clinical Notes

General Considerations

Each cerebellar hemisphere is connected by nervous pathways principally with the same side of the body; thus, a **lesion in one cerebellar hemisphere gives rise to signs and symptoms that are limited to the same side of the body**. The main connections of the cerebellum are summarized in Figure 6-14.

The essential function of the cerebellum is to coordinate, by synergistic action, all reflex and voluntary muscular activity. Thus, it graduates and harmonizes muscle tone and maintains normal body posture. It permits voluntary movements, such as walking, to take place smoothly with precision and economy of effort. It must be understood that although the cerebellum plays an important role in skeletal muscle activity, it is not able to initiate muscle movement.

Signs and Symptoms of Cerebellar Disease

While the importance of the cerebellum in the maintenance of muscle tone and the coordination of muscle movement has been emphasized, it should be remembered that the symptoms and signs of acute lesions differ from those produced by chronic lesions. Acute lesions produce sudden, severe symptoms and signs, but there is considerable clinical evidence to show that patients can recover completely from large cerebellar injuries. This suggests that other CNS areas can compensate for loss of cerebellar function. Chronic lesions, such as slowly enlarging tumors, produce symptoms and signs that are much less severe than those of acute lesions. The reason for this may be that other CNS areas have time to compensate for loss of cerebellar function. The following symptoms and signs are characteristic of cerebellar dysfunction.

Hypotonia

The muscles lose resilience to palpation. There is diminished resistance to passive movements of joints. Shaking the limb produces excessive movements at the terminal joints. The condition is attributable to loss of cerebellar influence on the simple stretch reflex.

Postural Changes and Alteration of Gait

The head is often rotated and flexed, and the shoulder on the side of the lesion is lower than on the normal side. The patient assumes a wide base when he or she stands and is often stiff legged to compensate for loss of muscle tone. When the individual walks, he or she lurches and staggers toward the affected side.

Disturbances of Voluntary Movement (Ataxia)

The muscles contract irregularly and weakly. **Tremor** occurs when fine movements, such as buttoning clothes, writing, and shaving, are attempted. Muscle groups fail to work harmoniously, and there is **decomposition of movement**. When the patient is asked to touch the tip of the nose with the index finger, the movements are not properly coordinated, and the finger either passes the nose (past-pointing) or hits the nose. A similar test can be performed on the lower limbs by asking the patient to place the heel of one foot on the shin of the opposite leg.

Dysdiadochokinesia

Dysdiadochokinesia is the inability to perform alternating movements regularly and rapidly. Ask the patient to pronate and supinate the forearms rapidly. On the side of

Figure 6-14 Some of the main connections of the cerebellum. The cerebellar peduncles are shown as *ovoid dashed lines.*

the cerebellar lesion, the movements are slow, jerky, and incomplete.

Disturbances of Reflexes

Movement produced by tendon reflexes tends to continue for a longer period of time than normal. The **pendular knee jerk**, for example, occurs following tapping of the patellar tendon. Normally, the movement occurs and is self-limited by the stretch reflexes of the agonists and antagonists. In cerebellar disease, because of loss of influence on the stretch reflexes, the movement continues as a series of flexion and extension movements at the knee joint; that is, the leg moves like a pendulum.

Disturbances of Ocular Movement

Nystagmus, which is essentially an ataxia of the ocular muscles, is a rhythmical oscillation of the eyes. It is more easily demonstrated when the eyes are deviated in a horizontal

direction. This rhythmic oscillation of the eyes may be of the same rate in both directions **(pendular nystagmus)** or quicker in one direction than in the other **(jerk nystagmus)**. In the latter situation, the movements are referred to as the slow phase away from the visual object, followed by a quick phase back toward the target. The quick phase is used to describe the form of nystagmus. For example, a patient is said to have a nystagmus to the left if the quick phase is to the left and the slow phase is to the right. The movement of nystagmus may be confined to one plane and may be horizontal or vertical, or it may be in many planes when it is referred to as rotatory nystagmus.

The posture of the eye muscles depends mainly on the normal functioning of two sets of afferent pathways. The first is the visual pathway whereby the eye views the object of interest, and the second pathway is much more complicated and involves the labyrinths, the vestibular nuclei, and the cerebellum.

Disorders of Speech

Dysarthria occurs in cerebellar disease because of ataxia of the muscles of the larynx. Articulation is jerky, and the syllables often are separated from one another. Speech tends to be explosive, and the syllables often are slurred.

In cerebellar lesions, paralysis and sensory changes are not present. Although muscle hypotonia and incoordination may be present, the disorder is not limited to specific muscles or muscle groups; rather, an entire extremity or the entire half of the body is involved. If both cerebellar hemispheres are involved, then the entire body may show disturbances of muscle action. Even though the muscular contractions may be weak and the patient may be easily fatigued, there is no atrophy.

Cerebellar Syndromes

Vermis Syndrome

The most common cause of vermis syndrome is a **medulloblastoma** of the vermis in children. Involvement of the flocculonodular lobe results in signs and symptoms related to the vestibular system. Since the vermis is unpaired and influences midline structures, muscle incoordination involves the head and trunk and not the limbs. There is a tendency to fall forward or backward. There is difficulty in holding the head steady and in an upright position. There also may be difficulty in holding the trunk erect.

Cerebellar Hemisphere Syndrome

Tumors of one cerebellar hemisphere may be the cause of cerebellar hemisphere syndrome. The symptoms and signs are usually unilateral and involve muscles on the side of the diseased cerebellar hemisphere. Movements of the limbs, especially the arms, are disturbed. Swaying and falling to the side of the lesion often occur. Dysarthria and nystagmus are also common findings. Disorders of the lateral part of the cerebellar hemispheres produce delays in initiating movements and inability to move all limb segments together in a coordinated manner but show a tendency to move one joint at a time.

Common Diseases Involving the Cerebellum

One of the most common diseases affecting cerebellar function is acute alcohol poisoning. This occurs as the result of alcohol acting on GABA receptors on the cerebellar neurons.

The following frequently involve the cerebellum: congenital agenesis or hypoplasia, trauma, infections, tumors, multiple sclerosis, vascular disorders such as thrombosis of the cerebellar arteries, and poisoning with heavy metals.

The many manifestations of cerebellar disease can be reduced to two basic defects: hypotonia and loss of influence of the cerebellum on the activities of the cerebral cortex.

Key Concepts

Cerebellum

- The cerebellum is composed of an outer covering of gray matter called the cortex and inner white matter. Embedded in the white matter of each hemisphere are three masses of gray matter forming the four intracerebellar nuclei.

- The gray matter of the cortex is divided into three layers: the external, molecular layer; the middle, Purkinje layer; and the inner, granular layer.

- Basket and stellate cells are found in the molecular layer and are scattered throughout the dendritic arborizations of the Purkinje cells, whose cell bodies are found within the Purkinje layer.

- Granule cells (and Golgi cells) are found throughout the granular layer and have synaptic contact with mossy fiber input (cerebellar afferent tracts). The axon of each granule cell branches and runs parallel to the long axis of the cerebellar folium.

- Climbing fibers are terminal fibers of the olivocerebellar tracts. A single Purkinje neuron makes synaptic contact with only one climbing fiber.

- Mossy fibers are the terminal fibers of all other cerebellar afferent tracts. Each mossy fiber communicates with thousands of Purkinje cells through the granule cells.

Cerebellar Afferent Fibers

- The cerebellum receives three afferent pathways from the cerebrum and is important for monitoring and control of voluntary movements.

- The cerebellum also receives three afferent pathways from the spinal cord, all of which supply the cerebellum with muscle and joint information of the limb and trunk.

Cerebellar Efferent Fibers

- The output of the cerebellum is through Purkinje cell axons, most of which synapse on the neurons of the deep cerebellar nuclei.

- The efferent fibers from the deep nuclei connect with the red nucleus (globose-emboliform-rubral), thalamus (dentatothalamic), vestibular complex (fastigial vestibular), and reticular formation (fastigial reticular).

Cerebellar Functions

- The cerebellum functions as a coordinator of precise movements by continually comparing the output of the motor area of cerebral cortex with the proprioceptive information received from the site of muscle action, and makes necessary adjustments.

Clinical Problem Solving

1. A 10-year-old girl is taken to a neurologist because her parents notice that her gait is becoming awkward. Six months previously, the child had complained that she felt her right arm is clumsy, and she had inadvertently knocked a teapot off the table. More recently, her family notices that her hand movements are becoming jerky and awkward; this is particularly obvious when she is eating with a knife and fork. The mother comments that her daughter has had problems with her right foot since birth and that she had a clubfoot. She also has scoliosis and is attending an orthopedic surgeon for treatment. The mother said she is particularly worried about her daughter because two other members of the family had similar signs and symptoms.

On physical examination, the child is found to have a lurching gait with a tendency to reel over to the right. Intention tremor is present in the right arm and the right leg. When the strength of the limb muscles is tested, those of the right leg are found to be weaker than those of the left leg. The muscles of the right arm and right lower leg are also hypotonic. She has severe pes cavus of the right foot and a slight pes cavus of the left foot. Kyphoscoliosis of the upper part of the thoracic vertebral column also is present.

On examination of her sensory system, she is found to have loss of muscle joint sense and vibratory sense of both legs. She also has loss of two-point discrimination of the skin of both legs. Her knee jerks are found to be exaggerated, but her ankle jerks are absent. The biceps and triceps jerks of both arms are normal. She has bilateral Babinski responses. Slight nystagmus is present in both eyes. Using your knowledge of neuroanatomy, explain the symptoms and signs listed for this patient. Did the disease process involve more than one area of the central nervous system? Explain.

2. Two physicians are talking in the street when one turns to the other and says, "Look at that man over there. Look at the way he is walking. He is not swinging his right arm at all; it is just hanging down by his side. I wonder if he has a cerebellar lesion." Does a person with a unilateral cerebellar hemisphere tumor tend to hold the arm limply at the side when he walks?

3. A 37-year-old man visits his physician because he has noticed clumsiness of his right arm. The symptoms started 6 months previously and are getting worse. He also notices that his right hand has a tremor when he attempts fine movements or tries to insert a key in a lock. When he walks, he notices that now and again he tends to reel over to the right, "as if he had too much alcohol to drink." On physical examination, the face is tilted slightly to the left, and the right shoulder is held lower than the left. Passive movements of the arms and legs reveal hypotonia and looseness on the right side. When asked to walk heel to toe along a straight line on the floor, the patient sways over to the right side. When he was asked to touch his nose with his right index finger, the right hand displays tremor, and the finger tends to overshoot the target. Speech is normal, and nystagmus is not present. Using your knowledge of neuroanatomy, explain each sign and symptom. Is the lesion of the cerebellum likely to be in the midline or to one side?

4. A 4½-year-old boy is taken to a neurologist because his mother is concerned about his attacks of vomiting on waking in the morning and his tendency to be unsteady on standing up. The mother also notices that the child walks with an unsteady gait and often falls backward. On physical examination, the child tends to stand with the legs well apart—that is, broad based. The head is larger than normal for his age, and the suture lines of the skull can be easily felt. A retinal examination with an ophthalmoscope shows severe papilledema in both eyes. The muscles of the upper and lower limbs show some degree of hypotonia. Nystagmus is not present, and the child showed no tendency to fall to one side or the other when asked to walk. Using your knowledge of neuroanatomy, explain the symptoms and signs. Is the lesion in the cerebellum likely to be in the midline or to one side?

5. During a ward round, a third-year student is asked to explain the phenomenon of nystagmus. How would you have answered that question? Why do patients with cerebellar disease exhibit nystagmus?

6. What is the essential difference between the symptoms and signs of acute and chronic lesions of the cerebellum? Explain these differences.

 Answers and Explanations to Clinical Problem Solving

1. This 10-year-old girl had the symptoms and signs of Friedreich ataxia, an inherited degenerative disease of the cerebellum and posterior and lateral parts of the spinal cord.

Degeneration of the cerebellum was revealed by the altered gait, clumsy movements of the right arm, tendency to fall to the right, intention tremor of the right arm and leg, hypotonicity of the right arm and right leg, and nystagmus of both eyes.

Involvement of the fasciculus gracilis was evidenced by loss of vibratory sense, loss of two-point discrimination, and loss of muscle joint sense of the lower limbs.

Corticospinal tract degeneration resulted in weakness of the legs and the presence of the Babinski plantar response. The exaggerated knee jerks were due to the involvement of the upper motor neurons other than the corticospinal tract.

The loss of the ankle jerks was due to the interruption of the reflex arcs at spinal levels S1–S2 by the degenerative process.

The clubfoot and scoliosis can be attributed to altered tone of the muscles of the leg and trunk over a period of many years.

2. Yes. A person who has a unilateral lesion involving one cerebellar hemisphere demonstrates absence of coordination between different groups of muscles on the same side of the body. This disturbance affects not only agonists and antagonists in a single joint movement but also all associated muscle activity. For example, a normal person when walking swings his or her arms at both sides; with cerebellar disease, this activity would be lost on the side of the lesion.

3. This man, at operation, was found to have an astrocytoma of the right cerebellar hemisphere. This fact explains the occurrence of unilateral symptoms and signs. The lesion was on the right side, and the clumsiness, tremor, muscle incoordination, and hypotonia occurred on the right side of the body. The progressive worsening of the clinical condition could be explained on the basis that more and more of the cerebellum was becoming destroyed as the tumor rapidly expanded. The flaccidity of the muscles of the right arm and leg was due to hypotonia, that is, a removal of the influence of the cerebellum on the simple stretch reflex involving the muscle spindles and tendon organs. The clumsiness, tremor, and overshooting on the finger-nose test were caused by the lack of cerebellar influence on the process of coordination between different groups of muscles. The falling to the right side, the tilting of the head, and the drooping of the right shoulder were due to loss of muscle tone and fatigue.

4. The diagnosis was medulloblastoma of the brain in the region of the roof of the fourth ventricle,

with involvement of the vermis of the cerebellum. The child died 9 months later after extensive deep x-ray therapy. The sudden onset of vomiting, the increased size of the head beyond normal limits, the sutural separation, and the severe bilateral papilledema could all be accounted for by the rapid rise in intracranial pressure owing to the rapid increase in size of the tumor. The broad-based, unsteady gait and the tendency to fall backward (or forward), and not to one side, indicate a tumor involving the vermis. The presence of bilateral hypotonia, especially during the later stages, was due to involvement of both cerebellar hemispheres. At autopsy, the tumor was found to have invaded the fourth ventricle extensively, and there was evidence of internal hydrocephalus because the cerebrospinal fluid had been unable to escape through the foramina in the roof of the fourth ventricle.

5. Nystagmus, an involuntary oscillation of the eyeball, may occur physiologically, as when a person watches rapidly moving objects, or by rapid rotation of the body. It commonly occurs in diseases of the nervous system, eye, and inner ear. In cerebellar disease, nystagmus is due to ataxia of the muscles moving the eyeball. There is lack of coordination between the agonists and antagonists involved in the eyeball movement. For full understanding of the different forms of nystagmus, a textbook of neurology should be consulted. Also see page 242.

6. Acute lesions, such as those resulting from a thrombosis of a cerebellar artery or a rapidly growing tumor, produce sudden severe symptoms and signs because of the sudden withdrawal of the influence of the cerebellum on muscular activity. Patients can recover quickly from large cerebellar injuries, and this can be explained by the fact that the cerebellum influences muscular activity not directly, but indirectly, through the vestibular nuclei, reticular formation, red nucleus, tectum, and corpus striatum and the cerebral cortex; it may be that these other areas of the central nervous system (CNS) take over this function. In chronic lesions, the symptoms and signs are much less severe, and there is enough time to allow other CNS areas to compensate for loss of cerebellar function.

 Review Questions

Directions: Each of the numbered items in this section is followed by answers. Select the ONE lettered answer that is CORRECT.

1. The following statements concern the gross appearance of the cerebellum:
   (a) It is separated from the occipital lobes of the cerebral hemispheres by the tentorium cerebelli.
   (b) It lies anterior to the medulla oblongata and the pons.
   (c) The anterior lobe is separated from the middle (posterior) lobe by the uvulonodular fissure.
   (d) The flocculonodular lobe is separated from the middle (posterior) lobe by the horizontal fissure.
   (e) The third ventricle lies anterior to the cerebellum.

2. The following general statements concern the cerebellum:
   (a) The cerebellum greatly influences the activity of smooth muscle.
   (b) The cerebellum has no influence on the skeletal muscles supplied by the cranial nerves.
   (c) Each cerebellar hemisphere controls the tone of skeletal muscles supplied by spinal nerves on the same side of the body.
   (d) The important Purkinje cells are Golgi type II neurons.
   (e) The Purkinje cells exert a stimulatory influence on the intracerebellar nuclei.

3. The following statements concern the structure of the cerebellum:
   (a) The cerebellum consists of two cerebellar hemispheres joined by a narrow median vermis.
   (b) The inferior surface of the cerebellum shows a deep groove formed by the superior surface of the vermis.
   (c) The inferior cerebellar peduncles join the cerebellum to the pons.
   (d) The gray matter is confined to the cerebellar cortex.
   (e) The gray matter of folia of the dentate nucleus has a branched appearance on the cut surface, called the arbor vitae.

4. The following statements concern the structure of the cerebellar cortex:
   (a) The cortex is folded by many vertical fissures into folia.
   (b) The structure of the cortex differs widely in different parts of the cerebellum.
   (c) The Purkinje cells are found in the most superficial layer of the cortex.
   (d) The Golgi cells are found in the most superficial layer of the cerebellar cortex.
   (e) The axons of the Purkinje cells form the efferent fibers from the cerebellar cortex.

5. The following statements concern the intracerebellar nuclei:
   (a) The nuclei are found within the superficial layers of the white matter.
   (b) The nuclei are located in the walls of the fourth ventricle.
   (c) The nuclei are composed of many small unipolar neurons.
   (d) The axons of the nuclei form the main cerebellar outflow.
   (e) From medial to lateral, the nuclei are named as follows: dentate, emboliform, globose, and fastigial.

6. The following statements concern the cerebellar peduncles:
   (a) In the superior cerebellar peduncle, most of the fibers are afferent and arise from the neurons of the spinal cord.
   (b) The anterior spinocerebellar tract enters the cerebellum through the superior cerebellar peduncle.

   (c) The inferior cerebellar peduncle is made up exclusively of fibers that pass from the inferior olivary nuclei to the middle lobe of the cerebellar hemisphere.
   (d) The middle cerebellar peduncle is formed of fibers that arise from the dentate nuclei.
   (e) The cerebellar peduncles are surface structures that are difficult to see even by brain dissection.

7. The following statements concern the afferent fibers entering the cerebellum:
   (a) The mossy fibers end by making synaptic contacts with the dendrites of the Purkinje cells.
   (b) The fibers enter the cerebellum mainly through the internal and external arcuate fibers.
   (c) The climbing and mossy fibers constitute the two main lines of input to the cerebellar cortex.
   (d) The afferent fibers are inhibitory to the Purkinje cells.
   (e) The afferent fibers to the cerebellum are nonmyelinated.

8. The following statements concern the functions of the cerebellum:
   (a) The cerebellum influences the actions of muscle tendons.
   (b) The cerebellum controls voluntary movement by coordinating the force and extent of contraction of different muscles.
   (c) The cerebellum stimulates the contraction of antagonistic muscles.
   (d) The cerebellum directly influences skeletal muscle activity without the assistance of the cerebral cortex.
   (e) The cerebellum coordinates the peristaltic waves seen in intestinal muscle.

9. The following statements concern the cerebellum:
   (a) The afferent climbing fibers make single synaptic contacts with individual Purkinje cells.
   (b) The afferent mossy fibers may stimulate many Purkinje cells by first stimulating the stellate cells.
   (c) The neurons of the intracerebellar nuclei send axons without interruption to the opposite cerebral hemisphere.
   (d) The output of the cerebellar nuclei influences muscle activity so that movements can progress in an orderly sequence from one movement to the next.
   (e) Past-pointing is caused by the failure of the cerebral cortex to inhibit the cerebellum after the movement has begun.

10. The following statements concern the cerebellum:
   (a) The cerebellar cortex has a different microscopic structure in different individuals.
   (b) The axons of the Purkinje cells exert an inhibitory influence on the neurons of the deep cerebellar nuclei.
   (c) Each cerebellar hemisphere principally influences movement on the opposite hand.
   (d) The part of the cerebellum that lies in the midline is called the flocculus.
   (e) Intention tremor is a sign of cerebellar disease.

Directions: Matching Questions. Following thrombosis of the posterior inferior cerebellar artery, a patient presents the numbered signs and symptoms listed below; match the signs and symptoms with the appropriate lettered structures involved. Each lettered option may be selected once, more than once, or not at all.

11. Loss of pain and temperature on the left side of the body
12. Nystagmus
13. Hypotonicity of the muscles on the right with a tendency to fall to the right
    (a) Right reticulospinal tract
    (b) Right inferior cerebellar peduncle
    (c) None of the above

Directions: Match the numbered nerve tracts listed below with the lettered pathways by which they leave the cerebellum. Each lettered option may be selected once, more than once, or not at all.

14. Corticopontocerebellar
15. Cuneocerebellar
16. Cerebellar reticular
17. Cerebellar rubral

(a) Superior cerebellar peduncle
(b) Corpus callosum
(c) Striae medullaris
(d) Inferior cerebellar peduncle
(e) Middle cerebellar peduncle
(f) None of the above

Directions: Each case history is followed by questions. Read the case history, then select the ONE BEST lettered answer.

A 45-year-old man, who was an alcoholic, started to develop a lurching, staggering gait even when he was not intoxicated. The condition became slowly worse over a period of several weeks and then appeared to stabilize. Friends noticed that he had difficulty in walking in tandem with another person and tended to become unsteady on turning quickly.

18. A thorough physical examination of this patient revealed the following findings **except**:
    (a) The patient exhibited instability of trunk movements and incoordination of leg movements.
    (b) While standing still, the patient stood with his feet together.
    (c) He had no evidence of polyneuropathy.
    (d) The ataxia of the legs was confirmed by performing the heel-to-shin test.
    (e) Magnetic resonance imaging showed evidence of atrophy of the cerebellar vermis.
19. The following additional abnormal signs might have been observed in this patient **except**:
    (a) Nystagmus in both eyes
    (b) Dysarthria
    (c) Tremor of the left hand when reaching for a cup
    (d) Paralysis of the right upper arm muscles
    (e) Dysdiadochokinesia

 Answers and Explanations to Review Questions

1. A is correct. The cerebellum is separated from the occipital lobes of the cerebral hemisphere by the tentorium cerebelli. B. The cerebellum lies posterior to the medulla oblongata (see Fig. 6-1). C. The anterior lobe is separated from the middle (posterior) lobe by the primary fissure (see Fig. 6-3). D. The flocculonodular lobe is separated from the middle (posterior) lobe by the uvulonodular fissure (see Fig. 6-3). E. The fourth ventricle lies anterior to the cerebellum (see Fig. 6-1).

2. C is correct. Each cerebellar hemisphere controls the tone of skeletal muscles supplied by spinal nerves on the same side of the body. A. The cerebellum has no effect on the activity of smooth muscle. B. The cerebellum has the same influence on the skeletal muscle supplied by cranial nerves as on that supplied by spinal nerves. D. The important Purkinje cells are Golgi type I neurons. E. The Purkinje cells exert an inhibitory influence on the intracerebellar nuclei.

3. A is correct. The cerebellum consists of two cerebellar hemispheres joined by a narrow median vermis (see Fig. 6-2). B. The inferior surface of the cerebellum shows a deep groove formed by the inferior surface of the vermis (see Fig. 6-2). C. The inferior cerebellar peduncle joins the cerebellum to the medulla oblongata (see Fig. 6-9). D. The gray matter of the cerebellum is found in the cortex and in the three masses forming the intracerebellar nuclei. E. The white matter and folia of the cortex have a branched appearance on the cut surface, called the arbor vitae (see Fig. 6-1).

4. E is correct. The axons of the Purkinje cells form the efferent fibers from the cerebellar cortex. A. The cerebellar cortex is folded by many transverse fissures into folia (see Fig. 6-1). B. The structure of the cortex is identical in different parts of the cerebellum. C. The Purkinje cells are found in the middle layer of the cerebellar cortex (see Fig. 6-4). D. The Golgi cells are found in the deepest (granular) layer of the cerebellar cortex (see Fig. 6-4).

5. D is correct. The axons from the neurons of the intracerebellar nuclei form the main cerebellar outflow. A. The intracerebellar nuclei are deeply embedded in the white matter (see Fig. 6-7). B. The nuclei are located posterior to the roof of the fourth ventricle (see Fig. 6-7). C. The nuclei are composed of large multipolar neurons. E. From medial to lateral, the nuclei are named as follows: fastigial, globose, emboliform, and dentate (see Fig. 6-7).

6. B is correct. The anterior spinocerebellar tract enters the cerebellum through the superior cerebellar

peduncle (see Fig. 6-11). A. In the superior cerebellar peduncle, most of the fibers are efferent and arise from the neurons of the intracerebellar nuclei (see Fig. 6-12). C. The inferior cerebellar peduncle contains afferent fibers of the posterior spinocerebellar tract, the cuneocerebellar tract, the vestibular nucleus, and the olivocerebellar tract (see Figs. 6-10 and 6-11). In addition, efferent fibers come from the cerebellum, including the fastigial vestibular pathway and the fastigial reticular pathway (see Fig. 6-12). D. The middle cerebellar peduncle is formed of fibers that arise from the pontine nuclei (see Fig. 6-10); other fibers connect the cerebellar hemispheres of the two sides together (see Fig. 6-12). E. The cerebellar peduncles are surface structures and are easily seen on dissection.

7. C is correct. The climbing and mossy fibers of the cerebellum constitute the two main lines of input to the cerebellar cortex. A. The mossy fibers end by making synaptic contacts with the dendrites of the granular cells and the Golgi cells (see Fig. 6-8). B. The afferent fibers enter the cerebellum through the superior, inferior, and middle cerebellar peduncles. D. The afferent fibers are excitatory to the Purkinje cells. E. The afferent fibers to the cerebellum are myelinated.

8. B is correct. The cerebellum controls voluntary movement by coordinating the force and extent of contraction of different muscles. A. The cerebellum influences the actions of muscles not tendons. C. The cerebellum inhibits the contraction of antagonistic muscles. D. The cerebellum indirectly influences skeletal muscle activity with the assistance of the cerebral cortex. E. The cerebellum has no effect on the control of smooth muscle in the wall of the intestine.

9. D is correct. The output of the cerebellar nuclei influences muscle activity so that movements can progress in an orderly sequence from one movement to the next. A. The afferent climbing fibers make multiple synaptic contacts with 1 to 10 Purkinje cells. B. The afferent mossy fibers may stimulate many Purkinje cells by first stimulating the granular cells. C. The neurons of the intracerebellar nuclei send axons to the ventrolateral nucleus of the thalamus, where they are relayed to the cerebral cortex (see Fig. 6-12). E. Past-pointing is caused by the failure of the cerebellum to inhibit the cerebral cortex after the movement has begun.

10. E is correct. Intention tremor is a sign of cerebellar disease. A. The cerebellar cortex has the same uniform microscopic structure in different individuals. B. The axons of the Purkinje cells exert a stimulatory influence on the neurons of the deep cerebellar nuclei. C. Each cerebellar hemisphere principally influences movement on the same side of the body. D. The part of the cerebellum that lies in the midline is called the vermis.

11. C is correct.

12. B is correct: right inferior cerebellar peduncle.

13. B is correct: right inferior cerebellar peduncle.

14. E is correct: middle cerebellar peduncle.

15. D is correct: inferior cerebellar peduncle.

16. D is correct: inferior cerebellar peduncle.

17. A is correct: superior cerebellar peduncle.

18. B is correct. Patients with cerebellar disease frequently exhibit poor muscle tone, and to compensate for this, they stand stiff legged with their feet wide apart.

19. D is correct. Although patients with cerebellar disease display disturbances of voluntary movement, none of the muscles are paralyzed or show atrophy.

7 Cerebrum

CHAPTER OBJECTIVES

- To introduce the student to the complexities of the forebrain

- To understand the definition of the diencephalon and accurately localize the thalamus and hypothalamus by studying the sagittal, coronal, and horizontal sections of the brain

- To understand the exact position of the main conduit of the ascending and descending tracts, namely the internal capsule, which is so often the site of pathologic lesions

A 23-year-old man is referred to a neurologist because of intermittent attacks of headaches, dizziness, and weakness and numbness of the left leg. On close questioning, the patient admits that the headache is made worse by changing the position of his head. A computed tomography (CT) scan reveals a small white opaque ball at the anterior end of the third ventricle. A diagnosis of a colloid cyst of the third ventricle is made.

The aggravation of the headache caused by changing the position of the head can be explained by the fact that the cyst is mobile and suspended from the choroid plexus. When the head is moved into certain positions, the ball-like cyst blocks the foramen of Monro on the right side, further raising the intracerebral pressure and increasing the hydrocephalus. The weakness and numbness of the left leg are due to pressure on the right thalamus and the tracts in the right internal capsule, produced by the slowly expanding tumor. The patient makes a complete recovery after surgical excision of the tumor.

The cerebral hemispheres are developed from the telencephalon and form the largest part of the brain. Each hemisphere has a covering of gray matter, the cortex and internal masses of gray matter, the basal nuclei, and a lateral ventricle. The basic anatomical structure of this area is described so that the student can be prepared for the complexities associated with functional localization.

SUBDIVISIONS

The cerebrum is the largest part of the brain, situated in the anterior and middle cranial fossae of the skull and occupying the whole concavity of the vault of the skull. It may be divided into two parts: the **diencephalon**, which forms the central core, and the **telencephalon**, which forms the **cerebral hemispheres**.

DIENCEPHALON

The diencephalon consists of the third ventricle and the structures that form its boundaries (Figs. 7-1 and 7-2).

It extends posteriorly to the point where the third ventricle becomes continuous with the cerebral aqueduct and anteriorly as far as the interventricular foramina (Fig. 7-3). Thus, the diencephalon is a midline structure with symmetrical right and left halves. Obviously, these subdivisions of the brain are made for convenience, and from a functional point of view, nerve fibers freely cross the boundaries.

Gross Features

The **inferior surface** of the diencephalon is the only area exposed to the surface in the intact brain (see Fig. 7-2; see also Atlas Plate 1). It is formed by hypothalamic and other structures, which include, from anterior to posterior, the **optic chiasma**, with the **optic tract** on either side; the **infundibulum**, with the **tuber cinereum**; and the **mammillary bodies**.

The **superior surface** of the diencephalon is concealed by the **fornix**, which is a thick bundle of fibers that originates in the **hippocampus** of the temporal lobe and arches posteriorly over the **thalamus** (see Fig. 7-3; see also Atlas Plate 8) to join the **mammillary body**.

249

Cortex of frontal lobe

Genu of corpus callosum

Cavity of septum pellucidum

Head of caudate nucleus

Fornix

Anterior commissure

Internal capsule

Cortex of temporal lobe

Choroid plexus of lateral ventricle

Stria medullaris thalami

Interthalamic connection

Putamen of lentiform nucleus

Posterior commissure

Cavity of third ventricle

Thalamus

Inferior horn of lateral ventricle

Region of habenular nucleus

Pulvinar of thalamus

Fimbria of fornix

Superior colliculus

Posterior horn of lateral ventricle

Cortex of occipital lobe

Inferior colliculus

Pineal body

Vermis of cerebellum

Figure 7-1 Horizontal section of the brain showing the third and lateral ventricles exposed by dissection from above.

The actual superior wall of the diencephalon is formed by the **roof of the third ventricle**. This consists of a layer of ependyma, which is continuous with the rest of the ependymal lining of the third ventricle. It is covered superiorly by a vascular fold of pia mater, called the **tela choroidea of the third ventricle**. From the roof of the third ventricle, a pair of vascular processes, the **choroid plexuses of the third ventricle**, project downward from the midline into the cavity of the third ventricle.

The **lateral surface** of the diencephalon is bounded by the **internal capsule** of white matter and consists of nerve fibers that connect the cerebral cortex with other parts of the brainstem and spinal cord (see Fig. 7-1).

Because the diencephalon is divided into symmetrical halves by the slitlike third ventricle, it also has a **medial surface**. The medial surface of the diencephalon (i.e., the lateral wall of the third ventricle) is formed in its superior part by the medial surface of the **thalamus** and in its inferior part by the **hypothalamus** (see Fig. 7-3; see also

Atlas Plate 8). These two areas are separated from one another by a shallow sulcus, the **hypothalamic sulcus**. A bundle of nerve fibers, which are afferent fibers to the habenular nucleus, forms a ridge along the superior margin of the medial surface of the diencephalon and is called the **stria medullaris thalami** (see Fig. 7-1).

The diencephalon can be divided into four major parts: (1) the thalamus, (2) the subthalamus, (3) the epithalamus, and (4) the hypothalamus.

Thalamus

The thalamus is a large ovoid mass of gray matter that forms the major part of the diencephalon. It is a region of great functional importance and serves as a cell station to all the main sensory systems (except the olfactory pathway). The activities of the thalamus are closely related to that of the cerebral cortex and damage to the thalamus causes great loss of cerebral function.

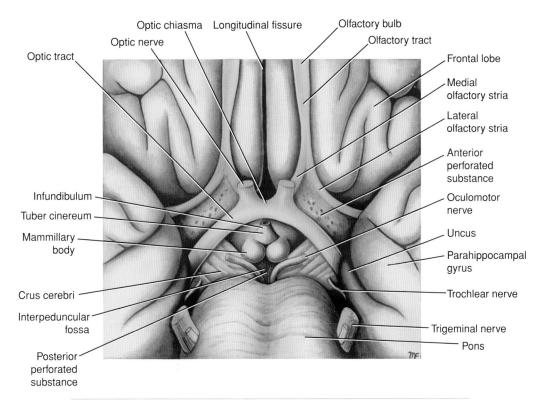

Optic chiasma   Longitudinal fissure   Olfactory bulb

Optic nerve   Olfactory tract

Optic tract   Frontal lobe

Medial
olfactory stria

Lateral
olfactory stria

Anterior
perforated
substance

Infundibulum   Oculomotor
nerve

Tuber cinereum   Uncus

Mammillary
body   Parahippocampal
gyrus

Crus cerebri   Trochlear nerve

Interpeduncular
fossa   Trigeminal nerve

Pons

Posterior
perforated
substance

Figure 7-2   Inferior surface of the brain showing parts of the diencephalon.

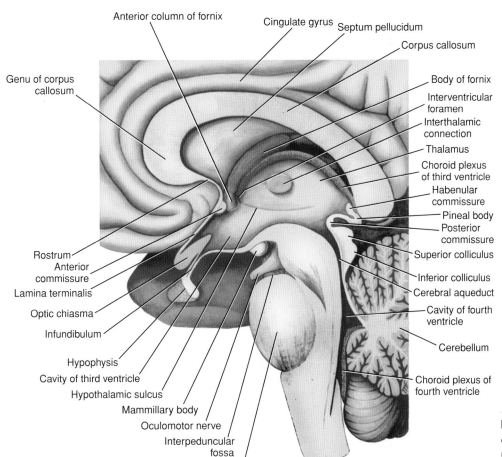

Anterior column of fornix   Cingulate gyrus   Septum pellucidum

Corpus callosum

Genu of corpus
callosum   Body of fornix

Interventricular
foramen

Interthalamic
connection

Thalamus

Choroid plexus
of third ventricle

Habenular
commissure

Pineal body

Posterior
commissure

Rostrum   Superior colliculus

Anterior
commissure   Inferior colliculus

Lamina terminalis   Cerebral aqueduct

Optic chiasma   Cavity of fourth
ventricle

Infundibulum   Cerebellum

Hypophysis

Cavity of third ventricle   Choroid plexus of
fourth ventricle

Hypothalamic sulcus

Mammillary body

Oculomotor nerve

Interpeduncular
fossa

Pons

Figure 7-3   Sagittal section
of the brain showing the
medial surface of the diencephalon.

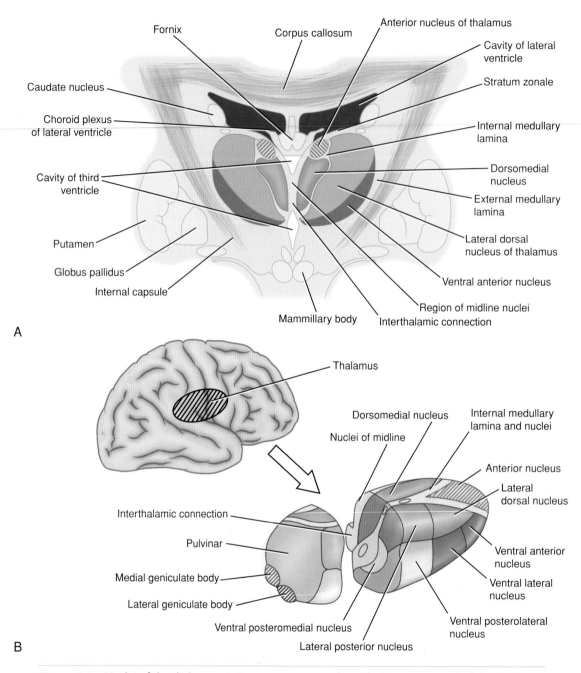

Figure 7-4   Nuclei of the thalamus. **A:** Transverse section through the anterior end of the thalamus. **B:** Diagram showing the position of the thalamus within the right cerebral hemisphere and the relative position of the thalamic nuclei to one another.

The thalamus is situated on each side of the third ventricle (see Fig. 7-3; see also Atlas Plate 5). The anterior end of the thalamus is narrow and rounded and forms the posterior boundary of the interventricular foramen. The posterior end (Fig. 7-4) is expanded to form the **pulvinar**, which overhangs the superior colliculus and the superior brachium. The **lateral geniculate body** forms a small elevation on the under aspect of the lateral portion of the pulvinar.

The superior surface of the thalamus is covered medially by the tela choroidea and the fornix, and laterally, it is covered by ependyma and forms part of the floor of the lateral ventricle; the lateral part is partially hidden by the choroid plexus of the lateral ventricle (see Fig. 7-1). The inferior surface is continuous with the tegmentum of the midbrain (see Fig. 7-3).

The medial surface of the thalamus forms the superior part of the lateral wall of the third ventricle and is usually connected to the opposite thalamus by a band of gray matter, the **interthalamic connection** (interthalamic adhesion) (see Fig. 7-3).

The lateral surface of the thalamus is separated from the lentiform nucleus by the very important band of white matter called the **internal capsule** (see Fig. 7-1).

The subdivisions of the thalamus (see Fig. 7-4) and the detailed description of the thalamic nuclei and their connections are given on first page of Chapter 12.

The thalamus is a very important cell station that receives the main sensory tracts (except the olfactory pathway). It should be regarded as a station where much of the information is integrated and relayed to the cerebral cortex and many other subcortical regions. It also plays a key role in the integration of visceral and somatic functions. For more information on the function of the thalamus, see Chapter 12.

Subthalamus

The subthalamus lies inferior to the thalamus and, therefore, is situated between the thalamus and the tegmentum of the midbrain; craniomedially, it is related to the hypothalamus.

The structure of the subthalamus is extremely complex, and only a brief description is given here. Among the collections of nerve cells found in the subthalamus are the cranial ends of the **red nuclei** and the **substantia nigra**. The **subthalamic nucleus** has the shape of a biconvex lens. The nucleus has important connections with the corpus striatum (see p. 310); as a result, it is involved in the control of muscle activity.

The subthalamus also contains many important tracts that pass up from the tegmentum to the thalamic nuclei; the cranial ends of the medial, spinal, and trigeminal lemnisci are examples.

Epithalamus

The epithalamus consists of the habenular nuclei and their connections and the pineal gland.

Habenular Nucleus

The habenular nucleus is a small group of neurons situated just medial to the posterior surface of the thalamus. Afferent fibers are received from the amygdaloid nucleus in the temporal lobe (see p. 261) through the stria medullaris thalami; other fibers pass from the hippocampal formation through the fornix. Some of the fibers of the stria medullaris thalami cross the midline and reach the habenular nucleus of the opposite side; these latter fibers form the **habenular commissure** (see Fig. 7-3). Axons from the habenular nucleus pass to the interpeduncular nucleus in the roof of the interpeduncular fossa, the tectum of the midbrain, the thalamus, and the reticular formation of the midbrain. The habenular nucleus is believed to be a center for integration of olfactory, visceral, and somatic afferent pathways.

Pineal Gland (Body)

The pineal gland is a small, conical structure that is attached by the pineal stalk to the diencephalon. It projects backward so that it lies posterior to the midbrain (see Fig. 7-3; see also Atlas Plate 8). The base of the pineal stalk possesses a recess that is continuous with the cavity of the third ventricle. The superior part of the base of the stalk contains the **habenular commissure**;

Figure 7-5 Photomicrograph of a section of the pineal gland stained with hematoxylin and eosin. (From Cui, D., Daley, W., Fratkin, J. D., Haines, D. E., Lynch, J. C., Naftel, J. P., Yang, G. Atlas of Histology with Functional and Clinical Correlations. Baltimore, MD: Wolters Kluwer, 2011.)

the inferior part of the base of the stalk contains the **posterior commissure**.

On microscopic section, the pineal gland is seen to be incompletely divided into lobules by connective tissue septa that extend into the substance of the gland from the capsule. Two types of cells are found in the gland, the **pinealocytes** and the **glial cells**. Concretions of calcified material called **brain sand** progressively accumulate within the pineal gland with age (Fig. 7-5).

The pineal gland possesses no nerve cells, but adrenergic sympathetic fibers derived from the superior cervical sympathetic ganglia enter the gland and run in association with the blood vessels and the pinealocytes.

Pineal Gland Functions

The pineal gland, once thought to be of little significance, is now recognized as an important endocrine gland capable of influencing the activities of the pituitary gland, the islets of Langerhans of the pancreas, the parathyroids, the adrenal cortex and the adrenal medulla, and the gonads. The pineal secretions, produced by the pinealocytes, reach their target organs via the bloodstream or through the cerebrospinal fluid (CSF). Their actions are mainly inhibitory and either directly inhibit the production of hormones or indirectly inhibit the secretion of releasing factors by the hypothalamus. Notably, the pineal gland does not possess a blood–brain barrier.

Animal experiments have shown that pineal activity exhibits a circadian rhythm that is influenced by light. The gland has been found to be most active during darkness. The probable nervous pathway from the retina runs to the suprachiasmatic nucleus of the hypothalamus, then to the tegmentum of the midbrain, and then to the pineal gland to stimulate its secretions. The latter part of this pathway may include the reticulospinal tract, the sympathetic outflow of the thoracic part of the spinal cord, and the superior cervical sympathetic ganglion and postganglionic nerve fibers that travel to the pineal gland on blood vessels.

Melatonin and the enzymes needed for its production are present in high concentrations within the pineal gland. Melatonin and other substances are released into the blood or into the CSF of the third ventricle where they pass to the anterior lobe of the pituitary gland and inhibit the release of the gonadotrophic hormone. In humans, as in animals, the plasma melatonin level rises in darkness and falls during the day. The pineal gland apparently plays an important role in the regulation of reproductive function.

Hypothalamus

The **hypothalamus** is that part of the diencephalon that extends from the region of the optic chiasma to the caudal border of the mammillary bodies (see Fig. 7-2; see also Atlas Plate 8). It lies below the hypothalamic sulcus on the lateral wall of the third ventricle. Thus, anatomically, the hypothalamus is a relatively small area of the brain that is strategically well placed close to the limbic system, the thalamus, the ascending and descending tracts, and the hypophysis. Microscopically, the hypothalamus is composed of small nerve cells that are arranged in groups or nuclei. The arrangement of these nuclei and their connections are fully described in Chapter 13.

Physiologically, nearly all the activities in the body are influenced by the hypothalamus. The hypothalamus controls and integrates the functions of the autonomic nervous system and the endocrine systems and plays a vital role in maintaining body homeostasis. It is involved in such activities as regulation of body temperature, body fluids, drives to eat and drink, sexual behavior, and emotion.

Hypothalamic Relations

Anterior to the hypothalamus is an area that extends forward from the optic chiasma to the lamina terminalis and the anterior commissure; it is referred to as the **preoptic area**. Caudally, the hypothalamus merges into the tegmentum of the midbrain. The thalamus lies superior to the hypothalamus, and the subthalamic region lies inferolaterally to the hypothalamus.

When observed from below, the hypothalamus is seen to be related to the following structures, from anterior to posterior: (1) the optic chiasma, (2) the tuber cinereum and the infundibulum, and (3) the mammillary bodies.

Optic Chiasma

The optic chiasma is a flattened bundle of nerve fibers situated at the junction of the anterior wall and floor of the third ventricle (see Figs. 7-2 and 7-3; see also Atlas Plate 8). The superior surface is attached to the **lamina terminalis**, and inferiorly, it is related to the **hypophysis cerebri**, from which it is separated by the **diaphragma sellae**. The anterolateral corners of the chiasma are continuous with the **optic nerves**, and the posterolateral corners are continuous with the **optic tracts**. A small recess, the **optic recess of the third ventricle**, lies on its superior surface.

Importantly, remember that the fibers originating from the nasal half of each retina cross the median plane at the chiasma to enter the optic tract of the opposite side.

Tuber Cinereum

The tuber cinereum is a convex mass of gray matter, as seen from the inferior surface (see Figs. 7-2 and 7-3; see also Atlas Plate 8). It is continuous inferiorly with the **infundibulum**. The infundibulum is hollow and becomes continuous with the posterior lobe of the **hypophysis cerebri**. The **median eminence** is a raised part of the tuber cinereum to which is attached the infundibulum. The median eminence, the infundibulum, and the posterior lobe (pars nervosa) of the hypophysis cerebri together form the **neurohypophysis**.

Mammillary Bodies

The mammillary bodies are two small hemispherical bodies situated side by side posterior to the tuber cinereum (see Figs. 7-2 and 7-3; see also Atlas Plate 8). They possess a central core of gray matter invested by a capsule of myelinated nerve fibers. Posterior to the mammillary bodies lies an area of the brain that is pierced by a number of small apertures and is called the posterior perforated substance. These apertures transmit the central branches of the posterior cerebral arteries.

Third Ventricle

The third ventricle, which is derived from the forebrain vesicle, is a slitlike cleft between the two thalami (see Figs. 7-1 and 7-3; see also Atlas Plates 5 and 8). It communicates anteriorly with the **lateral ventricles** through the **interventricular foramina** (foramina of Monro), and it communicates posteriorly with the **fourth ventricle** through the **cerebral aqueduct**. The third ventricle has anterior, posterior, lateral, superior, and inferior walls and is lined with ependyma.

The **anterior wall** is formed by a thin sheet of gray matter, the **lamina terminalis**, across which runs the **anterior commissure** (see Fig. 7-3). The anterior commissure is a round bundle of nerve fibers that are situated anterior to the **anterior columns of the fornix**; they connect the right and left temporal lobes.

The **posterior wall** is formed by the opening into the cerebral aqueduct. Superior to this opening is the small **posterior commissure**. Superior to the commissure is the **pineal recess**, which projects into the stalk of the **pineal body**. Superior to the pineal recess is the small **habenular commissure**.

The **lateral wall** is formed by the medial surface of the **thalamus** superiorly and the **hypothalamus** inferiorly. These two structures are separated by the **hypothalamic sulcus**. The lateral wall is limited superiorly by the **stria medullaris thalami**. The lateral walls are joined by the **interthalamic connection**.

The **superior wall** or **roof** is formed by a layer of ependyma that is continuous with the lining of the ventricle. Superior to this layer is a two-layered fold of pia mater called **the tela choroidea of the third ventricle**. The vascular tela choroidea projects downward on each side of the midline, invaginating the ependymal roof to form the **choroid plexuses of the third ventricle**. Within the tela choroidea lie the **internal cerebral veins**. Superiorly, the roof of the ventricle is related to the **fornix** and the **corpus callosum**.

The **inferior wall** or **floor** is formed by the **optic chiasma**, the **tuber cinereum**, the **infundibulum**, with its funnel-shaped recess, and the **mammillary bodies**

(see Figs. 7-2 and 7-3). The **hypophysis** is attached to the infundibulum. Posterior to these structures lies the **tegmentum of the cerebral peduncles**.

The ventricular system is fully described in Chapter 16.

GENERAL APPEARANCE OF THE CEREBRAL HEMISPHERES

The cerebral hemispheres are the largest part of the brain; they are separated by a deep midline sagittal fissure, the **longitudinal cerebral fissure** (Fig. 7-6; see also Atlas Plates 1 and 2). The fissure contains the sickle-shaped fold of dura mater, the **falx cerebri**, and the **anterior cerebral arteries**. In the depths of the fissure, the great commissure, the **corpus callosum**, connects the hemispheres across the midline. A second horizontal fold of dura mater separates the cerebral hemispheres

Figure 7-6 Superior view of the cerebral hemispheres.

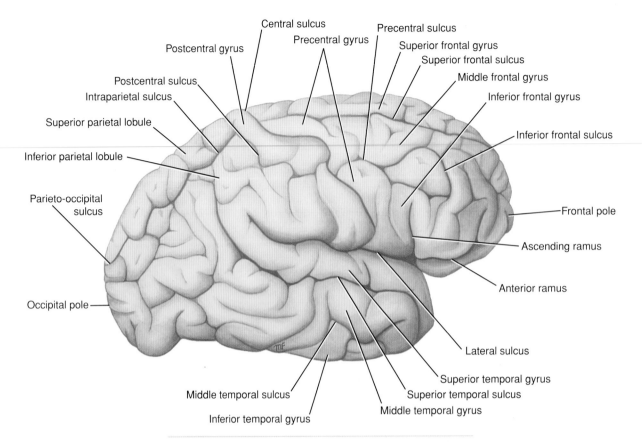

Figure 7-7 Lateral view of the right cerebral hemisphere.

from the cerebellum and is called the **tentorium cerebelli**.

To increase the surface area of the cerebral cortex maximally, the surface of each cerebral hemisphere is thrown into **folds** or **gyri**, which are separated from each other by **sulci** or **fissure**. For ease of description, each hemisphere is divided into **lobes**, which are named according to the cranial bones under which they lie. The **central** and **parieto-occipital sulci** and the **lateral** and **calcarine sulci** are boundaries used for the division of the cerebral hemisphere into **frontal**, **parietal**, **temporal**, and **occipital lobes** (Fig. 7-7; also see Fig. 7-10).

MAIN SULCI

The **central sulcus** (see Fig. 7-7; see also Atlas Plate 3) is of great importance because the gyrus that lies anterior to it contains the motor cells that initiate the movements of the opposite side of the body; posterior to it lies the general sensory cortex that receives sensory information from the opposite side of the body. The central sulcus indents the superior medial border of the hemisphere about 0.4 in (1 cm) behind the midpoint (Fig. 7-8). It runs downward and forward across the lateral aspect of the hemisphere, and its lower end is separated from the posterior ramus of the lateral sulcus by a narrow bridge of cortex. The central sulcus is the only

sulcus of any length on this surface of the hemisphere that indents the superomedial border and lies between two parallel gyri.

The **lateral sulcus** (see Fig. 7-7; see also Atlas Plate 3) is a deep cleft found mainly on the inferior and lateral surfaces of the cerebral hemisphere. It consists of a short stem that divides into three rami. The stem arises on the inferior surface, and on reaching the lateral surface, it divides into the **anterior horizontal ramus** and the **anterior ascending ramus** and continues as the **posterior ramus** (see Fig. 7-7). An area of cortex called the **insula** lies at the bottom of the deep lateral sulcus and cannot be seen from the surface unless the lips of the sulcus are separated (Fig. 7-9).

The **parieto-occipital sulcus** begins on the superior medial margin of the hemisphere about 2 in (5 cm) anterior to the occipital pole (see Fig. 7-8; see also Atlas Plate 3). It passes downward and anteriorly on the medial surface to meet the calcarine sulcus (see Fig. 7-8).

The **calcarine sulcus** is found on the medial surface of the hemisphere (see Fig. 7-8; see also Atlas Plate 3). It commences under the posterior end of the corpus callosum and arches upward and backward to reach the occipital pole, where it stops. In some brains, however, it continues for a short distance onto the lateral surface of the hemisphere. The calcarine sulcus is joined at an acute angle by the parieto-occipital sulcus about halfway along its length.

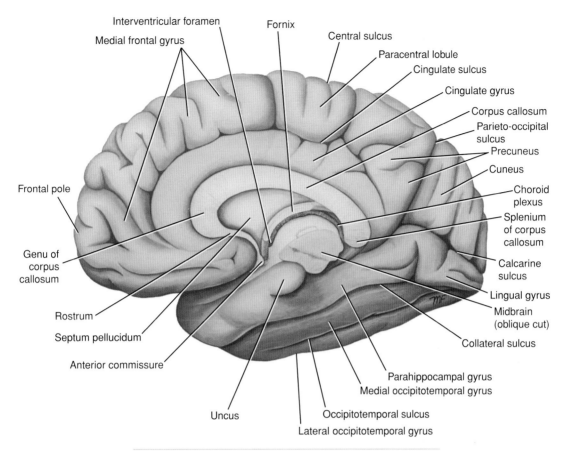

Figure 7-8 Medial view of the right cerebral hemisphere.

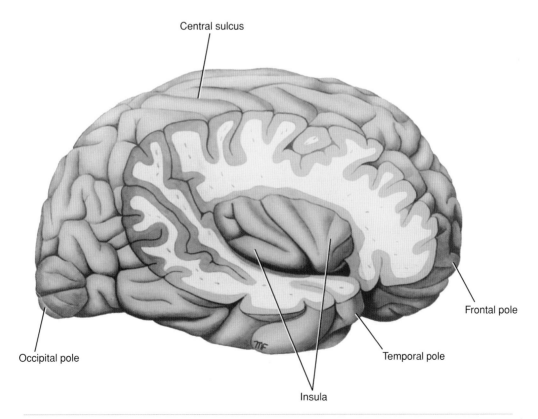

Figure 7-9 Lateral view of the right cerebral hemisphere dissected to reveal the right insula.

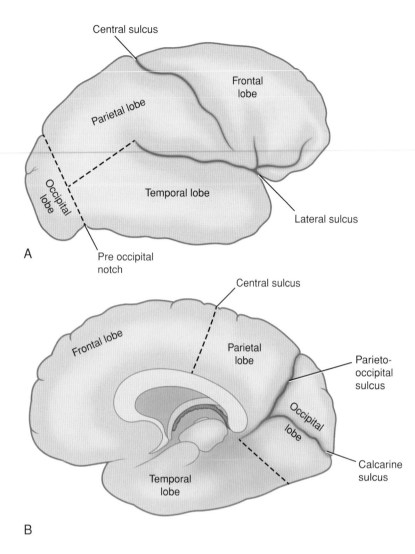

Figure 7-10 **A:** Lateral view of the right cerebral hemisphere showing the lobes. **B:** Medial view of the right cerebral hemisphere showing the lobes. Note that the *dashed lines* indicate the approximate position of the boundaries where no sulci are present.

CEREBRAL HEMISPHERE LOBES

Cerebral hemispheres are functionally divided into lobes, each of which are anatomically identified using specific gyri and sulci.

Superolateral Surface (Atlas Plate 3)

The **frontal lobe** occupies the area anterior to the central sulcus and superior to the lateral sulcus (Fig. 7-10). The superolateral surface of the frontal lobe is divided by three sulci into four gyri. The **precentral sulcus** runs parallel to the central sulcus, and the **precentral gyrus** lies between them (see Fig. 7-7). Extending anteriorly from the precentral sulcus are the **superior** and **inferior frontal sulci**. The **superior frontal gyrus** lies superior to the superior frontal sulcus, the **middle frontal gyrus** lies between the superior and inferior frontal sulci, and the **inferior frontal gyrus** lies inferior to the inferior frontal sulcus. The inferior frontal gyrus is invaded by the anterior and ascending rami of the lateral sulcus.

The **parietal lobe** occupies the area posterior to the central sulcus and superior to the lateral sulcus; it extends posteriorly as far as the parieto-occipital sulcus (see Figs. 7-7 to 7-10). The lateral surface of the parietal lobe is divided by two sulci into three gyri. The postcentral sulcus runs parallel to the central sulcus, and the postcentral gyrus lies between them. Running posteriorly from the middle of the postcentral sulcus is the **intraparietal sulcus** (see Fig. 7-7). Superior to the intraparietal sulcus is the **superior parietal lobule** (gyrus), and inferior to the intraparietal sulcus is the **inferior parietal lobule** (gyrus).

The **temporal lobe** occupies the area inferior to the lateral sulcus (see Figs. 7-7 to 7-10). The lateral surface of the temporal lobe is divided into three gyri by two sulci. The **superior** and **middle temporal sulci** run parallel to the posterior ramus of the lateral sulcus and divide the temporal lobe into the **superior**, **middle**, and **inferior temporal gyri**; the inferior temporal gyrus is continued onto the inferior surface of the hemisphere (see Fig. 7-7).

The **occipital lobe** occupies the small area behind the parieto-occipital sulcus (see Figs. 7-7 to 7-10).

Medial and Inferior Surfaces
(Atlas Plates 3, 6, and 8)

The lobes of the cerebral hemisphere are not clearly defined on the medial and inferior surfaces. However, many important areas should be recognized. The **corpus callosum**, which is the largest commissure of the brain, forms a striking feature on this surface (see Fig. 7-8). The **cingulate gyrus** begins beneath the anterior end of the corpus callosum and continues above the corpus callosum until it reaches its posterior end. The gyrus is separated from the corpus callosum by the **callosal sulcus**. The cingulate gyrus is separated from the superior frontal gyrus by the **cingulate sulcus** (see Fig. 7-8).

The **paracentral lobule** is the area of the cerebral cortex that surrounds the indentation produced by the central sulcus on the superior border. The anterior part of this lobule is a continuation of the precentral gyrus on the superior lateral surface, and the posterior part of the lobule is a continuation of the postcentral gyrus.

The **precuneus** is an area of cortex bounded anteriorly by the upturned posterior end of the cingulate sulcus and posteriorly by the parieto-occipital sulcus.

The **cuneus** is a triangular area of cortex bounded above by the parieto-occipital sulcus, inferiorly by the calcarine sulcus, and posteriorly by the superior medial margin.

The **collateral sulcus** is situated on the inferior surface of the hemisphere (Fig. 7-11; also see Fig. 7-8). This runs anteriorly below the calcarine sulcus. Between the collateral sulcus and the **calcarine sulcus** is the

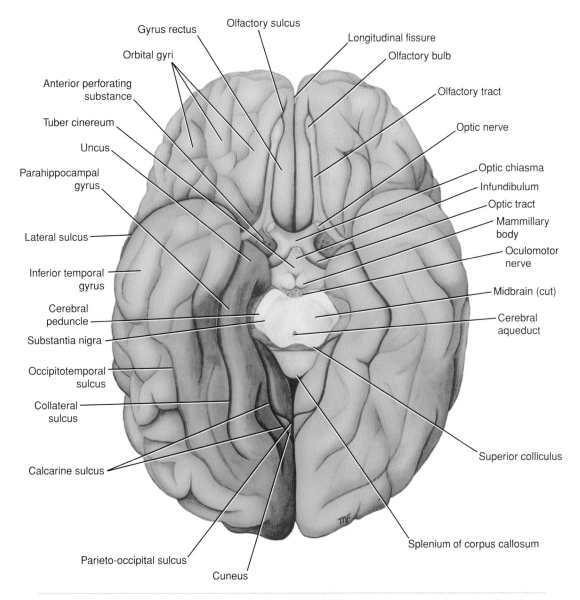

Figure 7-11 Inferior view of the brain; the medulla oblongata, the pons, and the cerebellum have been removed.

lingual gyrus. Anterior to the lingual gyrus is the **para-hippocampal gyrus**; the latter terminates in front as the hooklike **uncus** (see Fig. 7-11).

The **medial occipitotemporal gyrus** extends from the occipital pole to the temporal pole. It is bounded medially by the **collateral** and **rhinal sulci** and laterally by the **occipitotemporal sulcus**. The **occipitotemporal gyrus** lies lateral to the sulcus and is continuous with the inferior temporal gyrus.

On the inferior surface of the frontal lobe, the olfactory bulb and tract overlie a sulcus called the **olfactory sulcus**. Medial to the olfactory sulcus is the **gyrus rectus**, and lateral to the sulcus are a number of **orbital gyri**.

INTERNAL STRUCTURE OF THE CEREBRAL HEMISPHERES (ATLAS PLATES 4 AND 5)

The cerebral hemispheres are covered with a layer of gray matter, the cerebral cortex; the structure and function of the cerebral cortex are discussed in

Chapter 15. Located in the interior of the cerebral hemispheres are the **lateral ventricles**, masses of gray matter, the **basal nuclei**, and nerve fibers. The nerve fibers are embedded in neuroglia and constitute the **white matter** (Fig. 7-12).

Lateral Ventricles

The two lateral ventricles each occupy one cerebral hemisphere (Fig. 7-13; also see Fig. 7-12). Each ventricle is a roughly C-shaped cavity lined with ependyma and filled with CSF. The lateral ventricle may be divided into a **body**, which occupies the parietal lobe, and from which **anterior**, **posterior**, and **inferior horns** extend into the frontal, occipital, and temporal lobes, respectively. The lateral ventricle communicates with the cavity of the third ventricle through the **interventricular foramen** (see Figs. 7-8 and 7-13). This opening, which lies in the anterior part of the medial wall of the lateral ventricle, is bounded anteriorly by the anterior column of the fornix and posteriorly by the anterior end of the thalamus.

Figure 7-12 Horizontal section of the cerebrum, as seen from above, showing the relationship between the lentiform nucleus, the caudate nucleus, the thalamus, and the internal capsule.

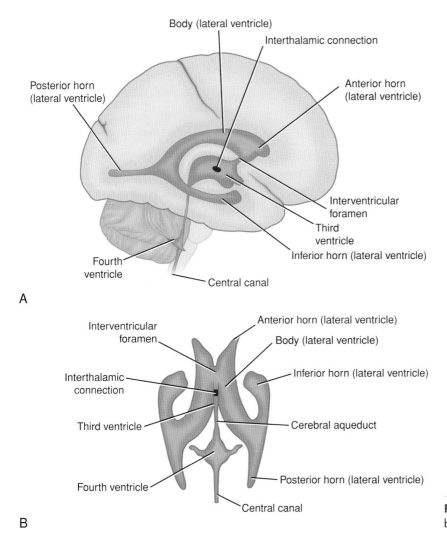

Figure 7-13 Ventricular cavities of the brain. **A:** Lateral view. **B:** Superior view.

Basal Nuclei

The term **basal nuclei** (**basal ganglia**) is applied to a collection of masses of gray matter situated within each cerebral hemisphere. They are the corpus striatum, the amygdaloid nucleus, and the claustrum.

Corpus Striatum

The corpus striatum is situated lateral to the thalamus. It is almost completely divided by a band of nerve fibers, the **internal capsule**, into the caudate nucleus and the lentiform nucleus (see Figs. 7-12 and 7-17).

The **caudate nucleus**, a large C-shaped mass of gray matter that is closely related to the lateral ventricle, lies lateral to the thalamus (Fig. 7-14). The lateral surface of the nucleus is related to the internal capsule, which separates it from the lentiform nucleus.

The **lentiform nucleus** is a wedge-shaped mass of gray matter whose broad convex base is directed laterally and its blade medially (see Figs. 7-12 and 7-14). It is buried deep in the white matter of the cerebral hemisphere and is related medially to the internal capsule, which separates it from the caudate nucleus and the thalamus. The lentiform nucleus is related laterally to a thin sheet of white matter, the **external capsule** (see Fig. 7-12), that separates it from a thin sheet of gray matter, called the **claustrum**. The claustrum, in turn, separates the external capsule from the subcortical white matter of the insula. Inferiorly at its anterior end, the lentiform nucleus is continuous with the caudate nucleus.

The detailed structure and connections of the corpus striatum are considered in Chapter 10. Briefly, it may be stated that the corpus striatum receives afferent fibers from different areas of the cerebral cortex, the thalamus, subthalamus, and brainstem. Efferent fibers then travel back to the same areas of the nervous system. The function of the corpus striatum is concerned with muscular movement, which is accomplished by controlling the cerebral cortex rather than through direct descending pathways to the brainstem and spinal cord.

Amygdaloid Nucleus

The amygdaloid nucleus is situated in the temporal lobe close to the uncus (see Fig. 7-14). The amygdaloid nucleus is considered part of the limbic system and is described in Chapter 9 (see p. 303).

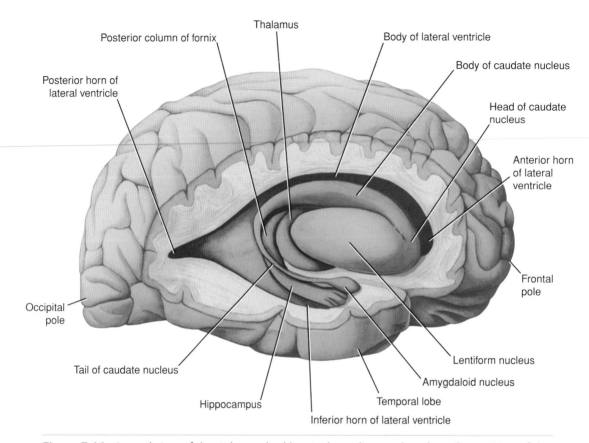

Figure 7-14 Lateral view of the right cerebral hemisphere dissected to show the position of the lentiform nucleus, the caudate nucleus, the thalamus, and the hippocampus.

Claustrum

The claustrum is a thin sheet of gray matter that is separated from the lateral surface of the lentiform nucleus by the **external capsule** (see Fig. 7-12). Lateral to the claustrum is the subcortical white matter of the insula. The function of the claustrum is unknown.

White Matter

The white matter is composed of myelinated nerve fibers of different diameters supported by neuroglia. The nerve fibers may be classified into three groups according to their connections: (1) commissural fibers, (2) association fibers, and (3) projection fibers.

Commissure Fibers

Commissure fibers essentially connect corresponding regions of the two hemispheres. They are as follows: the corpus callosum, the anterior commissure, the posterior commissure, the fornix, and the habenular commissure.

The **corpus callosum**, the largest commissure of the brain, connects the two cerebral hemispheres (Fig. 7-15; see also Fig. 7-8 and Atlas Plate 8). It lies at the bottom of the longitudinal fissure. For purposes of description, it is divided into the rostrum, the genu, the body, and the splenium.

The **rostrum** is the thin part of the anterior end of the corpus callosum, which is prolonged posteriorly to

be continuous with the upper end of the lamina terminalis (see Fig. 7-8).

The **genu** is the curved anterior end of the corpus callosum that bends inferiorly in front of the septum pellucidum (see Figs. 7-8 and 7-15).

The **body** of the corpus callosum arches posteriorly and ends as the thickened posterior portion called the **splenium** (see Fig. 7-15).

Traced laterally, the fibers of the genu curve forward into the frontal lobes and form the **forceps minor** (see Fig. 7-15B). The fibers of the body extend laterally as the **radiation of the corpus callosum**. They intersect with bundles of association and projection fibers as they pass to the cerebral cortex. Some of the fibers form the roof and lateral wall of the posterior horn of the lateral ventricle and the lateral wall of the inferior horn of the lateral ventricle; these fibers are referred to as the **tapetum**. Traced laterally, the fibers in the splenium arch backward into the occipital lobe and form the **forceps major**.

The **anterior commissure** is a small bundle of nerve fibers that crosses the midline in the **lamina terminalis** (see Fig. 7-8). When traced laterally, a smaller or anterior bundle curves forward on each side toward the anterior perforated substance and the olfactory tract. A larger bundle curves posteriorly on each side and grooves the inferior surface of the lentiform nucleus to reach the temporal lobes.

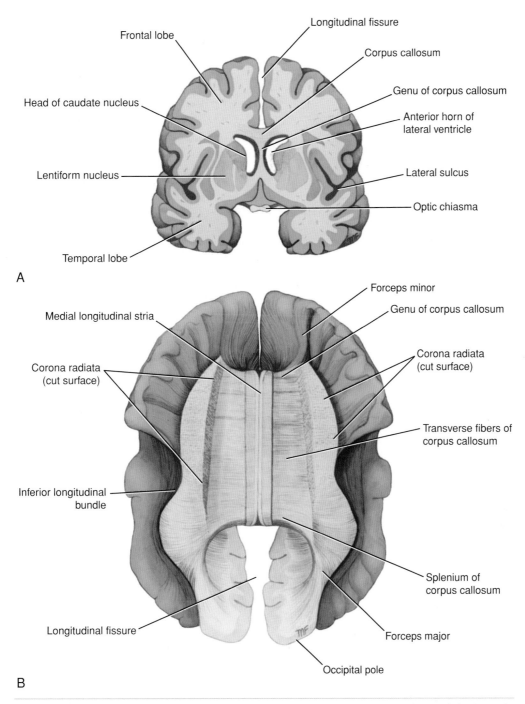

Figure 7-15 **A:** Coronal section of the brain passing through the anterior horn of the lateral ventricle and the optic chiasma. **B:** Superior view of the brain dissected to show the fibers of the corpus callosum and the corona radiata.

The **posterior commissure** is a bundle of nerve fibers that crosses the midline immediately above the opening of the cerebral aqueduct into the third ventricle (see Fig. 7-3); it is related to the inferior part of the stalk of the pineal gland. Various collections of nerve cells are situated along its length. The destinations and functional significance of many of the nerve fibers are not known. However, the fibers from the pretectal nuclei involved in the pupillary light reflex are believed

to cross in this commissure on their way to the parasympathetic part of the oculomotor nuclei.

The **fornix** is composed of myelinated nerve fibers and constitutes the efferent system of the hippocampus that passes to the mammillary bodies of the hypothalamus. The nerve fibers first form the **alveus** (see Fig. 9-5), which is a thin layer of white matter covering the ventricular surface of the hippocampus, and then converge to form the **fimbria**. The fimbriae of the two

Posterior columns of fornix

Commissure of fornix

Body of fornix

Anterior columns of fornix

Frontal poles

Occipital poles

Anterior horn of lateral ventricle

Interventricular foramen

Lentiform nucleus

Lateral ventricle

Thalamus

Figure 7-16 Horizontal section of the brain leaving the fornix in position.

sides increase in thickness and, on reaching the posterior end of the hippocampus, arch forward above the thalamus and below the corpus callosum to form the **posterior columns of the fornix**. The two columns then come together in the midline to form the **body of the fornix** (Fig. 7-16). The **commissure of the fornix** consists of transverse fibers that cross the midline from one column to another just before the formation of the body of the fornix. The function of the commissure of the fornix is to connect the hippocampal formations of the two sides.

The **habenular commissure** is a small bundle of nerve fibers that crosses the midline in the superior part of the root of the pineal stalk (see Fig. 7-3). The commissure is associated with the **habenular nuclei**, which are situated on either side of the midline in this region. The habenular nuclei receive many afferents from the amygdaloid nuclei and the hippocampus. These afferent fibers pass to the habenular nuclei in the **stria medullaris thalami**. Some of the fibers cross the midline to reach the contralateral nucleus through the habenular commissure. The function of the habenular nuclei and its connections in humans is unknown.

Association Fibers

Association fibers are nerve fibers that essentially connect various cortical regions within the same hemisphere and may be divided into short and long groups (Fig. 7-17). The **short association fibers** lie immediately beneath the cortex and connect adjacent gyri; these fibers run transversely to the long axis of the sulci. The **long association fibers** are collected into named bundles that can be dissected in a formalin-hardened brain. The **uncinate fasciculus** connects the first motor speech area and the gyri on the inferior surface of the frontal lobe

with the cortex of the pole of the temporal lobe. The **cingulum** is a long, curved fasciculus lying within the white matter of the cingulate gyrus (see Fig. 7-8). It connects the frontal and parietal lobes with parahippocampal and adjacent temporal cortical regions. The **superior longitudinal fasciculus** is the largest bundle of nerve fibers. It connects the anterior part of the frontal lobe to the occipital and temporal lobes. The **inferior longitudinal fasciculus** runs anteriorly from the occipital lobe, passing lateral to the optic radiation, and is distributed to the temporal lobe. The **fronto-occipital fasciculus** connects the frontal lobe to the occipital and temporal lobes. It is situated deep within the cerebral hemisphere and is related to the lateral border of the caudate nucleus.

Projection Fibers

Afferent and efferent nerve fibers passing to and from the brainstem to the entire cerebral cortex must travel between large nuclear masses of gray matter within the cerebral hemisphere. At the upper part of the brainstem, these fibers form a compact band known as the **internal capsule**, which is flanked medially by the caudate nucleus and the thalamus and laterally by the lentiform nucleus (see Fig. 7-12). Because of the wedge shape of the lentiform nucleus, as seen on horizontal section, the internal capsule is bent to form an **anterior limb** and a **posterior limb**, which are continuous with each other at the **genu** (Figs. 7-18 and 7-19). Once the nerve fibers have emerged superiorly from between the nuclear masses, they radiate in all directions to the cerebral cortex. These radiating projection fibers are known as the **corona radiata** (Fig. 7-19). Most of the projection fibers lie medial to the association fibers, but they intersect the commissural fibers of the corpus callosum and the anterior commissure. The nerve fibers lying within the most posterior

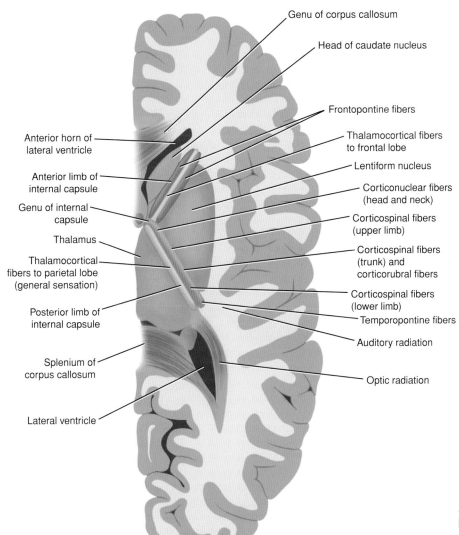

Figure 7-17 Horizontal section of the right cerebral hemisphere showing the relationships and different parts of the internal capsule.

part of the posterior limb of the internal capsule radiate toward the calcarine sulcus and are known as the **optic radiation** (Fig. 7-18). The detailed arrangement of the fibers within the internal capsule is shown in Figure 7-18.

Septum Pellucidum

The septum pellucidum is a thin vertical sheet of nervous tissue consisting of white and gray matter covered on either side by ependyma (see Figs. 7-8 and 7-12; see also Atlas Plate 8). It stretches between the fornix and the corpus callosum. Anteriorly, it occupies the interval between the body of the corpus callosum and the rostrum. It is essentially a double membrane with a closed, slitlike cavity between the membranes. The septum pellucidum forms a partition between the anterior horns of the lateral ventricles.

Tela Choroidea

The tela choroidea is a two-layered fold of pia mater. It is situated between the fornix superiorly and the roof of the third ventricle and the upper surfaces of the two thalami inferiorly. When seen from above, the anterior end is situated at the interventricular foramina (see Fig. 16-6). Its lateral edges are irregular and project laterally into the body of the lateral ventricles. Here, they are covered by ependyma and form the choroid plexuses of the lateral ventricle. Posteriorly, the lateral edges continue into the inferior horn of the lateral ventricle and are covered with ependyma so that the choroid plexus projects through the choroidal fissure.

On either side of the midline, the tela choroidea projects down through the roof of the third ventricle to form the choroid plexuses of the third ventricle.

The blood supply of the tela choroidea and, therefore, also of the choroid plexuses of the third and lateral ventricles is derived from the **choroidal branches of the internal carotid** and **basilar arteries**. The venous blood drains into the **internal cerebral veins**, which unite to form the **great cerebral vein**. The great cerebral vein joins the **inferior sagittal sinus** to form the **straight sinus**.

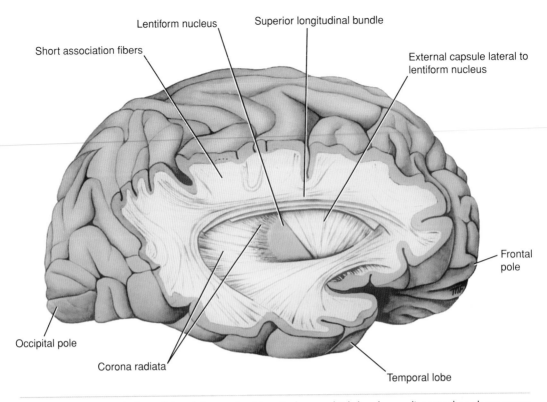

Figure 7-18 Lateral view of the right cerebral hemisphere, which has been dissected to show some of the principal association fibers.

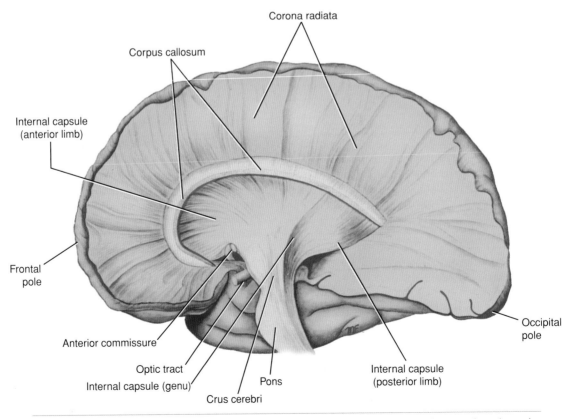

Figure 7-19 Medial view of the right cerebral hemisphere, which has been dissected to show the internal capsule and the corona radiata. The thalamus has been removed. Note the interdigitation of the horizontally running fibers of the corpus callosum and the vertical fibers of the corona radiata.

Clinical Notes

Thalamic Lesions

Lesions of the thalamus usually result from thrombosis or hemorrhage of one of the arteries that supply the thalamus. Because the thalamus is concerned with receiving sensory impulses from the opposite side of the body, the disability resulting from a lesion within it will be confined to the contralateral side of the body. There may be a major impairment of all forms of sensation, which could include light touch, tactile localization and discrimination, and loss of appreciation of joint movements.

Subthalamic Lesions

The subthalamus should be regarded as one of the extrapyramidal motor nuclei and has a large connection with the globus pallidus. Lesions of the subthalamus result in sudden, forceful involuntary movements in a contralateral extremity. The movements may be jerky (choreiform) or violent (ballistic).

Pineal Gland

The pineal gland consists essentially of pinealocytes and glial cells supported by a connective tissue framework. As the result of regressive changes that occur with age, calcareous concretions accumulate within the glial cells and connective tissue of the gland. These deposits are useful to the radiologist, since they serve as a landmark and assist in determining whether the pineal gland has been displaced laterally by a space-occupying lesion within the skull.

The functions of the pineal gland are mainly inhibitory and have been shown to influence the pituitary gland, the islets of Langerhans, the parathyroids, the adrenals, and the gonads.

Clinical observation of patients with pineal tumors or tumors of neighboring areas of nervous tissue that may press on the pineal gland has shown severe alteration of reproductive function.

Hypothalamus

The hypothalamus is an area of the nervous system that is of great functional importance. Not only does it control emotional states, but it also assists in the regulation of fat, carbohydrate, and water metabolism. Among its many other activities, it influences body temperature, genital functions, sleep, and food intake. The pituitary and the hypothalamus constitute a closely integrated unit, and the hypothalamus plays a role in the release of pituitary hormones.

Hypothalamic Syndromes

Lesions of the hypothalamus may result from infection, trauma, or vascular disorders. Tumors, such as a **craniopharyngioma** or **chromophobe adenoma of the pituitary** and **pineal tumors**, may interfere with the function of the hypothalamus. The most common abnormalities include **genital hypoplasia** or **atrophy**, **diabetes insipidus**, **obesity**, **disturbances of sleep**, **irregular pyrexia**, and **emaciation**. Some of these disorders may occur together, such as in the **adiposogenital dystrophy syndrome**.

Cerebral Cortex, Sulci, and Cerebral Hemisphere Lobes

The cerebral cortex is composed of gray matter. Only about a third lies on the exposed convexity of the gyri; the remaining two thirds form the walls of the sulci. Moreover, different areas of the cortex have different functions, and the anatomical division of the cortex into lobes and gyri by sulci enables the physician to localize loss of function or accurately place a brain lesion. For example, focal lesions of the precentral gyrus will produce contralateral hemiparesis, while lesions of the postcentral gyrus will result in contralateral hemisensory loss. More widespread lesions of the frontal lobe might cause symptoms and signs indicative of loss of attention span or change in social behavior. Widespread degeneration of the cerebral cortex gives rise to symptoms of dementia.

Lateral Ventricles

Each lateral ventricle contains about 7 to 10 mL of cerebrospinal fluid (CSF). This fluid is produced in the choroid plexus of the lateral ventricle and normally drains into the third ventricle through the interventricular foramen (foramen of Monro). Blockage of the foramen by a cerebral tumor would result in distention of the ventricle, thus producing a type of **hydrocephalus**.

The choroid plexus of the lateral ventricle is continuous with that of the third ventricle through the interventricular foramen. The choroid plexus is largest where the body and posterior and inferior horns join, where it may become calcified with age. Do not confuse this **calcification of the choroid plexus**, as seen on radiographs, with that of the pineal gland.

In the past, the size and shape of the lateral ventricle were investigated clinically by **pneumoencephalography** (Figs. 7-20 to 7-23). In this procedure, small amounts of air were introduced into the subarachnoid space by lumbar puncture with the patient in the sitting position. If the patient already had a raised intracranial pressure, this method was dangerous, and air or radiopaque fluid was injected directly into the lateral ventricles through a burr hole in the skull (this procedure was referred to as **ventriculography**). This procedure has now been replaced by CT and magnetic resonance imaging (MRI) (Figs. 7-24 to 7-27).

Basal Nuclei

The **basal nuclei**, in this discussion, refers to the masses of gray matter that are deeply placed within the cerebrum. They include the caudate nucleus, the lentiform nucleus, the amygdaloid nucleus, and the claustrum.

Because of the close relationship that exists between these nuclei and the internal capsule, tumors of the caudate or lentiform nuclei may cause severe motor or sensory symptoms on the opposite side of the body. Tumors pressing on the anterior two thirds of the posterior limb of the internal capsule will cause progressive spastic hemiplegia, while more posteriorly situated tumors will produce impairment of sensation on the opposite side.

Disorders of function of the basal nuclei are considered after the connections of these nuclei are discussed in Chapter 10.

Cerebral Commissures

The major commissure is the large corpus callosum. Most fibers within the corpus callosum interconnect symmetrical areas of the cerebral cortex. Because it transfers

Figure 7-20 Anteroposterior pneumoencephalogram of a 28-year-old man.

information from one hemisphere to another, the corpus callosum is essential for learned discrimination, sensory experience, and memory.

Occasionally, the corpus callosum fails to develop, and in these individuals, no definite signs or symptoms appear. Should the corpus callosum be destroyed by disease in later life, however, each hemisphere becomes isolated, and the patient responds as if he or she has two separate brains. The patient's general intelligence and behavior appear normal, since over the years both hemispheres have been trained to respond to different situations. If a pencil is placed in the patient's right hand (with the eyes closed), he or she will recognize the object by touch and be able to describe it. If the pencil is placed in the left hand, the tactile information will pass to the right postcentral gyrus. This information will not be able to travel through the corpus callosum to the speech area in the left hemisphere; therefore, the patient will be unable to describe the object in his or her left hand.

Section of the corpus callosum has been attempted surgically, with some success, in order to prevent the spread of seizures from one hemisphere to the other.

Internal Capsule Lesions

The internal capsule is an important compact band of white matter. It is composed of ascending and descending nerve fibers that connect the cerebral cortex to the brainstem and spinal cord. The internal capsule is flanked medially

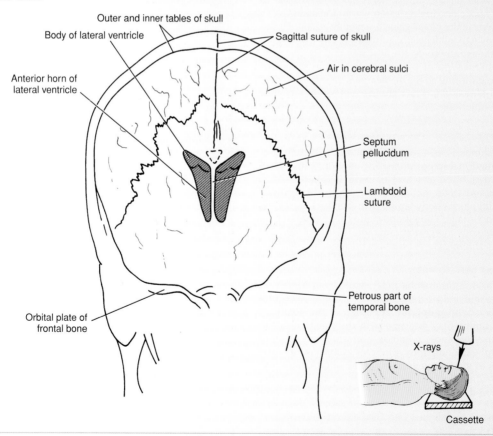

Figure 7-21 Explanation of the radiograph seen in Figure 7-20. Note the position of the x-ray gun relative to the head and the film cassette.

Figure 7-22 Lateral pneumoencephalogram of a 28-year-old man.

by the caudate nucleus and thalamus and laterally by the lentiform nucleus. The arrangement of the nerve fibers within the internal capsule is shown in Figure 7-18.

The internal capsule is frequently involved in vascular disorders of the brain. The most common cause of arterial hemorrhage is atheromatous degeneration in an artery in a patient with high blood pressure. Because of the high concentration of important nerve fibers within the internal capsule, even a small hemorrhage can cause widespread effects on the contralateral side of the body. Not only is the immediate neural tissue destroyed by the blood, which later clots, but also neighboring nerve fibers may be compressed or be edematous.

Alzheimer Disease

Alzheimer disease is a degenerative disease of the brain occurring in middle to late life, but an early form of the disease is now well recognized. The disease affects more than 4 million people in the United States, resulting in

Figure 7-23 Explanation of the radiograph seen in Figure 7-22. Note the position of the x-ray gun relative to the head and the film cassette.

Frontal lobe
White matter
Head of caudate nucleus
Lentiform nucleus
Body of lateral ventricle
Falx cerebri
Occipital lobe

Longitudinal fissure
Genu of corpus callosum
Septum pellucidum
Anterior horn of lateral ventricle
Fornix
Third ventricle
Thalamus
Posterior horn of lateral ventricle
Internal occipital protuberance

Figure 7-24 Horizontal (axial) CT scan of the brain.

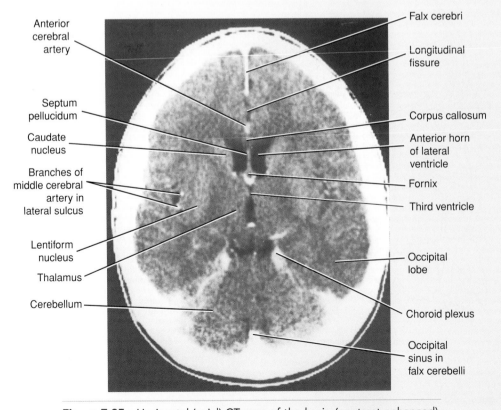

Anterior cerebral artery
Septum pellucidum
Caudate nucleus
Branches of middle cerebral artery in lateral sulcus
Lentiform nucleus
Thalamus
Cerebellum

Falx cerebri
Longitudinal fissure
Corpus callosum
Anterior horn of lateral ventricle
Fornix
Third ventricle
Occipital lobe
Choroid plexus
Occipital sinus in falx cerebelli

Figure 7-25 Horizontal (axial) CT scan of the brain (contrast enhanced).

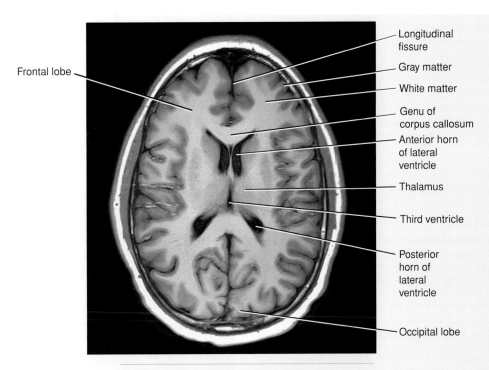

Longitudinal fissure

Gray matter

White matter

Genu of corpus callosum

Anterior horn of lateral ventricle

Thalamus

Third ventricle

Posterior horn of lateral ventricle

Occipital lobe

Frontal lobe

Figure 7-26   Horizontal (axial) MRI of the brain.

Gray matter

White matter

Cingulate gyrus

Cingulate sulcus

Corpus callosum

Hippocampus   Fornix   Pons   Midbrain   Lateral ventricle

Figure 7-27   Coronal MRI of the brain.

over 100,000 deaths per year. The risk of the disease rises sharply with advancing years.

The cause of Alzheimer disease is unknown, but evidence suggests a genetic predisposition. Several abnormal genes have been found, each of which leads to a similar clinical and pathologic syndrome, with only variations in the age of onset and the rate of progression to suggest that the pathogenetic mechanisms differ. Some cases of familial Alzheimer disease, for example, have been shown to have mutations in several genes (*App*, *presenilin 1*, and *presenilin 2*).

Early memory loss, a disintegration of personality, complete disorientation, deterioration in speech, and restlessness are common signs. In the late stages, the patient may become mute, incontinent, and bedridden and usually dies of some other disease.

Microscopically, changes eventually occur throughout the cerebral cortex, but to begin with, certain regions of the brain are selectively involved. The early sites include the hippocampus, the entorhinal cortex, and the associated areas of the cerebral cortex. Many so-called senile plaques are found in the atrophic cortex. The plaques result from the accumulation of several proteins around deposits of beta amyloid. In the center of each plaque is an extracellular collection of degenerating nervous tissue; surrounding the core is a rim of large abnormal neuronal processes, probably presynaptic terminals, filled with an excess of intracellular neurofibrils that are tangled and twisted, forming neurofibrillary tangles. The neurofibrillary tangles are aggregations of the microtubular protein tau, which is hyperphosphorylated. There is a marked loss of choline acetyltransferase, the biosynthetic enzyme for acetylcholine, in the areas of the cortex in which the senile plaques occur. This is thought to be due to loss of the ascending projection fibers rather than a loss of cortical cells. As these cellular changes occur, the affected neurons die.

At this time, there is no clinical test for making the definite diagnosis of Alzheimer disease. Reliance is placed on taking a careful history and carrying out numerous neurologic and psychiatric examinations spaced out over time. In this way, other causes of dementia can be excluded. Alterations in the levels of amyloid peptides or tau in the serum or CSF may be helpful. CT scans or MRIs are also used, and abnormalities in the medial part of the temporal lobe occur in this disease. In advanced cases, a thin, atrophied cerebral cortex and dilated lateral ventricles may be found. The recent use of positron emission tomography (PET) shows evidence of diminished cortical metabolism (Fig. 7-28).

The use of cholinesterase inhibitors for the treatment of Alzheimer disease has been found to be helpful. These drugs probably act by increasing the presence of acetylcholine at the sites of the disease where there is a deficiency of this neurotransmitter.

Figure 7-28 Axial (horizontal) PET scan of a male patient with Alzheimer disease, showing defects (*arrowheads*) in metabolism in the bitemporoparietal regions of the cerebral cortex, following the injection of 18-fluorodeoxyglucose. The yellow areas indicate regions of high metabolic activity. (*Courtesy Dr. Holley Dey.*)

Key Concepts

Cerebral Subdivisions

- The cerebrum is subdivided into the diencephalon (central core) and the telencephalon (cerebral hemispheres).

Diencephalon

- The diencephalon consists of the third ventricle and the structures that form its boundaries, including the thalamus, subthalamus, epithalamus, and hypothalamus.

Thalamus

- The thalamus is a very important cell station that receives the main sensory tracts. Sensory information is integrated and relayed to the cerebral cortex and other subcortical regions.

Subthalamus

- The subthalamus consists of nerve cells associated with the red nuclei and substantia nigra and is involved in control of muscle activity.

Epithalamus

- The epithalamus consists of the habenular nuclei (integration of visceral and somatic pathways) and the pineal gland (endocrine gland and melatonin).

Hypothalamus

- The hypothalamus controls and integrates the functions of the autonomic nervous system and endocrine systems and plays a vital role in maintaining body homeostasis.
- Physiologically, hardly any activity in the body is not influenced by the hypothalamus.

Main Sulci

- The central sulcus separates the frontal and parietal lobes. The gyrus anterior to it contains motor cells that initiate the movements of the contralateral side of the body; the gyrus posterior to it contains general sensory cortex that receives sensory information from the contralateral side of the body.
- The lateral sulcus is a deep cleft on the inferior lateral cerebral hemisphere, between frontal and temporal lobes. The insula lies deep to the lateral sulcus.
- The parieto-occipital sulcus is located on the medial side of the hemisphere, running inferiorly to intersect the calcarine sulcus.
- The calcarine sulcus is found on the medial surface of the hemispheres, in the occipital lobe. Primary visual cortex is located here.

Cerebral Hemisphere Lobes

- The frontal lobe occupies the area anterior to the central sulcus and is divided by three sulci into three gyri.
- The temporal lobe occupies the area inferior to the lateral sulcus and is divided into three gyri by two sulci.
- The occipital lobe occupies the area behind the parieto-occipital sulcus.

Internal Structures

- The two lateral ventricles are located one in each hemisphere. The lateral ventricles are large cavities that house CSF. Each are in communication with the third ventricle through the interventricular foramen.
- Basal nuclei are a collection of gray matter masses including the corpus striatum, amygdaloid nucleus, and the claustrum.
    - The corpus striatum is composed of the caudate nucleus and the lentiform nucleus, both separated by the internal capsule. These structures are involved in muscular movement control through communications with the cortex.
    - The claustrum is separated from the lentiform nucleus by the external capsule. The function of the claustrum is unknown.
    - The amygdaloid nucleus is located in the temporal lobe adjacent to the anterior horn of the lateral ventricle.
- Commissure fibers in the cerebrum are myelinated fibers connecting two corresponding regions of the two hemispheres.
- The largest commissure is the corpus callosum, which connects the two hemispheres. Other commissures include the fornix and the anterior and posterior commissures.

❓ Clinical Problem Solving

1. A 53-year-old woman is admitted to an emergency department after she collapses in the street. Apart from being confused and disoriented, she exhibits violent, uncoordinated movements of her right arm and right leg and slight spontaneous movements on the right side of her face. The physician is able to ascertain from a friend that the patient had been perfectly fit that morning and has no previous history of this condition. On examination, the involuntary movements of the right limbs are mainly confined to the muscles of the proximal part of the limbs. One week later, the patient dies of cardiac failure. What is the medical term used to describe this condition? Which area of the brain is likely to be involved in the production of this condition?

2. A 64-year-old man is admitted to a hospital on the suspicion that he has a cerebral tumor. One of the investigations asked for by the physician is a simple anteroposterior radiograph and lateral radiograph of the head. Using your knowledge of

neuroanatomy, name the structure that would assist the radiologist in this case in determining whether lateral displacement of the brain had occurred within the skull.

3. A 12-year-old boy is seen by a pediatrician because his parents are concerned about his excessive weight and lack of development of the external genitalia. On examination, the child is seen to be tall for his age and very obese. The excessive fat is concentrated especially in the lower part of the anterior abdominal wall and the proximal parts of the limbs. His penis and testes are small. Is it possible that disease of the diencephalon might account for this condition?

4. A neurosurgeon explains to her residents that she will attempt to remove a glioma located in the right middle frontal gyrus by turning back a flap of the scalp and removing a rectangular piece of the overlying skull. Where exactly is the right middle frontal gyrus in the brain? What are the names of the sulci that lie above and below this gyrus? Which skull bone overlays this gyrus?

5. While performing an autopsy, a pathologist has great difficulty in finding the central sulcus in each cerebral hemisphere. Because finding this sulcus is the key to localizing many other sulci and gyri, what landmarks would you use to identify the central sul-

cus? Are the sulci and gyri in the two hemispheres similar in size and shape? Do they exhibit individual variations in their arrangement?

6. A fourth-year medical student is shown coronal and horizontal MRIs of the brain and is asked to comment on his observations. The patient is a 55-year-old man. The student responds by saying that the left lateral ventricle is larger than normal and that there is an area of low signal intensity close to the left interventricular foramen suggesting the presence of a brain tumor. On looking at a standard lateral radiograph of the skull and brain, he notes a small area of "calcification" situated in the region of the posterior part of the left ventricle. Using your knowledge of neuroanatomy, describe the location of the lateral ventricle in the brain. What are the different parts of the lateral ventricle? Where is the cerebrospinal fluid produced, and what does it normally drain into? What is responsible for the calcification seen in the left lateral ventricle in this patient?

7. A medical student, while performing an autopsy, finds that the patient has no corpus callosum. On consulting the patient's clinical notes, she is surprised to find no reference to a neurologic disorder. Are you surprised that this patient had no recorded neurologic signs and symptoms?

 Answers and Explanations to Clinical Problem Solving

1. This woman exhibited continuous uncoordinated activity of the proximal musculature of the right arm and right leg, resulting in the limbs being flung violently about. The muscles of the right side of the face were also slightly affected. This condition is known as hemiballismus. It was caused by hemorrhage into the left subthalamic nucleus.

2. During the third decade of life, calcareous concretions appear in the neuroglia and connective tissue of the pineal gland. This provides a useful midline landmark to the radiologist. A lateral displacement of such a landmark would indicate the presence of an intracranial mass. In this patient, the pineal gland shadow was in the midline, and all the other investigations, including CT, showed no evidence of a cerebral tumor.

3. Yes. Adiposity alone or associated with genital dystrophy can occur with disease of the hypothalamus.

4. The right middle frontal gyrus is located on the lateral surface of the frontal lobe of the right cerebral hemisphere. It is bounded superiorly and inferiorly by the superior and inferior frontal sulci, respectively. The right middle frontal gyrus is overlaid by the frontal bone of the skull.

5. The important central sulcus is large and runs downward and forward across the lateral aspect of each hemisphere. Superiorly, it indents the superior medial border of the hemisphere about 1 cm behind the midpoint; it lies between two parallel gyri. It is

the only sulcus of any length that indents the superior medial border. The arrangement of the sulci and gyri is very similar on both sides of the brain. However, individual details of their arrangement vary greatly.

6. The lateral ventricle is a C-shaped cavity situated within each cerebral hemisphere. The lateral ventricle wraps itself around the thalamus, the lentiform nucleus, and the caudate nucleus. It is divided into a body that occupies the parietal lobe, an anterior horn that extends into the frontal lobe, a posterior horn that extends into the occipital lobe, and an inferior horn that runs forward and inferiorly into the temporal lobe. The cerebrospinal fluid is produced in the choroid plexus of the lateral ventricle and drains through the small interventricular foramen into the third ventricle. In later life, the choroid plexus, especially in its posterior part, sometimes shows calcified deposits, which are occasionally revealed on radiographs, as in this case. This patient later was found to have a cerebral tumor that was compressing the left interventricular foramen, hence the enlarged left ventricle.

7. No. The corpus callosum occasionally fails to develop, and in those patients, no definite neurologic signs and symptoms appear. If, however, the corpus callosum is divided during a surgical procedure in the adult, the loss of interconnections between the two hemispheres becomes apparent (see pp. 267–268).

? Review Questions

Directions: Each of the numbered items in this section is followed by answers. Select the ONE lettered answer that is CORRECT.

1. The following statements concern the diencephalon:
   (a) It extends anteriorly as far as the optic chiasma.
   (b) It is bounded laterally by the internal capsule.
   (c) The thalamus is located in the medial wall of the third ventricle.
   (d) The epithalamus is formed by the cranial end of the substantia nigra and the red nuclei.
   (e) It extends posteriorly as far as the interthalamic connection.

2. The following statements concern the pineal gland:
   (a) It produces a secretion that is opaque to x-rays.
   (b) It contains high concentrations of melatonin.
   (c) Melatonin stimulates the release of the gonadotrophic hormone from the anterior lobe of the pituitary gland.
   (d) Production of secretions of the pineal gland decreases during darkness.
   (e) The pinealocytes are inhibited by the sympathetic nerve endings.

3. The following statements concern the thalamus:
   (a) It is the largest part of the diencephalon and serves as a relay station to all the main sensory tracts (except the olfactory pathway).
   (b) It is separated from the lentiform nucleus by the external capsule.
   (c) It forms the anterior boundary of the interventricular foramen.
   (d) It is completely separate from the thalamus on the opposite side.
   (e) The thalamus is a small rectangular mass of gray matter.

4. The following statements concern the hypothalamus:
   (a) It is formed by the upper part of the lateral wall and roof of the third ventricle.
   (b) Caudally, the hypothalamus merges with the tectum of the midbrain.
   (c) The nuclei are composed of groups of large nerve cells.
   (d) Functionally, it plays a role in the release of pituitary hormones.
   (e) The mammillary bodies are not part of the hypothalamus.

5. The following statements concern the hypothalamus:
   (a) The hypothalamus has no influence on the activities of the autonomic and endocrine systems.
   (b) It receives few afferent visceral and somatic sensory fibers.
   (c) It gives off efferent fibers that pass to the sympathetic and parasympathetic outflows in the brain and spinal cord.
   (d) It does not assist in the regulation of water metabolism.

   (e) The hypothalamus plays no role in controlling emotional states.

6. The following statements concern the third ventricle:
   (a) The posterior wall is formed by the opening into the cerebral aqueduct and the pineal recess.
   (b) It does not communicate directly with the lateral ventricles.
   (c) The vascular tela choroidea projects from the floor to form the choroid plexus.
   (d) Lying in the floor of the ventricle, from posterior to anterior, are the optic chiasma, the tuber cinereum, and the mammillary bodies.
   (e) The wall of the ventricle is not lined with ependyma.

Matching Questions. Directions: The following questions apply to Figure 7-29. Match the numbers listed on the left with the appropriate lettered structure listed on the right. Each lettered option may be selected once, more than once, or not at all.

7. Number 1	(a) Genu of corpus callosum
8. Number 2	(b) Interventricular foramen
9. Number 3	(c) Body of fornix
10. Number 4	(d) Anterior commissure
11. Number 5	(e) None of the above
12. Number 6	
13. Number 7	

Figure 7-29 Sagittal section of the brain showing the medial surface of the diencephalon.

Directions: Each of the numbered items in this section is followed by answers. Select the ONE lettered answer that is CORRECT.

14. The following statements concern the longitudinal cerebral fissure:
    (a) The fissure contains the fold of dura mater, the falx cerebelli.
    (b) The fissure contains the middle cerebral arteries.
    (c) The superior sagittal sinus lies below it.
    (d) In the depths of the fissure, the corpus callosum crosses the midline.
    (e) The inferior sagittal sinus lies above it.
15. The following statements concern the central sulcus:
    (a) The central sulcus extends onto the medial surface of the cerebral hemisphere.
    (b) The frontal lobe lies posterior to it.
    (c) The parietal lobe lies anterior to it.
    (d) The central sulcus is continuous inferiorly with the lateral sulcus.
    (e) The arachnoid mater extends into the central sulcus.
16. The following statements concern the lateral ventricle:
    (a) Each ventricle is J shaped and filled with cerebrospinal fluid.
    (b) It communicates with the third ventricle through the interventricular foramen.
    (c) The body of the ventricle occupies the frontal lobe.
    (d) The lateral ventricle does not possess a choroid plexus.
    (e) The anterior horn occupies the parietal lobe.
17. The following statements concern the corpus callosum:
    (a) It is connected to the fornix by the lamina terminalis.
    (b) The rostrum connects the genu to the septum pellucidum.
    (c) Most of the fibers within the corpus callosum interconnect symmetrical areas of the cerebral cortex.
    (d) The fibers of the genu curve forward into the frontal lobes as the forceps major.
    (e) The corpus callosum is related inferiorly to the falx cerebri.
18. The following statements concern the anterior commissure:
    (a) It is embedded in the superior part of the septum pellucidum.
    (b) When traced laterally, an anterior bundle of fibers curves forward to join the olfactory tract.
    (c) Some of the fibers are concerned with the sensations of taste.
    (d) It forms the anterior boundary of the interventricular foramen.
    (e) It is formed by a large bundle of nerve fibers.
19. The following statements concerning the internal capsule are correct **except**:
    (a) It is continuous below with the tectum of the midbrain.
    (b) It has an anterior limb and a posterior limb, which are in a straight line.

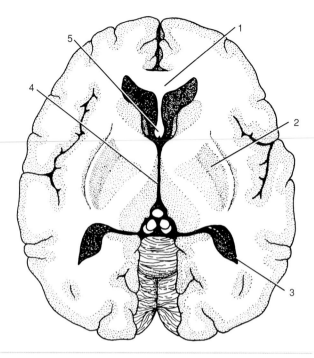

Figure 7-30 Horizontal section of the cerebrum, as seen from above.

    (c) The genu and the anterior part of the posterior limb contain the corticobulbar and corticospinal fibers.
    (d) It is related medially to the lentiform nucleus.
    (e) It is continuous below with the corona radiata.
20. The following statements concern the basal ganglia:
    (a) The caudate nucleus is not attached to the lentiform nucleus.
    (b) The corpus striatum is concerned with muscular movement.
    (c) The lentiform nucleus is related medially to the external capsule.
    (d) The lentiform nucleus is oval shaped, as seen on horizontal section.
    (e) The amygdaloid nucleus does not form one of the basal ganglia.

Matching Questions. Directions: The following questions apply to Figure 7-30. Match the numbers listed on the left with the appropriate lettered structure listed on the right. Each lettered option may be selected once, more than once, or not at all.

21. Number 1   (a) Optic radiation
22. Number 2   (b) Lateral sulcus
23. Number 3   (c) Lentiform nucleus
24. Number 4   (d) Anterior horn of lateral ventricle
25. Number 5   (e) None of the above

The following questions apply to Figure 7-31. Match the numbers listed on the left with the appropriate lettered structure listed on the right. Each lettered option may be selected once, more than once, or not at all.

26. Number 1   (a) Central sulcus
27. Number 2   (b) Postcentral gyrus

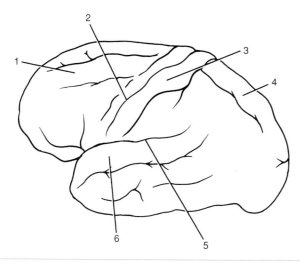

Figure 7-31 Lateral view of the left cerebral hemisphere.

28. Number 3
29. Number 4
30. Number 5
31. Number 6

(c) Superior temporal gyrus
(d) Superior parietal lobule
(e) None of the above

Directions: The case histories below are followed by questions. Select the ONE BEST lettered answer.

A 70-year-old man with hypertension was admitted to an emergency department, having suddenly developed hemiparesis on the right side and numbness of the right leg. Axial CT and MRI were undertaken. MRI revealed a small hemorrhage in the left thalamus, which passed horizontally through the lateral ventricles. After careful observation, 2 days later, the paresis was much improved, and the patient reported that his numbness had disappeared. The patient was discharged from the hospital 1 week later and made an uneventful recovery. His hypertension was brought under control with suitable medication.

32. Using your knowledge of the relationships of the left thalamus, select the statement that explains the transient right hemiparesis and numbness.
    (a) The hemorrhage occurred into the third ventricle.

(b) The hemorrhage into the thalamus extended laterally into the posterior limb of the left internal capsule.
(c) The hemorrhage was small and confined to the thalamus on the left side.
(d) The hemorrhage was small and occurred in the lateral part of the left thalamus, producing transient edema in the left internal capsule.
(e) The hemorrhage extended laterally into the left lateral ventricle.

33. This hypertensive patient had a small thalamic hemorrhage. Select the **most likely** cause for the hemorrhage:
    (a) One of the small diseased thalamic arteries may have ruptured.
    (b) One of the small veins draining the thalamus may have ruptured.
    (c) Vasoconstriction of the thalamic arteries could have occurred.
    (d) Softening of the neuronal tissue around the thalamic arteries might have taken place.
    (e) No relation exists between hypertension and the thalamic hemorrhage in this patient.

An 8-year-old boy with a severe earache on the right side was taken to a pediatrician. The symptoms had started 7 days ago, and the pain had progressively worsened. On examination, the boy was found to have severe right-sided otitis media with acute mastoiditis. On being questioned, the boy admitted that his head hurt badly all over and that he felt sick. While he was being examined, he vomited. His body temperature was slightly elevated. In view of the severity of the headache and the presence of nausea and vomiting, the pediatrician decided to have an MRI performed. The result showed a small, well-defined, right cerebral abscess.

34. The cerebral abscess in this patient was most likely located at which site in the right cerebral hemisphere:
    (a) Frontal lobe
    (b) Thalamus
    (c) Occipital lobe
    (d) Temporal lobe
    (e) Cuneus

Answers and Explanations to Review Questions

1. B is correct. The diencephalon is bounded laterally by the internal capsule (see Fig. 7-1). A. The diencephalon extends anteriorly as far as the interventricular foramen (see Fig. 7-3). C. The thalamus is situated on the lateral wall of the third ventricle (see Fig. 7-3). D. The epithalamus consists of the habenular nuclei and their connections and the pineal gland. E. The diencephalon extends posteriorly as far as the cerebral aqueduct (see Fig. 7-3).

2. B is correct. The pineal gland contains high concentrations of melatonin. A. The pineal secretions are translucent to x-rays. C. Melatonin inhibits the

release of the gonadotrophic hormone from the anterior lobe of the pituitary gland. D. There is an increased production of the secretions of the pineal gland during darkness. E. The pinealocytes are stimulated by the sympathetic nerve endings.

3. A is correct. The thalamus is the largest part of the diencephalon and serves as a relay station to all the main sensory tracts, except the olfactory pathway. B. The thalamus is separated from the lentiform nucleus by the internal capsule (see Fig. 7-1). C. The thalamus forms the posterior boundary of the interventricular foramen (see Fig. 7-3). D. The

thalamus may be joined to the thalamus of the opposite side by the interthalamic connection. E. The thalamus is a large ovoid mass of gray matter (see Fig. 7-4).

4. D is correct. The hypothalamus plays an important role in the release of pituitary hormones. A. The hypothalamus is formed by the lower part of the lateral wall and floor of the third ventricle, below the hypothalamic sulcus (see Fig. 7-3). B. Caudally, the hypothalamus merges with the tegmentum of the midbrain. C. The nuclei of the hypothalamus are composed of groups of small nerve cells. E. The mammillary bodies are part of the hypothalamus.

5. C is correct. The hypothalamus gives off efferent fibers that pass to the sympathetic and parasympathetic outflows in the brain and spinal cord. A. The hypothalamus has influence on the activities of the autonomic and endocrine systems. B. The hypothalamus receives many afferent visceral and somatic sensory nerve fibers. D. The hypothalamus assists in the regulation of water metabolism. E. The hypothalamus plays a role in controlling emotional states.

6. A is correct. The posterior wall of the third ventricle is formed by the opening into the cerebral aqueduct and the pineal recess (see Fig. 7-3). B. The third ventricle does communicate directly with the lateral ventricles through the interventricular foramina (see Fig. 7-13). C. The vascular tela choroidea projects from the roof of the third ventricle to form the choroid plexus (see Fig. 7-3). D. Lying in the floor of the third ventricle, from anterior to posterior, are the optic chiasma, the tuber cinereum, and the mammillary bodies. E. The wall of the third ventricle is lined with ependyma.

7. D is correct.

8. A is correct.

9. E is correct. The structure is the septum pellucidum.

10. B is correct.

11. C is correct.

12. E is correct. The structure is the thalamus.

13. E is correct. The structure is the splenium of the corpus callosum.

14. D is correct. In the depths of the longitudinal cerebral fissure, the corpus callosum crosses the midline (see Fig. 7-6). A. The longitudinal cerebral fissure contains a fold of dura mater, the falx cerebri. B. The longitudinal cerebral fissure does not contain the middle cerebral arteries; they are located in the lateral cerebral fissures. C. The superior sagittal venous sinus lies above the longitudinal cerebral fissure. E. The inferior sagittal venous sinus lies in the lower border of the falx cerebri in the longitudinal cerebral fissure.

15. A is correct. The central sulcus extends onto the medial surface of the cerebral hemisphere (see Fig. 7-8). B. The frontal lobe lies anterior to the central sulcus (see Fig. 7-10). C. The parietal lobe lies posterior to the central sulcus (see Fig. 7-10). D. The central sulcus is not continuous inferiorly with the lateral sulcus (see Fig. 7-10). E. The arachnoid mater does not extend into the central sulcus.

16. B is correct. The lateral ventricle communicates with the third ventricle through the interventricular foramen (see Fig. 7-3). A. Each lateral ventricle is C shaped

and filled with cerebrospinal fluid (see Fig. 7-13). C. The body of the lateral ventricle occupies the parietal lobe. D. The lateral ventricle does possess a choroid plexus (see Fig. 7-1). E. The anterior horn of the lateral ventricle occupies the frontal lobe (see Fig. 7-13).

17. C is correct. Most of the fibers within the corpus callosum interconnect symmetrical areas of the cerebral cortex. A. The corpus callosum is connected to the fornix by the septum pellucidum (see Fig. 7-3). B. The rostrum of the corpus callosum connects the genu to the lamina terminalis (see Fig. 7-3). D. The fibers of the genu of the corpus callosum curve forward into the frontal lobes of the cerebral hemisphere as the forceps minor (see Fig. 7-15). E. The corpus callosum is related superiorly to the falx cerebri.

18. B is correct. When the anterior commissure is traced laterally, an anterior bundle of nerve fibers is seen to curve forward to join the olfactory tract. A. The anterior commissure is embedded in the superior part of the lamina terminalis (see Fig. 7-3). C. Some of the fibers of the anterior commissure are concerned with the sensation of smell. D. The anterior boundary of the interventricular foramen is formed by the anterior pillar of the fornix and not the anterior commissure (see Fig. 7-3). E. The anterior commissure is formed by a small bundle of nerve fibers.

19. C is correct. The internal capsule contains the corticobulbar and corticospinal fibers in the genu and the anterior part of the posterior limb (see Fig. 7-18). A. The internal capsule is continuous below with the crus cerebri of the midbrain (see Fig. 7-19). B. The internal capsule is bent around the lentiform nucleus and has an anterior limb, the genu, and a posterior limb (see Fig. 7-18). D. The internal capsule is related laterally to the lentiform nucleus (see Fig. 7-18). E. The internal capsule is continuous above with the coronal radiata (see Fig. 7-19).

20. B is correct. The corpus striatum is concerned with the control of muscular movement. A. The head of the caudate nucleus is attached to the lentiform nucleus (see Fig. 7-14). C. The lentiform nucleus is related laterally to the external capsule (see Fig. 7-12). D. The lentiform nucleus is wedge shaped, as seen on horizontal section (see Fig. 7-12). E. The amygdaloid nucleus forms one of the basal ganglia.

21. E is correct. The structure is the genu of the corpus callosum.

22. C is correct.

23. E is correct. The structure is the posterior horn of the lateral ventricle.

24. E is correct. The structure is the third ventricle.

25. E is correct. The structure is the anterior column of the fornix.

26. E is correct. The structure is the middle frontal gyrus.

27. A is correct.

28. B is correct.

29. D is correct.

30. E is correct. The structure is the lateral sulcus.

31. C is correct.

32. D is correct.

33. A is correct.

34. D is correct.

8

The Structure and Functional Localization of the Cerebral Cortex

CHAPTER OBJECTIVES

- To describe the basic structure and functional localization of the highly complex cerebral cortex

- To describe behavioral consequences from regional damage of the different cortical regions

A 19-year-old woman is involved in an automobile accident. She is not wearing a seat belt and is thrown from the car and suffers severe head injuries. During examination by the emergency medical technicians, she is found to be unconscious and is admitted to the emergency department. After 5 hours, she recovers consciousness and makes a remarkable recovery over the next 2 weeks. She leaves the hospital 1 month after the accident, with very slight weakness of her right leg. Nothing else abnormal is noted. Four months later, she is seen by a neurologist because she is experiencing sudden attacks of jerking movements of her right leg and foot. The attacks last only a few minutes. One week later, the patient has a very severe attack, which involves her right leg and then spreads to her right arm. On this occasion, she loses consciousness during the attack. The neurologist diagnoses Jacksonian epileptic seizures, caused by cerebral scarring secondary to the automobile injury. The weakness of the right leg immediately after the accident is due to damage to the superior part of the left precentral gyrus. Her initial attacks of epilepsy are of the partial variety and are caused by irritation of the area of the left precentral gyrus corresponding to the leg. In her last attack, the epileptiform seizure spreads to other areas of the left precentral gyrus, thus involving most of the right side of her body, and she loses consciousness. Knowledge of the functional localization of the cerebral cortex enables the physician to make an accurate diagnosis and advise suitable treatment. The cerebral scar tissue is cleanly excised by a neurosurgeon, and, apart from a small residual weakness of the right leg, the patient has no further epileptiform seizures. The cerebral cortex is the highest level of the central nervous system and always functions in association with the lower centers. The cerebral cortex receives vast amounts of information and responds in a precise manner by bringing about appropriate changes. Many of the responses are influenced by inherited programs, whereas others are colored by programs learned during an individual's life and stored in the cerebral cortex. The clinician can use this information to locate hemispheric lesions based on clinical symptoms and signs.

STRUCTURE

The cerebral cortex forms a complete covering of the cerebral hemisphere. It is composed of gray matter and has been estimated to contain approximately 10 billion neurons. The surface area of the cortex has been increased by throwing it into convolutions, or gyri, which are separated by fissures or sulci. The thickness of the cortex varies from 1.5 to 4.5 mm. The cortex is thickest over the crest of a gyrus and thinnest in the depth of a sulcus. The cerebral cortex, like gray matter elsewhere in the central nervous system, consists of a mixture of nerve cells, nerve fibers, neuroglia, and blood vessels. The following types of nerve cells are present in the cerebral cortex: (1) pyramidal cells,

(2) stellate cells, (3) fusiform cells, (4) horizontal cells of Cajal, and (5) cells of Martinotti (Fig. 8-1).

Nerve Cells

The **pyramidal cells** are named from the shape of their cell bodies. Most of the cell bodies measure 10 to 50 μm long. However, giant pyramidal cells, also known as **Betz cells**, whose cell bodies measure as much as 120 μm, are found in the motor precentral gyrus of the frontal lobe.

The apices of the pyramidal cells are oriented toward the pial surface of the cortex. From the apex of each cell, a thick apical dendrite extends upward toward the pia, giving off collateral branches. From

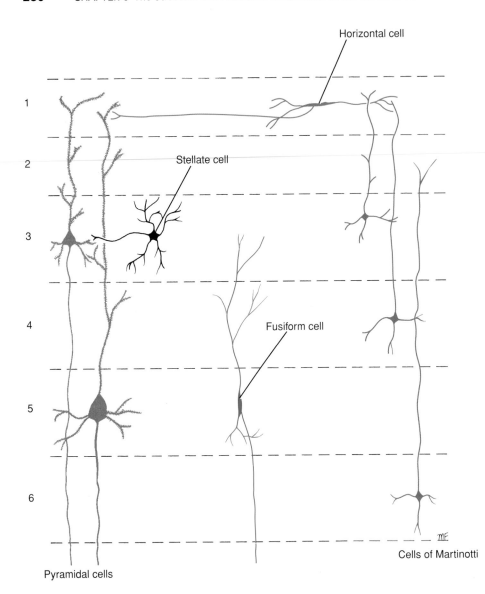

Figure 8-1 Main types of neurons found in the cerebral cortex.

the basal angles, several basal dendrites pass laterally into the surrounding neuropil. Each dendrite possesses numerous **dendritic spines** for synaptic junctions with axons of other neurons. The axon arises from the base of the cell body and either terminates in the deeper cortical layers or, more commonly, enters the white matter of the cerebral hemisphere as a projection, association, or commissural fiber.

The **stellate cells**, sometimes called granule cells because of their small size, are polygonal in shape, and their cell bodies measure about 8 µm in diameter. These cells have multiple branching dendrites and a relatively short axon, which terminates on a nearby neuron.

The **fusiform cells** have their long axis vertical to the surface and are concentrated mainly in the deepest cortical layers. Dendrites arise from each pole of the cell body. The inferior dendrite branches within the same cellular layer, while the superficial dendrite ascends toward the surface of the cortex and branches in the superficial layers. The axon arises from the inferior part

of the cell body and enters the white matter as a projection, association, or commissural fiber.

The **horizontal cells of Cajal** are small, fusiform, horizontally oriented cells found in the most superficial layers of the cortex. A dendrite emerges from each end of the cell, and an axon runs parallel to the surface of the cortex, making contact with the dendrites of pyramidal cells.

The **cells of Martinotti** are small, multipolar cells that are present throughout the levels of the cortex. The cell has short dendrites, but the axon is directed toward the pial surface of the cortex, where it ends in a more superficial layer, commonly the most superficial layer. The axon gives origin to a few short collateral branches en route.

Nerve Fibers

The nerve fibers of the cerebral cortex are arranged both radially and tangentially (Figs. 8-2 and 8-3). The **radial fibers** run at right angles to the cortical surface.

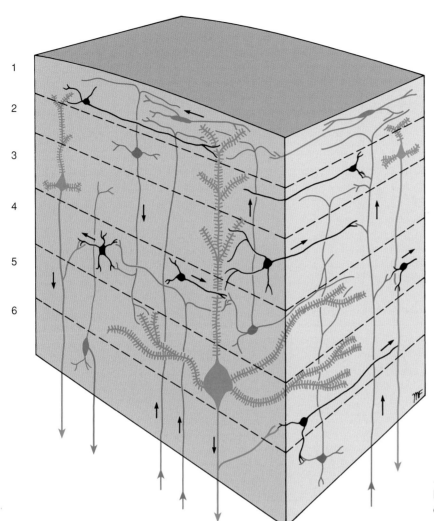

Figure 8-2 Neuronal connections of the cerebral cortex. Note the presence of the afferent and efferent fibers.

They include the afferent entering projection, association, and commissural fibers, which terminate within the cortex, and the axons of pyramidal, stellate, and fusiform cells, which leave the cortex to become projection, association, and commissural fibers of the white matter of the cerebral hemisphere.

The **tangential fibers** run parallel to the cortical surface and are, for the most part, collateral and terminal branches of afferent fibers. They also include the axons of horizontal and stellate cells and collateral branches of pyramidal and fusiform cells. The tangential fibers are most concentrated in layers 4 and 5, where they are referred to as the outer and inner **bands of Baillarger**, respectively. The bands of Baillarger are particularly well developed in the sensory areas due to the high concentration of the terminal parts of the thalamocortical fibers. In the visual cortex, the outer **band of Baillarger**, which is so thick that it can be seen with the naked eye, is known as the **stria of Gennari**. Because of this obvious band, or stria, the visual cortex in the walls of the calcarine sulcus is sometimes called the **striate cortex**.

Layers

Dividing the cerebral cortex into layers that may be distinguished by the type, density, and arrangement of their cells is convenient for descriptive purposes (see Figs. 8-1 and 8-3). The names and characteristic features of the layers are described here; regional differences are discussed later.

1. **Molecular layer (plexiform layer).** This is the most superficial layer; it consists mainly of a dense network of tangentially oriented nerve fibers. These fibers are derived from the apical dendrites of the pyramidal cells and fusiform cells, the axons of the stellate cells, and the cells of Martinotti. Afferent fibers originating in the thalamus and in association with commissural fibers also are present. Scattered among these nerve fibers are occasional horizontal cells of Cajal. This most superficial layer of the cortex clearly is where large numbers of synapses between different neurons occur.
2. **External granular layer.** This layer contains large numbers of small pyramidal cells and stellate cells.

1
Molecular layer

2
External
granular layer

3
External
pyramidal layer

4
Internal
granular layer

5
Ganglionic layer
(internal
pyramidal
layer)

6
Multiform layer
(layer of
polymorphic
cells)

External band
of Baillarger

Inner band
of Baillarger

Efferent cortical fibers   Afferent cortical fibers

Figure 8-3 Layers of the cerebral cortex showing the neurons on the left and the nerve fibers on the right.

The dendrites of these cells terminate in the molecular layer, and the axons enter deeper layers, where they terminate or pass on to enter the white matter of the cerebral hemisphere.

3. **External pyramidal layer.** This layer is composed of pyramidal cells, whose cell body size increases from the superficial to the deeper borders of the layer. The apical dendrites pass into the molecular layer, and the axons enter the white matter as projection, association, or commissural fibers.

4. **Internal granular layer.** This layer is composed of closely packed stellate cells with a high concentration of horizontally arranged fibers known collectively as the **external band of Baillarger**.

5. **Ganglionic layer (internal pyramidal layer).** This layer contains very large and medium-size pyramidal cells. Scattered among the pyramidal cells are stellate cells and cells of Martinotti. In addition, a large number of horizontally arranged fibers form the **inner band of Baillarger** (see Fig. 8-3). In the motor

cortex of the precentral gyrus, the pyramidal cells of this layer are very large and are known as Betz cells. These cells account for about 3% of the projection fibers of the **corticospinal** or **pyramidal tract**.

6. **Multiform layer (layer of polymorphic cells).** Although the majority of the cells are fusiform, many of the cells are modified pyramidal cells, whose cell bodies are triangular or ovoid. The cells of Martinotti also are conspicuous in this layer. Many nerve fibers are present that are entering or are leaving the underlying white matter.

Cortical Structure Variations

The system of numbering and nomenclature of the cortical layers used above is similar to that distinguished by Brodmann (1909). However, recognize that not all areas of the cerebral cortex possess six layers (see Fig. 8-3). Those areas of the cortex in which the basic six layers cannot be recognized are referred to as **heterotypical**, as opposed to the majority, which are **homotypical** and possess six layers. Two heterotypical areas are described: the granular and the agranular type.

In the **granular type**, the granular layers are well developed and contain densely packed stellate cells. Thus, layers 2 and 4 are well developed, and layers 3 and 5 are poorly developed, so layers 2 through 5 merge into a single layer of predominantly granular cells. These cells receive thalamocortical fibers. The granular type of cortex is found in the postcentral gyrus, in the superior temporal gyrus, and in parts of the hippocampal gyrus.

In the **agranular type** of cortex, the granular layers are poorly developed, so layers 2 and 4 are practically absent. The pyramidal cells in layers 3 and 5 are densely packed and are very large. The agranular type of cortex is found in the precentral gyrus and other areas in the frontal lobe. These areas give rise to large numbers of efferent fibers that are associated with motor function.

CORTICAL MECHANISMS

Extensive research in recent years involving electrophysiology, histochemistry, immunocytochemistry, and other microscopic techniques has resulted in a vast increase in our knowledge of the connections of the neurons of the cerebral cortex. This information combined with new methods of studying the functions of the human cerebral cortex in the living using electroencephalograms (EEGs), positron emission tomography (PET), and magnetic resonance imaging (MRI) have led to a new understanding of the functions of the different areas and the different layers of the cerebral cortex. Much of the new information, however, is still merely factual data and cannot be used in the clinical setting.

The cerebral cortex is organized into vertical units or columns of functional activity (see Fig. 8-2) measuring about 300 to 600 μm wide. In the sensory cortex, for example, each column serves a single specific sensory function. Such a functional unit extends through all six layers from the cortical surface to the white matter. Each unit possesses afferent fibers, internuncial neurons, and efferent fibers. An afferent fiber may synapse directly with an efferent neuron or may involve vertical chains of internuncial neurons. A single vertical chain of neurons may be involved in isolation, or the wave of excitation may spread to adjacent vertical chains through short axon granular cells. The horizontal cells of Cajal permit activation of vertical units that lie some distance away from the incoming afferent fiber. The spread of incoming information serving one sensory modality laterally from one column to an adjacent column, or to columns some distance away, may permit the individual to start the process of understanding the nature of the sensory input.

CORTICAL AREAS

Over the past century, clinicopathologic studies in humans and electrophysiologic and ablation studies in animals have produced evidence that different areas of the cerebral cortex are functionally specialized. However, the precise division of the cortex into different areas of specialization, as described by Brodmann, oversimplifies and misleads the reader. The simple division of cortical areas into motor and sensory is erroneous because many of the sensory areas are far more extensive than originally described and because motor responses can be obtained by stimulation of sensory areas. Until a satisfactory terminology has been devised to describe the various cortical areas, the main cortical areas will be named by their anatomical location.

Some of the main anatomical connections of the cerebral cortex are summarized in Table 8-1.

Frontal Lobe

The **precentral area** is situated in the precentral gyrus and includes the anterior wall of the central sulcus and the posterior parts of the superior, middle, and inferior frontal gyri; it extends over the superomedial border of the hemisphere into the paracentral lobule (Fig. 8-4). Histologically, the characteristic feature of this area is the almost complete absence of the granular layers and the prominence of the pyramidal nerve cells. The giant pyramidal cells of Betz, which can measure as much as 120 μm long and 60 μm wide, are concentrated most highly in the superior part of the precentral gyrus and the paracentral lobule; their numbers diminish as one passes anteriorly in the precentral gyrus or inferiorly toward the lateral fissure. The great majority of the corticospinal and corticobulbar fibers originate from the small pyramidal cells in this area. The number of Betz cells present is estimated to be between 25,000 and 30,000 and accounts for only about 3% of the corticospinal fibers. Notably, the postcentral gyrus and the second somatosensory areas, as well as the occipital and temporal lobes, give origin to descending tracts as well; they are involved in controlling the sensory input to the nervous system and are not involved in muscular movement.

The precentral area may be divided into posterior and anterior regions. The posterior region, which is referred to as the **motor area**, **primary motor area**, or Brodmann area 4, occupies the precentral gyrus extending over the superior border into the paracentral lobule. The anterior region is known as the **premotor area**, **secondary motor area**, or Brodmann area 6 and parts of areas 8, 44, and 45. It occupies the anterior part of the precentral gyrus and the posterior parts of the superior, middle, and inferior frontal gyri.

The primary motor area, if electrically stimulated, produces isolated movements on the opposite side of the body as well as contraction of muscle groups concerned with the performance of a specific movement. Although isolated ipsilateral movements do not occur, bilateral movements of the extraocular muscles, the muscles of the upper part of the face, the tongue, and the mandible, and the larynx and the pharynx do occur.

The movement areas of the body are represented in inverted form in the precentral gyrus (Fig. 8-5). Starting from below and passing superiorly are structures

Table 8-1   Main Anatomical Connections of the Cerebral Cortex

Function	Origin	Cortical Area	Destination
Sensory			
Somatosensory (most to contralateral side of body; oral to same side; pharynx, larynx, and perineum bilateral)	Ventral posterior lateral and ventral posterior medial nuclei of thalamus	Primary somesthetic area (B3, 1, and 2), posterior central gyrus	Secondary somesthetic area; primary motor area
Vision	Lateral geniculate body	Primary visual area (B17)	Secondary visual area (B18 and 19)
Auditory	Medial geniculate body	Primary auditory area (B41 and 42)	Secondary auditory area (B22)
Taste	Nucleus solitarius	Posterior central gyrus (B43)	
Smell	Olfactory bulb	Primary olfactory area; periamygdaloid and prepiriform areas	Secondary olfactory area (B28)
Motor			
Fine movements (most to contralateral side of body; extraocular muscles, upper face, tongue, mandible, larynx, bilateral)	Thalamus from cerebellum, basal ganglia; somatosensory area; premotor area	Primary motor area (B4)	Motor nuclei of brainstem and anterior horn cells of spinal cord; corpus striatum

B, Brodmann area.

involved in swallowing and the tongue, jaw, lips, larynx, eyelid, and brow. The next area is an extensive region for movements of the fingers, especially the thumb, hand, wrist, elbow, shoulder, and trunk. The movements of the hip, knee, and ankle are represented in the highest areas of the precentral gyrus; the movements of the toes are situated on the medial surface of the cerebral hemisphere in the paracentral lobule. The movements of the anal and vesical sphincters are also located in the paracentral lobule. The area of cortex controlling a particular movement is proportional to the skill involved in performing the movement and is unrelated to the mass of muscle participating in the movement.

Thus, the function of the primary motor area is to carry out the individual movements of different parts of the body. To assist in this function, it receives numerous afferent fibers from the premotor area, the sensory cortex, the thalamus, the cerebellum, and the basal ganglia. The primary motor cortex is not responsible for the design of the pattern of movement but is the final station for conversion of the design into execution of the movement.

The premotor area, which is wider superiorly than below and narrows down to be confined to the anterior part of the precentral gyrus, has no giant pyramidal cells of Betz. Electrical stimulation of the premotor area produces muscular movements similar to those obtained by stimulation of the primary motor area; however, stronger stimulation is necessary to produce the same degree of movement.

The premotor area receives numerous inputs from the sensory cortex, the thalamus, and the basal ganglia. The function of the premotor area is to store programs of motor activity assembled as the result of past experience. Thus, the premotor area programs the activity of the primary motor area. It is particularly involved in controlling coarse postural movements through its connections with the basal ganglia.

The **supplementary motor area** is situated in the medial frontal gyrus on the medial surface of the hemisphere and anterior to the paracentral lobule. Stimulation of this area results in movements of the contralateral limbs, but a stronger stimulus is necessary than when the primary motor area is stimulated. Removal of the supplementary motor area produces no permanent loss of movement.

The **frontal eye field** (see Fig. 8-4A) extends forward from the facial area of the precentral gyrus into the middle frontal gyrus (parts of Brodmann areas 6, 8, and 9). Electrical stimulation of this region causes conjugate movements of the eyes, especially toward the opposite side. The exact pathway taken by nerve fibers from this area is not known, but they are thought to pass to the superior colliculus of the midbrain. The superior colliculus is connected to the nuclei of the extraocular muscles by the reticular formation. The frontal eye field is considered to control voluntary scanning movements of the eye and is independent of visual stimuli. The involuntary following of moving objects by the eyes involves the visual area of the occipital cortex to which the frontal eye field is connected by association fibers.

The **motor speech area of Broca** is located in the inferior frontal gyrus between the anterior and ascending rami and the ascending and posterior rami of the lateral fissure (Brodmann areas 44 and 45). In the majority of

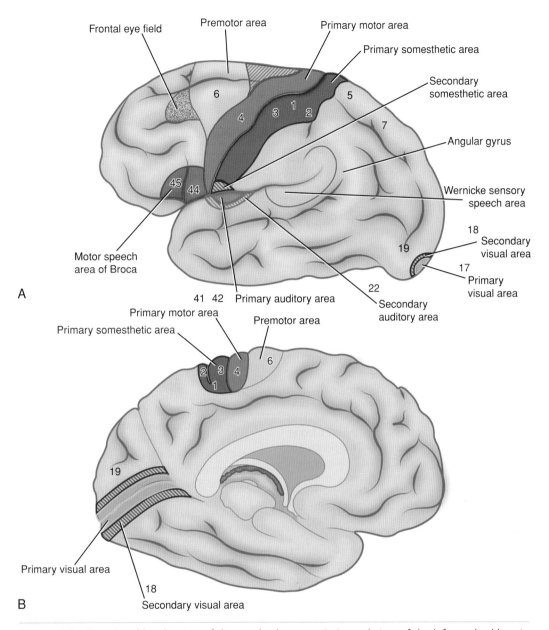

Figure 8-4 Functional localization of the cerebral cortex. **A:** Lateral view of the left cerebral hemisphere. **B:** Medial view of the left cerebral hemisphere.

individuals, this area is important on the left or dominant hemisphere, and ablation will result in paralysis of speech. In those individuals in whom the right hemisphere is dominant, the area on the right side is of importance. The ablation of this region in the nondominant hemisphere has no effect on speech.

The Broca speech area brings about the formation of words by its connections with the adjacent primary motor areas; the muscles of the larynx, mouth, tongue, soft palate, and the respiratory muscles are appropriately stimulated.

The **prefrontal cortex** is an extensive area that lies anterior to the precentral area. It includes the greater parts of the superior, middle, and inferior frontal gyri; the orbital gyri; most of the medial frontal gyrus; and the anterior half of the cingulate gyrus (Brodmann areas 9, 10, 11, and 12). Large numbers of afferent and efferent pathways connect the prefrontal area with other areas of the cerebral cortex, the thalamus, the hypothalamus, and the corpus striatum. The frontopontine fibers also connect this area to the cerebellum through the pontine nuclei. The commissural fibers of the forceps minor and genu of the corpus callosum unite these areas in both cerebral hemispheres.

The prefrontal area is concerned with the makeup of the individual's personality. As the result of the input from many cortical and subcortical sources, this area plays a role as a regulator of the person's depth of feeling. It also exerts its influence in determining the initiative and judgment of an individual.

Figure 8-5   Motor homunculus on the precentral gyrus.

Parietal Lobe

The **primary somesthetic area** (primary somatic sensory cortex S1) occupies the postcentral gyrus (see Fig. 8-4) on the lateral surface of the hemisphere and the posterior part of the paracentral lobule on the medial surface (Brodmann areas 3, 1, and 2). Histologically, the anterior part of the postcentral gyrus is the area that borders the central sulcus (area 3), is granular in type, and contains only scattered pyramidal cells. The **outer layer of Baillarger** is broad and very obvious. The posterior part of the postcentral gyrus (areas 1 and 2) possesses fewer granular cells. The primary somesthetic areas of the cerebral cortex receive projection fibers from the ventral posterior lateral and ventral posterior medial nuclei of the thalamus. The opposite half of the body is represented as inverted. The pharyngeal region, tongue, and jaws are represented in the most inferior part of the postcentral gyrus; this is followed by the face, fingers, hand, arm, trunk, and thigh. The leg and the foot areas are found on the medial surface of the hemisphere in the posterior part of the paracentral lobule. The anal and genital regions are also found in this latter area. The apportioning of the cortex for a particular part of the body is related to its functional importance rather than to its size. The face, lips, thumb, and index finger have particularly large areas assigned to them. In fact, the size of the cortical area allocated to each part of the body is directly proportional to the number of sensory receptors present in that part of the body.

Although most sensations reach the cortex from the contralateral side of the body, some from the oral region go to the same side, and those from the pharynx, larynx, and perineum go to both sides. On entering the cortex, the afferent fibers excite the neurons in layer IV, and then the signals spread toward the surface of the cerebral unit and toward the deeper layers. From layer VI, large numbers of axons leave the cortex and pass to lower sensory relay stations of the thalamus, medulla oblongata, and the spinal cord, providing feedback. This sensory feedback is largely inhibitory and serves to modulate the intensity of the sensory input.

The anterior part of the postcentral gyrus situated in the central sulcus receives a large number of afferent fibers from muscle spindles, tendon organs, and joint receptors. This sensory information is analyzed in the vertical columns of the sensory cortex; it is then passed forward beneath the central sulcus to the primary motor cortex, where it greatly influences the control of skeletal muscle activity.

The **secondary somesthetic area** (secondary somatic sensory cortex S2) is in the superior lip of the posterior limb of the lateral fissure. The secondary sensory area is much smaller and less important than the primary sensory area. The face area lies most anterior, and the leg area is posterior. The body is bilaterally represented with the contralateral side dominant. The detailed connections of this area are unknown. Many sensory impulses come from the primary area, and many signals are transmitted from the brainstem. The functional significance of this area is not understood. It has been shown that the neurons respond particularly to transient cutaneous stimuli, such as brush strokes or tapping of the skin.

The **somesthetic association area** occupies the superior parietal lobule extending onto the medial surface of the hemisphere (Brodmann areas 5 and 7). This area has many connections with other sensory areas of the cortex, and its main function is probably to receive and integrate different sensory modalities. For example, it enables one to recognize objects placed in the hand without the help of vision. In other words, it not only receives information concerning the size and shape of an object but also relates this to past sensory experiences; thus, the information may be interpreted, and recognition may occur. A quarter placed in the hand can be distinguished from a dime or a nickel by the size, shape, and feel of the coin without having to use one's eyes.

Occipital Lobe

The **primary visual area** (Brodmann area 17) is situated in the walls of the posterior part of the calcarine sulcus and occasionally extends around the occipital pole onto the lateral surface of the hemisphere (see

Fig. 8-4). Macroscopically, this area can be recognized by the thinness of the cortex and the visual stria; microscopically, it is seen to be a granular type of cortex with only a few pyramidal cells present.

The visual cortex receives afferent fibers from the lateral geniculate body. The fibers first pass forward in the white matter of the temporal lobe and then turn back to the primary visual cortex in the occipital lobe. The visual cortex receives fibers from the temporal half of the ipsilateral retina and the nasal half of the contralateral retina. The right half of the field of vision, therefore, is represented in the visual cortex of the left cerebral hemisphere and vice versa. Note that the superior retinal quadrants (inferior field of vision) pass to the superior wall of the calcarine sulcus, while the inferior retinal quadrants (superior field of vision) pass to the inferior wall of the calcarine sulcus.

The macula lutea, which is the central area of the retina and the area for most perfect vision, is represented on the cortex in the posterior part of area 17 and accounts for one-third of the visual cortex. The visual impulses from the peripheral parts of the retina terminate in concentric circles anterior to the occipital pole in the anterior part of area 17.

The **secondary visual area** (Brodmann areas 18 and 19) surrounds the primary visual area on the medial and lateral surfaces of the hemisphere. This area receives afferent fibers from area 17 and other cortical areas as well as from the thalamus. The function of the secondary visual area is to relate the visual information received by the primary visual area to past visual experiences, thus enabling the individual to recognize and appreciate what he or she is seeing.

The **occipital eye field** is thought to exist in the secondary visual area in humans. Stimulation produces conjugate deviation of the eyes, especially to the opposite side. The function of this eye field is believed to be reflex and associated with movements of the eye when it is following an object. The occipital eye fields of both hemispheres are connected by nervous pathways and also are thought to be connected to the superior colliculus. By contrast, the frontal eye field controls voluntary scanning movements of the eye and is independent of visual stimuli.

Temporal Lobe

The **primary auditory area** (Brodmann areas 41 and 42) includes the gyrus of Heschl and is situated in the inferior wall of the lateral sulcus (see Fig. 8-4A). Area 41 is a granular type of cortex; area 42 is homotypical and is mainly an auditory association area.

Projection fibers to the auditory area arise principally in the medial geniculate body and form the **auditory radiation of the internal capsule**. The anterior part of the primary auditory area is concerned with the reception of sounds of low frequency, and the posterior part of the area is concerned with the sounds of high frequency. A unilateral lesion of the auditory area produces partial deafness in both ears, the greater loss being in the contralateral ear. This can be explained

on the basis that the medial geniculate body receives fibers mainly from the organ of Corti of the opposite side as well as some fibers from the same side.

The **secondary auditory area** (auditory association cortex) is situated posterior to the primary auditory area in the lateral sulcus and in the superior temporal gyrus (Brodmann area 22). It receives impulses from the primary auditory area and from the thalamus. The secondary auditory area is thought to be necessary for the interpretation of sounds and for the association of the auditory input with other sensory information.

The **sensory** speech area of Wernicke is localized in the left dominant hemisphere, mainly in the superior temporal gyrus, with extensions around the posterior end of the lateral sulcus into the parietal region. The Wernicke area is connected to the Broca area by a bundle of nerve fibers called the **arcuate** fasciculus. It receives fibers from the visual cortex in the occipital lobe and the auditory cortex in the superior temporal gyrus. The Wernicke area permits understanding of written and spoken language and enables a person to read a sentence, understand it, and say it out loud (Figs. 8-6 and 8-7).

Because the Wernicke area represents the site on the cerebral cortex where somatic, visual, and auditory association areas all come together, it should be regarded as an area of very great importance.

Other Cortical Areas

The **taste area** is situated at the lower end of the postcentral gyrus in the superior wall of the lateral sulcus and in the adjoining area of the insula (Brodmann area 43). Ascending fibers from the nucleus solitarius probably ascend to the ventral posteromedial nucleus of the thalamus, where they synapse on neurons that send fibers to the cortex.

The **vestibular area** is believed to be situated near the part of the postcentral gyrus concerned with sensations of the face. Its location lies opposite the auditory area in the superior temporal gyrus. The vestibular area and the vestibular part of the inner ear are concerned with appreciation of the positions and movements of the head in space. Through its nerve connections, the movements of the eyes and the muscles of the trunk and limbs are influenced in the maintenance of posture.

The **insula** is an area of the cortex that is buried within the lateral sulcus and forms its floor (see Fig. 7-9). It can be examined only when the lips of the lateral sulcus are separated widely. Histologically, the posterior part is granular and the anterior part is agranular, thus resembling the adjoining cortical areas. Its fiber connections are incompletely known. This area is thought to be important for planning or coordinating the articulatory movements necessary for speech.

Association Cortex

The primary sensory areas with their granular cortex and the primary motor areas with their agranular cortex form only a small part of the total cortical surface area. The remaining areas have all six cellular layers

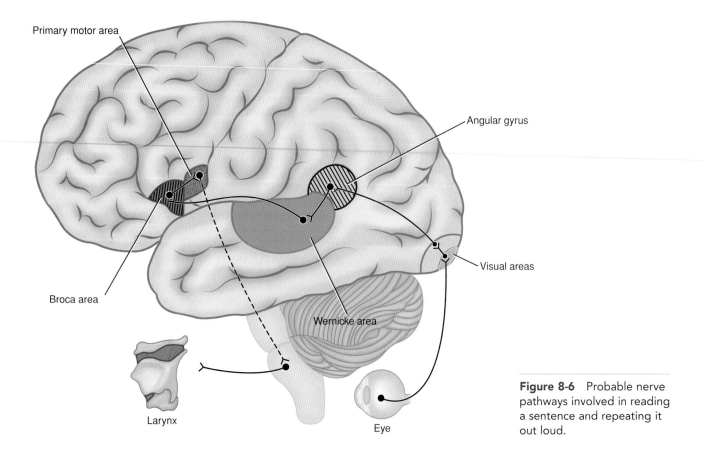

Primary motor area

Angular gyrus

Broca area

Visual areas

Wernicke area

Larynx

Eye

Figure 8-6 Probable nerve pathways involved in reading a sentence and repeating it out loud.

Primary motor area

Auditory area

Wernicke area

Broca area

Ear

Larynx

Figure 8-7 Probable nerve pathways involved with hearing a question and answering it.

and, therefore, are referred to as homotypical cortex. Classically, these large remaining areas were known as association areas, although precisely what they associate is not known. The original concept—that they receive information from the primary sensory areas that is to be integrated and analyzed in the association cortex and then fed to the motor areas—has not been established. As the result of clinical studies and animal experimentation, it has now become apparent that these areas of the cortex have multiple inputs and outputs and are very much concerned with behavior, discrimination, and interpretation of sensory experiences. Three main association areas are recognized: prefrontal, anterior temporal, and posterior parietal. The prefrontal cortex is discussed on page 291.

The anterior temporal cortex is thought to play a role in the storage of previous sensory experiences. Stimulation may cause the individual to recall objects seen or music heard in the past.

In the posterior parietal cortex, visual information from the posterior occipital cortex and the sensory input of touch and pressure and proprioception from the anterior parietal cortex is integrated into concepts of size, form, and texture. This ability is known as **stereognosis**. A conscious appreciation of the body image is also assembled in the posterior parietal cortex. The brain knows at all times where each part of the body is located in relation to its environment. This information is so important when performing body movements. The right side of the body is represented in the left hemisphere, and the left side of the body is represented in the right hemisphere.

CEREBRAL DOMINANCE

Anatomical examination of the two cerebral hemispheres shows that the cortical gyri and fissures are almost identical. Moreover, nervous pathways projecting to the cortex do so largely contralaterally and equally to identical cortical areas. In addition, the cerebral commissures, especially the corpus callosum and the anterior commissure, provide a pathway for information that is received in one hemisphere to be transferred to the other. Nevertheless, certain nervous activity is predominantly performed by one of the two cerebral hemispheres. Handedness, perception of language, and speech are functional areas of behavior that are controlled by the dominant hemisphere in most individuals. By contrast, spatial perception, recognition of faces, and music are interpreted by the nondominant hemisphere (Fig. 8-8).

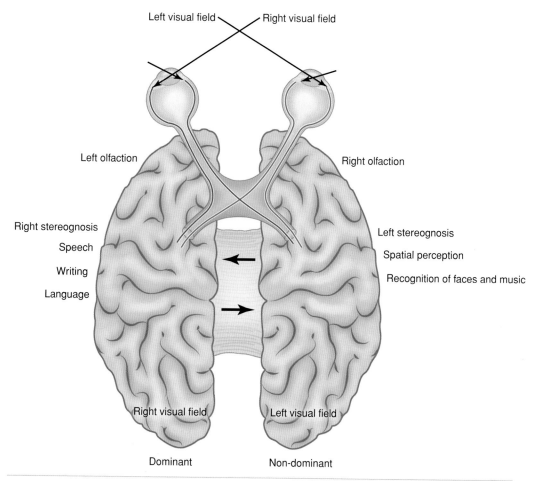

Figure 8-8 Nervous activities performed predominantly by dominant and nondominant hemispheres.

More than 90% of the adult population is right handed and, therefore, is left-hemisphere dominant. About 96% of the adult population is left-hemisphere dominant for speech.

In their work on human fetuses and neonates, Yakolev and Rakic have shown that more descending fibers in the left pyramid cross over the midline in the decussation than vice versa. This would suggest that the anterior horn cells on the right side of the spinal cord have a greater corticospinal innervation than those on the left side in most individuals, which might explain the dominance of the right hand.

Other researchers have shown that the speech area of the adult cortex is larger on the left than on the right, whereas the two hemispheres of the newborn are believed to have equipotential capabilities. During childhood, one hemisphere slowly comes to dominate the other, and only after the first decade does the dominance become fixed. This would explain why a 5-year-old child with damage to the dominant hemisphere can easily learn to become left-handed and speak well, whereas this is almost impossible in the adult.

Clinical Notes

General Considerations

The cerebral cortex should be regarded as the last receiving station involved along a line of stations receiving information from the eyes and ears and organs of general sensation. The function of the cortex is, in simple terms, to discriminate, and it relates the received information to past memories. The enriched sensory input is then presumably discarded, stored, or translated into action. In this whole process, interplay between the cortex and basal nuclei is provided by the many cortical and subcortical nervous connections.

Cerebral Cortex Lesions

In humans, the effect of destruction of different areas of the cerebral cortex has been studied by examining patients with lesions resulting from cerebral tumors, vascular accidents, surgery, or head injuries. Moreover, electrical recordings have been taken from different areas of the cortex during surgical exposure of the cerebral cortex or when stimulating different parts of the cortex in the conscious patient. One thing that has emerged from these studies is that the human cerebral cortex possesses, in a remarkable degree, the ability to reorganize the remaining intact cortex so that a certain amount of cerebral recovery is possible after brain lesions.

Motor Cortex

Lesions of the primary **motor cortex** in one hemisphere result in paralysis of the contralateral extremities, with the finer and more skilled movements suffering most. Destruction of the **primary motor area** (area 4) produces more severe paralysis than destruction of the **secondary motor area** (area 6). Destruction of both areas produces the most complete form of contralateral paralysis.

Lesions of the **secondary motor area** alone produce difficulty in the performance of skilled movements, with little loss of strength.

The **Jacksonian epileptic seizure** is due to an irritative lesion of the primary motor area (area 4). The convulsion begins in the part of the body represented in the primary motor area that is being irritated. The convulsive movement may be restricted to one part of the body, such as the face or the foot, or it may spread to involve many regions, depending on the spread of irritation of the primary motor area.

MUSCLE SPASTICITY

A discrete lesion of the primary motor cortex (area 4) results in little change in the muscle tone. However, larger lesions involving the primary and secondary motor areas (areas 4 and 6), which are the most common, result in muscle spasm. The explanation for this is that the primary motor cortex gives origin to corticospinal and corticonuclear tracts, and the secondary motor cortex gives origin to extrapyramidal tracts that pass to the basal ganglia and the reticular formation. The corticospinal and corticonuclear tracts tend to increase muscle tone, but the extrapyramidal fibers transmit inhibitory impulses that lower muscle tone (see pp. 167-168). Destruction of the secondary motor area removes the inhibitory influence, and consequently, the muscles are spastic.

Frontal Eye Field

Destructive lesions of the frontal eye field of one hemisphere cause the two eyes to deviate to the side of the lesion and an inability to turn the eyes to the opposite side. The involuntary tracking movement of the eyes when following moving objects is unaffected, because the lesion does not involve the visual cortex in the occipital lobe.

Irritative lesions of the frontal eye field of one hemisphere cause the two eyes to periodically deviate to the opposite side of the lesion.

Broca Motor Speech Area

Destructive lesions in the left inferior frontal gyrus result in the loss of ability to produce speech, that is, **expressive aphasia**. The patients, however, retain the ability to think the words they wish to say, they can write the words, and they can understand their meaning when they see or hear them.

Wernicke Sensory Speech Area

Destructive lesions restricted to the Wernicke speech area in the dominant hemisphere produce a loss of ability to understand the spoken and written word, that is, **receptive aphasia**. Since the Broca area is unaffected, speech is unimpaired, and the patient can produce fluent speech. However, the patient is unaware of the meaning of the words he or she uses and uses incorrect words or even nonexistent words. The patient is also unaware of any mistakes.

Motor and Sensory Speech Areas

Destructive lesions involving both the Broca and Wernicke speech areas result in loss of the production of speech and the understanding of the spoken and written word, that is, **global aphasia**.

Patients who have lesions involving the **insula** have difficulty in pronouncing phonemes in their proper order and usually produce sounds that are close to the target word but are not exactly correct.

Dominant Angular Gyrus

Destructive lesions in the angular gyrus in the posterior parietal lobe (often considered a part of the Wernicke area) divide the pathway between the visual association area and the anterior part of the Wernicke area. This results in the patient being unable to read (**alexia**) or write (**agraphia**).

Prefrontal Cortex

Destruction of the prefrontal region does not produce any marked loss of intelligence. It is an area of the cortex that is capable of associating experiences that are necessary for the production of abstract ideas, judgment, emotional feeling, and personality. Tumors or traumatic destruction of the prefrontal cortex result in the person's losing initiative and judgment. Emotional changes that occur include a tendency to euphoria. The patient no longer conforms to the accepted mode of social behavior and becomes careless of dress and appearance.

Prefrontal Cortex and Schizophrenia

The prefrontal cortex has a rich dopaminergic innervation. A failure of this innervation may be responsible for some of the symptoms of schizophrenia, which include important disorders of thought. PET scans have shown that the blood flow in the prefrontal cortex in schizophrenic patients challenged with executive type functions is much less than in normal individuals.

Frontal Leukotomy and Frontal Lobectomy

Frontal leukotomy (cutting the fiber tracts of the frontal lobe) and frontal lobectomy (removal of the frontal lobe) are surgical procedures that have been used to reduce the emotional responsiveness of patients with obsessive emotional states and intractable pain. The surgical technique was developed to remove the frontal association activity so that past experience is not recalled and the possibilities of the future are not considered; thus, introspection is lessened.

A patient suffering severe pain, such as may be experienced in the terminal stages of cancer, will still feel the pain following frontal lobectomy, but he or she will no longer worry about the pain and, therefore, will not suffer. It should be pointed out that the introduction of effective tranquilizing and mood-elevating drugs has made these operative procedures largely obsolete.

Sensory Cortex

The lower centers of the brain, principally the thalamus, relay a large part of the sensory signals to the cerebral cortex for analysis. The sensory cortex is necessary for the appreciation of spatial recognition, recognition of relative intensity, and recognition of similarity and difference.

Lesions of the **primary somesthetic area** of the cortex result in contralateral sensory disturbances, which are most severe in the distal parts of the limbs. Crude painful, tactile, and thermal stimuli often return, but this is believed to be due to the function of the thalamus. The patient remains unable to judge degrees of warmth, unable to localize tactile stimuli accurately, and unable to judge weights of objects. Loss of muscle tone may also be a symptom of lesions of the sensory cortex.

Lesions of the secondary somesthetic area of the cortex do not cause recognizable sensory defects.

Somesthetic Association Area

Lesions of the superior parietal lobule interfere with the patient's ability to combine touch, pressure, and proprioceptive impulses, so he or she is unable to appreciate texture, size, and form. This loss of integration of sensory impulses is called **astereognosis**. For example, with the eyes closed, the individual would be unable to recognize a key placed in the hand.

Destruction of the posterior part of the parietal lobe, which integrates somatic and visual sensations, will interfere with the appreciation of body image on the opposite side of the body. The individual may fail to recognize the opposite side of the body as his or her own. The patient may fail to wash it or dress it or to shave that side of the face or legs.

Primary Visual Area

Lesions involving the walls of the posterior part of one calcarine sulcus result in a loss of sight in the opposite visual field, that is, **crossed homonymous hemianopia**. Interestingly, the central part of the visual field is apparently normal when tested. This so-called macular sparing is probably due to the patient's shifting the eyes very slightly while the visual fields are being examined. The following clinical defects should be understood. Lesions of the upper half of one primary visual area—the area above the calcarine sulcus—result in **inferior quadrantic hemianopia**, whereas lesions involving one visual area below the calcarine sulcus result in **superior quadrantic hemianopia**. Lesions of the occipital pole produce central scotomas. The most common causes of these lesions are vascular disorders, tumors, and injuries from gunshot wounds.

Secondary Visual Area

Lesions of the secondary visual area result in a loss of ability to recognize objects seen in the opposite field of vision. The reason for this is that the area of cortex that stores past visual experiences has been lost.

Primary Auditory Area

Because the primary auditory area in the inferior wall of the lateral sulcus receives nerve fibers from both cochleae, a lesion of one cortical area will produce slight bilateral loss of hearing, but the loss will be greater in the opposite ear. The main defect noted is a loss of ability to locate the source of the sound. Bilateral destruction of the primary auditory areas causes complete deafness.

Secondary Auditory Area

Lesions of the cortex posterior to the primary auditory area in the lateral sulcus and in the superior temporal gyrus result in an inability to interpret sounds. The patient may experience **word deafness (acoustic verbal agnosia)**.

Cerebral Dominance and Cerebral Damage

Although both hemispheres are almost identical in structure, handedness, perception of language, speech, spatial judgment, and areas of behavior are controlled by one hemisphere and not the other in the majority of the adult population. About 90% of people are right-handed, and the control resides in the left hemisphere. The remainder are left-handed, and a few individuals are ambidextrous. In 96% of individuals, speech and understanding of spoken and written language are controlled by the left hemisphere. Thus, in most adults, the left cerebral hemisphere is dominant.

From a clinical point of view, the age at which cerebral dominance comes into effect is important. For example, when cerebral damage occurs before the child has learned to speak, speech usually develops and is maintained in the remaining intact hemisphere. This transference of speech control is much more difficult in older persons.

Cerebral Cortical Potentials

Electrical recordings taken from inside neurons of the cerebral cortex show a negative resting potential of about 60 mV. The action potentials overshoot the zero potential. Note that resting potential shows marked fluctuation, which is probably due to the continuous but variable reception of afferent impulses from other neurons. Spontaneous electrical activity can be recorded from the cortical surface rather than intracellularly; such recordings are known as **electrocorticograms**. Similar recordings can be made by placing the electrodes on the scalp. The result of this latter procedure is referred to as the **electroencephalogram**. The changes of electrical potential recorded usually are very small and in the order of 50 mV. Characteristically, three frequency bands may be recognized in the normal individual; they are referred to as **alpha**, **beta**, and **delta rhythms**. Abnormalities of the electroencephalogram may be of great value clinically in helping to diagnose cerebral tumors, epilepsy, and cerebral abscess. An electrically silent cortex indicates cerebral death.

Consciousness

A conscious person is awake and aware of himself or herself and the surroundings. For normal consciousness, active functioning of two main parts of the nervous system, the reticular formation (in the brainstem) and the cerebral cortex, is necessary. The reticular formation is responsible for the state of wakefulness. The cerebral cortex is necessary for the state of awareness, that is, the state in which the individual can respond to stimuli and interact with the environment. Eye opening is a brainstem function; speech is a cerebral cortex function. Drugs that produce unconsciousness, such as anesthetics, selectively depress the **reticular alerting mechanism**, while those that cause wakefulness have a stimulating effect on this mechanism.

A physician should be able to recognize the different signs and symptoms associated with different stages of consciousness, namely, **lethargy**, **stupor**, and **coma** (unconsciousness). In a lethargic individual, the speech is slow, and voluntary movement is diminished and slow. The movement of the eyes is slow. A stupored patient will speak only if stimulated with painful stimuli. The voluntary movements are nearly absent, the eyes are closed, and very little spontaneous eye movement occurs. A deeply stupored patient will not speak; severe pain will elicit mass movements of different parts of the body. The eyes will show even less spontaneous movement.

An unconscious patient will not speak and will respond only reflexly to painful stimuli, or not at all; the eyes are closed and do not move.

Clinicians commonly observe a patient with, for example, intracranial bleeding pass progressively from consciousness to lethargy, stupor, and coma, and then, if recovery occurs, pass in the reverse direction. For these altered states of unconsciousness to occur, the thalamocortical system and the reticular formation must be either directly involved bilaterally or indirectly affected by distortion or pressure.

Persistent Vegetative State

A person can have an intact reticular formation but a nonfunctioning cerebral cortex. That person is awake (i.e., the eyes are open and move around) and has sleep–wake cycles; however, the person has no awareness and, therefore, cannot respond to stimuli such as a verbal command or pain. This condition, known as a **persistent vegetative state**, is usually seen following severe head injuries or an anoxic cerebral insult. Unfortunately, the lay observer thinks the patient is "conscious."

To be wakeful without having awareness is possible; however, having awareness without wakefulness is not. The cerebral cortex requires the input from the reticular formation in order to function.

Sleep

Sleep is a changed state of consciousness. The pulse rate, respiratory rate, and blood pressure fall; the eyes deviate upward; the pupils contract but react to light; the tendon reflexes are lost; and the plantar reflex may become extensor. A sleeping person is not, however, unconscious, because he or she may be awakened quickly by the cry of a child, for example, even though he or she has slept through the background noise of an air-conditioner.

Sleep is facilitated by reducing the sensory input and by fatigue. This results in decreased activity of the reticular formation and the thalamocortical activating mechanism. Whether this decreased activity is a passive phenomenon or whether the reticular formation is actively inhibited is not known.

Epilepsy

Epilepsy is a symptom in which a sudden transitory disturbance of the normal physiology of the brain occurs, usually the cerebral cortex, that ceases spontaneously and tends to recur. The condition is usually associated with a disturbance of normal electrical activity and, in its most typical form, is accompanied by seizures. In partial seizures, the abnormality occurs in only one part of the brain and the patient does not lose consciousness. In generalized seizures, the abnormal activity involves large areas of the brain bilaterally, and the individual loses consciousness.

In some patients with generalized seizures, nonconvulsive attacks may occur, in which the patient suddenly stares blankly into space. This syndrome is referred to as **petit mal**. The majority of patients with generalized seizures have a sudden loss of consciousness, with accompanying tonic muscle spasm and clonic contraction as well as transient apnea and often loss of bowel and bladder control. The convulsions usually last from a few seconds to a few minutes.

In most patients with epilepsy, the cause is unknown. Some patients appear to have a hereditary predisposition; in a few patients, a local lesion, such as a cerebral tumor or scarring of the cortex following trauma, is the cause.

Key Concepts

Cerebral Cortex Structure

- The cerebral cortex forms a complete covering of the cerebral hemisphere. It is composed of gray matter thrown into convolutions, or gyri, to increase surface area.
- Pyramidal and fusiform cells are found in the cortex and have axons that either terminates in the deeper cortical layers, or more commonly, enters the white matter of the cerebral hemisphere as a projection, association, or commissural fiber.
- Stellate, horizontal, and cells of Martinotti typically terminate on dendrites or axons of cells found within other layers of the cortex.
- From superficial to deep, the six cortical layers are molecular, external granular, external pyramidal, internal granular, internal pyramidal, and multiform layers.

Cortical Areas

- Within each cerebral lobe, there are specialized regions of cortex with unique behavioral functions.

Frontal Lobe

- The precentral area of the frontal lobe can be divided into posterior and anterior regions. The posterior region, occupying the precentral gyrus, is referred to as the primary motor area because activation of the cells in this region results in isolated movements of muscles on the contralateral side of the body.
- The movement areas in the motor cortex are organized with the lower limb structures represented on the medial aspect of the gyrus and ascending to trunk, upper limb, and face, laterally on the gyrus.
- The supplementary motor area and frontal eye field are both associated with the middle frontal gyrus. The latter is associated with conjugate movements of the eyes.
- Broca area is responsible for speech production and is located in the inferior frontal gyrus; paralysis of this area results in speech paralysis.

Parietal Lobe

- The primary somesthetic (primary sensory) area occupies the postcentral gyrus of the parietal lobe. Sensations for parts of the body are organized in a somatotopic map beginning with feet on the medial most aspect of the gyrus and the head on the most lateral aspect of the gyrus.

Occipital Lobe

- The primary visual area is found within the cortex of the calcarine sulcus. This cortex receives afferent information from the lateral geniculate body, which received information from the retina.

Temporal Lobe

- The primary auditory area includes the gyrus of Heschl and is situated in the inferior wall of the lateral sulcus. The sensory speech area of Wernicke is localized in the left dominate hemisphere, in the superior temporal gyrus. This area permits the understanding of written and spoken language.

 Clinical Problem Solving

1. During a pathology class, a student is shown a slide illustrating a particular form of cerebral tumor. A small area of the cerebral cortex is visible at the edge of the section. The instructor asks the student whether the tissue has been removed from a motor or sensory area of the cortex. What is the main difference in structure between the motor and sensory areas of the cerebral cortex?
2. A 43-year-old man is examined by a neurologist for a suspected brain tumor. The patient is tested for stereognosis, that is, the appreciation of form in three dimensions. With the patient's eyes closed, a hairbrush is placed in his right hand, and he is asked to recognize the object. He is unable to recognize the brush even after the neurologist moves the brush about in the patient's hand. On opening his eyes, the patient immediately recognizes the brush. (a) Name the area of the cerebral cortex likely to be diseased in this patient. (b) Do you think moving the object around in the patient's hand is necessary?
3. A 65-year-old man visits his physician because he notices that he has been dragging his right foot when walking for the past 3 weeks. On physical examination, he is found to have an increase in tone of the

flexor muscles of the right arm, and, when he walks, he tends to hold his right arm adducted and flexed. He also holds his right fist tightly clenched. On study of the patient's gait, he is seen to have difficulty in flexing his right hip and knee. Slight but definite weakness and increased tone of the muscles of the right leg is noted. As the patient walks, he moves his right leg in a semicircle and places his forefoot on the ground before the heel. Examination of the right shoe shows evidence of increased wear beneath the right toes. Given that this patient had a cerebrovascular lesion involving the cerebral cortex, which area of the cortex was involved to cause these symptoms?

4. While examining an unconscious patient, a clinician notes that when the patient's head is gently rotated to the right, the two eyes deviated to the left. On rotation of the patient's head to the left, the patient's eyes still look to the left. Which area of the cortex is likely to be damaged in this patient?

5. A 25-year-old soldier is wounded in combat by an explosive device. A small piece of shrapnel enters the right side of his skull over the precentral gyrus. Five years later, he is examined by a physician during a routine physical checkup and is found to have weakness of the left leg. The physician cannot detect any increase in muscle tone in his left leg. Explain why most patients with damage to the motor area of the cerebral cortex have spastic muscle paralysis, while a few patients retain normal muscle tone.

6. A distinguished neurobiologist gives a lecture on the physiology of the cerebral cortex to the freshman medical student class. After reviewing the structure of the different areas of the cerebral cortex and the functional localization of the cerebral cortex, he states that our knowledge of the cytoarchitecture of the human cerebral cortex has contributed very little to our understanding of the normal functional activity of the cerebral cortex. Do you agree with his statement? What do you understand by the term *vertical chain theory*?

7. An 18-year-old boy receives a gunshot wound that severely damages his left precentral gyrus. On recovering from the incident, he leaves the hospital with spastic paralysis of the right arm and leg. However, he still possesses some coarse voluntary movements of the right shoulder, hip, and knee. Explain the presence of these residual movements on the right side.

8. A 53-year-old professor and chairman of an anatomy department sustains a severe head injury while rock climbing. During the ascent of a crevasse, his companion's ice axe falls from his belt and struck the professor's head, causing a depressed fracture of the frontal bone. After convalescing from his accident, the professor returns to his position in the medical school, but faculty and the student body quickly notice that the professor's social behavior has changed dramatically. His lectures, although amusing, no longer have direction. Although previously a smartly dressed man, he now has an unkempt appearance. The organization of the department started to deteriorate rapidly. Finally, he is removed from office after urinating into the trash basket in one of the classrooms. Use your knowledge of neuroanatomy to explain the professor's altered behavior.

9. A 50-year-old woman with a cerebrovascular lesion is found to experience difficulty in understanding spoken speech, although she fully understands written speech. Which area of the cerebral cortex was damaged?

10. A 62-year-old man, on recovering from a stroke, is found to have difficulty in understanding written speech (alexia) but can easily understand spoken speech and written symbols. Which area of the cerebral cortex is damaged in this patient?

11. What is understood by the following terms: (a) *coma*, (b) *sleep*, and (c) *electroencephalogram*? Name three neurologic conditions in which the diagnosis may be assisted by an electroencephalogram.

 Answers and Explanations to Clinical Problem Solving

1. The cerebral cortex is made up of six identifiable layers. In the motor cortex in the precentral gyrus, the second and fourth layers lack of granular cells, and the third and fifth layers in the somesthetic cortex in the postcentral gyrus lack of pyramidal cells. The motor cortex is thicker than the sensory cortex.

2. (a) The area likely to be diseased is the left parietal lobe with advanced destruction of the superior parietal lobule. This is the somesthetic association area, where the sensations of touch, pressure, and proprioception are integrated. (b) Yes, the patient must be allowed to finger the object so that these different sensations can be appreciated.

3. This patient had a cerebrovascular lesion involving the left precentral gyrus. The damage to the pyramidal cells that give origin to the corticospinal

fibers was responsible for the right-sided paralysis. The increased tone of the paralyzed muscles was due to the loss of inhibition caused by involvement of the extrapyramidal fibers (see p. 290).

4. Destructive lesions of the frontal eye field of the left cerebral hemisphere caused the two eyes to deviate to the side of the lesion and an inability to turn the eyes to the opposite side. The frontal eye field is thought to control voluntary scanning movements of the eye and is independent of visual stimuli.

5. A small discrete lesion of the primary motor cortex results in little change in muscle tone. Larger lesions involving the primary and secondary motor areas, which are the most common, result in muscle spasm. The explanation for this is given on page 290.

6. The extensive histologic research of Brodmann, Campbell, Economo, and the Vogts has allowed the cerebral cortex to be divided into areas that have a different microscopic arrangement and different types of cells. These cortical maps are fundamentally similar, and the one proposed by Brodmann is used widely. Because the functional significance of many areas of the human cerebral cortex is not known, closely correlating structure with function has not been possible. In general, the motor cortices are thicker than the sensory cortices, and the motor cortex has less prominent second and fourth granular layers and has large pyramidal cells in the fifth layer. Other areas with a different structure may have similar functional roles. More recent studies using electrophysiologic techniques have indicated that dividing the cerebral cortex according to its thalamocortical projections is more accurate. The vertical chain mechanism of the cerebral cortex is fully described on page 283.

7. In this patient, the persistence of coarse voluntary movements of the right shoulder, hip, and knee joints can be explained on the basis that coarse postural movements are controlled by the premotor area of the cortex and the basal ganglia, and these areas were spared in this patient.

8. The professor's altered behavior was due to a severe lesion involving both frontal lobes of the cerebrum secondary to the depressed fracture of the frontal bone. While destruction of the prefrontal cortex does not cause a marked loss of intelligence, it does result in the individual losing initiative and drive, and often the patient no longer conforms to the accepted modes of social behavior.

9. The understanding of spoken speech requires the normal functioning of the secondary auditory area, which is situated posterior to the primary auditory area in the lateral sulcus and in the superior temporal gyrus. This area is believed to be necessary for the interpretation of sounds, and the information is passed on to the sensory speech area of Wernicke.

10. The understanding of written speech requires the normal functioning of the secondary visual area of the cerebral cortex, which is situated in the walls of the posterior part of the calcarine sulcus on the medial and lateral surfaces of the cerebral hemisphere. The function of the secondary visual area is to relate visual information received by the primary visual area to past visual experiences. This information is then passed on to the dominant angular gyrus and relayed to the anterior part of the Wernicke speech area (see p. 283).

11. (a) *Coma* is the term applied to an unconscious patient. The patient will not speak and will respond only reflexly to painful stimuli. Deeply comatose individuals will make no response. The eyes are closed and do not move. (b) *Sleep* is a changed state of consciousness; it is discussed on page 292. (c) An *electroencephalogram* is a recording of the electrical activity of the cerebral cortex made by placing electrodes on the scalp. Detection of abnormalities of the alpha, beta, and delta rhythms may assist in the diagnosis of cerebral tumors, epilepsy, and cerebral abscesses.

? Review Questions

Directions: Each of the numbered items in this section is followed by answers. Select the ONE lettered answer that is CORRECT.

1. The following statements concern the cerebral cortex:
   (a) The cerebral cortex is thinnest over the crest of a gyrus and thickest in the depth of a sulcus.
   (b) The largest giant pyramidal cells are found in the postcentral gyrus.
   (c) In the visual cortex, the outer band of Baillarger is thin and can only be seen under a microscope.
   (d) The molecular layer is the most superficial layer of the cerebral cortex and is composed of the small cell bodies of the granular cells.
   (e) From a functional point of view, the cerebral cortex is organized into vertical units of activity.

2. The following statements concern the precentral area of the frontal lobe of the cerebral cortex:
   (a) The anterior region is known as the *primary motor area.*
   (b) The primary motor area is responsible for skilled movements on the opposite side of the body.
   (c) The function of the primary motor area is to store programs of motor activity, which are conveyed to the premotor area for the execution of movements.
   (d) Individual skeletal muscles are represented in the primary motor area.
   (e) The area of cortex controlling a particular movement is not proportional to the skill involved.

3. The following statements concern the motor speech area of Broca:
   (a) In most individuals, this area is important on the left or dominant hemisphere.
   (b) The Broca speech area brings about the formation of words by its connections with the secondary motor area.
   (c) It is not connected to the sensory speech area of Wernicke.
   (d) It is located in the superior frontal gyrus between the anterior and ascending rami and

the ascending and posterior rami of the lateral fissure.

(e) Brodmann areas 34 and 35 represent the motor speech area.

4. The following statements concern the primary somesthetic area:

(a) It occupies the lower part of the precentral gyrus.

(b) Histologically, it contains large numbers of pyramidal cells and few granular cells.

(c) The opposite half of the body is represented inverted.

(d) Although most sensations reach the cortex from the contralateral side of the body, sensations from the hand go to both sides.

(e) The area extends onto the anterior part of the paracentral lobule.

5. The following statements concern the visual areas of the cortex:

(a) The primary visual area is located in the walls of the parieto-occipital sulcus.

(b) The visual cortex receives afferent fibers from the medial geniculate body.

(c) The right half of the visual field is represented in the visual cortex of the right cerebral hemisphere.

(d) The superior retinal quadrants pass to the inferior portion of the visual cortex.

(e) The secondary visual area (Brodmann areas 18 and 19) is surrounded by the primary visual area on the medial and lateral surfaces of the hemisphere.

6. The following statements concern the superior temporal gyrus:

(a) The primary auditory area is situated in the inferior wall of the lateral sulcus.

(b) The main projection fibers to the primary auditory area arise from the thalamus.

(c) The sensory speech area of Wernicke is localized in the inferior temporal gyrus in the dominant hemisphere.

(d) A unilateral lesion of the auditory area produces complete deafness in both ears.

(e) The secondary auditory area is sometimes referred to as Brodmann areas 41 and 42.

7. The following statements concern the association areas of the cerebral cortex:

(a) They form a small area of the cortical surface.

(b) The prefrontal area is concerned with the makeup of the individual's personality.

(c) They are concerned with the interpretation of motor experiences.

(d) Appreciation of the body image is assembled in the anterior parietal cortex, and the right side of the body is represented in the left hemisphere.

(e) The association areas have only four layers of cortex.

8. The following statements concern cerebral dominance:

(a) The cortical gyri of the dominant and nondominant hemispheres are arranged differently.

(b) More than 90% of the adult population is right-handed and, therefore, is left-hemisphere dominant.

(c) About 96% of the adult population is right-hemisphere dominant for speech.

(d) The nondominant hemisphere interprets handedness, perception of language, and speech.

(e) After puberty, the dominance of the cerebral hemispheres becomes fixed.

Matching Questions. Directions: The following questions apply to Figure 8-9. Match the numbers listed on the left with the most likely words designating lettered

Figure 8-9 Lateral view of the left cerebral hemisphere.

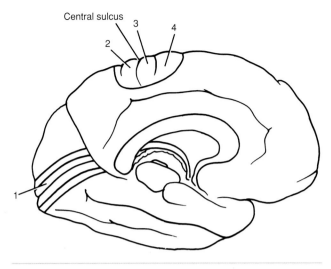

Central sulcus

Figure 8-10 Medial view of the left cerebral hemisphere.

functional areas of the cerebral cortex listed on the right. Each lettered option may be selected once, more than once, or not at all.

9.	Number 1	(a) Primary motor area
10.	Number 2	(b) Secondary auditory area
11.	Number 3	(c) Frontal eye field
12.	Number 4	(d) Primary somesthetic area
		(e) None of the above

The following questions apply to Figure 8-10. Match the numbers listed on the left with the most likely lettered words designating functional areas of the cerebral cortex listed on the right. Each lettered option may be selected once, more than once, or not at all.

13.	Number 1	(a) Premotor area
14.	Number 1	(b) Primary somesthetic area
15.	Number 1	(c) Primary visual area
16.	Number 1	(d) Primary motor area
		(e) None of the above

Directions: Each case history is followed by questions. Read the case history, then select the ONE BEST lettered answer.

A 54-year-old woman was seen by a neurologist because her sister had noticed a sudden change in her behavior. On questioning, the patient stated that after waking up from a deep sleep about a week ago, she noticed that the left side of her body did not feel as if it belonged to her. Later, the feeling worsened, and she became unaware of the existence of her left side. Her sister told the neurologist that the patient now neglects to wash the left side of her body.

17. The neurologist examined the patient and found the following most likely signs **except**:
    (a) The patient did not look toward her left side.
    (b) She readily reacted to sensory stimulation of her skin on the left side.
    (c) On being asked to move her left leg, she promptly did so.
    (d) Muscular weakness of the upper and lower limbs on the left side was evident.
    (e) On being asked to walk across the examining room, she tended not to use her left leg as much as her right leg.

18. The neurologist made the following likely conclusions **except**:
    (a) The diagnosis of left hemiasomatognosia (loss of appreciation of the left side of the body) was made.
    (b) This condition probably resulted from a lesion of the left parietal lobe.
    (c) In addition, the patient exhibited left hemiakinesia (unilateral motor neglect).
    (d) A lesion was likely in areas 6 and 8 of the medial and lateral premotor regions of the right frontal lobe.
    (e) The failure to look toward the left side (visual extinction) suggested a lesion existed in the right parieto-occipital lobes.

 Answers and Explanations to Review Questions

1. E is correct. From a functional standpoint, the cerebral cortex is organized into vertical units of activity. A. The cerebral cortex is thickest over the crest of a gyrus and thinnest in the depth of a sulcus. B. The largest giant pyramidal cells are found in the precentral gyrus (see Fig. 8-1). C. In the visual cortex, the outer band of Baillarger is so thick that it can be seen with the naked eye (see Fig. 8-3). D. The molecular layer is the most superficial layer of the cerebral cortex and is composed mainly of a dense network of tangentially oriented nerve fibers (see Fig. 8-2).

2. B is correct. The primary motor area of the frontal lobe is responsible for skilled movements on the opposite side of the body. A. In the frontal lobe of the cerebral hemisphere, the posterior region

is known as the primary motor area (see Fig. 8-4). C. The function of the premotor area is to store programs of motor activity, which are conveyed to the primary motor area for the execution of movements. D. The individual skeletal muscles are not represented in the primary motor area. E. The area of cerebral cortex controlling a particular movement is proportional to the skill of the movement.

3. A is correct. In most individuals, the speech area of Broca is important on the left or dominant hemisphere. B. The Broca speech area brings about the formation of words by its connections with the primary motor area. C. The Broca speech area is connected to the sensory speech area of Wernicke. D. The speech area of Broca is in the inferior frontal gyrus between the anterior and ascending rami

and the ascending and posterior rami of the lateral fissure (see Fig. 8-4). E. Brodmann areas 44 and 45 represent the motor speech area (see Fig. 8-4).

4. C is correct. In the primary somesthetic area, the opposite half of the body is represented inverted. A. The primary somesthetic area occupies the postcentral gyrus (see Fig. 8-4). B. Histologically, the primary somesthetic area contains large numbers of granular cells and few pyramidal cells. D. Most sensations from different parts of the body reach the cortex from the contralateral side of the body; those from the hand also only go to the contralateral side. E. The primary somesthetic area extends onto the posterior part of the paracentral lobule (see Fig. 8-4).

5. D is correct. The superior retinal quadrants pass to the inferior portion of the visual cortex. A. The primary visual cortex is located in the walls of the posterior part of the calcarine sulcus (see Fig. 8-4). B. The visual cortex receives afferent fibers from the lateral geniculate body. C. The right half of the visual field is represented in the visual cortex of the left cerebral hemisphere. E. The secondary visual area (Brodmann areas 18 and 19) surrounds the primary visual area on the medial and lateral surfaces of the hemisphere (see Fig. 8-4).

6. A is correct. The primary auditory area is situated in the inferior wall of the lateral sulcus (see Fig. 8-4). B. The main projection fibers to the primary auditory area arise from the medial geniculate body. C. The sensory speech area of Wernicke is localized in the superior temporal gyrus in the dominant hemisphere (see Fig. 8-4). D. A unilateral lesion of the auditory area produces partial deafness in both ears. E. The primary auditory area is sometimes referred to as Brodmann areas 41 and 42.

7. B is correct. The prefrontal area is concerned with the makeup of the individual's personality. A. The association areas of the cerebral cortex form a large area of the cortical surface. C. The association areas are concerned with the interpretations of sensory experiences. D. Appreciation of the body image is assembled in the posterior parietal cortex, and the right side of the body is represented in the left hemisphere. E. The association areas have all six cellular layers and are referred to as *homotypical cortex.*

8. B is correct. More than 90% of the adult population is right-handed and, therefore, is left-hemisphere dominant. A. The cortical gyri of the dominant and nondominant hemispheres are arranged in the same way. C. About 96% of the adult population is left-hemisphere dominant for speech. D. The nondominant hemisphere interprets spatial perception, recognition of faces, and music. E. After the first decade of life, the dominance of the cerebral hemispheres becomes fixed.

The answers for Figure 8-9, which shows the lateral view of the left cerebral hemisphere, are as follows:

9. C is correct; 1 is the frontal eye field.
10. E is correct; 2 is the secondary somesthetic area (see Fig. 8-4).
11. E is correct; 3 is the Wernicke sensory speech area (see Fig. 8-4).
12. B is correct; 4 is the secondary auditory area (see Fig. 8-4).

The answers for Figure 8-10, which shows the medial view of the left cerebral hemisphere, are as follows:

13. C is correct; 1 is the primary visual area (see Fig. 8-4).
14. B is correct; 2 is the primary somesthetic area (see Fig. 8-4).
15. D is correct; 3 is the primary motor area (see Fig. 8-4).
16. A is correct; 4 is the premotor area (see Fig. 8-4).
17. D is correct. The patient exhibited no weakness of her muscles on the left side despite the fact that her sister stated that she tended not to use her left leg.
18. B is correct. An MRI revealed a tumor in the right parieto-occipital lobes; a further lesion was present in the right frontal lobe.

9 Reticular Formation and Limbic System

CHAPTER OBJECTIVE

CHAPTER OBJECTIVE

- To provide a brief overview of the structure and function of the reticular formation

- To present the parts of the limbic system and its functions

A 24-year-old medical student is rushed by ambulance to the emergency department after an accident on his motorcycle. On examination, he is found to be unconscious and shows evidence of severe injury to the right side of his head. He fails to respond when spoken to, and he does not make any response to deep painful pressure applied over his supraorbital nerve. The plantar reflex is extension, and the corneal, tendon, and pupillary reflexes are absent. The patient is clearly in a deep coma. Further neurologic examination reveals nothing that might add to the diagnosis. A computed tomography scan shows a large depressed fracture of the right parietal bone of the skull.

After a week in the intensive care unit, the patient's condition changes. He suddenly shows signs of being awake but not aware of his environment or inner needs. To the delight of his family, he follows them with his eyes and responds in a limited manner to primitive postural and reflex movements; he does not, however, speak and does not respond to commands. Although he has sleep–wake cycles, he does not respond appropriately to pain. The patient's neurologic condition is unchanged 6 months later.

The neurologist determines that the patient is awake but not aware of his surroundings. He explains to the family that the part of the brain referred to as the *reticular formation* in the brainstem had survived the accident and is responsible for the patient apparently being awake and able to breathe without assistance. However, because his cerebral cortex is dead, the patient will remain in this vegetative state.

Not very long ago, the reticular system was believed to be a vague network of nerve cells and fibers occupying the central core of the brainstem with no particular function. Today, it is known to play a key role in many important activities of the nervous system.

Limbic system was a term loosely used to describe the part of the brain between the cerebral cortex and the hypothalamus, a little understood area of the brain. Today, it is known to play a vital role in emotion, behavior, drive, and memory.

RETICULAR FORMATION

The reticular formation, as its name suggests, resembles a net (reticular) that is made up of nerve cells and nerve fibers. The net extends up through the axis of the central nervous system (CNS) from the spinal cord to the cerebrum. It is strategically placed among the important nerve tracts and nuclei. It receives input from most of the sensory systems and has efferent fibers that descend and influence nerve cells at all CNS levels. The exceptionally long dendrites of the neurons of the reticular formation permit input from widely placed ascending and descending pathways. Through its many connections, it can influence skeletal muscle activity, somatic and visceral sensations, the autonomic and endocrine systems, and even the level of consciousness.

General Arrangement

The reticular formation consists of a deeply placed continuous network of nerve cells and fibers that extend from the spinal cord through the medulla, the pons, the midbrain, the subthalamus, the hypothalamus, and the thalamus. The diffuse network may be divided into three longitudinal columns: the first occupying the median plane, called the **median column**, and consisting of intermediate-size neurons; the second, called the **medial column**, containing large neurons; and the third, or **lateral column**, containing mainly small neurons (Fig. 9-1).

With classic neuronal staining techniques, the groups of neurons are poorly defined; therefore, tracing an anatomical pathway through the network is difficult. However, with the new techniques of neurochemistry

Figure 9-1 Diagram showing the approximate positions of the median, medial, and lateral columns of the reticular formation in the brainstem.

and cytochemical localization, the reticular formation is shown to contain highly organized groups of transmitter-specific cells that can influence functions in specific CNS areas. The monoaminergic groups of cells, for example, are located in well-defined areas throughout the reticular formation.

Polysynaptic pathways exist, and both crossed and uncrossed ascending and descending pathways are present, involving many neurons that serve both somatic and visceral functions.

Inferiorly, the reticular formation is continuous with the interneurons of the gray matter of the spinal cord, while superiorly, impulses are relayed to the cerebral cortex; a substantial projection of fibers also leaves the reticular formation to enter the cerebellum.

Afferent Projections

Many different afferent pathways project onto the reticular formation from most parts of the CNS (Fig. 9-2). Spinoreticular and spinothalamic tracts and the medial lemniscus project from the spinal cord. Ascending afferent tracts including the vestibular, acoustic, and visual pathways project from the cranial nerve nuclei. The cerebelloreticular pathway projects from the cerebellum,

Figure 9-2 Diagram showing the afferent fibers of the reticular formation.

and further afferent tracts project from the subthalamic, hypothalamic, and thalamic nuclei and from the corpus striatum and limbic system. Other important afferent fibers arise in the primary motor cortex of the frontal lobe and from the somesthetic cortex of the parietal lobe.

Efferent Projections

Multiple efferent pathways extend down to the brainstem and spinal cord through the reticulobulbar and reticulospinal tracts to neurons in the motor nuclei of the cranial nerves and the anterior horn cells of the spinal cord. Other descending pathways extend to the sympathetic outflow and the craniosacral parasympathetic outflow of the autonomic nervous system (ANS). Additional pathways extend to the corpus striatum, the cerebellum, the red nucleus, the substantia nigra, the tectum, and the nuclei of the thalamus, subthalamus, and hypothalamus. Most regions of the cerebral cortex receive efferent fibers as well.

Functions

Given the vast number of connections of the reticular formation to all parts of the nervous system, not surprisingly, it serves many functions. A few of the more important functions are considered here.

1. **Control of skeletal muscle.** Through the reticulospinal and reticulobulbar tracts, the reticular formation can influence the activity of the α and γ motor neurons. Thus, the reticular formation can modulate muscle tone and reflex activity. It can also bring about reciprocal inhibition; for example, when the flexor muscles contract, the antagonistic extensors relax. The reticular formation, assisted by the vestibular apparatus of the inner ear and the vestibular spinal tract, plays an important role in maintaining the tone of the antigravity muscles when standing. The so-called respiratory centers of the brainstem, described by neurophysiologists as being in the control of the respiratory muscles, are now considered part of the reticular formation.

2. **Control of facial expression muscles.** The reticular formation is important in controlling the muscles of facial expression when associated with emotion. For example, when a person smiles or laughs in response to a joke, the motor control is provided by the reticular formation on both sides of the brain. The descending tracts are separate from the corticobulbar fibers. This means that a person who has suffered a stroke that involves the corticobulbar fibers and exhibits facial paralysis on the lower part of the face is still able to smile symmetrically (see Fig. 11-25).

3. **Control of somatic and visceral sensations.** By virtue of its central location in the cerebrospinal axis, the reticular formation can influence all ascending pathways that pass to supraspinal levels. The influence may be facilitative or inhibitory. In particular, the reticular formation may have a key role in the "gating mechanism" for the control of pain perception (see p. 146).

4. **Control of the ANS.** Higher control of the ANS, from the cerebral cortex, hypothalamus, and other subcortical nuclei, can be exerted by the reticulobulbar and reticulospinal tracts, which descend to the sympathetic outflow and the parasympathetic craniosacral outflow.

5. **Control of the endocrine system.** Either directly or indirectly through the hypothalamic nuclei, the reticular formation can influence the synthesis or release of releasing or release-inhibiting factors and thereby control the activity of the hypophysis cerebri.

6. **Influence on biologic clocks.** By means of its multiple afferent and efferent pathways to the hypothalamus, the reticular formation probably influences the biologic rhythms.

7. **Reticular activating system.** Arousal and the level of consciousness are controlled by the reticular formation. Multiple ascending pathways carrying sensory information to higher centers are channeled through the reticular formation, which, in turn, projects this information to different parts of the cerebral cortex, causing a sleeping person to awaken. In fact, state of consciousness is now thought to be dependent on the continuous projection of sensory information to the cortex. Different degrees of wakefulness seem to depend on the degree of activity of the reticular formation. Incoming pain sensations strongly increase the activity of the reticular formation, which, in turn, greatly excites the cerebral cortex. Acetylcholine plays a key role as an excitatory neurotransmitter in this process.

Thus, the reticular formation, almost totally ignored in the past, is now being shown to influence practically all activities of the body.

LIMBIC SYSTEM

The word *limbic* means border or margin, and the term *limbic* system was loosely used to include a group of structures that lie in the border zone between the cerebral cortex and the hypothalamus. Research has now shown that the limbic system is involved with many other structures beyond the border zone in the control of emotion, behavior, and drive; it also appears to be important to memory.

Anatomically, the limbic structures include the subcallosal, the cingulate, and the parahippocampal gyri, the hippocampal formation, the amygdaloid nucleus, the mammillary bodies, and the anterior thalamic nucleus (Fig. 9-3). The alveus, the fimbria, the fornix, the mammillothalamic tract, and the stria terminalis constitute the connecting pathways of this system.

Hippocampal Formation

The hippocampal formation consists of the hippocampus, the dentate gyrus, and the parahippocampal gyrus.

The **hippocampus** is a curved elevation of gray matter that extends throughout the entire length of the floor of the inferior horn of the lateral ventricle (Fig. 9-4). Its anterior end is expanded to form the **pes hippocampus.** It is named *hippocampus* because it resembles a seahorse in coronal section. The convex ventricular

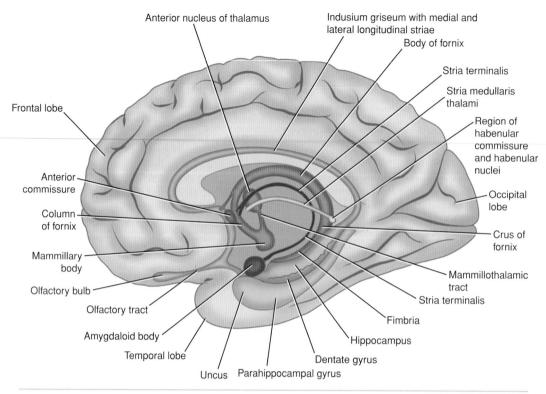

Figure 9-3 Medial aspect of the right cerebral hemisphere showing structures that form the limbic system.

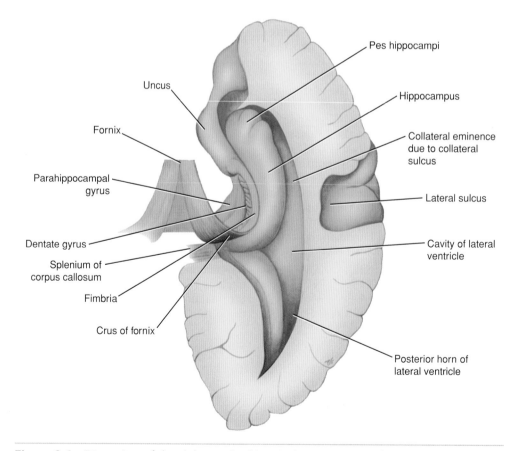

Figure 9-4 Dissection of the right cerebral hemisphere exposing the cavity of the lateral ventricle, showing the hippocampus, the dentate gyrus, and the fornix.

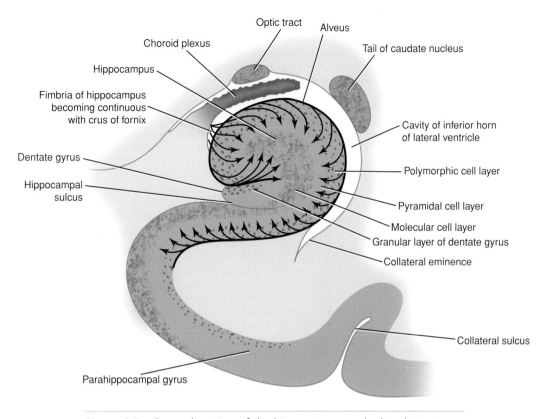

Figure 9-5 Coronal section of the hippocampus and related structures.

surface is covered with ependyma, beneath which lies a thin layer of white matter called the **alveus** (Fig. 9-5). The alveus consists of nerve fibers that have originated in the hippocampus, and these converge medially to form a bundle called the **fimbria**. The fimbria, in turn, becomes continuous with the crus of the fornix. The hippocampus terminates posteriorly beneath the splenium of the corpus callosum.

The **dentate** gyrus is a narrow, notched band of gray matter that lies between the fimbria of the hippocampus and the parahippocampal gyrus (see Fig. 9-4). Posteriorly, the gyrus accompanies the fimbria almost to the splenium of the corpus callosum and becomes continuous with the **indusium** griseum. The indusium griseum is a thin, vestigial layer of gray matter that covers the superior surface of the corpus callosum (Fig. 9-6). Embedded in the superior surface of the indusium griseum are two slender bundles of white fibers on each side called the **medial** and **lateral** longitudinal striae. The striae are the remains of the white matter of the vestigial indusium griseum. Anteriorly, the dentate gyrus is continued into the **uncus**.

The **parahippocampal gyrus** lies between the hippocampal fissure and the collateral sulcus and is continuous with the hippocampus along the medial edge of the temporal lobe (see Figs. 9-4 and 9-5).

Amygdaloid Nucleus

The amygdaloid nucleus is so named because it resembles an almond. It is situated partly anterior and partly superior to the tip of the inferior horn of the lateral ventricle (see Fig. 7-14). It is fused with the tip of the tail of the caudate nucleus, which has passed anteriorly in the roof of the inferior horn of the lateral ventricle. The stria terminalis emerges from its posterior aspect. The amygdaloid nucleus consists of a complex of nuclei that can be grouped into a larger **basolateral group** and smaller **corticomedial group**.

The mammillary bodies and the anterior nucleus of the thalamus are considered elsewhere in this text.

Connecting Pathways of the Limbic System

The connecting pathways of the limbic system are the alveus, the fimbria, the fornix, the mammillothalamic tract, and the stria terminalis.

The **alveus** consists of a thin layer of white matter that lies on the superior or ventricular surface of the hippocampus (see Fig. 9-5). It is composed of nerve fibers that originate in the hippocampal cortex. The fibers converge on the medial border of the hippocampus to form a bundle called the **fimbria**.

The fimbria now leaves the posterior end of the hippocampus as the **crus of the fornix** (see Fig. 9-4). The crus from each side curves posteriorly and superiorly beneath the splenium of the corpus callosum and around the posterior surface of the thalamus. The two crura now converge to form the **body of the fornix**, which is applied closely to the undersurface of the corpus callosum (see Fig. 9-3). As the two crura come together, they are connected by transverse fibers called

Figure 9-6 Dissection of both cerebral hemispheres showing the superior surface of the corpus callosum.

the **commissure of the fornix** (see Fig. 7-16). These fibers decussate and join the hippocampi of the two sides.

Anteriorly, the body of the fornix is connected to the undersurface of the corpus callosum by the **septum pellucidum**. Inferiorly, the body of the fornix is related to the tela choroidea and the ependymal roof of the third ventricle.

The body of the fornix splits anteriorly into two anterior **columns of the fornix**, each of which curves anteriorly and inferiorly over the interventricular foramen (foramen of Monro). Then, each column disappears into the lateral wall of the third ventricle to reach the **mammillary body** (see Fig. 9-3).

The **mammillothalamic tract** provides important connections between the mammillary body and the anterior nuclear group of the thalamus.

The **stria terminalis** emerges from the posterior aspect of the amygdaloid nucleus and runs as a bundle of nerve fibers posteriorly in the roof of the inferior horn of the lateral ventricle on the medial side of the tail of the caudate nucleus. It follows the curve of the caudate nucleus and comes to lie in the floor of lthe body of the lateral ventricle.

Hippocampal Structure and the Dentate Gyrus

The cortical structure of the parahippocampal gyrus is six layered (see Fig. 9-5). As the cortex is traced into the hippocampus, there is a gradual transition from a six- to a three-layered arrangement. These three layers are the superficial **molecular layer**, consisting of nerve fibers and scattered small neurons; the **pyramidal layer**, consisting of many large pyramid-shaped neurons; and the inner **polymorphic layer**, which is similar in structure to the polymorphic layer of the cortex seen elsewhere.

The dentate gyrus also has three layers, but the pyramidal layer is replaced by the granular layer. The granular layer is composed of densely arranged rounded or oval neurons that give rise to axons that terminate on the dendrites of the pyramidal cells in the hippocampus. A few of the axons join the fimbria and enter the fornix.

Afferent Connections of the Hippocampus

Afferent connections of the hippocampus may be divided into six groups (Fig. 9-7):

1. Fibers arising in the cingulate gyrus pass to the hippocampus.

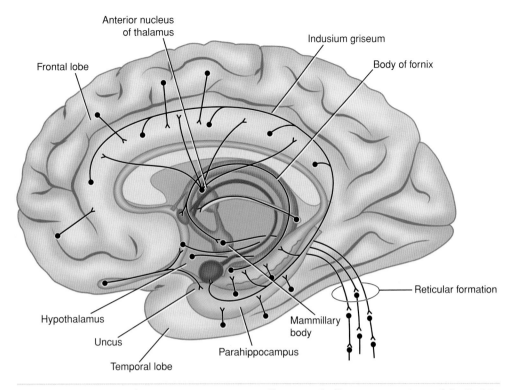

Figure 9-7 Diagram showing some important afferent and efferent connections of the limbic system.

2. Fibers arising from the septal nuclei (nuclei lying within the midline close to the anterior commissure) pass posterior in the fornix to the hippocampus.
3. Fibers arising from one hippocampus pass across the midline to the opposite hippocampus in the commissure of the fornix.
4. Fibers from the indusium griseum pass posteriorly in the longitudinal striae to the hippocampus.
5. Fibers from the entorhinal area or olfactory-associated cortex pass to the hippocampus.
6. Fibers arising from the dentate and parahippocampal gyri travel to the hippocampus.

Efferent Connections of the Hippocampus

Axons of the large pyramidal cells of the hippocampus emerge to form the alveus and the fimbria. The fimbria continues as the crus of the fornix. The two crura converge to form the body of the fornix. The body of the fornix splits into the two columns of the fornix, which curve downward and forward in front of the interventricular foramina. The fibers within the fornix are distributed to the following regions (see Fig. 9-7):

1. Fibers pass posterior to the anterior commissure to enter the mammillary body, where they end in the medial nucleus.
2. Fibers pass posterior to the anterior commissure to end in the anterior nuclei of the thalamus.
3. Fibers pass posterior to the anterior commissure to enter the tegmentum of the midbrain.
4. Fibers pass anterior to the anterior commissure to end in the septal nuclei, the lateral preoptic area, and the anterior part of the hypothalamus.

5. Fibers join the stria medullaris thalami to reach the habenular nuclei.

Consideration of the above complex anatomical pathways indicates that the structures comprising the limbic system not only are interconnected but also send projection fibers to many different parts of the nervous system. Physiologists now recognize the importance of the hypothalamus as being the major output pathway of the limbic system.

Limbic System Functions

The limbic system, via the hypothalamus and its connections with outflow of the ANS and its control of the endocrine system, is able to influence many aspects of emotional behavior. These include particularly the reactions of fear and anger and the emotions associated with sexual behavior.

Evidence also suggests that the hippocampus is concerned with converting recent memory to long-term memory. A lesion of the hippocampus results in the individual being unable to store long-term memory. Memory of remote past events before the lesion developed is unaffected. This condition is called **antero-grade amnesia**. Note that injury to the amygdaloid nucleus and the hippocampus produces greater memory loss than injury to either one of these structures alone.

Evidence does not show that the limbic system has an olfactory function. Its various afferent and efferent connections provide pathways for the integration and effective homeostatic responses to a wide variety of environmental stimuli.

Clinical Notes

Reticular Formation

The reticular formation is a continuous network of nerve cells and fibers that extend through the neuroaxis from the spinal cord to the cerebral cortex. The reticular formation not only modulates the control of motor systems but also influences sensory systems. By means of its multiple ascending pathways, which project to different parts of the cerebral cortex, it is believed to influence the state of consciousness.

Loss of Consciousness

In experimental animals, damage to the reticular formation, which spares the ascending sensory pathways, causes persistent unconsciousness. Pathologic lesions of the reticular formation in humans can result in loss of consciousness and even coma. It has been suggested that the loss of consciousness that occurs in epilepsy may be due to inhibition of the activity of the reticular formation in the upper part of the diencephalon.

Limbic System

Because the anatomical connections of the limbic system are extremely complex and their significance is not fully understood, committing all of them to memory is unnecessary. The results of neurophysiologic experiments, which have included stimulation and ablation of different parts of the limbic system in animals, are not entirely clear. Nevertheless, certain important roles have been inferred: (1) The limbic structures are involved in the development of sensations of emotion and with the visceral responses accompanying those emotions, and (2) the hippocampus is concerned with recent memory.

Schizophrenia

The symptoms of schizophrenia include chronically disordered thinking, blunted affect, and emotional withdrawal. Paranoid delusions and auditory hallucinations may also be present. Clinical research has shown that if the limbic receptors to dopamine are blocked by a pharmacologic agent, the worst symptoms of schizophrenia are lessened. Phenothiazine administration, for example, blocks the dopamine receptors in the limbic system. Unfortunately, this drug, as well as most other antipsychotic drugs, has major motor side effects on the dopaminergic receptors within the extrapyramidal system, producing abnormal involuntary movements. Research is now concentrating on finding a drug that will block the limbic dopamine receptors but without effect on the receptors of the extrapyramidal system (substantia nigra–corpus striatum).

Clearly, no direct evidence exists to suggest that excessive production of dopamine by certain neurons actually contributes to schizophrenia.

Amygdaloid Complex Destruction

Unilateral or bilateral destruction of the amygdaloid nucleus and the para-amygdaloid area in patients suffering from aggressive behavior in many cases results in a decrease in aggressiveness, emotional instability, and restlessness; increased interest in food; and hypersexuality but no memory disturbance. Monkeys that have been subjected to bilateral removal of the temporal lobes demonstrate what is known as **Klüver–Bucy syndrome**. They become docile and show no evidence of fear or anger and are unable to appreciate objects visually. They have increased appetite and sexual activity. Moreover, the animals indiscriminately seek partnerships with male and female animals.

Precise stereotactic lesions in the amygdaloid complex in humans reduce emotional excitability and bring about normalization of behavior in patients with severe disturbances. No loss of memory occurs.

Temporal Lobe Dysfunction

Temporal lobe epilepsy may be preceded by an aura of acoustic or olfactory experience. The olfactory aura is usually an unpleasant odor. The patient is often confused, anxious, and docile and may perform automatic and complicated movements, such as undressing in public or driving a car, and then, following the seizure, may have no memory of what occurred previously.

Key Concepts

Reticular Formation

- The reticular formation consists of a deeply placed, continuous network of nerve cells and fibers that extend throughout the medulla, pons, midbrain, subthalamus, hypothalamus, and thalamus.

- It is organized into three longitudinal columns: median, medial, and lateral.

- These columns can modulate 1) muscle tone and reflex activity, 2) somatic and visceral sensations, 3) autonomic nervous system, 4) endocrine functions, 5) biologic clocks, and 6) the reticular activating system (arousal and consciousness).

Limbic System

- This group of structures controls emotion, behavior, drive, and memory and includes the subcallosal, cingulate, and parahippocampal gyri, the hippocampal formation, the amygdaloid nucleus, the mammillary bodies, and the anterior thalamic nucleus.

- The hippocampal formation consists of the hippocampus, dentate gyrus, and parahippocampal gyrus.

Clinical Problem Solving

1. While discussing the neurologic basis of emotions during a ward round, a neurologist asks a third-year medical student what she knows about the Klüver–Bucy syndrome. What would be your answer to that question? Does Klüver–Bucy syndrome ever occur in humans?
2. A 23-year-old woman with a 4-year history of epileptic attacks visits her neurologist. A friend of hers vividly describes one of her attacks. For a few seconds before the convulsions begin, the patient complains of an unpleasant odor, similar to that encountered in a cow shed. This is followed by a shrill cry as she falls to the floor unconscious. Her whole body immediately becomes involved in generalized tonic and clonic movements. Clearly, this patient has a generalized form of epileptic seizure. Using your knowledge of neuroanatomy, suggest which lobe of the brain was initially involved in the epileptic discharge.
3. A 54-year-old man dies in the hospital with a cerebral tumor. He had always been intellectually very bright and could easily recall events in his childhood. For the past 6 months, his family had noticed that he had difficulty in recalling where he had placed things, such as his pipe. He also had difficulty in recalling recent news events, and, just before he died, he could not remember that his brother had visited him the day before. Using your knowledge of neuroanatomy, suggest which part of the brain was being affected by the expanding and highly invasive tumor.

Answers and Explanations to Clinical Problem Solving

1. The Klüver–Bucy syndrome consists of the signs and symptoms found in monkeys following bilateral removal of the temporal lobe. The monkeys become docile and unresponsive and display no signs of fear or anger. They have increased appetite and sexual activity, which is often disinhibited. They are able to see objects but are unable to recognize the objects. Humans in whom the amygdaloid area is destroyed do not usually demonstrate this syndrome. It has, however, been described in humans following the bilateral removal of large areas of the temporal lobes.
2. The olfactory aura that preceded the general convulsions of the epileptic attack would indicate that the temporal lobe of the cerebral cortex was initially involved.
3. An autopsy study revealed extensive invasion of the hippocampus, fornix, and mammillary bodies in both cerebral hemispheres. The hippocampus is apparently involved in the storage and categorizing of afferent information related to recent memory.

 Review Questions

Directions: Each of the numbered items in this section is followed by answers. Select the ONE lettered answer that is CORRECT.

1. The following statements concern the reticular formation:
   (a) Reticulobulbar and reticulospinal tracts form the afferent pathways from the reticular formation to the motor nuclei of the cranial nerves and the anterior horn cells of the spinal cord, respectively.
   (b) The reticular formation extends through the neuroaxis from the spinal cord to the midbrain.
   (c) The main pathways through the reticular formation may easily be traced from one part of the CNS to another using silver stains.
   (d) Superiorly, the reticular formation is relayed to the cerebral cortex.
   (e) Afferent pathways project into the reticular formation from only a few parts of the CNS.
2. The following statements concern the functions of the reticular formation:
   (a) It influences the activity of the α and γ motor neurons.
   (b) It opposes the actions of the vestibular spinal tract.
   (c) It does not bring about reciprocal inhibition during contraction of the prime mover muscles.
   (d) It plays no part in maintaining the tone of the antigravity muscles.
   (e) It cannot modulate reflex activity.

Figure 9-8 Medial aspect of the right cerebral hemisphere showing structures that form the limbic system.

3. The following statements concern the functions of the reticular formation:
   (a) It does not affect the reception of pain.
   (b) It cannot influence all ascending pathways to the supraspinal levels.
   (c) By means of its reticulobulbar and reticulospinal tracts, it can control parasympathetic and sympathetic outflows.
   (d) It has no effect on biologic rhythms.
   (e) It does not influence the degree of wakefulness of an individual.
4. Anatomically, the following structures collectively form the limbic system:
   (a) Amygdaloid nucleus, red nucleus, and vestibular nuclei
   (b) Pulvinar of the thalamus and the substantia nigra
   (c) Hippocampal formation
   (d) Cingulate gyrus and uncus
   (e) Subcallosal, cingulate, and parahippocampal gyri, hippocampal formation, amygdaloid nucleus, mammillary bodies, and anterior thalamic nuclei
5. The following statements concern the efferent connections of the hippocampus:
   (a) They arise from the small granular cells of the cortex.
   (b) They travel through the fornix.

   (c) None of the fibers enter the mammillary body.
   (d) The fibers within the fornix pass posterior to the interventricular foramen.
   (e) Some of the fibers end in thalamic posterior nuclei.
6. The following statements concern the functions of the limbic system:
   (a) It is not concerned with fear and anger.
   (b) It is concerned with visual experiences.
   (c) The hippocampus is concerned with recent memory.
   (d) The limbic system plays an important role in olfactory function.
   (e) It directly influences the activity of the endocrine system.

Matching Questions. Directions: The following questions apply to Figure 9-8. Match the numbers listed on the left with the appropriate lettered structure listed on the right. Each lettered option may be selected once, more than once, or not at all.

7. Number 1	(a) Uncus
8. Number 2	(b) Body of fornix
9. Number 3	(c) Parahippocampal gyrus
10. Number 4	(d) Dentate gyrus
	(e) None of the above

 Answers and Explanations to Review Questions

1. D is correct. The reticular formation is relayed superiorly to the cerebral cortex. A. The retrobulbar and reticulospinal tracts form the efferent pathways from the reticular formation to the motor nuclei of the cranial nerves and the anterior horn cells of the spinal cord, respectively. B. The reticular formation extends through the neuroaxis from the spinal cord to the thalamus. C. The main pathways through the reticular formation are poorly defined and difficult to trace from one part of the CNS to another using silver stains. E. Afferent pathways project into the reticular formation from most parts of the CNS.

2. A is correct. The reticular formation influences the activity of the α and γ motor neurons. B. The reticular formation does not oppose the actions of the vestibular spinal tract. C. The reticular formation brings about reciprocal inhibition during contraction of the prime mover muscles. D. The reticular formation helps maintain the tone of the antigravity muscles. E. The reticular formation can modulate reflex activity.

3. C is correct. The reticular formation by means of its reticulobulbar and reticulospinal tracts can control the parasympathetic and sympathetic outflows. A. The reticular formation does affect the reception of pain. B. The reticular formation can influence all ascending pathways to the supraspinal levels. D. The reticular formation can affect the biologic rhythms. E. The reticular formation can influence the degree of wakefulness of an individual.

4. E is correct. The limbic system is made up of the subcallosal, the cingulate, and the parahippocampal gyri, the hippocampal formation, the amygdaloid nucleus, the mammillary bodies, and the anterior thalamic nuclei (see Fig. 9-3).

5. B is correct. The efferent connections of the hippocampus travel through the fornix. A. The efferent connections of the hippocampus arise from large pyramidal cells of the cortex. C. Some of the efferent fibers from the hippocampus enter the mammillary bodies. D. The efferent fibers in the fornix pass anterior to the interventricular foramen. E. Some of the efferent fibers from the hippocampus end in the anterior nuclei of the thalamus.

6. C is correct. The hippocampus is concerned with recent memory. A. The limbic system is concerned with the reactions of fear and anger. B. The limbic system is not concerned with visual experiences. D. The limbic system plays no part in olfactory function. E. The limbic system indirectly influences the activity of the endocrine system.

The answers for Figure 9-8 are as follows:

7. B is correct. Number 1 is the body of the fornix.
8. D is correct. Number 2 is the dentate gyrus.
9. C is correct. Number 3 is the parahippocampal gyrus.
10. A is correct. Number 4 is the uncus.

10 Basal Nuclei (Basal Ganglia)

CHAPTER OBJECTIVE

- To describe the basal nuclei and their connections

- To relate basal nuclei functions to diseases commonly affecting this area of the nervous system

A 58-year-old man goes to a neurologist because he has noticed the development of a slight tremor of his left hand. The tremors involve all of the fingers and the thumb and are present at rest but cease during voluntary movement.

On examination, the patient tends to perform all his movements slowly, and his face has very little expression and is almost masklike. On passively moving the patient's arms, the neurologist finds that the muscles show increased tone, with a slight jerky resistance to the movements. When asked to stand up straight, the patient does so but with a stooped posture, and, when he walks, he does so by shuffling across the examining room.

The neurologist makes the diagnosis of Parkinson disease, based on her knowledge of the structure and function of the basal ganglia and their connections to the substantia nigra of the midbrain. She is able to prescribe appropriate drug therapy, which results in a great improvement in the hand tremors.

The basal nuclei play an important role in the control of posture and voluntary movement. Unlike many other parts of the nervous system concerned with motor control, the basal nuclei have no direct input or output connections with the spinal cord.

TERMINOLOGY

The term **basal nuclei** is applied to a collection of masses of gray matter situated within each cerebral hemisphere. They are the corpus striatum, the amygdaloid nucleus, and the claustrum.

Clinicians and neuroscientists use a variety of different terminologies to describe the basal nuclei. A summary of the terminologies commonly used is shown in Table 10-1. The subthalamic nuclei, the substantia nigra, and the red nucleus are functionally closely related to the basal nuclei, but they should not be included with them.

The interconnections of the basal nuclei are complex, but in this account, only the more important pathways are considered. The basal nuclei play an important role in the control of posture and voluntary movement.

CORPUS STRIATUM

The corpus striatum (Fig. 10-1; see also Atlas Plate 5) is situated lateral to the thalamus and is almost completely divided by a band of nerve fibers, the **internal capsule**, into the caudate nucleus and the lentiform nucleus. The term *striatum* is used here because of the striated appearance produced by the strands of gray matter passing through the internal capsule and connecting the caudate nucleus to the putamen of the lentiform nucleus (see below).

Table 10-1   Terminology Commonly Used to Describe the Basal Nuclei

Neurologic Structure	Basal Nucleus (Nuclei)[a]
Caudate nucleus	Caudate nucleus
Lentiform nucleus	Globus pallidus plus putamen
Claustrum	Claustrum
Corpus striatum	Caudate nucleus plus lentiform nucleus
Neostriatum (striatum)	Caudate nucleus plus putamen
Amygdaloid body	Amygdaloid nucleus

[a]The term *basal* has been used in the past to denote the position of the nuclei at the base of the forebrain.

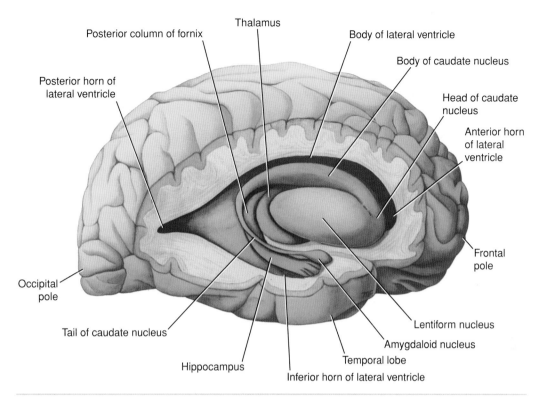

Figure 10-1   Lateral view of the right cerebral hemisphere dissected to show the position of the different basal nuclei.

Caudate Nucleus

The caudate nucleus is a large C-shaped mass of gray matter that is closely related to the lateral ventricle and lies lateral to the thalamus. The lateral surface of the nucleus is related to the internal capsule, which separates it from the lentiform nucleus (Fig. 10-2). For purposes of description, it can be divided into a head, a body, and a tail.

The **head** of the caudate nucleus is large and rounded and forms the lateral wall of the anterior horn of the lateral ventricle (see also Atlas Plate 5). The head is continuous inferiorly with the putamen of the lentiform nucleus (the caudate nucleus and the putamen are sometimes referred to as the **neostriatum** or **striatum**). Just superior to this point of union, strands of gray matter pass through the internal capsule, giving the region a striated appearance, hence the term **corpus striatum.**

The **body** of the caudate nucleus is long and narrow and is continuous with the head in the region of the interventricular foramen. The body of the caudate nucleus forms part of the floor of the body of the lateral ventricle.

The **tail** of the caudate nucleus is long and slender and is continuous with the body in the region of the posterior end of the thalamus. It follows the contour of the lateral ventricle and continues forward in the roof of the inferior horn of the lateral ventricle. It terminates anteriorly in the **amygdaloid nucleus** (see Fig. 10-1).

Lentiform Nucleus

The lentiform nucleus is a wedge-shaped mass of gray matter whose broad convex base is directed laterally and whose blade is directed medially (see Fig. 10-2; see also Atlas Plate 5). It is buried deep in the white matter of the cerebral hemisphere and is related medially to the internal capsule, which separates it from the caudate nucleus and the thalamus. The lentiform nucleus is related laterally to a thin sheet of white matter, the **external capsule**, which separates it from a thin sheet of gray matter, called the **claustrum**. The claustrum, in turn, separates the external capsule from the subcortical white matter of the insula. A vertical plate of white matter divides the nucleus into a larger, darker lateral portion, the **putamen**, and an inner lighter portion, the **globus pallidus**. The paleness of the globus pallidus is due to the presence of a high concentration of myelinated nerve fibers. Inferiorly at its anterior end, the putamen is continuous with the head of the caudate nucleus (see Fig. 10-1).

AMYGDALOID NUCLEUS

The amygdaloid nucleus is situated in the temporal lobe close to the uncus (see Fig. 10-1). The amygdaloid nucleus is considered to be part of the limbic system and is described in Chapter 9. Through its connections, it can influence the body's response to environmental changes. In the sense of fear, for example, it can change

Figure 10-2   Horizontal section of the cerebrum, as seen from above, showing the relationships of the different basal nuclei.

the heart rate, blood pressure, skin color, and rate of respiration.

SUBSTANTIA NIGRA AND SUBTHALAMIC NUCLEI

The substantia nigra of the midbrain and the subthalamic nuclei of the diencephalon are functionally closely related to the activities of the basal nuclei and are described elsewhere (see pp. 211 and 253). The neurons of the substantia nigra are dopaminergic and inhibitory and have many connections to the corpus striatum. The neurons of the subthalamic nuclei are glutaminergic and excitatory and have many connections to the globus pallidus and substantia nigra.

CLAUSTRUM

The claustrum is a thin sheet of gray matter that is separated from the lateral surface of the lentiform nucleus by the external capsule (see Fig. 10-2). Lateral to the claustrum is the subcortical white matter of the insula. The function of the claustrum is unknown.

CONNECTIONS OF THE CORPUS STRIATUM AND GLOBUS PALLIDUS

The caudate nucleus and the putamen form the main sites for receiving input to the basal nuclei. The globus pallidus forms the major site from which the output leaves the basal nuclei.

They receive no direct input from or output to the spinal cord.

Corpus Striatum Afferent Fibers

Projections to the corpus striatum include corticostriate, thalamostriate, nigrostriatal, and brainstem striatal fibers.

Corticostriate Fibers

All parts of the cerebral cortex send axons to the caudate nucleus and the putamen (Fig. 10-3). Each part of the cerebral cortex projects to a specific part of the caudate–putamen complex. Most of the projections are from the cortex of the same side. The largest input is from the sensory motor cortex. Glutamate is the neurotransmitter of the corticostriate fibers (Fig. 10-4).

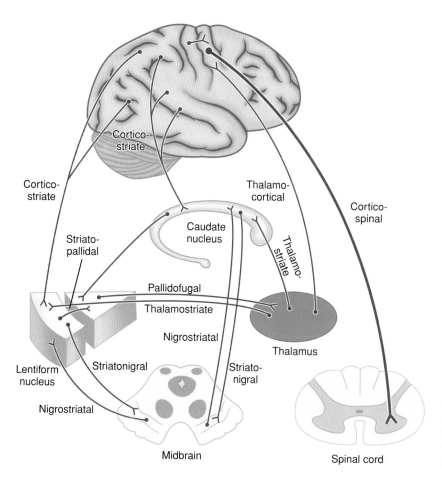

Figure 10-3 Some of the main connections between the cerebral cortex, the basal nuclei, the thalamic nuclei, the brainstem, and the spinal cord.

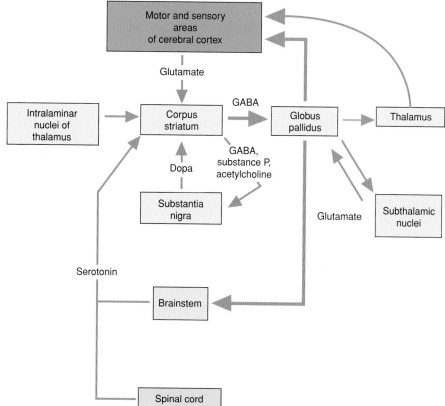

Figure 10-4 Basal nuclei pathways showing the known neurotransmitters.

Thalamostriate Fibers

The intralaminar nuclei of the thalamus send large numbers of axons to the caudate nucleus and the putamen (see Fig. 10-3).

Nigrostriatal Fibers

Neurons in the substantia nigra send axons to the caudate nucleus and the putamen (see Figs. 10-3 and 10-4) and liberate dopamine at their terminals as the neurotransmitter. These fibers are believed to be inhibitory in function.

Brainstem Striatal Fibers

Ascending fibers from the brainstem end in the caudate nucleus and putamen and liberate serotonin at their terminals as the neurotransmitter. These fibers are thought to be inhibitory in function.

Corpus Striatum Efferent Fibers

Projections from the corpus striatum include striatopallidal and striatonigral fibers.

Striatopallidal Fibers

Striatopallidal fibers pass from the caudate nucleus and putamen to the globus pallidus (see Fig. 10-3). They have γ-aminobutyric acid (GABA) as their neurotransmitter (see Fig. 10-4).

Striatonigral Fibers

Striatonigral fibers pass from the caudate nucleus and putamen to the substantia nigra (see Fig. 10-3). Some of the fibers use GABA or acetylcholine as the neurotransmitter, while others use substance P (see Fig. 10-4).

Globus Pallidus Afferent Fibers

Striatopallidal fibers pass from the caudate nucleus and putamen to the globus pallidus. As noted previously, these fibers have GABA as their neurotransmitter (Fig. 10-4).

Globus Pallidus Efferent Fibers

Pallidofugal fibers are complicated and can be divided into groups: (1) the **ansa lenticularis**, which pass to the thalamic nuclei; (2) the **fasciculus lenticularis**, which pass to the subthalamus; (3) the **pallidotegmental** fibers, which terminate in the caudal tegmentum of the midbrain; and (4) the **pallidosubthalamic fibers**, which pass to the subthalamic nuclei.

BASAL NUCLEI FUNCTIONS

The basal nuclei (Fig. 10-5) are joined together and connected with many different regions of the nervous system by a very complex number of neurons.

Basically, the corpus striatum receives afferent information from most of the cerebral cortex, the thalamus,

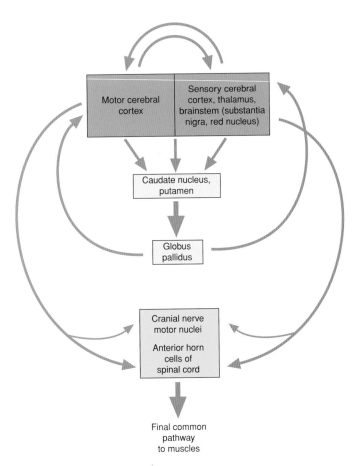

Figure 10-5 Diagram showing the main functional connections of the basal nuclei and how they can influence muscle activity.

the subthalamus, and the brainstem, including the substantia nigra. The information is integrated within the corpus striatum, and the outflow passes back to the areas listed above. This circular pathway is believed to function as follows.

The activity of the basal nuclei is initiated by information received from the premotor and supplemental areas of the motor cortex, the primary sensory cortex, the thalamus, and the brainstem. The outflow from the basal nuclei is channeled through the globus pallidus, which then influences the activities of the motor areas of the cerebral cortex or other motor centers in the brainstem. Thus, the basal nuclei control muscular movements by influencing the cerebral cortex and have no direct control through descending pathways to the brainstem and spinal cord. In this way, the basal nuclei assist in the regulation of voluntary movement and the learning of motor skills.

Writing the letters of the alphabet, drawing a diagram, passing a football, using the vocal cords in talking and singing, and using the eye muscles when looking at an object are a few examples where the basal nuclei influence the skilled cortical motor activities.

Destruction of the primary motor cerebral cortex prevents the individual from performing fine discrete movements of the hands and feet on the opposite side of the body (see p. 290). However, the individual is still capable of performing gross crude movements of the opposite limbs. If destruction of the corpus striatum then takes place, paralysis of the remaining movements of the opposite side of the body occurs.

The basal nuclei not only influence the execution of a particular movement of, say, the limbs but also help prepare for the movements. This may be achieved by controlling the axial and girdle movements of the body and the positioning of the proximal parts of the limbs. The activity in certain neurons of the globus pallidus increases before active movements take place in the distal limb muscles. This important preparatory function enables the trunk and limbs to be placed in appropriate positions before the primary motor part of the cerebral cortex activates discrete movements in the hands and feet.

Clinical Notes

Disorders of the basal nuclei are of two general types. **Hyperkinetic disorders** involve excessive and abnormal movements, such as seen with chorea, athetosis, and ballism. **Hypokinetic disorders** involve a lack or slowness of movement. Parkinson disease includes both types of motor disturbances.

Chorea

In chorea, the patient exhibits involuntary, quick, jerky, irregular movements that are nonrepetitive. Swift grimaces and sudden movements of the head or limbs are good examples.

Huntington Disease

Huntington disease is an autosomal dominant inherited disease, with the onset occurring most often in adult life. Death occurs 15 to 20 years after onset. The disease has been traced to a single gene defect on chromosome 4. This gene encodes a protein, **huntingtin**, the function of which is not known. The codon (CAG) that encodes glutamine is repeated many more times than normal. The disease affects men and women with equal frequency and unfortunately often reveals itself only after they have had children.

Patients have the following characteristic signs and symptoms:

1. **Choreiform movements** first appear as involuntary movements of the extremities and twitching of the face (facial grimacing). Later, more muscle groups are involved, so the patient becomes immobile and unable to speak or swallow.
2. **Progressive dementia** occurs with loss of memory and intellectual capacity.

In this disease, the GABA-secreting, substance P–secreting, and acetylcholine-secreting neurons of the striatonigral-inhibiting pathway degenerate. This results in the dopa-secreting neurons of the substantia nigra becoming overactive; thus, the nigrostriatal pathway inhibits the caudate nucleus and the putamen (Fig. 10-6). This inhibition produces the abnormal movements seen in this disease. Computed tomography scans show enlarged lateral ventricles due to degeneration of the caudate nuclei. Medical treatment of Huntington chorea has been disappointing.

Sydenham Chorea

Sydenham chorea (St. Vitus dance) is a disease of childhood in which rapid, irregular, involuntary movements of the limbs, face, and trunk occur. The condition is associated with rheumatic fever. The antigens of the streptococcal bacteria are similar in structure to the proteins present in the membranes of striatal neurons. The host's antibodies not only combine with the bacterial antigens but also attack the membranes of the neurons of the basal ganglia. This results in the production of choreiform movements, which are fortunately transient, and full recovery is made.

Hemiballismus

Hemiballismus is a form of involuntary movement confined to one side of the body. It usually involves the proximal extremity musculature, and the limb suddenly flies about out of control in all directions. The lesion, which is usually a small stroke, occurs in the opposite subthalamic nucleus or its connections; smooth movements of different parts of the body are integrated in the subthalamic nucleus.

Parkinson Disease

Parkinson disease is a progressive disease of unknown cause that commences between the ages of 45 and 55 years. It is associated with neuronal degeneration in the **substantia nigra** and, to a lesser extent, in the **globus pallidus**, **putamen**, and **caudate nucleus**. The disease affects about 1 million people in the United States.

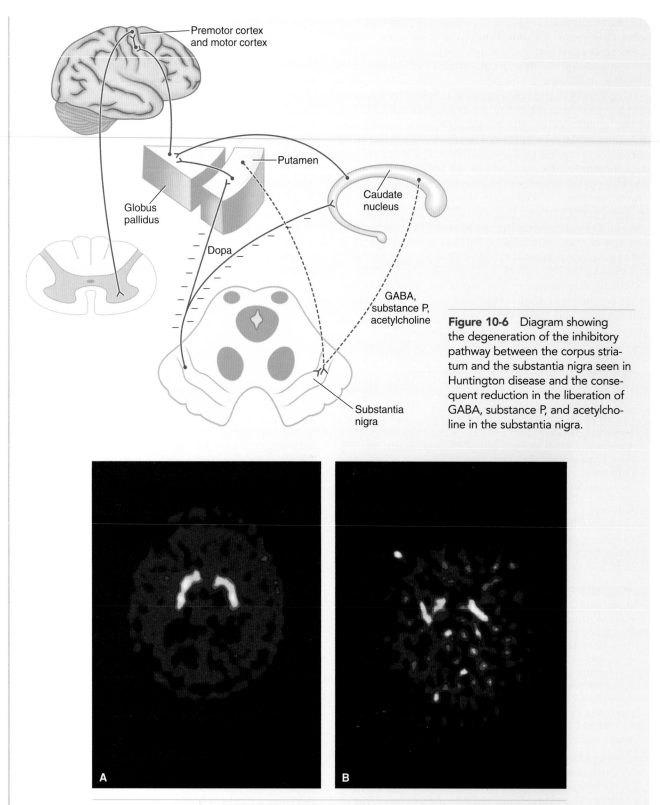

Figure 10-6 Diagram showing the degeneration of the inhibitory pathway between the corpus striatum and the substantia nigra seen in Huntington disease and the consequent reduction in the liberation of GABA, substance P, and acetylcholine in the substantia nigra.

Figure 10-7 Axial (horizontal) positron emission tomography (PET) scans of a normal brain (**A**) and the brain of a patient with early Parkinson disease (**B**) following the injection of 18-F-fluorodopa. The normal brain image shows large amounts of the compound (yellow areas) distributed throughout the corpus striatum in both cerebral hemispheres. In the patient with Parkinson disease, the brain image shows that the total amount of the compound is low, and it is unevenly distributed in the corpus striatum. (Courtesy Dr. Holley Dey.)

Figure 10-8 Diagram showing the degeneration of the inhibitory pathway between the substantia nigra and the corpus striatum in Parkinson disease and the consequent reduction in the release of the neurotransmitter dopamine in the striatum.

The degeneration of the neurons of the substantia nigra that send their axons to the corpus striatum results in a reduction in the release of the neurotransmitter dopamine within the corpus striatum (Figs. 10-7 and 10-8). This leads to hypersensitivity of the dopamine receptors in the postsynaptic neurons in the striatum.

Patients have the following characteristic signs and symptoms:

1. **Tremor.** This is the result of the alternating contraction of agonists and antagonists. The tremor is slow and occurs most obviously when the limbs are at rest. It disappears during sleep. It should be distinguished from the intention tremor seen in cerebellar disease, which only occurs when purposeful active movement is attempted.
2. **Rigidity.** This differs from the rigidity caused by lesions of the upper motor neurons in that it is present to an equal extent in opposing muscle groups. If the tremor is absent, the rigidity is felt as resistance to passive movement and is sometimes referred to as **plastic** rigidity. If the tremor is present, the muscle resistance is overcome as a series of jerks, called **cogwheel** rigidity.
3. **Bradykinesis.** Initiating (**akinesia**) and performing new movements is difficult. The movements are slow, the face is expressionless, and the voice is slurred and unmodulated. Swinging of the arms in walking is lost.
4. **Postural disturbances.** The patient stands with a stoop, and his or her arms are flexed. The patient walks by taking short steps and often is unable to stop. In fact, he or she may break into a shuffling run to maintain balance.
5. Neither loss of muscle power nor loss of sensibility occurs. Since the corticospinal tracts are normal, the superficial abdominal reflexes are normal, and no Babinski response is seen. The deep tendon reflexes are normal.

In a few types of Parkinson disease, the cause is known. **Postencephalitic** parkinsonism developed following the viral encephalitis outbreak of 1916 to 1917, in which damage occurred to the basal nuclei. **Iatrogenic** parkinsonism can be a side effect of antipsychotic drugs (e.g., phenothiazines). Meperidine analogues (used by drug addicts) and poisoning from carbon monoxide and manganese can also produce the symptoms of parkinsonism. **Atherosclerotic** parkinsonism can occur in elderly hypertensive patients.

Parkinson disease may be treated by elevating the brain dopamine level. Unfortunately, dopamine cannot cross the blood–brain barrier, but its immediate precursor L-dopa can and is used in its place. L-Dopa is taken up by the dopaminergic neurons in the basal nuclei and converted to dopamine. Selegiline, a drug that inhibits monoamine oxidase, which is responsible for destroying dopamine, is also of benefit in the treatment of the disease. Evidence shows that selegiline can slow the process of degeneration of the dopa-secreting neurons in the substantia nigra.

Transplantation of human embryonic dopamine-producing neurons into the caudate nucleus and putamen has been

Figure 10-9 Change in 18-F-fluorodopa uptake in the brains of patients with Parkinson disease after transplantation, as shown in fluorodopa PET scans. In the panel on the far left, an axial (horizontal) section through the caudate nucleus and putamen of a normal subject shows intense uptake of 18-F-fluorodopa (red). On the right side, the upper panels show preoperative and 12-month postoperative scans in a patient in the transplantation group. Before surgery, the uptake of 18-F-fluorodopa was restricted to the region of the caudate nucleus. After transplantation, there was increased uptake of 18-F-fluorodopa in the putamen bilaterally. The lower panels show 18-F-fluorodopa scans in a patient in the sham-surgery group. There was no postoperative change in 18-F-fluorodopa uptake. (Courtesy of Freed, C. R., Greene, P. E., Breeze, R. E., et al. (2001). Transplantation of embryonic dopamine neurons for severe Parkinson's disease. *New England Journal of Medicine, 344*(10), 710–719.)

shown to lead to improvement in motor function in Parkinson disease (Fig. 10-9). Evidence shows that the grafts can survive, and synaptic contacts are made. Unfortunately, many of the grafted neurons do not survive, and in many cases, the clinical improvement is counteracted by the continuing degeneration of the patient's own dopa-producing neurons. Autotransplantation of suprarenal medullary cells can be a source of dopa-producing cells, but in the future, genetically engineered cells could be another source of dopa.

Since most of the symptoms of Parkinson disease are caused by an increased inhibitory output from the basal nuclei to the thalamus and the precentral motor cortex, surgical lesions in the globus pallidus (**pallidotomy**) have been shown to be effective in alleviating parkinsonian signs. At the present time, such procedures are restricted to patients who are no longer responding to medical treatment.

Drug-Induced Parkinsonism

Although Parkinson disease (primary parkinsonism) is the most common type of parkinsonism found in clinical practice, drug-induced parkinsonism is becoming very prevalent. Drugs that block striatal dopamine receptors (D2) are often given for psychotic behavior (e.g., phenothiazines and butyrophenones). Other drugs may deplete striatal dopamine (e.g., tetrabenazines). Drug-induced parkinsonism disappears once the agent is withdrawn.

Athetosis

Athetosis consists of slow, sinuous, writhing movements that most commonly involve the distal segments of the limbs. Degeneration of the globus pallidus occurs with a breakdown of the circuitry involving the basal nuclei and the cerebral cortex.

Key Concepts

- The corpus striatum comprises gray matter that sits lateral to the thalamus and is divided by the internal capsule into the caudate nucleus and lentiform nucleus.

- The caudate nucleus is a large C-shaped structure, forming the lateral wall and floor of the lateral ventricle, and is divided into a head, body, and tail. It terminates anteriorly in the amygdaloid nucleus.

- The lentiform nucleus consists of two nuclei, the putamen and globus pallidus. The paleness of the globus pallidus is due to the high concentration of myelinated nerve fibers.

- The corpus striatum, along with amygdaloid nucleus, substantia nigra, subthalamic nuclei, and claustrum, forms numerous complex afferent and efferent pathways.

- This circular process is initiated by motor information from the cortex, thalamus, and brainstem, processed by structures of the basal ganglia, and then channeled through the globus pallidus to influence muscular movements by returning and influencing the cerebral cortex.

- The basal nuclei not only influence the execution of a particular movement but also help prepare for movements (i.e., placing the trunk in the appropriate position in preparation for the movement by the lower limbs).

? Clinical Problem Solving

1. A 10-year-old girl is seen by a neurologist because of the gradual development of involuntary movements. To begin with, the movements are regarded by her parents as general restlessness, but later, abnormal facial grimacing and jerking movements of the arms and legs occur. The child is now having difficulty in performing normal movements of the arms, and walking is becoming increasingly difficult. The abnormal movements appear to be worse in the upper limbs and are more exaggerated on the right side of the body. The movements are made worse when the child becomes excited but disappear completely when she sleeps. The child is recently treated for rheumatic fever. Is there any possible connection between this child's symptoms and the basal nuclei in the cerebral hemispheres?

2. A 40-year-old man complaining of rapid and jerky involuntary movements involving the upper and lower limbs is seen by his physician. The condition started about 6 months ago and is getting progressively worse. He says that he is extremely worried about his health because his father had developed similar symptoms 20 years ago and had died in a mental institution. His wife tells the physician that her husband also suffers from episodes of extreme depression and that she has noticed that he has periods of irritability and impulsive behavior. The physician makes the diagnosis of Huntington chorea. Using your knowledge of neuroanatomy, explain how this disease involves the basal nuclei.

3. A 61-year-old man suddenly develops uncoordinated movements of the trunk and right arm. The right upper limb will suddenly, vigorously, and aimlessly be thrown about, knocking over anything in its path. The patient is recovering from a right-sided hemiplegia, secondary to a cerebral hemorrhage. What is the name given to this clinical sign? Does this condition involve the basal nuclei?

Answers and Explanations to Clinical Problem Solving

1. This child is suffering from Sydenham chorea (see p. 315). This condition occurs, in the majority of cases, in female children between the ages of 5 and 15 years. It is characterized by the presence of rapid, irregular, involuntary movements that are purposeless. The disease is associated with rheumatic fever, and complete recovery is the rule.

2. Huntington chorea is a progressive inherited disease that usually appears between the ages of 30 and

45 years. The involuntary movements are usually more rapid and jerky than those seen in patients with Sydenham chorea. Progressive mental changes lead to dementia and death. The GABA-secreting, substance P–secreting, and acetylcholine-secreting neurons of the striatonigral pathway progressively degenerate. This results in the dopamine-secreting neurons of the substantia nigra becoming overactive; thus, the nigrostriatal pathway inhibits the caudate nucleus and the putamen. This causes the involuntary movements. Atrophy of the caudate nucleus and putamen occurs.

3. The clinical sign is known as hemiballismus. The sudden onset is usually caused by vascular impairment due to hemorrhage or occlusion. Yes, hemiballismus does involve the basal nuclei; it is the result of destruction of the contralateral subthalamic nucleus or its neuronal connections, causing the violent, uncoordinated movements of the axial and proximal limb muscles.

 Review Questions

Directions: Each of the numbered items in this section is followed by answers. Select the ONE lettered answer that is CORRECT.

1. The following statements concern the basal nuclei (ganglia):
   (a) The caudate nucleus and the red nucleus form the neostriatum (striatum).
   (b) The head of the caudate nucleus is connected to the putamen.
   (c) The tegmentum of the midbrain forms part of the basal nuclei.
   (d) The internal capsule lies lateral to the globus pallidus.
   (e) The basal nuclei are formed of white matter.

2. The following statements concern the basal nuclei (ganglia):
   (a) The amygdaloid nucleus is connected to the caudate nucleus.
   (b) The lentiform nucleus is completely divided by the external capsule into the globus pallidus and the putamen.
   (c) The claustrum does not form part of the basal nuclei.
   (d) The corpus striatum lies medial to the thalamus.
   (e) The function of the claustrum is well known.

3. The following statements concern the basal nuclei (ganglia):
   (a) The corpus striatum is made up of the caudate nucleus and the amygdaloid nucleus.
   (b) The head of the caudate nucleus lies lateral to the internal capsule.
   (c) The insula forms part of the basal nuclei.
   (d) The tail of the caudate nucleus lies in the roof of the lateral ventricle.
   (e) The subthalamic nuclei are functionally closely related to the basal nuclei and are considered to be part of them.

4. The following statements concern the caudate nucleus:
   (a) It is divided into a head, neck, trunk, and tail.
   (b) It is an M-shaped mass of gray matter.
   (c) The body of the caudate nucleus forms part of the roof of the body of the lateral ventricle.
   (d) The head lies medial to the anterior horn of the lateral ventricle.
   (e) The tail terminates anteriorly in the amygdaloid nucleus.

5. The following statements concern the afferent corticostriate fibers to the corpus striatum:
   (a) Each part of the cerebral cortex is randomly projected to different parts of the corpus striatum.
   (b) Glutamate is not the neurotransmitter.
   (c) All parts of the cerebral cortex send fibers to the caudate nucleus and putamen.
   (d) The smallest input is from the sensory motor part of the cerebral cortex.
   (e) Most of the projections are from the cortex of the opposite side.

6. The following statements concern the nigrostriatal fibers:
   (a) The neurons in the substantia nigra send axons to the putamen.
   (b) Acetylcholine is the neurotransmitter.
   (c) The nigrostriatal fibers are stimulatory in function.
   (d) The caudate nucleus does not receive axons from the substantia nigra.
   (e) Parkinson disease is caused by an increase in the release of dopamine within the corpus striatum.

7. The following statements concern the efferent fibers of the corpus striatum:
   (a) Many of the efferent fibers descend directly to the motor nuclei of the cranial nerves.
   (b) Some of the striatopallidal fibers have GABA as the neurotransmitter.
   (c) The striatonigral fibers pass from the red nucleus to the substantia nigra.
   (d) Many of the efferent fibers pass directly to the cerebellum.
   (e) The anterior horn cells of the spinal cord are influenced directly by the efferent fibers from the corpus striatum.

8. The following statements concern the functions of the basal nuclei (ganglia):
   (a) The corpus striatum integrates information received directly from the cerebellar cortex.
   (b) The outflow of the basal nuclei is channeled through the globus pallidus to the sensory areas of the cerebral cortex, thus influencing muscular activities.
   (c) The globus pallidus only influences the movements of the axial part of the body.
   (d) The activities of the globus pallidus precede the activities of the motor cortex concerned with discrete movements of the hands and feet.
   (e) The activities of the basal nuclei are suppressed by information received from the sensory cortex, the thalamus, and the brainstem.

Matching Questions. Directions: The following questions apply to Figure 10-10. Match the numbers listed below on the left with the appropriate lettered structure listed on the right. Each lettered option may be selected once, more than once, or not at all.

9.	Number 1	(a)	Anterior horn of lateral ventricle
10.	Number 2	(b)	Internal capsule
11.	Number 3	(c)	Claustrum
12.	Number 4	(d)	Putamen
13.	Number 5	(e)	External capsule
14.	Number 6	(f)	Globus pallidus
		(g)	None of the above

Figure 10-10 Horizontal section of the cerebrum.

 Answers and Explanations to Review Questions

1. B is correct. The head of the caudate nucleus is connected to the putamen of the lentiform nucleus (see Fig. 10-1). A. The caudate nucleus and the putamen form the neostriatum. C. The tegmentum of the midbrain does not form part of the basal nuclei. D. The internal capsule lies medial to the apex of the globus pallidus (see Fig. 10-2). E. The basal nuclei are formed of gray matter.

2. A is correct. The amygdaloid nucleus is connected to the caudate nucleus (see Fig. 10-1). B. The lentiform nucleus is not divided by the external capsule into the globus pallidus and the putamen (see Fig. 10-2). C. The claustrum forms part of the basal nuclei. D. The corpus striatum lies lateral to the thalamus (see Fig. 10-2). E. The function of the claustrum is unknown.

3. D is correct. The tail of the caudate nucleus lies in the roof of the lateral ventricle (see Fig. 10-2). A. The corpus striatum is made up of the caudate nucleus and the lentiform nucleus. B. The head of the caudate nucleus lies medial to the internal capsule (see Fig. 10-2). C. The insula does not form part of the basal nuclei. E. The subthalamic nuclei are functionally closely related to the basal nuclei but are not considered to be part of them.

4. E is correct. The tail of the caudate nucleus terminates anteriorly in the amygdaloid nucleus (see Fig. 10-1). A. The caudate nucleus is divided into the head, body, and tail (see Fig. 10-1). B. The caudate nucleus is a C-shaped mass of gray matter (see Fig. 10-1). C. The body of the caudate nucleus forms part of the floor of the body of the lateral ventricle (see Fig. 10-1). D. The head of the caudate nucleus lies lateral to the anterior horn of the lateral ventricle (see Fig. 10-2).

5. C is correct. All parts of the cerebral cortex send fibers to the caudate nucleus and putamen. A. Each part of the cerebral cortex is projected to specific parts of the corpus striatum. B. Glutamate is the neurotransmitter at the nerve endings of the corticostriate fibers to the corpus striatum (see Fig. 10-4). D. The largest input to the different parts of the corpus striatum is from the sensory motor part of the cerebral cortex. E. Most of the projection fibers are from the cerebral cortex of the same side.

6. A is correct. The neurons in the substantia nigra send axons to the putamen (see Fig. 10-3). B. Dopamine is the neurotransmitter at the nerve endings of the nigrostriatal fibers. C. The nigrostriatal fibers are inhibitory in function. D. The caudate nucleus

does receive axons from the substantia nigra. E. Parkinson disease is caused by a reduction in the release of dopamine within the corpus striatum.

7. B is correct. Some of the striatopallidal fibers have GABA as the neurotransmitter. A. None of the efferent fibers from the corpus striatum descend directly to the motor nuclei of the cranial nerves. C. The striatonigral fibers pass from the caudate nucleus to the substantia nigra (see Fig. 10-3). D. No efferent fibers from the corpus striatum pass directly to the cerebellum. E. The anterior horn cells of the spinal cord are not influenced directly by the efferent fibers from the corpus striatum.

8. D is correct. The activities of the globus pallidus precede the activities of the motor cerebral cortex concerned with discrete movements of the hands and feet. A. The corpus striatum does not integrate information received directly from the cerebellar cortex.

B. The outflow of the basal nuclei is channeled through the globus pallidus to the motor areas of the cerebral cortex, thus influencing muscular activities. C. The globus pallidus influences movements of the entire body. E. The activities of the basal nuclei are initiated by information received from the sensory cortex, the thalamus, and the brainstem.

The answers for Figure 10-10, which shows a horizontal section of the cerebrum, are as follows:

9. F is correct. Structure 1 is the globus pallidus.
10. B is correct. Structure 2 is the internal capsule.
11. D is correct. Structure 3 is the putamen.
12. E is correct. Structure 4 is the external capsule.
13. C is correct. Structure 5 is the claustrum.
14. A is correct. Structure 6 is the anterior horn of the lateral ventricle.

11 Cranial Nerve Nuclei

See Atlas Plates 1, 6, and 8.

CHAPTER OBJECTIVES

- To learn the basic information regarding the motor and sensory nuclei of the cranial nerves, including their locations and central connections

- Understand the functional ramifications of lesions to cranial nerve nuclei versus damage of the cranial nerve proper

A 49-year-old man wakes up one morning to find the right side of his face paralyzed. When examined by his local medical practitioner, he is found to have complete paralysis of the entire right side of the face. He is also found to have severe hypertension. The patient talks with slightly slurred speech. The physician tells the patient that he has suffered a mild stroke, and he is admitted to the hospital.

The patient is later seen by a neurologist who disagrees with the diagnosis. The original physician grouped together the facial paralysis, the slurred speech, and the hypertension and, in the absence of other findings, made the incorrect diagnosis of cerebral hemorrhage. A lesion of the corticonuclear fibers on one side of the brain will cause paralysis only of the muscles of the lower part of the opposite side of the face. This patient has complete paralysis of the entire right side of the face, which could only be caused by a lesion of the lower motor neuron. The correct diagnosis was Bell palsy, an inflammation of the connective tissue sheath of the facial nerve, which temporarily interfered with the functions of the axons of the right facial nerve. This case provides a good example of how knowledge of the central connections of a cranial nerve enables a physician to make the correct diagnosis.

The cranial nerves are commonly damaged by trauma or disease, and testing for their integrity forms part of every physical examination.

CRANIAL NERVES

The 12 pairs of cranial nerves (CNs) leave the brain and pass through foramina and fissures in the skull. All the nerves are distributed in the head and neck, except CN X, which also supplies structures in the thorax and abdomen. The CNs are named as follows:

1. Olfactory
2. Optic
3. Oculomotor
4. Trochlear
5. Trigeminal
6. Abducens
7. Facial
8. Vestibulocochlear
9. Glossopharyngeal
10. Vagus
11. Accessory
12. Hypoglossal

See Atlas Plates 1, 6, and 8.

CRANIAL NERVE ORGANIZATION

The olfactory, optic, and vestibulocochlear nerves are entirely sensory. The oculomotor, trochlear, abducens, accessory, and hypoglossal nerves are entirely motor. The trigeminal, facial, glossopharyngeal, and vagus nerves are both sensory and motor nerves. The letter symbols commonly used to indicate the functional components of each cranial nerve are shown in Table 11-1. The cranial nerves have central motor and/or sensory nuclei within the brain and peripheral nerve fibers that emerge from the brain and exit from the skull to reach their effector or sensory organs.

The different components of the cranial nerves, their functions, and the openings in the skull through which the nerves leave the cranial cavity are summarized in Table 11-2.

Cranial Nerve Motor Nuclei

The motor nuclei of the cranial nerves receive impulses from the cerebral cortex through the corticonuclear

Table 11-1 The Letter Symbols Commonly Used to Indicate the Functional Components of Each Cranial Nerve

Component	Function	Letter Symbols
Afferent Fibers	**Sensory**	
General somatic afferent	General sensations	GSA
Special somatic afferent	Hearing, balance, vision	SSA
General visceral afferent	Viscera	GVA
Special visceral afferent	Smell, taste	SVA
Efferent Fibers		
General somatic efferent	Somatic striated muscles	GSE
General visceral efferent	Glands and smooth muscles (parasympathetic innervation)	GVE
Special visceral efferent	Branchial arch striated muscles	SVE

Table 11-2 Cranial Nerves

Number	Name	Components[a]	Function	Opening in Skull
I	Olfactory	Sensory (SVA)	Smell	Openings in cribriform plate of ethmoid
II	Optic	Sensory (SSA)	Vision	Optic canal
III	Oculomotor	Motor (GSE, GVE)	Raises upper eyelid, turns eyeball upward, downward, and medially; constricts pupil; accommodates eye	Superior orbital fissure
IV	Trochlear	Motor (GSE)	Assists in turning eyeball downward and laterally	Superior orbital fissure
V	Trigeminal[b]			
	Ophthalmic division	Sensory (GSA)	Cornea, skin of forehead, scalp, eyelids, and nose; also mucous membrane of paranasal sinuses and nasal cavity	Superior orbital fissure
	Maxillary division	Sensory (GSA)	Skin of face over maxilla; teeth of upper jaw; mucous membrane of nose, the maxillary sinus, and palate	Foramen rotundum
	Mandibular division	Motor (SVE)	Muscles of mastication, mylohyoid, anterior belly of digastric, tensor veli palatini, and tensor tympani	Foramen ovale
		Sensory (GSA)	Skin of cheek, skin over mandible and side of head, teeth of lower jaw and temporomandibular joint; mucous membrane of mouth and anterior part of tongue	
VI	Abducent	Motor (GSE)	Lateral rectus muscle turns eyeball laterally	Superior orbital fissure
VII	Facial	Motor (SVE)	Muscles of face and scalp, stapedius muscle, posterior belly of digastric, and stylohyoid muscles	Internal acoustic meatus, facial canal, stylomastoid foramen
		Sensory (SVA)	Taste from anterior two-thirds of tongue, from floor of mouth and palate	
		Secretomotor (GVE) parasympathetic	Submandibular and sublingual salivary glands, the lacrimal gland, and glands of nose and palate	

(continued)

Table 11-2   Cranial Nerves (*Continued*)

Number	Name	Components[a]	Function	Opening in Skull
VIII	Vestibulocochlear			
	Vestibular	Sensory (SSA)	From utricle and saccule and semicircular canals—position and movement of head	Internal acoustic meatus
	Cochlear	Sensory (SSA)	Organ of Corti—hearing	
IX	Glossopharyngeal	Motor (SVE)	Stylopharyngeus muscle—assists swallowing	Jugular foramen
		Secretomotor (GVE) parasympathetic	Parotid salivary gland	
		Sensory (GVA, SVA, GSA)	General sensation and taste from posterior third of tongue and pharynx; carotid sinus (baroreceptor); and carotid body (chemoreceptor)	
X	Vagus	Motor (GVE, SVE) Sensory (GVA, SVA, GSA)	Heart and great thoracic blood vessels; larynx, trachea, bronchi, and lungs; alimentary tract from pharynx to splenic flexure of colon; liver, kidneys, and pancreas	Jugular foramen
XI	Accessory			
	Cranial root	Motor (SVE)	Muscles of soft palate (except tensor veli palatini), pharynx (except stylopharyngeus), and larynx (except cricothyroid) in branches of vagus	Jugular foramen
	Spinal root	Motor (SVE)	Sternocleidomastoid and trapezius muscles	
XII	Hypoglossal	Motor (GSE)	Muscles of tongue (except palatoglossus) controlling its shape and movement	Hypoglossal canal

[a]The letter symbols are explained in Table 11-1.
[b]The trigeminal nerve also carries proprioceptive impulses from the muscles of mastication and the facial and extraocular muscles.

(corticobulbar) fibers. These fibers originate from the pyramidal cells in the inferior part of the precentral gyrus (area 4) and from the adjacent part of the postcentral gyrus. The corticonuclear fibers descend through the **corona radiata** and the **genu of the internal capsule**. They pass through the midbrain just medial to the corticospinal fibers in the **basis pedunculi** and end by synapsing either directly with the lower motor neurons within the cranial nerve nuclei or indirectly through the **internuncial neurons**. The corticonuclear fibers thus constitute the **first-order neuron** of the descending pathway, the internuncial neuron constitutes the **second-order neuron**, and the lower motor neuron constitutes the **third-order neuron**.

The majority of the corticonuclear fibers to the motor cranial nerve nuclei cross the median plane before reaching the nuclei. Bilateral connections are present for all the cranial motor nuclei except for part of the facial nucleus that supplies the muscles of the lower part of the face and a part of the hypoglossal nucleus that supplies the genioglossus muscle.

Somatic Motor and Branchiomotor Nuclei

The somatic motor and branchiomotor nerve fibers of a cranial nerve are the axons of nerve cells situated within the brain. These nerve cell groups form motor nuclei and innervate striated muscle. Each nerve cell with its processes is referred to as a **lower motor neuron**. Such a nerve cell is, therefore, equivalent to the motor cells in the anterior gray columns of the spinal cord.

General Visceral Motor Nuclei

The general visceral motor nuclei form the cranial outflow of the parasympathetic portion of the autonomic nervous system. They are the **Edinger–Westphal nucleus** of the oculomotor nerve, the **superior salivatory** and **lacrimal nuclei** of the facial nerve, the **inferior salivatory nucleus** of the glossopharyngeal nerve, and the **dorsal motor nucleus** of the vagus. These nuclei receive numerous afferent fibers, including descending pathways from the hypothalamus.

Cranial Nerve Sensory Nuclei

Sensory nuclei of the cranial nerves include somatic and visceral afferent nuclei. The sensory or afferent parts of a cranial nerve are the axons of nerve cells outside the brain and are situated in ganglia on the nerve trunks (equivalent to posterior root ganglion of a spinal nerve) or may be situated in a sensory organ, such as the nose, eye, or ear. These cells and their processes form the **first-order neuron**. The central processes of these cells enter the brain and terminate by synapsing with cells forming the sensory nuclei. These cells and their processes form the **second-order neuron**. Axons from these nuclear cells now cross the midline and ascend to other sensory nuclei, such as the thalamus, where they synapse. The nerve cells of these nuclei form the **third-order neuron**, and their axons terminate in the cerebral cortex.

OLFACTORY NERVES (CRANIAL NERVE I)

The olfactory nerves arise from the olfactory receptor nerve cells in the olfactory mucous membrane located in the upper part of the nasal cavity above the level of the superior concha (Fig. 11-1). The **olfactory receptor cells** are scattered among supporting cells. Each receptor cell consists of a small bipolar nerve cell with

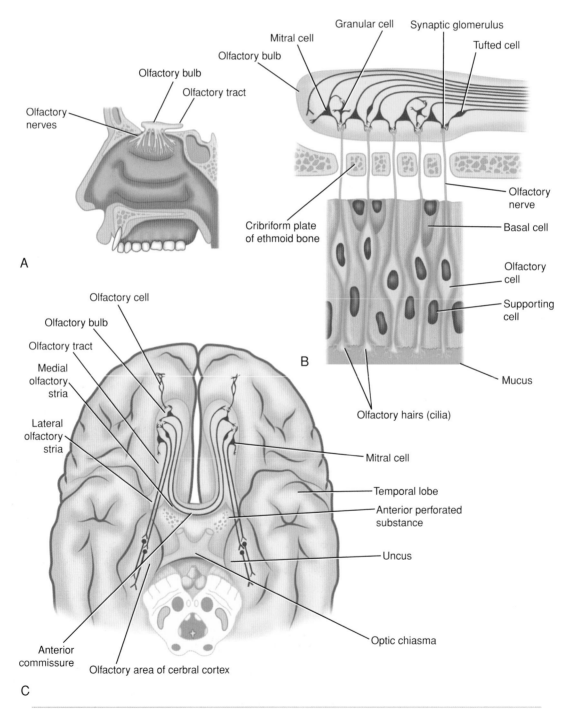

Figure 11-1   A: Distribution of olfactory nerves on the lateral wall of the nose. **B:** Connections between the olfactory cells and the neurons of the olfactory bulb. **C:** Connections between the olfactory cell and the rest of the olfactory system.

a coarse peripheral process that passes to the surface of the membrane and a fine central process. From the coarse peripheral process, a number of short cilia arise, the **olfactory hairs**, which project into the mucus covering the surface of the mucous membrane. These projecting hairs react to odors in the air and stimulate the olfactory cells.

The fine central processes form the **olfactory nerve fibers** (see Fig. 11-1A,B). Bundles of these nerve fibers pass through the openings of the cribriform plate of the ethmoid bone to enter the olfactory bulb. The olfactory nerve fibers are unmyelinated and are covered with Schwann cells.

Olfactory Bulb

This ovoid structure possesses several types of nerve cells, the largest of which is the **mitral cell** (see Fig. 11-1C). The incoming olfactory nerve fibers synapse with the dendrites of the mitral cells and form rounded areas known as **synaptic glomeruli**. Smaller nerve cells, called **tufted cells** and **granular cells**, also synapse with the mitral cells. The olfactory bulb, in addition, receives axons from the contralateral olfactory bulb through the olfactory tract.

Olfactory Tract

This narrow band of white matter runs from the posterior end of the olfactory bulb beneath the inferior surface of the frontal lobe of the brain (see Fig. 11-1B). It consists of the axons of the mitral and tufted cells of the bulb and some centrifugal fibers from the opposite olfactory bulb.

As the olfactory tract reaches the **anterior perforated substance**, it divides into **medial** and **lateral olfactory striae**. The lateral stria carries the axons to the **olfactory area of the cerebral cortex**, namely, the **periamygdaloid** and **prepiriform areas** (see Fig. 11-1C). The medial olfactory stria carries the fibers that cross the median plane in the anterior commissure to pass to the olfactory bulb of the opposite side.

The periamygdaloid and prepiriform areas of the cerebral cortex are often known as the **primary olfactory cortex**. The **entorhinal area** (**area 28**) of the parahippocampal gyrus, which receives numerous connections from the primary olfactory cortex, is called the **secondary olfactory cortex**. These areas of the cortex are responsible for the appreciation of olfactory sensations. Note that in contrast to all other sensory pathways, the olfactory afferent pathway has only two neurons and reaches the cerebral cortex without synapsing in one of the thalamic nuclei.

The primary olfactory cortex sends nerve fibers to many other centers within the brain to establish connections for emotional and autonomic responses to olfactory sensations.

OPTIC NERVE (CRANIAL NERVE II)

The fibers of the optic nerve are the axons of the cells in the **ganglionic layer** of the retina. They converge on the **optic disc** and exit from the eye, about 3 or 4 mm to the nasal side of its center, as the optic nerve (Fig. 11-2). The fibers of the optic nerve are myelinated, but the sheaths are formed from oligodendrocytes rather than Schwann cells, since the optic nerve is comparable to a tract within the central nervous system.

The optic nerve leaves the orbital cavity through the optic canal and unites with the optic nerve of the opposite side to form the **optic chiasma**.

Optic Chiasma

The optic chiasma is situated at the junction of the anterior wall and floor of the third ventricle. Its anterolateral angles are continuous with the optic nerves, and the posterolateral angles are continuous with the optic tracts. In the chiasma, the fibers from the nasal (medial) half of each retina, including the nasal half of the **macula**, cross the midline and enter the optic tract of the opposite side, while the fibers from the temporal (lateral) half of each retina, including the temporal half of the **macula**, pass posteriorly in the optic tract of the same side.

Optic Tract

The optic tract emerges from the optic chiasma and passes posterolaterally around the cerebral peduncle. Most of the fibers now terminate by synapsing with nerve cells in the **lateral geniculate body**, which is a small projection from the posterior part of the thalamus. A few of the fibers pass to the **pretectal nucleus** and the **superior colliculus** of the midbrain and are concerned with light reflexes (Fig. 11-3).

Lateral Geniculate Body

The lateral geniculate body is a small, oval swelling projecting from the **pulvinar of the thalamus**. It consists of six layers of cells, on which synapse the axons from the optic tract. The axons of the nerve cells within the geniculate body leave it to form the **optic radiation** (see Fig. 11-2).

Optic Radiation

The fibers of the optic radiation are the axons of the nerve cells of the lateral geniculate body. The tract passes posteriorly through the retrolenticular part of the **internal capsule** and terminates in the **visual cortex (area 17)**, which occupies the upper and lower lips of the calcarine sulcus on the medial surface of the cerebral hemisphere. The visual association cortex (areas 18 and 19) is responsible for recognition of objects and perception of color.

Visual Pathway and Binocular Vision Neurons

Four neurons conduct visual impulses to the visual cortex: (1) **rods** and **cones**, which are specialized receptor neurons in the retina; (2) **bipolar neurons**, which connect the rods and cones to the ganglion cells; (3) **ganglion**

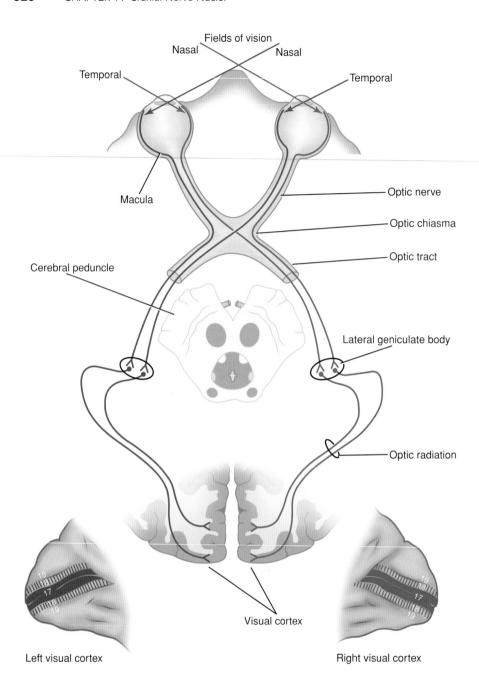

Figure 11-2   Optic pathway.

cells, whose axons pass to the lateral geniculate body; and (4) **neurons of the lateral geniculate body**, whose axons pass to the cerebral cortex.

In binocular vision, the right and left fields of vision are projected on portions of both retinae. The image of an object in the right field of vision is projected on the nasal half of the right retina and the temporal half of the left retina. In the optic chiasma, the axons from these two retinal halves are combined to form the left optic tract. The lateral geniculate body neurons now project the complete right field of vision on the visual cortex of the left hemisphere and the left visual field on the visual cortex of the right hemisphere. The lower retinal quadrants (upper field of vision) project on the lower wall of the calcarine sulcus, while the upper

retinal quadrants (lower field of vision) project on the upper wall of the sulcus. Note also that the **macula lutea** is represented on the posterior part of area 17, and the periphery of the retina is represented anteriorly.

Visual Reflexes

Several unique neuronal pathways exert involuntary control over our vision for optimal visual function, protection, and cognitive processing.

Direct and Consensual Light Reflexes

If a light is shone into one eye, the pupils of both eyes normally constrict. The constriction of the pupil on which the light is shone is called the **direct light reflex**;

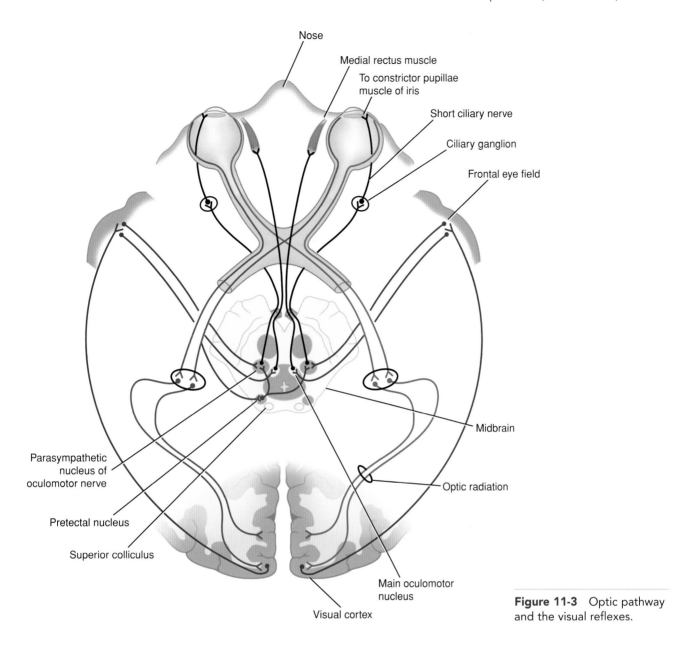

Nose

Medial rectus muscle

To constrictor pupillae muscle of iris

Short ciliary nerve

Ciliary ganglion

Frontal eye field

Midbrain

Optic radiation

Main oculomotor nucleus

Visual cortex

Superior colliculus

Pretectal nucleus

Parasympathetic nucleus of oculomotor nerve

Figure 11-3 Optic pathway and the visual reflexes.

the constriction of the opposite pupil, even though no light fell on that eye, is called the **consensual light reflex** (see Fig. 11-3).

The afferent impulses travel through the optic nerve, optic chiasma, and optic tract. Here, a small number of fibers leave the optic tract and synapse on nerve cells in the **pretectal nucleus**, which lies close to the superior colliculus. The impulses are passed by axons of the pretectal nerve cells to the parasympathetic nuclei (**Edinger–Westphal nuclei**) of the third cranial nerve on **both sides**. Here, the fibers synapse and the parasympathetic nerves travel through the third cranial nerve to the **ciliary ganglion** in the orbit. Finally, postganglionic parasympathetic fibers pass through the **short ciliary nerves** to the eyeball and the **constrictor pupillae muscle** of the iris. Both pupils constrict in the consensual light reflex because the pretectal nucleus sends fibers to the parasympathetic nuclei on both

sides of the midbrain. The fibers that cross the median plane do so close to the cerebral aqueduct in the posterior commissure.

Accommodation Reflex

When the eyes are directed from a distant to a near object, contraction of the medial recti brings about convergence of the ocular axes; the lens thickens to increase its refractive power by contraction of the ciliary muscle; and the pupils constrict to restrict the light waves to the thickest central part of the lens. The afferent impulses travel through the optic nerve, the optic chiasma, the optic tract, the lateral geniculate body, and the optic radiation to the visual cortex. The visual cortex is connected to the eye field of the frontal cortex. From here, cortical fibers descend through the internal capsule to the oculomotor nuclei in the midbrain. The oculomotor nerve travels to the medial recti muscles. Some of the descending cortical fibers synapse with the parasympathetic nuclei (Edinger–Westphal nuclei) of the third cranial nerve on **both sides**. Here, the fibers synapse, and the parasympathetic nerves travel through the third cranial nerve to the ciliary ganglion in the orbit. Finally, postganglionic parasympathetic fibers pass through the short ciliary nerves to the **ciliary muscle** and the **constrictor pupillae muscle** of the iris.

Corneal Reflex

Light touching of the cornea or conjunctiva results in blinking of the eyelids. Afferent impulses from the cornea or conjunctiva travel through the ophthalmic division of the trigeminal nerve to the sensory nucleus of the trigeminal nerve (Fig. 11-4A). Internuncial neurons connect with the motor nucleus of the facial nerve on both sides through the medial longitudinal fasciculus. The facial nerve and its branches supply the orbicularis oculi muscle, which causes closure of the eyelids.

Visual Body Reflexes

The automatic scanning movements of the eyes and head that are made when reading, the automatic movement of the eyes, head, and neck toward the source of

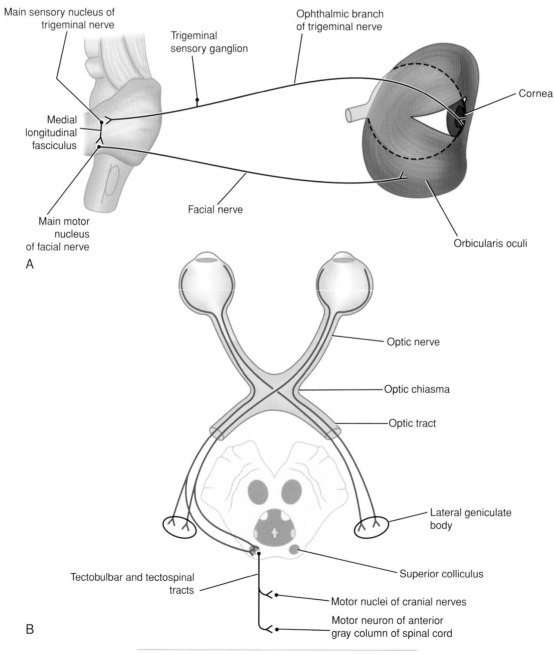

Figure 11-4 A: Corneal reflex. **B:** Visual body reflex.

the visual stimulus, and the protective closing of the eyes and even the raising of the arm for protection are reflex actions that involve the following reflex arcs (see Fig. 11-4B). The visual impulses follow the optic nerves, optic chiasma, and optic tracts to the superior colliculi. Here, the impulses are relayed to the tectospinal and tectobulbar (tectonuclear) tracts and to the neurons of the anterior gray columns of the spinal cord and cranial motor nuclei.

Pupillary Skin Reflex

The pupil will dilate if the skin is painfully stimulated by pinching. The afferent sensory fibers are believed to have connections with the efferent preganglionic sympathetic neurons in the lateral gray columns of the first and second thoracic segments of the spinal cord. The **white rami communicantes** of these segments pass to the sympathetic trunk, and the preganglionic fibers ascend to the superior **cervical sympathetic ganglion**. The postganglionic fibers pass through the **internal carotid plexus**, **long ciliary nerves**, and **short ciliary nerves** to the dilator pupillae muscle of the iris.

OCULOMOTOR NERVE (CRANIAL NERVE III)

The oculomotor nerve is entirely motor in function.

Oculomotor Nerve Nuclei

The oculomotor nerve has two motor nuclei: (1) the main motor nucleus and (2) the accessory parasympathetic nucleus.

The **main oculomotor nucleus** is situated in the anterior part of the gray matter that surrounds the **cerebral aqueduct of the midbrain** (Fig. 11-5). It lies at the level of the **superior colliculus**. The nucleus consists of groups of nerve cells that supply all the extrinsic muscles of the eye except the superior oblique and the lateral rectus. The outgoing nerve fibers pass anteriorly through the red nucleus and emerge on the anterior surface of the midbrain in the **interpeduncular fossa**. The main oculomotor nucleus receives corticonuclear fibers from both cerebral hemispheres. It receives tectobulbar fibers from the superior colliculus and, through this route, receives information from the visual cortex. It also receives fibers from the medial longitudinal fasciculus, by which it is connected to the nuclei of the fourth, sixth, and eighth cranial nerves.

The **accessory** parasympathetic nucleus (**Edinger–Westphal** nucleus) is situated posterior to the main oculomotor nucleus (see Fig. 11-5A). The axons of the nerve cells, which are preganglionic, accompany the other oculomotor fibers to the orbit. Here, they synapse in the **ciliary** ganglion, and postganglionic fibers pass through the **short** ciliary nerves to the constrictor pupillae of the iris and the ciliary muscles. The accessory parasympathetic nucleus receives corticonuclear

fibers for the accommodation reflex, and fibers from the pretectal nucleus for the direct and consensual light reflexes (see Fig. 11-3).

Oculomotor Nerve Course

The oculomotor nerve emerges on the anterior surface of the midbrain (see Fig. 11-5A). It passes forward between the posterior cerebral and the superior cerebellar arteries. It then continues into the middle cranial fossa in the lateral wall of the cavernous sinus. Here, it divides into a superior and an inferior ramus, which enter the orbital cavity through the superior orbital fissure.

The oculomotor nerve supplies the following extrinsic muscles of the eye: the levator palpebrae superioris, superior rectus, medial rectus, inferior rectus, and inferior oblique. It also supplies, through its branch to the ciliary ganglion and the short ciliary nerves, parasympathetic nerve fibers to the following intrinsic muscles: the constrictor pupillae of the iris and ciliary muscles.

Therefore, the oculomotor nerve is entirely motor and is responsible for lifting the upper eyelid; turning the eye upward, downward, and medially; constricting the pupil; and accommodating the eye.

TROCHLEAR NERVE (CRANIAL NERVE IV)

The trochlear nerve is entirely motor in function.

Trochlear Nerve Nucleus

The trochlear nucleus is situated in the anterior part of the gray matter that surrounds the **cerebral aqueduct of the midbrain** (Fig. 11-6). It lies inferior to the oculomotor nucleus at the level of the **inferior colliculus**. The nerve fibers, after leaving the nucleus, pass posteriorly around the central gray matter to reach the posterior surface of the midbrain.

The trochlear nucleus receives corticonuclear fibers from both cerebral hemispheres. It receives the tectobulbar fibers, which connect it to the visual cortex through the superior colliculus (see Fig. 11-6A). It also receives fibers from the **medial longitudinal fasciculus**, by which it is connected to the nuclei of the third, sixth, and eighth cranial nerves.

Trochlear Nerve Course

The trochlear nerve, the most slender of the cranial nerves and the only one to leave the posterior surface of the brainstem, emerges from the midbrain and **immediately decussates with the nerve of the opposite side**. The trochlear nerve passes forward through the middle cranial fossa in the lateral wall of the cavernous sinus and enters the orbit through the superior orbital fissure. The nerve supplies the superior oblique muscle of the eyeball. The trochlear nerve is entirely

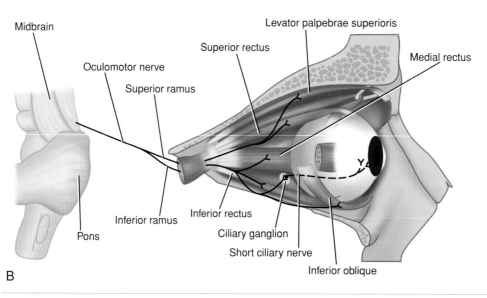

Figure 11-5 **A:** Oculomotor nerve nuclei and their central connections. **B:** The distribution of the oculomotor nerve.

motor and assists in turning the eye downward and laterally.

TRIGEMINAL NERVE (CRANIAL NERVE V)

The trigeminal nerve is the largest cranial nerve and contains both sensory and motor fibers (Fig. 11-7). It is the sensory nerve to the greater part of the head and the motor nerve to several muscles, including the muscles of mastication.

Trigeminal Nerve Nuclei

The trigeminal nerve has four nuclei: (1) the main sensory nucleus, (2) the spinal nucleus, (3) the mesencephalic nucleus, and (4) the motor nucleus.

Main Sensory Nucleus

The main sensory nucleus lies in the posterior part of the pons, lateral to the motor nucleus (see Fig. 11-7A). It is continuous below with the spinal nucleus.

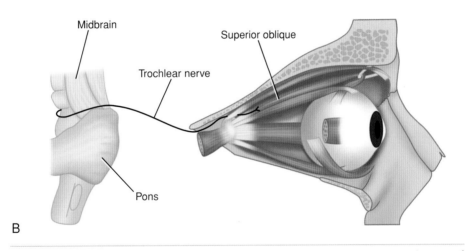

Figure 11-6 **A:** Trochlear nerve nucleus and its central connections. **B:** Distribution of the trochlear nerve.

Spinal Nucleus

The spinal nucleus is continuous superiorly with the main sensory nucleus in the pons and extends inferiorly through the whole length of the medulla oblongata and into the upper part of the spinal cord as far as the second cervical segment (see Fig. 11-7B).

Mesencephalic Nucleus

The mesencephalic nucleus is composed of a column of unipolar nerve cells situated in the lateral part of the gray matter around the cerebral aqueduct. It extends inferiorly into the pons as far as the main sensory nucleus (see Fig. 11-7).

Motor Nucleus

The motor nucleus is situated in the pons, medial to the main sensory nucleus (see Fig. 11-7).

Trigeminal Nerve Sensory Components

The sensations of pain, temperature, touch, and pressure from the skin of the face and mucous membranes travel along axons whose cell bodies are situated in the **semilunar** or **trigeminal** sensory ganglion (see Fig. 11-7B). The central processes of these cells form the large sensory root of the trigeminal nerve. About half the fibers divide into ascending and descending branches when they enter the pons; the remainder ascend or descend without division. The ascending branches terminate in the main sensory nucleus, and the descending branches terminate in the spinal nucleus. The sensations of touch and pressure are conveyed by nerve fibers that terminate in the main sensory nucleus. The sensations of pain and temperature pass to the spinal nucleus. The sensory fibers from the ophthalmic division of the trigeminal nerve terminate in the inferior part of the spinal nucleus;

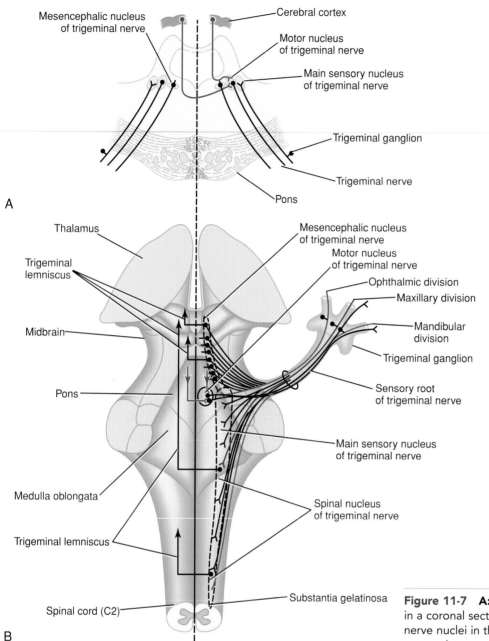

Figure 11-7 A: Trigeminal nerve nuclei seen in a coronal section of the pons. **B:** Trigeminal nerve nuclei in the brainstem and their central connections.

fibers from the maxillary division terminate in the middle of the spinal nucleus; and fibers from the mandibular division end in the superior part of the spinal nucleus.

Proprioceptive impulses from the muscles of mastication and from the facial and extraocular muscles are carried by fibers in the sensory root of the trigeminal nerve that have bypassed the semilunar or trigeminal ganglion. The fibers' cells of origin are the unipolar cells of the mesencephalic nucleus.

The axons of the neurons in the main sensory and spinal nuclei and the central processes of the cells in the mesencephalic nucleus now cross the median plane and ascend as the trigeminal lemniscus to terminate on

the nerve cells of the ventral posteromedial nucleus of the thalamus. The axons of these cells now travel through the internal capsule to the postcentral gyrus (areas 3, 1, and 2) of the cerebral cortex.

Trigeminal Nerve Motor Component

The motor nucleus receives corticonuclear fibers from both cerebral hemispheres (see Fig. 11-7). It also receives fibers from the reticular formation, the red nucleus, the tectum, and the medial longitudinal fasciculus. In addition, it receives fibers from the mesencephalic nucleus, thereby forming a monosynaptic reflex arc.

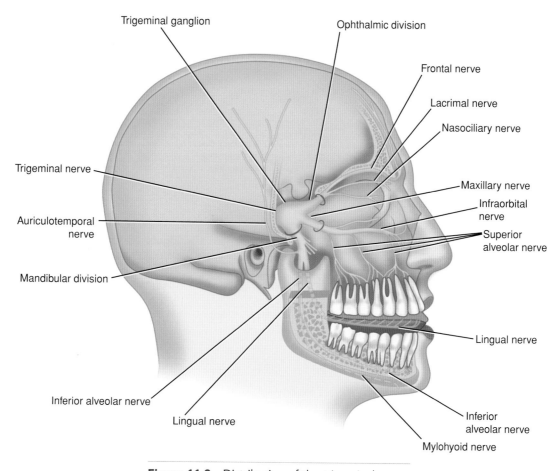

Figure 11-8 Distribution of the trigeminal nerve.

The cells of the motor nucleus give rise to the axons that form the motor root. The motor nucleus supplies the **muscles of mastication**, the **tensor tympani**, the **tensor veli palatini**, and the **mylohyoid** and the **anterior belly of the digastric muscle**.

Trigeminal Nerve Course

The trigeminal nerve leaves the anterior aspect of the pons as a small motor root and a large sensory root. The nerve passes forward out of the posterior cranial fossa and rests on the upper surface of the apex of the petrous part of the temporal bone in the middle cranial fossa. The large sensory root now expands to form the crescent-shaped **trigeminal ganglion**, which lies within a pouch of dura mater called the **trigeminal** or **Meckel cave**. The ophthalmic, maxillary, and mandibular nerves arise from the anterior border of the ganglion (Fig. 11-8). The ophthalmic nerve (V_1) contains only sensory fibers and leaves the skull through the superior orbital fissure to enter the orbital cavity. The maxillary nerve (V_2) also contains only sensory fibers and leaves the skull through the foramen rotundum. The mandibular nerve (V_3) contains both sensory and motor fibers and leaves the skull through the foramen ovale.

The sensory fibers to the skin of the face from each division supply a distinct zone (Fig. 11-9), there being little or no overlap of the dermatomes (compared with the overlap of the dermatomes of the spinal nerves). As noted previously, the motor fibers in the mandibular division are mainly distributed to muscles of mastication.

ABDUCENS NERVE (CRANIAL NERVE VI)

The abducens nerve is a small motor nerve that supplies the **lateral rectus muscle** of the eyeball.

Abducens Nerve Nucleus

The small motor nucleus is situated beneath the floor of the upper part of the fourth ventricle, close to the midline and beneath the **colliculus facialis** (Fig. 11-10A). The nucleus receives afferent corticonuclear fibers from both cerebral hemispheres. It receives the tectobulbar tract from the superior colliculus, by which the visual cortex is connected to the nucleus. It also receives fibers from the medial longitudinal fasciculus, by which it is connected to the nuclei of the third, fourth, and eighth cranial nerves (see Fig. 11-9).

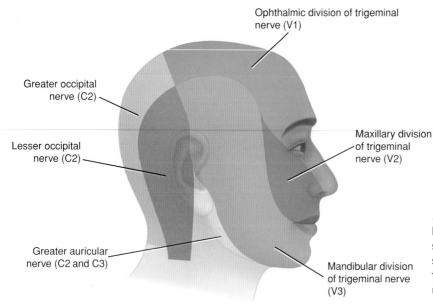

Figure 11-9 Sensory nerve supply to the skin of the head and neck. Note that the skin over the angle of the jaw is supplied by the great auricular nerve (C2 and C3) and not by branches of the trigeminal nerve.

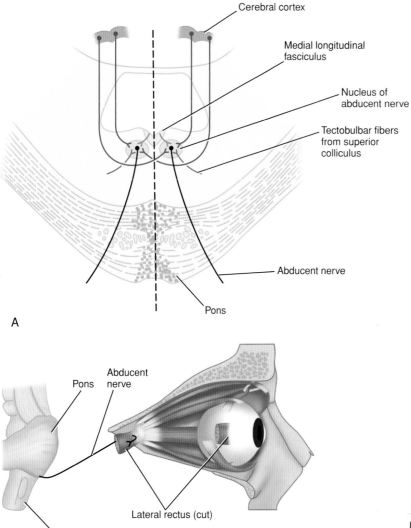

Figure 11-10 A: Abducens nerve nucleus and its central connections. **B:** Distribution of the abducens nerve.

Abducens Nerve Course

The fibers of the abducens nerve pass anteriorly through the pons and emerge in the groove between the lower border of the pons and the medulla oblongata (see Fig. 11-10B). It passes forward through the cavernous sinus, lying below and lateral to the internal carotid artery. The nerve then enters the orbit through the superior orbital fissure. The abducens nerve is entirely a motor nerve and supplies the lateral rectus muscle and, therefore, is responsible for turning the eye laterally.

FACIAL NERVE (CRANIAL NERVE VII)

The facial nerve is both a motor and a sensory nerve.

Facial Nerve Nuclei

The facial nerve has three nuclei: (1) the main motor nucleus, (2) the parasympathetic nuclei, and (3) the sensory nucleus.

Main Motor Nucleus

The main motor nucleus lies deep in the reticular formation of the lower part of the pons (Fig. 11-11). The part of the nucleus that supplies the muscles of the upper part of the face receives corticonuclear fibers from both cerebral hemispheres. The part of the nucleus that supplies the muscles of the lower part of the face receives only corticonuclear fibers from the opposite cerebral hemisphere.

These pathways explain the voluntary control of facial muscles. However, another involuntary pathway exists; it is separate and controls **mimetic or emotional changes in facial expression**. This other pathway forms part of the reticular formation (see p. 301).

Parasympathetic Nuclei

Parasympathetic nuclei lie posterolateral to the main motor nucleus. They are the **superior salivatory** and **lacrimal nuclei** (see Fig. 11-11). The superior salivatory nucleus receives afferent fibers from the hypothalamus through the **descending autonomic pathways**. Information concerning taste also is received from the **nucleus of the solitary tract** from the mouth cavity.

The lacrimal nucleus receives afferent fibers from the hypothalamus for emotional responses and from the sensory nuclei of the trigeminal nerve for reflex lacrimation secondary to irritation of the cornea or conjunctiva.

Sensory Nucleus

The sensory nucleus is the upper part of the **nucleus of the tractus solitarius** and lies close to the motor nucleus (see Fig. 11-11). Sensations of taste travel through the peripheral axons of nerve cells situated in the **geniculate ganglion** on the seventh cranial nerve. The central processes of these cells synapse on nerve cells in the nucleus. Efferent fibers cross the median plane and ascend to the ventral posteromedial nucleus of the opposite thalamus and to a number of hypothalamic nuclei. From the thalamus, the axons of the thalamic cells pass through the internal capsule and

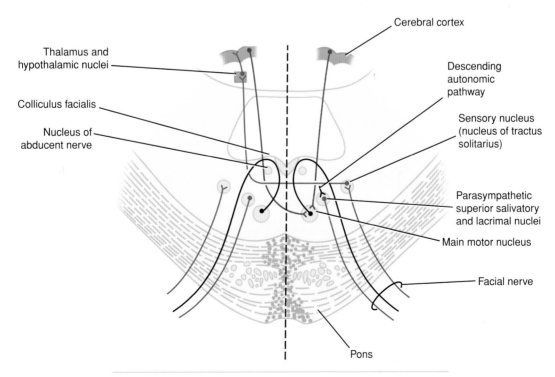

Figure 11-11   Facial nerve nuclei and their central connections.

corona radiata to end in the taste area of the cortex in the lower part of the postcentral gyrus.

Facial Nerve Course

The facial nerve consists of a motor and a sensory root. The fibers of the motor root first travel posteriorly around the medial side of the abducens nucleus (see Fig. 11-11). They then pass around the nucleus beneath the **colliculus facialis** in the floor of the fourth ventricle and, finally, pass anteriorly to emerge from the brainstem.

The sensory root (**nervus intermedius**) is formed of the central processes of the unipolar cells of the geniculate ganglion. It also contains the efferent preganglionic parasympathetic fibers from the parasympathetic nuclei.

The two roots of the facial nerve emerge from the anterior surface of the brain between the pons and the medulla oblongata. They pass laterally in the posterior cranial fossa with the vestibulocochlear nerve and enter the internal acoustic meatus in the petrous part of the temporal bone. At the bottom of the meatus, the nerve enters the facial canal and runs laterally through the inner ear. On reaching the medial wall of the tympanic cavity, the nerve expands to form the sensory **geniculate ganglion** (Fig. 11-12) and turns sharply backward above the promontory. At the posterior wall of the tympanic cavity, the facial nerve turns downward on the medial side of the aditus to the mastoid antrum, descends behind the pyramid, and emerges from the stylomastoid foramen.

A

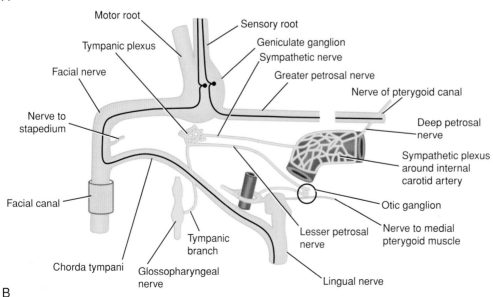

B

Figure 11-12 **A:** Distribution of the facial nerve. **B:** Branches of the facial nerve within the petrous part of the temporal bone; the taste fibers are shown in black. The glossopharyngeal nerve is also shown.

Facial Nerve Distribution

The **motor nucleus** supplies the muscles of facial expression, the auricular muscles, the stapedius, the posterior belly of the digastric, and the stylohyoid muscles (see Fig. 11-12).

The **superior salivatory nucleus** supplies the submandibular and sublingual salivary glands and the nasal and palatine glands. The **lacrimal nucleus** supplies the lacrimal gland.

The **sensory nucleus** receives taste fibers from the anterior two-thirds of the tongue, the floor of the mouth, and the palate.

VESTIBULOCOCHLEAR NERVE (CRANIAL NERVE VIII)

This nerve consists of two distinct parts, the **vestibular nerve** and the **cochlear nerve**, which are concerned with the transmission of afferent information from the internal ear to the central nervous system (Figs. 11-13 and 11-14).

Vestibular Nerve

The vestibular nerve conducts nerve impulses from the utricle and saccule that provide information concerning the position of the head; the nerve also conducts impulses from the semicircular canals that provide information concerning movements of the head.

The nerve fibers of the vestibular nerve are the central processes of nerve cells located in the **vestibular ganglion**, which is situated in the **internal acoustic meatus**. They enter the anterior surface of the brainstem in a groove between the lower border of the pons and the upper part of the medulla oblongata (see Fig. 11-13). When they enter the vestibular nuclear complex, the fibers divide into short ascending and long descending fibers; a small number of fibers pass directly to the cerebellum through the inferior cerebellar peduncle, bypassing the vestibular nuclei.

Vestibular Nuclear Complex

This complex consists of a group of nuclei situated beneath the floor of the fourth ventricle (see Fig. 11-13). Four nuclei may be recognized: (1) the **lateral** vestibular nucleus, (2) the **superior** vestibular nucleus, (3) the **medial** vestibular nucleus, and (4) the **inferior** vestibular nucleus (see Fig. 5-14).

The vestibular nuclei receive afferent fibers from the **utricle** and **saccule** and the **semicircular canals** through the vestibular nerve and fibers from the cerebellum through the inferior cerebellar peduncle (see Fig. 11-13). Efferent fibers from the nuclei pass to the

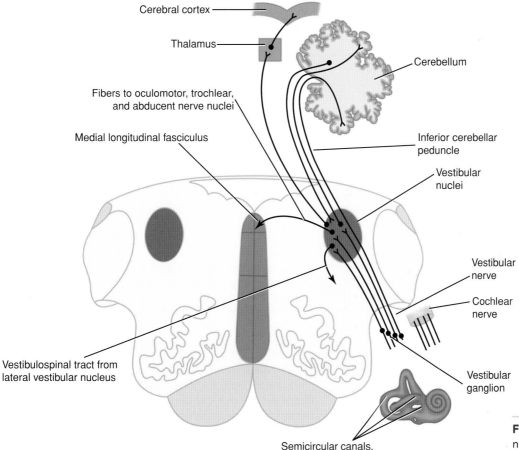

Figure 11-13 Vestibular nerve nuclei and their central connections.

Figure 11-14 Cochlear nerve nuclei and their central connections. The descending pathways have been omitted.

cerebellum through the inferior cerebellar peduncle. Efferent fibers also descend uncrossed to the spinal cord from the lateral vestibular nucleus and form the **vestibulospinal tract**. In addition, efferent fibers pass to the nuclei of the oculomotor, trochlear, and abducens nerves through the medial longitudinal fasciculus.

These connections enable the movements of the head and the eyes to be coordinated so that visual fixation on an object can be maintained. In addition, information received from the internal ear can assist in maintaining balance by influencing the muscle tone of the limbs and trunk.

Ascending fibers also pass upward from the vestibular nuclei to the cerebral cortex, to the vestibular area in the postcentral gyrus just above the lateral fissure. These fibers are thought to relay in the ventral posterior nuclei of the thalamus. The cerebral cortex probably serves to orient the individual consciously in space.

Cochlear Nerve

The cochlear nerve conducts nerve impulses concerned with sound from the organ of Corti in the cochlea. The fibers of the cochlear nerve are the central processes of nerve cells located in the **spiral ganglion of the cochlea** (Fig. 11-15). They enter the anterior surface of the brainstem at the lower border of the pons on the lateral side of the emerging facial nerve by the vestibular nerve

Vestibular ganglion

Pons

Cochlear nerve

Ampulla of superior semicircular duct

Ampulla of lateral semicircular duct

Utricle

Vestibular nerve

Spiral ganglion of cochlea

Medulla oblongata

Cochlear duct

Ampulla of posterior semicircular duct

Figure 11-15 Distribution of the vestibulocochlear nerve.

(see Fig. 11-14). On entering the pons, the nerve fibers divide, with one branch entering the **posterior cochlear nucleus** and the other branch entering the **anterior cochlear nucleus**.

Cochlear Nuclei

The anterior and posterior cochlear nuclei are situated on the surface of the inferior cerebellar peduncle (see Fig. 11-14). They receive afferent fibers from the cochlea through the cochlear nerve. The cochlear nuclei send axons (second-order neuron fibers) that run medially through the pons to end in the **trapezoid body** and the olivary nucleus. Here, they are relayed in the **posterior nucleus of the trapezoid body** and the superior olivary nucleus on the same or the opposite side. The axons now ascend through the posterior part of the pons and midbrain and form a tract known as the **lateral lemniscus**. Each lateral lemniscus, therefore, consists of third-order neurons from both sides. As these fibers ascend, some of them relay in small groups of nerve cells, collectively known as the **nucleus of the lateral lemniscus**.

On reaching the midbrain, the fibers of the lateral lemniscus either terminate in the **nucleus of the inferior colliculus** or are relayed in the **medial geniculate body** and pass to the **auditory cortex** of the cerebral hemisphere through the **acoustic radiation of the internal capsule**.

The primary auditory cortex (areas 41 and 42) includes the gyrus of Heschl on the upper surface of the superior temporal gyrus. The recognition and interpretation of sounds, on the basis of past experience, take place in the secondary auditory area.

Nerve impulses from the ear are transmitted along auditory pathways on both sides of the brainstem, with more being projected along the contralateral pathway. Many collateral branches are given off to the reticular activating system of the brainstem (see p. 301). The tonotopic organization present in the organ of Corti is preserved within the cochlear nuclei, the inferior colliculi, and the primary auditory area.

Descending Auditory Pathways

Descending fibers originating in the auditory cortex and in other nuclei in the auditory pathway accompany the ascending pathway. These fibers are bilateral and end on nerve cells at different levels of the auditory pathway and on the hair cells of the organ of Corti. These fibers are believed to serve as a feedback mechanism and inhibit the reception of sound. They may also have a role in the process of auditory sharpening, suppressing some signals and enhancing others.

Vestibulocochlear Nerve Course

The vestibular and cochlear parts of the nerve leave the anterior surface of the brain between the lower border of the pons and the medulla oblongata (see Fig. 11-15). They run laterally in the posterior cranial fossa and enter the internal acoustic meatus with the facial nerve. The fibers are then distributed to the different parts of the internal ear.

GLOSSOPHARYNGEAL NERVE (CRANIAL NERVE IX)

The glossopharyngeal nerve is a motor and a sensory nerve.

Glossopharyngeal Nerve Nuclei

The glossopharyngeal nerve has three nuclei: (1) the main motor nucleus, (2) the parasympathetic nucleus, and (3) the sensory nucleus.

Main Motor Nucleus

The main motor nucleus lies deep in the reticular formation of the medulla oblongata and is formed by the superior end of the nucleus ambiguus (Fig. 11-16). It receives corticonuclear fibers from both cerebral

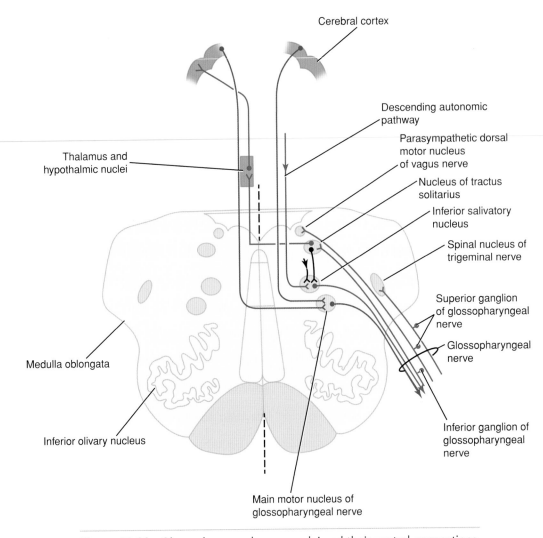

Figure 11-16 Glossopharyngeal nerve nuclei and their central connections.

hemispheres. The efferent fibers supply the **stylopharyngeus muscle**.

Parasympathetic Nucleus

The parasympathetic nucleus is also called the **inferior salivatory nucleus**. It receives afferent fibers from the hypothalamus through the **descending autonomic pathways**. It also is thought to receive information from the olfactory system through the reticular formation. Information concerning taste also is received from the nucleus of the solitary tract from the mouth cavity.

The efferent preganglionic parasympathetic fibers reach the otic ganglion through the **tympanic branch of the glossopharyngeal nerve**, the **tympanic plexus**, and the **lesser petrosal nerve** (Fig. 11-17). The postganglionic fibers pass to the **parotid salivary gland**.

Sensory Nucleus

The sensory nucleus is part of the **nucleus of the tractus solitarius** (see Fig. 11-16). Sensations of taste

travel through the peripheral axons of nerve cells situated in the **ganglion** on the glossopharyngeal nerve. The central processes of these cells synapse on nerve cells in the nucleus. Efferent fibers cross the median plane and ascend to the ventral group of nuclei of the opposite thalamus and a number of hypothalamic nuclei. From the thalamus, the axons of the thalamic cells pass through the internal capsule and corona radiata to end in the lower part of the postcentral gyrus.

Afferent information that concerns common sensation enters the brainstem through the superior ganglion of the glossopharyngeal nerve but ends in the **spinal nucleus of the trigeminal nerve**. Afferent impulses from the **carotid sinus**, a baroreceptor situated at the bifurcation of the common carotid artery, also travel with the glossopharyngeal nerve. They terminate in the **nucleus of the tractus solitarius** and are connected to the **dorsal motor nucleus of the vagus nerve**. The carotid sinus reflex that involves the glossopharyngeal and vagus nerves assists in the regulation of arterial blood pressure.

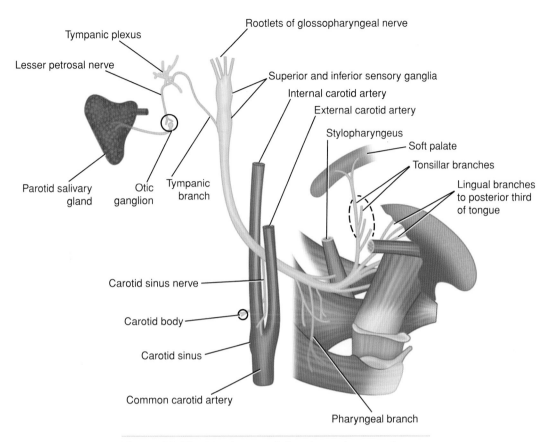

Figure 11-17 Distribution of the glossopharyngeal nerve.

Glossopharyngeal Nerve Course

The glossopharyngeal nerve leaves the anterolateral surface of the upper part of the medulla oblongata as a series of rootlets in a groove between the olive and the inferior cerebellar peduncle (see Fig. 11-16). It passes laterally in the posterior cranial fossa and leaves the skull through the jugular foramen. The superior and inferior glossopharyngeal sensory ganglia are situated on the nerve here. The nerve then descends through the upper part of the neck in company with the internal jugular vein and the internal carotid artery to reach the posterior border of the stylopharyngeus muscle, which it supplies. The nerve then passes forward between the superior and middle constrictor muscles of the pharynx to give sensory branches to the mucous membrane of the pharynx and the posterior third of the tongue (see Fig. 11-17).

VAGUS NERVE (CRANIAL NERVE X)

The vagus nerve is a motor and a sensory nerve.

Vagus Nerve Nuclei

The vagus nerve has three nuclei: (1) the main motor nucleus, (2) the parasympathetic nucleus, and (3) the sensory nucleus.

Main Motor Nucleus

The main motor nucleus lies deep in the reticular formation of the medulla oblongata and is formed by the nucleus ambiguus (Fig. 11-18). It receives corticonuclear fibers from both cerebral hemispheres. The efferent fibers supply the constrictor muscles of the pharynx and the intrinsic muscles of the larynx (Fig. 11-19).

Parasympathetic Nucleus

The parasympathetic nucleus forms the dorsal nucleus of the vagus and lies beneath the floor of the lower part of the fourth ventricle posterolateral to the hypoglossal nucleus (see Fig. 11-18). It receives afferent fibers from the hypothalamus through the descending autonomic pathways. It also receives other afferents, including those from the glossopharyngeal nerve (carotid sinus reflex). The efferent fibers are distributed to the involuntary muscle of the bronchi, heart, esophagus, stomach, small intestine, and large intestine as far as the distal third of the transverse colon (see Fig. 11-19).

Sensory Nucleus

The sensory nucleus is the lower part of the **nucleus of the tractus solitarius**. Sensations of taste travel through the peripheral axons of nerve cells situated in the **inferior ganglion on the vagus nerve**. The central

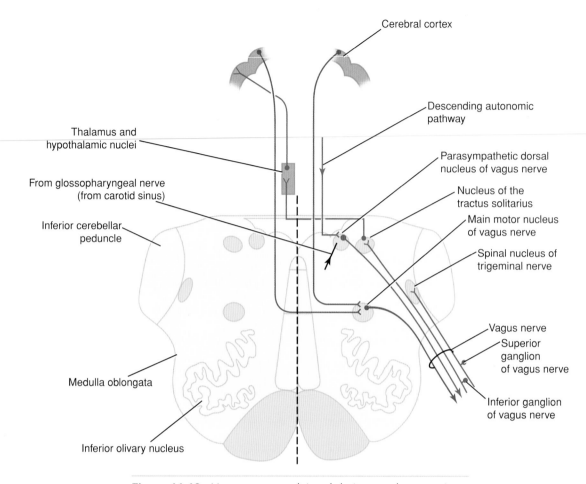

Figure 11-18 Vagus nerve nuclei and their central connections.

processes of those cells synapse on nerve cells in the nucleus (see Fig. 11-18). Efferent fibers cross the median plane and ascend to the ventral group of nuclei of the opposite thalamus as well as to a number of hypothalamic nuclei. From the thalamus, the axons of the thalamic cells pass through the internal capsule and corona radiata to end in the postcentral gyrus.

Afferent information concerning common sensation enters the brainstem through the superior ganglion of the vagus nerve but ends in the **spinal nucleus of the trigeminal nerve**.

Vagus Nerve Course

The vagus nerve leaves the anterolateral surface of the upper part of the medulla oblongata as a series of rootlets in a groove between the olive and the inferior cerebellar peduncle (see Fig. 11-18). The nerve passes laterally through the posterior cranial fossa and leaves the skull through the jugular foramen. The vagus nerve possesses two sensory ganglia, a rounded superior ganglion, situated on the nerve within the jugular foramen, and a cylindrical **inferior ganglion**, which lies on the nerve just below the foramen. Below the inferior ganglion, the cranial root of the accessory nerve joins the

vagus nerve and is distributed mainly in its pharyngeal and recurrent laryngeal branches.

The vagus nerve descends vertically in the neck within the carotid sheath with the internal jugular vein and the internal and common carotid arteries.

The **right vagus nerve** enters the thorax and passes posterior to the root of the right lung, contributing to the pulmonary plexus. It then passes on to the posterior surface of the esophagus and contributes to the **esophageal plexus**. It enters the abdomen through the esophageal opening of the diaphragm. The posterior vagal trunk (which is the name now given to the right vagus) is distributed to the posterior surface of the stomach and, by a large celiac branch, to the duodenum, liver, kidneys, and small and large intestines as far as the distal third of the transverse colon. This wide distribution is accomplished through the celiac, superior mesenteric, and renal plexuses.

The **left vagus nerve** enters the thorax and crosses the left side of the aortic arch and descends behind the root of the left lung, contributing to the **pulmonary plexus**. The left vagus then descends on the anterior surface of the esophagus, contributing to the **esophageal plexus**. It enters the abdomen through the esophageal opening of the diaphragm. The anterior vagal trunk (which is the

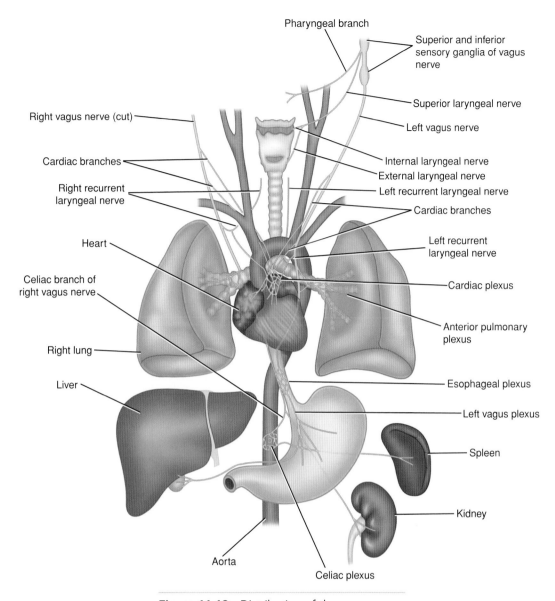

Figure 11-19   Distribution of the vagus nerve.

name now given to the left vagus) divides into several branches, which are distributed to the stomach, liver, upper part of the duodenum, and head of the pancreas.

ACCESSORY NERVE (CRANIAL NERVE XI)

The accessory nerve is a motor nerve that is formed by the union of a cranial and a spinal root.

Cranial Root

The cranial root (part) is formed from the axons of nerve cells of the nucleus ambiguus (Fig. 11-20). The nucleus receives corticonuclear fibers from both cerebral hemispheres. The efferent fibers of the nucleus emerge from the anterior surface of the medulla oblongata between the olive and the inferior cerebellar peduncle.

Cranial Root Course

The nerve runs laterally in the posterior cranial fossa and joins the spinal root. The two roots unite and leave the skull through the jugular foramen. The roots then separate, and the cranial root joins the vagus nerve and is distributed in its pharyngeal and recurrent laryngeal branches to the muscles of the soft palate, pharynx, and larynx.

Spinal Root

The spinal root (part) is formed from axons of nerve cells in the **spinal nucleus**, which is situated in the anterior gray column of the spinal cord in the upper five

Figure 11-20   Cranial and spinal nuclei of the accessory nerve and their central connections.

cervical segments (see Fig. 11-20). The spinal nucleus is thought to receive corticospinal fibers from both cerebral hemispheres.

Spinal Root Course

The nerve fibers emerge from the spinal cord midway between the anterior and posterior nerve roots of the cervical spinal nerves. The fibers form a nerve trunk that ascends into the skull through the foramen magnum. The spinal root passes laterally and joins the cranial root as they pass through the jugular foramen. After a short distance, the spinal root separates from the cranial root and runs downward and laterally and enters the deep surface of the sternocleidomastoid (SCM) muscle, which it supplies (Fig. 11-21). The nerve then crosses the posterior triangle of the neck and passes beneath the trapezius muscle, which it supplies.

The accessory nerve thus brings about movements of the soft palate, pharynx, and larynx and controls the movement of two large muscles in the neck.

Figure 11-21 Distribution of the accessory nerve.

HYPOGLOSSAL NERVE (CRANIAL NERVE XII)

The hypoglossal nerve is a motor nerve that supplies all the intrinsic muscles of the tongue as well as the styloglossus, the hyoglossus, and the genioglossus muscles.

Hypoglossal Nucleus

The hypoglossal nucleus is situated close to the midline immediately beneath the floor of the lower part of the fourth ventricle (Fig. 11-22). It receives corticonuclear fibers from both cerebral hemispheres. However, the cells responsible for supplying the genioglossus muscle

Figure 11-22 Hypoglossal nucleus and its central connections.

Figure 11-23 Distribution of the hypoglossal nerve.

(Fig. 11-23) only receive corticonuclear fibers from the opposite cerebral hemisphere.

The hypoglossal nerve fibers pass anteriorly through the medulla oblongata and emerge as a series of roots in the groove between the pyramid and the olive (see Fig. 11-22).

Hypoglossal Nerve Course

The hypoglossal nerve fibers emerge on the anterior surface of the medulla oblongata between the pyramid and the olive (see Fig. 11-22). The nerve crosses the posterior cranial fossa and leaves the skull through the hypoglossal canal. The nerve passes downward and forward in the neck between the internal carotid artery and the internal jugular vein until it reaches the lower border of the posterior belly of the digastric muscle. Here, it turns forward and crosses the internal and external carotid arteries and the loop of the lingual artery. It passes deep to the posterior margin of the mylohyoid muscle lying on the lateral surface of the hyoglossus muscle. The nerve then sends branches to the muscles of the tongue (see Fig. 11-23).

In the upper part of its course, the hypoglossal nerve is joined by C1 fibers from the cervical plexus. The delicate cervical nerve fibers merely run with the hypoglossal nerve for support and later leave it to supply muscles in the neck.

Thus, the hypoglossal nerve controls the movements and shape of the tongue.

 # Clinical Notes

General Considerations

The 12 pairs of cranial nerves supply information to the brain from outlying receptor organs and bring about changes in peripheral effector organs by means of appropriate motor nerves. Unfortunately for the student, the nerve cells are not arranged simply, as in the spinal cord, but are grouped together to form **nuclei** that are found in different situations at different levels of the brainstem. Moreover, whereas spinal nerves possess afferent somatic fibers, afferent visceral fibers, efferent somatic fibers, and efferent visceral fibers, cranial nerves, in addition, possess special somatic afferent fibers (e.g., visual and auditory) and special visceral afferent fibers (e.g., taste).

When the central connections of the different cranial nerve nuclei were discussed in the previous section, a simplified practical version was given, since many of the precise connections of the cranial nerve nuclei are still not known. Because the delicate movements of the eyes, the larynx, and the face require carefully integrated muscle action and the fine control of muscle tone, it must be assumed that the motor nuclei of the various cranial nerves receive input from the cerebellum, the red nucleus, the reticular formation, and the corpus striatum in the same manner as the lower motor neurons of the spinal cord.

Three points of clinical value should be remembered:

1. Bilateral corticonuclear connections are present for all the cranial motor nuclei **except** that part of the facial nucleus that supplies the muscles of the lower part of the face and that part of the hypoglossal nucleus that supplies the genioglossus muscle.
2. The cranial nerves that possess afferent sensory fibers have cell bodies that are found in ganglia along the course of the nerves; these are equivalent to the posterior root ganglia. In the case of the olfactory nerves, the cells are the olfactory receptors.
3. In situations in which the cranial nerve nuclei are close together, it is very rare for a disease process to affect one nucleus only. For example, the cell groups of the nucleus ambiguus serve the glossopharyngeal, the vagus, and the cranial root of the accessory nerve, and functional loss involving all three nerves is a common finding.

Clinical Examination

The systematic examination of the 12 cranial nerves is an important part of the examination of every neurologic patient. It may reveal a lesion of a cranial nerve nucleus or its central connections, or it may show an interruption of the lower motor neurons.

Olfactory Nerve

First, determine that the nasal passages are clear. Then, apply some easily recognizable aromatic substance, such as oil of peppermint, oil of clove, or tobacco, to each nostril in turn. Ask the patient whether he or she can smell anything; if so, ask the patient to identify the smell. It should be remembered that food flavors depend on the sense of smell and not on the sense of taste.

Bilateral anosmia can be caused by disease of the olfactory mucous membrane, such as the common cold or allergic rhinitis. **Unilateral anosmia** can result from disease affecting the olfactory nerves, bulb, or tract. A lesion of the olfactory cortex on one side is unlikely to produce complete anosmia, because fibers from each olfactory tract travel to both cerebral hemispheres. Fractures of the anterior cranial fossa involving the cribriform plate of the ethmoid could tear the olfactory nerves. Cerebral tumors of the frontal lobes or meningiomas of the anterior cranial fossa can produce anosmia by pressing on the olfactory bulb or tract.

Optic Nerve

First, ask the patient whether he or she has noted any change in eyesight. **Visual acuity** should be tested for near and distant vision. Near vision is tested by asking the patient to read a card with a standard size of type. Each eye is tested in turn, with or without spectacles. Distant vision is tested by asking the patient to read Snellen type at a distance of 20 ft.

The **visual fields** should then be tested. The patient and the examiner sit facing each other at a distance of 2 ft. The patient is asked to cover the right eye, and the examiner covers his own left eye. The patient is asked to look into the pupil of the examiner's right eye. A small object is then moved in an arc around the periphery of the field of vision, and the patient is asked whether he or she can see the object. The extent of the patient's field of vision is compared with the normal examiner's field. Then, the other eye is tested. The clinician must be careful not to miss loss or impairment of vision in the central area of the field (central scotoma).

VISUAL PATHWAY LESIONS

Lesions of the optic pathway may have many pathologic causes. Expanding tumors of the brain and neighboring structures, such as the pituitary gland and the meninges, and cerebrovascular accidents are commonly responsible. The most widespread effects on vision occur where the nerve fibers of the visual pathway are tightly packed together, such as in the optic nerve or the optic tract.

CIRCUMFERENTIAL BLINDNESS

Circumferential blindness may be caused by hysteria or optic neuritis (Fig. 11-24 [1]). Optic neuritis may occur following spread of infection from the sphenoid and ethmoid sinuses; the optic nerve is infected as it passes through the optic canal to enter the orbital cavity.

TOTAL BLINDNESS OF ONE EYE

Total blindness of one eye would follow complete section of one optic nerve (Fig. 11-24 [2]).

NASAL HEMIANOPIA

Nasal hemianopia would follow a partial lesion of the optic chiasma on its lateral side (Fig. 11-24 [3]).

BITEMPORAL HEMIANOPIA

Bitemporal hemianopia would follow a sagittal section of the optic chiasma (Fig. 11-24 [4]). This condition is most commonly produced by a tumor of the pituitary gland exerting pressure on the optic chiasma.

CONTRALATERAL HOMONYMOUS HEMIANOPIA

Contralateral homonymous hemianopia would follow division of the optic tract or optic radiation or destruction of the visual cortex on one side; the lesion would produce the same hemianopia for both eyes—that is, homonymous hemianopia (Fig. 11-24 [5–7]). If the right optic tract is divided, for example, a left temporal hemianopia and a right nasal hemianopia will occur.

FUNDUS EXAMINATION

The ocular fundus should be examined with an ophthalmoscope. The patient is asked to look at a distant object. When the right eye is examined, the physician should use his or her right eye and hold the ophthalmoscope in his or her right hand. The physician should systematically examine the fundus, looking first at the optic disc, then at the retina, then at the blood vessels, and finally at the macula.

The **optic disc** is creamy pink, and the lateral margin is seen clearly. The center of the disc is paler and hollowed out.

The **retina** is pinkish red, and there should be no hemorrhages or exudates.

The **blood vessels** should consist of four main arteries with their accompanying veins. Carefully examine the arteriovenous crossings. The veins should not be indented by the arteries.

The **macula** is examined by asking the patient to look directly at the light of the ophthalmoscope. It should look slightly darker than the surrounding retina.

EXTRAOCULAR MUSCLE EXAMINATION

To examine the extraocular muscles, the patient's head is fixed, and he or she is asked to move the eyes, in turn, to the

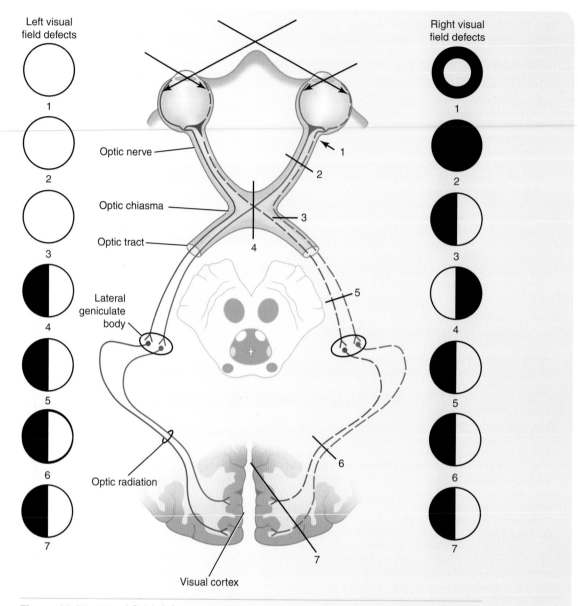

Figure 11-24 Visual field defects associated with lesions of the optic pathways. **1.** Right-sided circumferential blindness due to retrobulbar neuritis. **2.** Total blindness of the right eye due to division of the right optic nerve. **3.** Right nasal hemianopia due to a partial lesion of the right side of the optic chiasma. **4.** Bitemporal hemianopia due to a complete lesion of the optic chiasma. **5.** Left temporal hemianopia and right nasal hemianopia due to a lesion of the right optic tract. **6.** Left temporal and right nasal hemianopia due to a lesion of the right optic radiation. **7.** Left temporal and right nasal hemianopia due to a lesion of the right visual cortex.

left, to the right, upward, and downward, as far as possible in each direction. The patient should then be asked to look upward and laterally, upward and medially, downward and medially, and downward and laterally.

The pupillary reactions to convergence associated with accommodation and the direct and consensual pupillary reactions to light are tested. The nervous pathways involved in the pupillary reflexes are described on pages 328-329.

Oculomotor Nerve

The oculomotor nerve supplies all the extraocular muscles except the superior oblique and the lateral rectus. It also supplies the striated muscle of the levator palpebrae superioris and the smooth muscle concerned with accommodation, namely, the sphincter pupillae and the ciliary muscle.

In a complete lesion of the oculomotor nerve, the eye cannot be moved upward, downward, or inward. At rest, the eye looks laterally (external strabismus), owing to the activity of the lateral rectus, and downward, owing to the activity of the superior oblique. The patient sees double (diplopia). The upper eyelid droops (ptosis) due to paralysis of the levator palpebrae superioris. The pupil is widely dilated and nonreactive to light, owing to paralysis of the sphincter pupillae and unopposed action of the dilator (supplied by the sympathetic). Accommodation of the eye is paralyzed.

Incomplete lesions of the oculomotor nerve are common and may spare the extraocular muscles or the intraocular muscles. The condition in which the innervation of the extraocular muscles is spared with selective loss of the autonomic innervation of the sphincter pupillae and ciliary muscle is called **internal ophthalmoplegia**. The condition in which the sphincter pupillae and the ciliary muscle are spared with paralysis of the extraocular muscles is called **external ophthalmoplegia**.

The possible explanation for the involvement of the autonomic nerves and the sparing of the remaining fibers is that the parasympathetic autonomic fibers are superficially placed within the oculomotor nerve and are likely to be first affected by compression. The nature of the disease also plays a role. For example, in cases of diabetes with impaired nerve conduction (diabetic neuropathy), the autonomic fibers are unaffected, whereas the nerves to the extraocular muscles are paralyzed.

The conditions most commonly affecting the oculomotor nerve are diabetes, aneurysm, tumor, trauma, inflammation, and vascular disease. See lesions of the oculomotor nerve in the midbrain (Benedikt syndrome) on page 217.

Trochlear Nerve

The trochlear nerve supplies the superior oblique muscle, which rotates the eye downward and laterally.

In lesions of the trochlear nerve, the patient complains of double vision on looking straight downward, because the images of the two eyes are tilted relative to each other. This is because the superior oblique is paralyzed, and the eye turns medially as well as downward. In fact, the patient has great difficulty in turning the eye downward and laterally.

The conditions most often affecting the trochlear nerve include stretching or bruising as a complication of head injuries (the nerve is long and slender), cavernous sinus thrombosis, aneurysm of the internal carotid artery, and vascular lesions of the dorsal part of the midbrain. See lesions of the trochlear nerve in the midbrain on page 217.

Abducens Nerve

The abducens nerve supplies the lateral rectus muscle, which rotates the eye laterally. In a lesion of the abducens nerve, the patient cannot turn the eye laterally. When the patient is looking straight ahead, the lateral rectus is paralyzed, and the unopposed medial rectus pulls the eyeball medially, causing **internal strabismus**. Diplopia is also seen.

Lesions of the abducens nerve include damage due to head injuries (the nerve is long and slender), cavernous sinus thrombosis or aneurysm of the internal carotid artery, and vascular lesions of the pons.

INTERNUCLEAR OPHTHALMOPLEGIA

Lesions of the medial longitudinal fasciculus will disconnect the oculomotor nucleus that innervates the medial rectus muscle from the abducens nucleus that innervates the lateral rectus muscle. When the patient is asked to look laterally to the right or left, the ipsilateral lateral rectus contracts, turning the eye laterally, but the contralateral medial rectus fails to contract, and the eye looks straight forward.

Bilateral internuclear ophthalmoplegia can occur with multiple sclerosis, occlusive vascular disease, trauma, or brainstem tumors. Unilateral internuclear ophthalmoplegia can follow an infarct of a small branch of the basilar artery.

Trigeminal Nerve

The trigeminal nerve has sensory and motor roots. The sensory root passes to the trigeminal ganglion, from which emerge the ophthalmic (V_1), maxillary (V_2), and mandibular (V_3) divisions. The motor root joins the mandibular division.

The sensory function may be tested by using cotton and a pin over each area of the face supplied by the divisions of the trigeminal nerve (see Fig. 11-9). Note that the dermatomes overlap very little and that the skin covering the angle of the jaw is innervated by branches from the cervical plexus (C2 and C3). In lesions of the ophthalmic division, the cornea and conjunctiva will be insensitive to touch.

The motor function may be tested by asking the patient to clench his or her teeth. The masseter and the temporalis muscles can be palpated and felt to harden as they contract.

TRIGEMINAL NEURALGIA

In trigeminal neuralgia, the severe, stabbing pain over the face is of unknown cause and involves the pain fibers of the trigeminal nerve. Pain is felt most commonly over the skin areas innervated by the mandibular and maxillary divisions of the trigeminal nerve; only rarely is pain felt in the area supplied by the ophthalmic division.

Facial Nerve

The facial nerve supplies the muscles of facial expression, supplies the anterior two-thirds of the tongue with taste fibers, and is secretomotor to the lacrimal, submandibular, and sublingual glands.

To test the facial nerve, the patient is asked to show the teeth by separating the lips with the teeth clenched. Normally, equal areas of the upper and lower teeth are revealed on both sides. If a lesion of the facial nerve is present on one side, the mouth is distorted. A greater area of teeth is revealed on the side of the intact nerve, since the mouth is pulled up on that side. Another useful test is to ask the patient to close both eyes firmly. The examiner then attempts to open the eyes by gently raising the patient's upper lids. On the side of the lesion, the orbicularis oculi is paralyzed so that the eyelid on that side is easily raised.

The sensation of taste on each half of the anterior two-thirds of the tongue can be tested by placing small amounts of sugar, salt, vinegar, and quinine on the tongue for the sweet, salty, sour, and bitter sensations.

FACIAL NERVE LESIONS

The facial nerve may be injured or may become dysfunctional anywhere along its long course from the brainstem to the face. Its anatomical relationship to other structures greatly assists in the localization of the lesion. If the abducens nerve (supplies the lateral rectus muscle) and the facial nerve are not functioning, this would suggest a lesion in the pons of the brain. If the vestibulocochlear nerve (for balance and hearing) and the facial nerve are not functioning, this suggests a lesion in the internal acoustic meatus. If the patient is excessively sensitive to sound in one ear, the lesion probably involves the nerve to the stapedius muscle, which arises from the facial nerve in the facial canal.

Loss of taste over the anterior two-thirds of the tongue indicates that the facial nerve is damaged proximal to the point where it gives off the chorda tympani branch in the facial canal.

A firm swelling of the parotid salivary gland associated with impaired function of the facial nerve is strongly indicative of a cancer of the parotid gland with involvement of the nerve within the gland.

Deep lacerations of the face may involve branches of the facial nerve.

The part of the facial nucleus that controls the muscles of the upper part of the face receives corticonuclear fibers from both cerebral hemispheres. Therefore, it follows that with a lesion involving the upper motor neurons, only the muscles of the lower part of the face will be paralyzed (Fig. 11-25 [1]). However, in patients with a lesion of the facial nerve motor nucleus or the facial nerve itself—that is, a lower motor neuron lesion—all the muscles on the affected side of the face will be paralyzed (Fig. 11-25 [2]). The lower eyelid will droop, and the angle of the mouth will sag. Tears will flow over the lower eyelid, and saliva will dribble from the corner of the mouth. The patient will be unable to close the eye and will be unable to expose the teeth fully on the affected side.

In patients with hemiplegia, the emotional movements of the face are usually preserved. This indicates that the upper motor neurons controlling these **mimetic** movements have a course separate from that of the main corticobulbar fibers. A lesion involving this separate pathway alone results in a loss of emotional movements, but voluntary movements are preserved. A more extensive lesion will produce both mimetic and voluntary facial paralysis.

BELL PALSY

Bell palsy is a dysfunction of the facial nerve, as it lies within the facial canal; it is usually unilateral. The site of the dysfunction will determine the aspects of facial nerve function that do not work.

The swelling of the nerve within the bony canal causes pressure on the nerve fibers; this results in a temporary loss of function of the nerve, producing a lower motor neuron type of facial paralysis. The cause of Bell palsy is not known; it sometimes follows exposure of the face to a cold draft.

Vestibulocochlear Nerve

The vestibulocochlear nerve innervates the utricle and saccule, which are sensitive to static changes in equilibrium;

Figure 11-25 Facial expression defects associated with lesions of the upper motor neurons (*1*) and lower motor neurons (*2*).

the semicircular canals, which are sensitive to changes in dynamic equilibrium; and the cochlea, which is sensitive to sound.

VESTIBULAR NERVE FUNCTION DISTURBANCE

Disturbances of vestibular nerve function include dizziness (**vertigo**) and **nystagmus** (see p. 242). Vestibular nystagmus is an uncontrollable rhythmic oscillation of the eyes, and the fast phase is away from the side of the lesion. This form of nystagmus is essentially a disturbance in the reflex control of the extraocular muscles, which is one of the functions of the semicircular canals. Normally, the nerve impulses pass reflexly from the canals through the vestibular nerve, the vestibular nuclei, and the medial longitudinal fasciculus, to the third, fourth, and sixth cranial nerve nuclei, which control the extraocular muscles; the cerebellum assists in coordinating the muscle movements.

Vestibular function can be investigated with **caloric tests**. These involve the raising and lowering of the temperature in the external auditory meatus, which induces convection currents in the endolymph of the semicircular canals (principally, the lateral semicircular canal) and stimulates the vestibular nerve endings.

The causes of vertigo include diseases of the labyrinth, such as Ménière disease. Lesions of the vestibular nerve, the vestibular nuclei, and the cerebellum can also be responsible. Multiple sclerosis, tumors, and vascular lesions of the brainstem also cause vertigo.

COCHLEAR NERVE FUNCTION DISTURBANCE

Disturbances of cochlear function are manifested as **deafness** and **tinnitus**. The patient's ability to hear a whispered voice or a vibrating tuning fork should be tested; each ear should be tested separately.

Loss of hearing may be due to a defect of the auditory-conducting mechanism in the middle ear, damage to the receptor cells in the spiral organ of Corti in the cochlea, a lesion of the cochlear nerve, a lesion of the central auditory pathways, or a lesion of the cortex of the temporal lobe. Lesions of the internal ear include **Ménière disease**, **acute labyrinthitis**, and **trauma** following head injury. Lesions of the cochlear nerve include **tumor (acoustic neuroma)** and **trauma**. Lesions in the central nervous system include **tumors of the midbrain** and **multiple sclerosis**. Only bilateral temporal lobe lesions cause deafness.

Glossopharyngeal Nerve

The glossopharyngeal nerve supplies the stylopharyngeus muscle and sends secretomotor fibers to the parotid gland. Sensory fibers innervate the posterior third of the tongue for general sensation and taste.

The integrity of this nerve may be evaluated by testing the patient's general sensation and that of taste on the posterior third of the tongue.

Isolated lesions of the glossopharyngeal nerve are rare and usually also involve the vagus nerve.

Vagus Nerve

The vagus nerve innervates many important organs, but the examination of this nerve depends on testing the function of the branches to the pharynx, soft palate, and larynx. The **pharyngeal** or **gag reflex** may be tested by touching the lateral wall of the pharynx with a spatula. This should immediately cause the patient to gag; that is, the pharyngeal muscles will contract. The afferent neuron of the pharyngeal reflex runs in the glossopharyngeal nerve, and the efferent neurons run in the glossopharyngeal (to the stylopharyngeus muscle) and vagus nerves (pharyngeal constrictor muscles). Unilateral lesions of the vagus will show little or no gag reflex on that side.

The innervation of the soft palate may be tested by asking the patient to say "ah." Normally, the soft palate rises and the uvula moves backward in the midline.

All the muscles of the larynx are supplied by the recurrent laryngeal branch of the vagus, except the cricothyroid muscle, which is supplied by the external laryngeal branch of the superior laryngeal branch of the vagus. Hoarseness or absence of the voice may occur as a symptom of vagal nerve palsy. The movements of the vocal cords may be tested by means of a laryngoscopic examination. Lesions involving the vagus nerve in the posterior cranial fossa commonly involve the glossopharyngeal, accessory, and hypoglossal nerves as well.

Accessory Nerve

The accessory nerve supplies the SCM and the trapezius muscles by means of its spinal root. The patient should be asked to rotate the head to one side against resistance, causing the SCM of the opposite side to come into action. Then, the patient should be asked to shrug the shoulders, causing the trapezius muscles to come into action.

Lesions of the spinal part of the accessory nerve will result in paralysis of the SCM and trapezius muscles. The SCM muscle will atrophy, causing weakness in turning the head to the opposite side. The trapezius muscle will also atrophy, causing the shoulder to droop on that side as well as weakness and difficulty in raising the arm above the horizontal.

Lesions of the spinal part of the accessory nerve may occur anywhere along its course and may result from tumors or trauma from stab or gunshot wounds in the neck.

Hypoglossal Nerve

The hypoglossal nerve supplies the intrinsic muscles of the tongue and the styloglossus, hyoglossus, and genioglossus muscles. To test the integrity of the nerve, the patient is asked to put out the tongue; in the setting of a lower motor neuron lesion, the tongue will be observed to deviate toward the paralyzed side. The tongue will be smaller on the side of the lesion, owing to muscle atrophy, and fasciculation may accompany or precede the atrophy. Remember that the greater part of the hypoglossal nucleus receives corticonuclear fibers from both cerebral hemispheres. However, the part of the nucleus that supplies the genioglossus receives corticonuclear fibers only from the opposite cerebral hemisphere. If a patient has a lesion of the corticonuclear fibers, there will be no atrophy or fibrillation of the tongue, and on protrusion, the tongue will deviate to the side opposite the lesion. (Note that the genioglossus is the muscle that pulls the tongue forward.)

Lesions of the hypoglossal nerve may occur anywhere along its course and may result from tumor, demyelinating diseases, syringomyelia, and vascular accidents. Injury of the nerve in the neck may also follow stab and gunshot wounds.

Key Concepts

Cranial Nerve Organization

- The 12 pairs of cranial nerves leave the brain or superior spinal cord and pass through foramina and fissures in the skull. All nerves are distributed in the head and neck except for cranial nerve X, which also supplies structures in the thorax and abdomen.

- Olfactory, optic, and vestibulocochlear nerves are entirely sensory. Oculomotor, trochlear, abducens, accessory, and hypoglossal are entirely motor. All others cranial nerves are both sensory and motor.

Cranial Nerve I

- The olfactory nerves are a series of bipolar cells located in the mucous membrane of the nasal cavity roof. The projecting olfactory hairs react to odors in the air, stimulating the olfactory nerves.

- Nerves are myelinated by Schwann cells and project through the cribriform plate to synapse on mitral and tufted cells located in the olfactory bulb.

- Axons from the mitral and tufted cells form the olfactory tract and project to the primary olfactory cortex, accomplishing the function of smell.

- Secondary connections throughout the cortex are responsible for appreciation or triggering of emotional and autonomic responses to the detected smell.

Cranial Nerve II

- Fibers of the optic nerve are the axons of ganglion cells from the retina. The optic nerve leaves the orbital cavity through the optic canal and unites with the nerve of the opposite side to form the optic chiasma.

- The optic tract arises from the optic chiasma, carrying axons from the complementary half of each eye (i.e., ipsilateral nasal with contralateral temporal).

- Most fibers of optic tract synapse in the lateral geniculate body of the thalamus, which projects to the primary visual cortex via the optic radiations.

- A smaller number of fibers do not synapse in the lateral geniculate nucleus, but instead, project to the pretectal nucleus and the superior colliculus, and are concerned with light reflexes.

Cranial Nerve III

- Oculomotor nerve carries somatic and visceral motor fibers from the main oculomotor and Edinger–Westphal nuclei, respectively.

- This nerve controls the movement of extraocular muscles and the smooth muscle of the iris and ciliary muscles for the actions of constriction and accommodation.

- The nerve fibers exit the midbrain in the interpeduncular fossa and exit the cranial cavity through the superior orbital fissure.

Cranial Nerve IV

- The motor fibers from the trochlear nucleus exit the midbrain posteriorly and immediately decussate with the nerve on the opposite side.

- The trochlear nerves pass anteriorly around the midbrain and exit the cranial cavity via the superior orbital fissure to innervate the superior oblique muscle of the eyeball.

Cranial Nerve V

- The trigeminal nerve is the largest cranial nerve, carrying sensation to the head and motor control to the muscles of mastication.

- The trigeminal nerve has four nuclei: main (sensory), spinal (sensory), mesencephalic (sensory), and motor.

- Pain, temperature, touch, and pressure travel along axons whose cell bodies are located in the semilunar or trigeminal sensory ganglion.

  - The sensations of touch and pressure are conveyed by fibers that synapse in the main sensory nucleus.

  - The sensations of pain and temperature are conveyed by fibers that synapse in the spinal nucleus.

  - Proprioceptive fibers from the muscles of the face, orbit, mouth, and mastication, synapse in the mesencephalic nucleus

- The trigeminal nerve is formed from three major nerves: ophthalmic (V_1), maxillary (V_2), and mandibular (V_3).

Cranial Nerve VI

- The motor fibers from the abducens nerve nucleus exit the brainstem at the junction of the pons and medulla oblongata.

- The abducens nerve exits the cranial cavity through the superior orbital fissure, to the orbit, where it innervates the lateral rectus muscle of the eyeball.

Cranial Nerve VII

- The fibers of the facial nerve originate from the main motor nucleus, superior salivatory (parasympathetic) and lacrimal (parasympathetic), and nucleus of the tractus solitarious (sensory).
- The motor fibers exit the cranial cavity through the internal acoustic meatus where they join the sensory root stemming from the geniculate ganglion.
- The fibers from the motor nucleus innervate the muscles of facial expression, the stapedius, the posterior belly of the digastric, and the stylohyoid muscles.
- Fibers from the superior salivatory nucleus supply the submandibular and sublingual salivary glands. The lacrimal nucleus supplies the lacrimal gland.
- The sensory nucleus receives taste fibers from the anterior two-thirds of the tongue.

Cranial Nerve VIII

- The vestibulocochlear nerve consists of two parts, vestibular nerve and cochlear nerve.
- The vestibular nerve conducts head positioning information from the utricle, saccule, and semicircular canals.
- The cells bodies of these fibers are positioned in the vestibular ganglion and project to the vestibular nuclear complex, a group of nuclei that transmit vestibular information to the cortex and spinal cord.
- The cochlear nerve consists of bipolar cell bodies in the spiral nucleus of the cochlear, with fibers conducting cochlear sensations to the anterior and posterior cochlear nuclei.
- Second-order neurons from the cochlear nuclei communicate with the posterior nucleus of the trapezoid body, which sends a bundle of third-order fibers, called the lateral lemniscus, to the inferior colliculus and medial geniculate body. From here, axons project to the primary auditory cortex of the superior temporal gyrus.

Cranial Nerve IX

- The glossopharyngeal nerve has three nuclei: the main motor, inferior salivatory (parasympathetic), spinal trigeminal (sensory), and nucleus of the tractus solitarius (sensory).
- The motor fibers innervate the stylopharyngeus muscles.
- The parasympathetic fibers innervate the parotid salivary gland.

- The sensory fibers from the pharynx and posterior third of the tongue synapse in the spinal trigeminal nucleus, while the taste and carotid sinus and body reflexes synapse in the nucleus solitarius.
- The glossopharyngeal nerve exits the cranial cavity through the jugular foramen.

Cranial Nerve X

- The vagus has four nuclei: nucleus ambiguus (motor), dorsal nucleus (parasympathetic), spinal trigeminal (sensory), and nucleus of the tractus solitarius (sensory).
- The motor fibers from the nucleus ambiguus innervate the constrictor muscles of the pharynx and the intrinsic muscles of the larynx.
- The sensory fibers conveying taste from the epiglottis and visceral afferents from the organs synapse in the nucleus solitarius. Sensation from the mucosa of the larynx ends in the spinal nucleus of the trigeminal.
- Parasympathetic fibers from the dorsal nucleus of the vagus are distributed to the involuntary muscle of the bronchi, heart, esophagus, stomach, small intestine, and up to a third of the transverse colon.
- The vagus nerve exits the cranial cavity through the jugular foramen.

Cranial Nerve XI

- The accessory nerve is a motor nerve that receives efferent fibers from the nucleus ambiguus and the anterior gray column of the first five segments of the spinal cord.
- The fibers originating in the gray columns bring about movement of the SCM and trapezius muscles.
- Fibers from the nucleus ambiguus run with the vagus nerve and are usually attributed to the functions of CN X.
- The accessory nerve exits the cranial cavity through the jugular foramen.

Cranial Nerve XII

- The hypoglossal nerve is a motor nerve that receives its efferent fibers from the hypoglossal nucleus and innervates the muscles of the tongue.
- The hypoglossal nerve exits the medulla oblongata between the pyramid and the olive and traverses the hypoglossal canal to exit the cranial cavity.

? Clinical Problem Solving

1. A 60-year-old woman is seen as an outpatient because she has suddenly developed double vision. She is watching her favorite television program when it suddenly occurs. She has no other symptoms. A complete physical examination shows that her right eye, when at rest, is turned medially, and she is unable to turn it laterally. A moderate amount of glucose is found in her urine, and she has an abnormally elevated blood glucose level. When closely questioned, she admits that recently she has noticed having to pass water more frequently, especially at night. She also says she often feels thirsty. She has lost 28 lb during the past 2 years. Using your knowledge of neuroanatomy, explain the problem in her right eye. Do you think a connection exists between her glucosuria, high blood glucose, polyuria, polydipsia, and weight loss and her eye condition?

2. An 18-year-old man is admitted to the hospital unconscious after a serious motorcycle accident. A complete physical examination is performed and lateral and anteroposterior radiographs of the skull taken, which show that the patient has a fracture involving the anterior cranial fossa. It also is noted that he has a slight but continuous blood-stained watery discharge from his left nostril. Three days later, he regains consciousness, and a further physical examination reveals that he can no longer smell. This is tested by asking him to recognize the smell of coffee, oil of clove, and oil of peppermint. Using your knowledge of neuroanatomy, diagnose what is wrong with this patient. Is it possible for normal individuals with an acute sense of smell to be unable to recognize common scents? Could a tumor that had destroyed the olfactory cortex of one cerebral hemisphere be responsible for the anosmia in this patient?

3. A 72-year-old man with a known history of cerebrovascular problems visits his physician because 3 days previously, he had begun to have trouble reading the paper. He complains that the print started to tilt and that he is beginning to see double. He also says that he finds it difficult to see the steps when he descends the staircase to the physician's office. On physical examination, the patient has weakness of movement of the right eye both downward and laterally. Using your knowledge of neuroanatomy, explain this patient's signs and symptoms. If we assume that a cranial nerve nucleus is the site of the lesion, is it the right one or the left one that is involved?

4. A 73-year-old man consults his physician because he is becoming deaf. His only other complaints are that he did not think he was as tall as he used to be, and he is annoyed to find that each year he has to buy a size larger hat. The physician diagnoses osteitis deformans (Paget disease) and explains to the medical students that this is a disease of bones involving bone absorption and new bone formation. These bony changes lead to enlargement of the skull, deformities of the vertebral column, and bowing of the long bones of the legs. The physician asks the students whether a connection exists between the bone disease and the patient's deafness and which other cranial nerve they would be particularly interested in testing. How would you have answered these questions?

5. A neurologist is visited by a 25-year-old man who complains of a feeling of heaviness in both legs and giddiness on walking. On examination, the patient has widely disseminated lesions involving the corticospinal tracts, the posterior white column, and the optic nerves. A diagnosis of multiple sclerosis is made. This disease of unknown origin primarily involves the white matter of the brain and spinal cord. Do you think this patient's symptoms of vertigo could be accounted for by this disease?

6. A 54-year-old woman with left-sided hemiplegia is examined by a fourth-year medical student. He very carefully tests each cranial nerve and notes any defects. During the examination, he stands behind the patient and gently grasps the trapezius muscles between his fingers and thumbs and asks the patient to shrug her shoulders against resistance. He is surprised to find no evidence of weakness in either trapezius muscle and no muscle wasting. Would you expect to find evidence of weakness or wasting in the trapezius muscles of a patient with hemiplegia?

7. A 35-year-old man is admitted to the hospital with a complaint of severe pain of the right side of the forehead and the right eye. The pain started 3 weeks previously and has progressively increased since then. One week ago, he started to see double, and this morning, his wife notices that his right eye is turning out laterally. The physician in charge makes a careful neurologic workup on this patient and finds a lateral deviation of the right eye, dilatation of the right pupil with loss of direct and consensual light reflexes, paralysis of accommodation on the right, and paralysis of all right-sided ocular movement, except laterally. He initially advises the patient to have computed tomography and magnetic resonance imaging scans of the skull and later orders a right-sided carotid arteriogram. The film shows an aneurysm of the internal carotid artery on the right side. Explain the signs and symptoms of this patient. Relate the signs and symptoms to the aneurysm.

8. During ward rounds, a neurologist demonstrates the signs and symptoms of neurosyphilis to a group of students. The patient is a 62-year-old man. The physician asks the students to note that both the patient's pupils are small and fixed and are not altered by shining a light in the eyes or shading the

eyes. However, the pupils narrow when the patient is asked to look from a distant object to the tip of his nose. Moreover, the pupils dilate again when he is looking into the distance. "This is a good example of the Argyll Robertson pupil," said the physician. Using your knowledge of neuroanatomy, explain this curious pupillary reaction.

9. Describe the effects of a lesion at the following points along the visual pathway of the right eye:
   (a) Section of the right optic nerve
   (b) Midline section of the optic chiasma
   (c) Section of the right optic tract
   (d) Section of the right optic radiation
   (e) Destruction of the cortex of the right occipital pole
10. A 58-year-old woman is diagnosed as having an advanced carcinoma of the nasopharynx with neoplastic infiltration of the posterior cranial fossa. How do you test for the integrity of the 9th, 10th, and 11th cranial nerves?
11. A 32-year-old woman with syringomyelia is found on physical examination to have impairment of appreciation of pain and temperature of the face but preservation of light touch. Using your knowledge of neuroanatomy, explain this dissociated sensory loss in the face.

12. A 51-year-old man complaining of an agonizing, stabbing pain over the middle part of the right side of his face is seen in the emergency department. The stabs last a few seconds and are repeated several times. "The pain is the worst I have ever experienced," he tells the physician. A draft of cold air on the right side of his face or the touching of a few hairs in the right temporal region of his scalp can trigger the pain. The patient has no other complaints and says he feels otherwise very fit. A complete physical examination of the cranial nerves reveals nothing abnormal. In particular, no evidence of sensory or motor loss of the right trigeminal nerve is seen. The patient indicates the area on the right side of his face in which he is experiencing the pain; it is seen to be in the distribution of the maxillary division of the trigeminal nerve. Using your knowledge of neuroanatomy, make the diagnosis.
13. A physician turned to a group of students and says, "I think this patient has an advanced neoplasm in the posterior cranial fossa with involvement of the medulla oblongata and in particular the nuclei of the vagus nerve." What are the nuclei of the vagus nerve? Is it possible to have abnormal movements of the vocal cords in a patient with hemiplegia? Is it possible to have a solitary lesion of the vagal nuclei without involvement of other cranial nerve nuclei?

 Answers and Explanations to Clinical Problem Solving

1. The medial strabismus of her right eye, the diplopia, and the inability to turn the right eye laterally were due to paralysis of the right lateral rectus muscle caused by a lesion of the abducens nerve. Yes, a connection exists between the eye condition and the other symptoms. The glucosuria, high blood glucose, polyuria, polydipsia, and weight loss are the classic signs and symptoms of diabetes mellitus. The lesion of the abducens nerve was an example of diabetic neuropathy, a complication of untreated or poorly treated diabetes. Once the patient's diabetes was carefully controlled, the right lateral rectus palsy disappeared after 3 months.
2. This man suffered from anosmia secondary to a lesion involving both olfactory tracts. The watery discharge from the nose was due to a leak of cerebrospinal fluid through the fractured cribriform plate of the ethmoid bone. It was the fracture and the associated hemorrhage that had damaged both olfactory tracts. Yes, many normal persons with an acute sense of smell cannot name common scents. No, a lesion of one olfactory cortex cannot produce complete anosmia because both olfactory tracts communicate with each other through the anterior commissure.
3. This patient has a paralysis of the right superior oblique muscle resulting from a lesion of the trochlear nerve. Since the trochlear nerves decussate on emergence from the midbrain, the left trochlear nucleus is the site of the lesion. This patient had a thrombosis of a small artery supplying the left

trochlear nucleus. The difficulty in reading, the diplopia, and the difficulty in walking down stairs were due to the paralysis of the right superior oblique muscle.
4. As the result of the great increase in the thickness of the bones due to new bone formation in osteitis deformans, mental deterioration may occur owing to compression of the cerebral hemispheres. Those cranial nerves that pass through relatively small foramina in the skull are likely to be compressed by the new bone growth. The nerves commonly involved are the vestibulocochlear and facial nerves, following narrowing of the internal acoustic meatus. The olfactory and optic nerves also may be compressed as they pass through the cribriform plate and the optic canal, respectively.
5. Yes. Multiple sclerosis may affect white matter in widely disseminated areas of the central nervous system. Although remissions may occur, it is inevitably progressive. Thirty years later, when this patient died, numerous areas of sclerosis were found throughout the brainstem and white matter of the spinal cord. It was noted that the region of the vestibular nuclei beneath the floor of the fourth ventricle was involved in the disease process.
6. No. The trapezius muscle is supplied by the spinal part of the accessory nerve. The spinal nucleus of this nerve in the upper five cervical segments of the spinal cord receives cortical fibers from both cerebral hemispheres. This would account for the absence of muscular weakness in this patient with

a left-sided hemiplegia. For a muscle to atrophy (except for disuse atrophy), the integrity of the monosynaptic reflex arc must be destroyed. This was not the case in this patient.

7. The severe pain over the forehead and the right eye was due to irritation of the ophthalmic division of the trigeminal nerve by the slowly expanding aneurysm of the internal carotid artery as it was lying in the cavernous sinus. The double vision (diplopia) and the lateral deviation of the right eye were due to the unopposed action of the lateral rectus muscle (supplied by the abducens nerve). The dilatation of the right pupil with loss of direct and consensual light reflexes, paralysis of accommodation, and paralysis of all right-sided ocular movement except laterally were due to pressure on the right oculomotor nerve by the aneurysm. The nerve at this point is situated in the lateral wall of the cavernous sinus. Note that the lateral movement of the eyeball was accomplished by contracting the lateral rectus muscle (abducens nerve) and that the inferolateral movement was due to the contraction of the superior oblique muscle (trochlear nerve).

8. The Argyll Robertson pupil is a common finding in neurosyphilis, although it may occur in other diseases. The lesion is believed to be located where the pretectal fibers pass to the parasympathetic oculomotor nuclei on both sides of the midbrain. This lesion effectively destroys the direct and consensual light reflexes of both eyes but leaves the pathway for the accommodation reflex intact. (For details of pathway, see p. 329.)

9. A lesion will have the following effects along the visual pathway of the right eye:
   (a) Complete blindness of the right eye
   (b) Bitemporal hemianopia
   (c) Left homonymous hemianopia
   (d) Left homonymous hemianopia
   (e) Left homonymous hemianopia, usually with some macular sparing owing to the very large area of the cortex allotted to the macula

10. The glossopharyngeal nerve supplies the posterior third of the tongue with fibers that subserve common sensations and taste. This may be tested easily. The vagus nerve, by means of its pharyngeal branch, supplies many muscles of the soft palate, and these may be tested by asking the patient to say "ah" and observing that normally the uvula is elevated in the midline. A lesion of the vagus nerve would result in the uvula being elevated to the opposite side. Additional tests may be carried out by observing the movements of the vocal cords through a laryngoscope.

The spinal part of the accessory nerve may be tested by asking the patient to shrug her shoulders by using the trapezius muscles or to rotate her head so that she looks upward to the opposite side by contracting the sternocleidomastoid muscles. Both muscles are innervated by the spinal part of the accessory nerve.

11. The afferent fibers entering the central nervous system through the trigeminal nerve pass either to the main sensory nucleus in the pons or to the spinal nucleus situated in the medulla oblongata and the first two cervical segments of the spinal cord. The sensations of touch and pressure are served by the main sensory nucleus, while those of pain and temperature are served by the more inferiorly placed spinal nucleus. In this patient, the lesion of syringomyelia was situated in the medulla oblongata and the cervical part of the spinal cord, and the main sensory nucleus in the pons was intact.

12. This patient exhibited the classic history of right-sided trigeminal neuralgia involving the maxillary division of that cranial nerve. The temporal region of the scalp, supplied by the auriculotemporal branch of the mandibular division of that nerve, was the trigger area for the initiation of the intense pain. Clearly, knowledge of the distribution of the branches of the trigeminal nerve and the diseases that can affect this nerve is essential for a physician to be able to make the diagnosis.

13. The vagal nuclei are the (a) main motor nucleus, (b) parasympathetic nucleus, and (c) sensory nucleus. The main motor and parasympathetic nuclei are controlled by both cerebral hemispheres; thus, hemiplegia will have no effect on the movement of the vocal cords. The vagal nuclei are practically continuous with the nuclei of the glossopharyngeal and accessory nerves, and these usually are involved together in lesions of the medulla oblongata.

 Review Questions

Directions: Each of the numbered items in this section is followed by answers. Select the ONE lettered answer that is CORRECT.

1. The cranial nerve nuclei listed below have the following descending tracts terminating on them:
   (a) The inferior salivatory nucleus of the glossopharyngeal nerve receives descending tracts from the thalamus.
   (b) The nucleus of the abducens nerve receives only crossed corticobulbar tracts.
   (c) The nucleus of the facial nerve supplying the muscles of the lower part of the face receives only crossed corticobulbar tracts.
   (d) The trigeminal motor nucleus receives only uncrossed corticobulbar tracts.
   (e) The nucleus of the trochlear nerve receives only crossed corticobulbar tracts.

2. The nuclei associated with the facial nerve include the following:
   (a) Spinal nucleus
   (b) Inferior salivatory nucleus
   (c) Nucleus ambiguus
   (d) Main sensory nucleus
   (e) Lacrimal nucleus
3. A patient with unilateral upper motor neuron paralysis of the facial muscles can smile with both sides of his face in response to a joke but not voluntarily. This can be explained by the following facts:
   (a) The main corticobulbar fibers controlling voluntary movement of the facial muscles have been preserved.
   (b) Reticular fibers, possibly originating in the hypothalamus and descending to the motor nuclei of the facial nerves, are damaged.
   (c) The facial nerves are damaged.
   (d) The muscles producing mimetic movements of the face are innervated by corticobulbar fibers that have a course separate from the main corticobulbar fibers.
   (e) A lesion involving the lower motor neurons is present.

Directions: Each of the numbered items or incomplete statements in this section is followed by answers or by completions of the statement. Select the ONE lettered answer or completion that is BEST in each case.

4. Which of the following structures participates in the reception of sound?
   (a) Trapezoid body
   (b) Medial lemniscus
   (c) Nucleus of the trigeminal lemniscus
   (d) Inferior temporal gyrus
   (e) Lateral geniculate body
5. The cerebral cortex is necessary for which of the following visual reflexes?
   (a) Corneal reflex
   (b) Accommodation reflex
   (c) Consensual light reflex
   (d) Pupillary light reflex
   (e) Visual body reflex
6. The nasal field of the right eye is projected to the:
   (a) left lateral geniculate body.
   (b) both banks of the left calcarine fissure.
   (c) left optic tract.
   (d) temporal retina of the right eye.
   (e) left optic radiation.
7. Right pupillary constriction associated with light directed at the left eye requires the:
   (a) right optic radiation.
   (b) left optic nerve.
   (c) left Edinger–Westphal nucleus.
   (d) left oculomotor nerve.
   (e) right optic nerve.
8. Select the lettered statement concerning the hypoglossal nerve that is correct:
   (a) A lesion involving the hypoglossal nerve will result in deviation of the tongue toward the same side as the lesion when the tongue is protruded.
   (b) The hypoglossal nerve conducts taste impulses from the posterior third of the tongue.
   (c) The hypoglossal nerve emerges from the brainstem between the olive and the inferior cerebellar peduncle.
   (d) The hypoglossal nerve carries with it fibers from the third and fourth cervical nerves.
   (e) The fibers of the accessory nerve wind around the motor nucleus of the hypoglossal nerve beneath the floor of the fourth ventricle.
9. Select the lettered statement concerning the trigeminal nuclei that is correct:
   (a) The main sensory nucleus lies within the medulla oblongata.
   (b) The spinal nucleus extends inferiorly as far as the fifth cervical segment.
   (c) Proprioceptive impulses from the muscles of mastication reach the mesencephalic nucleus along fibers that are part of the unipolar neurons of the nucleus.
   (d) The sensations of pain and temperature terminate in the main sensory nucleus.
   (e) The trigeminal lemniscus contains only efferent fibers from the ipsilateral sensory nuclei of the trigeminal nerve.

Directions: Each of the numbered items in this section is followed by answers. Select the ONE lettered answer that is CORRECT.

10. The cranial nerves listed below are associated with the following functions:
    (a) The spinal part of the accessory nerve shrugs the shoulder.
    (b) The oculomotor nerve closes the eye.
    (c) The trigeminal nerve is responsible for swallowing.
    (d) The facial nerve receives the sensation of taste from the posterior two-thirds of the tongue.
    (e) The glossopharyngeal nerve receives the sensation of touch from the anterior third of the tongue.
11. The following statements concern the cranial nerves involved in the process of vision:
    (a) The nerve fibers of the optic nerve are surrounded by Schwann cells.
    (b) The optic nerve is surrounded by an extension of the subarachnoid space.
    (c) Internal ophthalmoplegia is a condition in which the oculomotor nerve supply to the dilator pupillae is lost, but the innervation of the extraocular muscles is spared.
    (d) External ophthalmoplegia is a condition in which the oculomotor nerve supply to the extraocular muscles is spared, but the innervation of the sphincter pupillae and the ciliary muscle is lost.
    (e) The optic nerve leaves the orbital cavity through the optic canal in the greater wing of the sphenoid bone.

12. The following statements concern the cranial nerves listed below:
    (a) The main sensory nucleus of the trigeminal nerve lies in the brainstem medial to the motor nucleus.
    (b) Proprioceptive impulses from the facial muscles end in the mesencephalic nucleus of the facial nerve.
    (c) The facial nerve leaves the posterior cranial fossa with the vestibulocochlear nerve by passing through the stylomastoid foramen.
    (d) The superior salivatory nucleus of the facial nerve innervates the parotid salivary gland.
    (e) The olfactory receptor cells are located in the mucous membrane of the nasal cavity above the level of the superior concha.

Directions: Each case history is followed by questions. Read the case history, then select the ONE BEST lettered answer.

A 64-year-old man visited his physician because he had noticed a swelling on the right side of his neck. He mentioned that he had suffered from a chronic cough for 6 months and was rapidly losing weight.

13. On physical examination, the following possible signs emerged except:
    (a) The right half of his tongue was wrinkled and wasted.
    (b) When he was asked to protrude his tongue, it turned to the right.
    (c) The swelling on the right side of his neck was high up deep to the right sternocleidomastoid muscle and was hard and fixed.
    (d) A chest radiograph revealed an advanced bronchogenic carcinoma of the right lung.
    (e) The patient had no taste sensation on the anterior two-thirds of the tongue on the right side.
14. The physician made the following correct conclusions except:
    (a) The patient had numerous lung metastases in the deep cervical lymph nodes on the right side.
    (b) A lesion of the right hypoglossal nerve existed at some point between the nucleus in the medulla oblongata and the tongue muscles supplied.
    (c) One of the metastases had invaded the right hypoglossal nerve in the neck.
    (d) The loss of weight could be explained by the presence of the advanced carcinoma in the lung.
    (e) The tongue was wrinkled because the mucous membrane was atrophied.

Directions: Each of the numbered incomplete statements in this section is followed by completions of the statement. Select the ONE lettered completion that is BEST in each case. For questions 15 through 23, study Figure 11-26, showing the inferior view of the brain.

15. Structure number 1 is the:
    (a) olfactory tract.
    (b) olfactory nerve.

Figure 11-26   Inferior view of the brain.

    (c) anterior cerebral artery.
    (d) olfactory bulb.
    (e) inferior frontal gyrus.
16. Structure number 2 is the:
    (a) inferior frontal gyrus.
    (b) lateral olfactory stria.
    (c) olfactory nerve.
    (d) olfactory bulb.
    (e) olfactory tract.
17. Structure number 3 is the:
    (a) optic nerve.
    (b) optic chiasma.
    (c) anterior perforating substance.
    (d) optic tract.
    (e) oculomotor nerve.
18. Structure number 4 is the:
    (a) optic nerve.
    (b) optic tract.
    (c) optic chiasma.
    (d) hypophysis cerebri.
    (e) interpeduncular fossa.
19. Structure number 5 is the:
    (a) anterior perforated substance.
    (b) oculomotor nerve.
    (c) maxillary nerve.
    (d) middle cerebral artery.
    (e) optic tract.
20. Structure number 6 is the:
    (a) vertebral artery.
    (b) spinal part of the accessory nerve.
    (c) hypoglossal nerve.
    (d) glossopharyngeal nerve.
    (e) first cervical nerve.

21. Structure number 7 is the:
    (a) ophthalmic nerve.
    (b) motor root of the trigeminal nerve.
    (c) sensory root of the trigeminal nerve.
    (d) flocculus of the cerebellum.
    (e) vestibulocochlear nerve.
22. Structure number 8 is the:
    (a) motor root of the trigeminal nerve.
    (b) sensory root of the trigeminal nerve.
    (c) vestibular part of the eighth cranial nerve.
    (d) maxillary nerve.
    (e) abducens nerve.
23. Structure number 9 is the:
    (a) trochlear nerve.
    (b) abducens nerve.
    (c) facial nerve.
    (d) oculomotor nerve.
    (e) vestibulocochlear nerve.

For questions 24 through 29, study Figure 11-27, showing a medial view of the right side of the brain following a median sagittal section.

24. Structure number 1 is the location of the nucleus of the:
    (a) abducens nerve.
    (b) trochlear nerve.
    (c) trigeminal nerve.
    (d) facial nerve.
    (e) oculomotor nerve.
25. Structure number 2 is the location of the nucleus of the:
    (a) trigeminal nerve.
    (b) trochlear nerve.
    (c) abducens nerve.
    (d) oculomotor nerve.
    (e) vestibulocochlear nerve.
26. Structure number 3 is the:
    (a) oculomotor nerve.
    (b) trochlear nerve.
    (c) trigeminal nerve.

Figure 11-27   Medial view of the right side of the brain following a median sagittal section.

    (d) abducens nerve.
    (e) facial nerve.
27. Structure number 4 is the:
    (a) trochlear nerve.
    (b) oculomotor nerve.
    (c) trigeminal nerve.
    (d) facial nerve.
    (e) abducens nerve.
28. Structure number 5 is the:
    (a) lamina terminalis.
    (b) oculomotor nerve.
    (c) trochlear nerve.
    (d) abducens nerve.
    (e) optic chiasma.
29. Structure number 6 is the:
    (a) olfactory bulb.
    (b) crista galli.
    (c) olfactory stria.
    (d) anterior cerebral artery.
    (e) inferior frontal gyrus.

 Answers and Explanations to Review Questions

1. C is correct. The nucleus of the facial nerve supplying the muscles of the lower part of the face receives only crossed corticobulbar tracts (see Fig. 11-25). A. The inferior salivatory nucleus of the glossopharyngeal nerve receives descending tracts from the hypothalamus. B. The nucleus of the abducens nerve receives crossed and uncrossed corticobulbar tracts. D. The trigeminal motor nucleus receives crossed and uncrossed corticobulbar tracts. E. The nucleus of the trochlear nerve receives crossed and uncrossed corticobulbar tracts.

2. E is correct. The lacrimal nucleus forms part of the group of facial nuclei. A. The trigeminal nerve has a spinal nucleus. B. The inferior salivatory nucleus forms part of the glossopharyngeal nuclei. C. The

nucleus ambiguus is the motor nucleus associated with the 9th, 10th, and cranial part of the 11th cranial nerves. D. The facial nerve has a sensory nucleus for taste.

3. D is correct. In this patient, the muscles producing the mimetic movements of the face are innervated by corticobulbar fibers that have a course separate from that of the main corticobulbar fibers. A. The main corticobulbar fibers controlling the movements of the voluntary facial muscles in this patient have been destroyed. B. The reticular fibers, possibly originating in the hypothalamus and descending to the motor nuclei of the facial nerves, are intact. C. The facial nerves are intact since this patient is able to move the facial muscles.

E. The lower motor neurons of the facial nerve supplying the facial muscles are intact.

4. A is correct. The trapezoid body participates in the reception of sound.

5. B is correct. The cerebral cortex is necessary for the accommodation reflex.

6. D is correct. The nasal field of the right eye is projected to the temporal retina of the right eye. A. The nasal field of the right eye is projected to the right lateral geniculate body (see Fig. 11-2). B. The nasal field of the right eye is projected to both banks of the right calcarine fissure (see Fig. 11-2). C. The nasal field of the right eye is projected through the right optic tract (see Fig. 11-2). E. The nasal field of the right eye is projected through the right optic radiation (see Fig. 11-2).

7. B is correct. The right pupillary constriction associated with light directed at the left eye requires the left optic nerve (see Fig. 11-3). A. The right optic radiation is not required (see Fig. 11-3). C. The left Edinger–Westphal nucleus is not required (see Fig. 11-3). D. The right oculomotor nerve is required (see Fig. 11-3). E. The right optic nerve is not required (see Fig. 11-3).

8. A is correct.

9. C is correct.

10. A is correct. The spinal part of the accessory nerve supplies the trapezius muscle, which shrugs the shoulder. B. The facial nerve supplies the orbicularis oculi muscle, which closes the eye. C. The trigeminal nerve supplies the muscles of mastication responsible for chewing. D. The facial nerve receives the sensation of taste from the anterior two-thirds of the tongue. E. The glossopharyngeal nerve receives the sensation of touch from the posterior third of the tongue.

11. B is correct. The optic nerve is surrounded by an extension of the subarachnoid space. A. The nerve fibers of the optic nerve are surrounded by oligodendrocytes. C. Internal ophthalmoplegia is a condition in which the oculomotor nerve supply to the sphincter pupillae and the ciliary muscle is lost, but the innervation of the extraocular muscles is spared. D. External ophthalmoplegia is a condition in which the oculomotor nerve supply to the extraocular muscles is lost, but the innervation of the sphincter pupillae and the ciliary muscle is spared. E. The optic nerve leaves the orbital cavity through the optic canal in the lesser wing of the sphenoid bone.

12. E is correct. The olfactory receptor cells are located in the mucous membrane of the nasal cavity above the level of the superior concha. A. The main sensory nucleus of the trigeminal nerve lies in the brainstem lateral to the motor nucleus (see Fig. 11-7). B. Proprioceptive impulses from the facial muscles end in the mesencephalic nucleus of the trigeminal nerve. C. The facial nerve leaves the posterior cranial fossa with the vestibulocochlear nerve and enters the internal acoustic meatus. D. The superior salivatory nucleus of the facial nerve innervates the submandibular and sublingual salivary glands.

13. E is correct. The taste sensation from the mucous membrane covering the anterior two-thirds of the tongue is conducted in the facial nerves and the chorda tympani nerves, which are a considerable distance from the metastases in the deep cervical lymph nodes in the neck.

14. E is correct. The wasted right half of the tongue and the pointing of the protruded tongue to the right side indicated a lesion of the right hypoglossal nerve. The tongue muscles on the right side had atrophied and diminished in size, resulting in the wrinkling of the overlying normal mucous membrane.

The answers to questions 15 through 23 pertain to Figure 11-26, which shows the inferior view of the brain.

15. D is correct. Structure number 1 is the olfactory bulb.

16. E is correct. Structure number 2 is the olfactory tract.

17. A is correct. Structure number 3 is the optic nerve.

18. D is correct. Structure number 4 is the hypophysis cerebri.

19. E is correct. Structure number 5 is the optic tract.

20. B is correct. Structure number 6 is the spinal part of the accessory nerve.

21. C is correct. Structure number 7 is the sensory root of the trigeminal nerve.

22. A is correct. Structure number 8 is the motor root of the trigeminal nerve.

23. D is correct. Structure number 9 is the oculomotor nerve.

The answers to questions 24 through 29 pertain to Figure 11-27, showing a medial view of the right side of the brain following a median sagittal section.

24. E is correct. Structure number 1 is the nucleus of the oculomotor nerve in the tegmentum of the midbrain at the level of the superior colliculus.

25. B is correct. Structure number 2 is the nucleus of the trochlear nerve in the tegmentum of the midbrain at the level of the inferior colliculus.

26. C is correct. Structure number 3 is the trigeminal nerve emerging on the anterior surface of the pons.

27. B is correct. Structure number 4 is the oculomotor nerve emerging from the anterior surface of the midbrain in the interpeduncular fossa.

28. E is correct. Structure number 5 is the optic chiasma.

29. A is correct. Structure number 6 is the olfactory bulb.

12 Thalamus

CHAPTER OBJECTIVE

- To review the thalamus, a very complex area of the nervous system

- To emphasize that the thalamus lies at the center of many afferent and efferent neuronal loops to other parts of the nervous system

- To review some of the common clinical problems involving the thalamus

A 61-year-old man with hypertension is seen in the emergency department, having apparently suffered a stroke. A neurologist is called and makes a complete examination of the patient. The patient is conscious and is unable to feel any sensation down the right side of his body. No evidence of paralysis is noted on either side of the body, and the reflexes are normal. The patient is admitted to the hospital for observation.

Three days later, the patient appears to be improving, and return of sensation is evident on the right side of his body. The patient, however, seems to be excessively sensitive to testing for sensory loss. On light pinprick on the lateral side of the right leg, the patient suddenly shouts out because of excruciating burning pain, and he asks that the examination be stopped. Although the patient experiences very severe pain with the mildest stimulation, the threshold for pain sensitivity is raised, and the interval between applying the pinprick and the start of the pain is longer than normal; also, the pain persists after the stimulus has been removed. Moreover, the patient volunteers the information that the pain appears to be confined to the skin and does not involve deeper structures. Later, heat and cold stimulation are found to cause the same degree of discomfort.

The neurologist makes the diagnosis of analgesia dolorosa or Dejerine–Roussy syndrome involving the left thalamus. This condition of thalamic overreaction is most commonly caused by infarction of the lateral nuclei of the thalamus due to hypertensive vascular disease or thrombosis. Understanding the functional role of the thalamus in the sensory system and knowing the central connections of the thalamus are necessary in making a diagnosis of thalamic disease.

The thalamus is situated at the rostral end of the brainstem and functions as an important relay and integrative station for information passing to all areas of the cerebral cortex, the basal ganglia, the hypothalamus, and the brainstem.

GENERAL APPEARANCE

The thalamus is a large, egg-shaped mass of gray matter that forms the major part of the diencephalon. There are two thalami, and one is situated on each side of the third ventricle (Fig. 12-1; see also Fig. 7-3 and Atlas Plates 4, 5, and 8). The anterior end of the thalamus is narrow and rounded and forms the posterior boundary of the interventricular foramen. The posterior end is expanded to form the **pulvinar**, which overhangs the superior colliculus (Fig. 12-2). The inferior surface is continuous with the tegmentum of the midbrain. The medial surface of the thalamus forms part of the lateral wall of the third ventricle and is usually connected to the opposite thalamus by a band of gray matter, the **interthalamic connection** (interthalamic adhesion).

SUBDIVISIONS

The thalamus is covered on its superior surface by a thin layer of white matter, called the **stratum zonale**, and on its lateral surface by another layer, the **external medullary lamina** (see Fig. 12-1). The gray matter of the thalamus is divided by a vertical sheet of white matter,

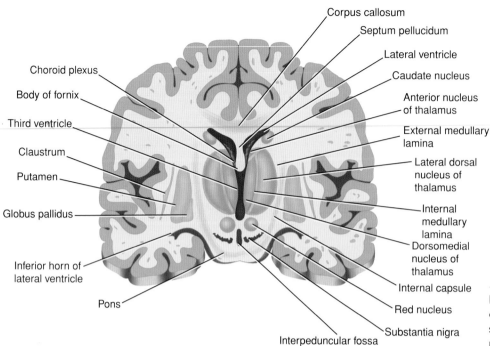

Corpus callosum
Septum pellucidum
Lateral ventricle
Caudate nucleus
Anterior nucleus of thalamus
External medullary lamina
Lateral dorsal nucleus of thalamus
Internal medullary lamina
Dorsomedial nucleus of thalamus
Internal capsule
Red nucleus
Substantia nigra
Interpeduncular fossa
Pons
Inferior horn of lateral ventricle
Globus pallidus
Putamen
Claustrum
Third ventricle
Body of fornix
Choroid plexus

Figure 12-1 Coronal section of the cerebral hemispheres showing the position and relations of the thalamus.

Cerebral cortex
Third ventricle
Stria medullaris thalami
Habenula
Pineal gland
Superior colliculus
Inferior colliculus
Trochlear nerve
Superior cerebellar peduncle
Sulcus limitans
Middle cerebellar peduncle
Facial colliculus
Floor of fourth ventricle
Cuneate tubercle
Gracile tubercle
Lentiform nucleus
Internal capsule
Caudate nucleus
Stria terminalis
Thalamus
Pulvinar of thalamus
Entrance into cerebral aqueduct
Medial eminence
Median sulcus
Striae medullares
Vestibular area
Hypoglossal triangle
Vagal triangle
Entrance into central canal
Posterior median sulcus
Central canal

Figure 12-2 Posterior view of the brainstem showing the thalamus and the tectum of the midbrain.

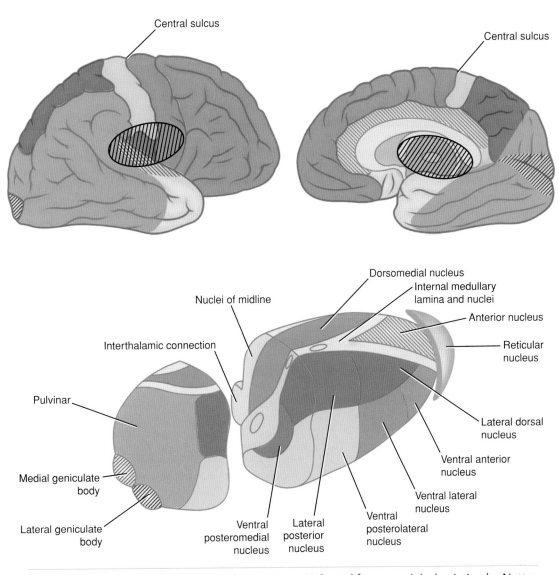

Figure 12-3 Important thalamocortical projections. (Adapted from an original painting by Netter, F. H. (1948). *The CIBA collection of medical illustrations*, copyright by CIBA Pharmaceutical Company, Division of CIBA-GEIGY Corporation.)

the **internal medullary lamina**, into medial and lateral halves (Fig. 12-3; also see Fig. 12-1). The internal medullary lamina consists of nerve fibers that pass from one thalamic nucleus to another. Anterosuperiorly, the internal medullary lamina splits, resembling a Y shape. The thalamus thus is subdivided into three main parts; the **anterior part** lies between the limbs of the Y, and the **medial** and **lateral parts** lie on the sides of the stem of the Y (see Fig. 12-3).

Each of the three parts of the thalamus contains a group of thalamic nuclei. Moreover, smaller nuclear groups are situated within the internal medullary lamina, and some are located on the medial and lateral surfaces of the thalamus.

Anterior Part

The anterior part of the thalamus contains the **anterior thalamic nuclei**. They receive the mammillothalamic tract from the mammillary nuclei. These anterior

thalamic nuclei also receive reciprocal connections with the cingulate gyrus and hypothalamus. The function of the anterior thalamic nuclei is closely associated with that of the limbic system and is concerned with emotional tone and the mechanisms of recent memory.

Medial Part

The medial part of the thalamus contains the large **dorsomedial nucleus** and several smaller nuclei. The dorsomedial nucleus has two-way connections with the whole prefrontal cortex of the frontal lobe of the cerebral hemisphere. It also has similar connections with the hypothalamic nuclei. It is interconnected with all other groups of thalamic nuclei. The medial part of the thalamus is responsible for the integration of a large variety of sensory information, including somatic, visceral, and olfactory information, and the relation of this information to one's emotional feelings and subjective states.

Lateral Part

The nuclei are subdivided into a dorsal tier and a ventral tier.

Dorsal Tier

The dorsal tier includes the **lateral dorsal nucleus**, the **lateral posterior nucleus**, and the **pulvinar**. The details of the connections of these nuclei are not clear. They are known, however, to have interconnections with other thalamic nuclei and with the parietal lobe, cingulate gyrus, and occipital and temporal lobes.

Ventral Tier

The ventral tier consists of the following nuclei in a craniocaudal sequence:

1. **Ventral anterior nucleus.** This nucleus is connected to the reticular formation, the substantia nigra, the corpus striatum, and the premotor cortex as well as to many of the other thalamic nuclei. Since this nucleus lies on the pathway between the corpus striatum and the motor areas of the frontal cortex, it probably influences the activities of the motor cortex.
2. **Ventral lateral nucleus.** This nucleus has connections similar to those of the ventral anterior nucleus but, in addition, has a major input from the cerebellum and a minor input from the red nucleus. Its main projections pass to the motor and premotor regions of the cerebral cortex. Here again, this thalamic nucleus probably influences motor activity.
3. **Ventral posterior nucleus.** This nucleus is subdivided into the **ventral posteromedial nucleus** and the **ventral posterolateral nucleus**. The ventral posteromedial nucleus receives the ascending trigeminal and gustatory pathways, while the ventral posterolateral nucleus receives the important ascending sensory tracts, the medial and spinal lemnisci. The thalamocortical projections from these important nuclei pass through the posterior limb of the internal capsule and corona radiata to the primary somatic sensory areas of the cerebral cortex in the postcentral gyrus (areas 3, 1, and 2).

Other Nuclei

Other thalamic nuclei include the intralaminar nuclei, the midline nuclei, the reticular nucleus, and the medial and lateral geniculate bodies.

The **intralaminar nuclei** are small collections of nerve cells within the internal medullary lamina. They receive afferent fibers from the reticular formation as well as fibers from the spinothalamic and trigeminothalamic tracts; they send efferent fibers to other thalamic nuclei, which in turn project to the cerebral cortex, and fibers to the corpus striatum. The nuclei are believed to influence the levels of consciousness and alertness in an individual.

The **midline nuclei** consist of groups of nerve cells adjacent to the third ventricle and in the interthalamic connection. They receive afferent fibers from the reticular formation. Their precise functions are unknown.

The **reticular nucleus** is a thin layer of nerve cells sandwiched between the external medullary lamina and the posterior limb of the internal capsule. Afferent fibers converge on this nucleus from the cerebral cortex and the reticular formation, and its output is mainly to other thalamic nuclei. The function of this nucleus is not fully understood, but it may be concerned with a mechanism by which the cerebral cortex regulates thalamic activity.

The **medial geniculate body** forms part of the auditory pathway and is a swelling on the posterior surface of the thalamus beneath the pulvinar. Afferent fibers to the medial geniculate body form the **inferior brachium** and come from the inferior colliculus. It should be remembered that the inferior colliculus receives the termination of the fibers of the lateral lemniscus. The medial geniculate body receives auditory information from both ears but predominantly from the opposite ear.

The efferent fibers leave the medial geniculate body to form the auditory radiation, which passes to the auditory cortex of the superior temporal gyrus. The **lateral geniculate body** forms part of the visual pathway and is a swelling on the undersurface of the pulvinar of the thalamus. The nucleus consists of six layers of nerve cells and is the terminus of all but a few fibers of the optic tract (except the fibers passing to the pretectal nucleus). The fibers are the axons of the ganglion cell layer of the retina and come from the temporal half of the ipsilateral eye and from the nasal half of the contralateral eye, the latter's fibers crossing the midline in the optic chiasma. Each lateral geniculate body, therefore, receives visual information from the opposite field of vision.

The efferent fibers leave the lateral geniculate body to form the visual radiation, which passes to the visual cortex of the occipital lobe.

CONNECTIONS

The following important neuronal loops exist between the thalamic nuclei and other areas of the central nervous system:

1. Every thalamic nucleus (except the reticular nucleus) sends axons to specific parts of the cerebral cortex (see Fig. 12-3), and every part of the cerebral cortex sends reciprocal fibers back to the thalamic nuclei. This would indicate that information received by the thalamus is always shared with the cerebral cortex and that the cortex and thalamus can modify each other's activities.
2. The thalamus is an important relay station for two sensory motor axonal loops involving the cerebellum and the basal nuclei: (1) the cerebellar–rubro–thalamic–cortical–ponto–cerebellar loop and (2) the corticostriatal–pallidal–thalamic–cortical loop, both of which are necessary for normal voluntary movement.

A summary of the various thalamic nuclei, their nervous connections, and their functions is provided in Table 12-1. The main connections of the various thalamic nuclei are summarized in Figure 12-4.

Table 12-1   Thalamic Nuclei: Connections and Functions

Thalamic Nucleus	Afferent Neuronal Loop	Efferent Neuronal Loop	Function
Anterior	Mammillothalamic tract, cingulate gyrus, hypothalamus	Cingulate gyrus, hypothalamus	Emotional tone, mechanisms of recent memory
Dorsomedial	Prefrontal cortex, hypothalamus, other thalamic nuclei	Prefrontal cortex, hypothalamus, other thalamic nuclei	Integration of somatic, visceral, and olfactory information and relation to emotional feelings and subjective states
Lateral dorsal, lateral posterior, pulvinar	Cerebral cortex, other thalamic nuclei	Cerebral cortex, other thalamic nuclei	Unknown
Ventral anterior	Reticular formation, substantia nigra, corpus striatum, premotor cortex, other thalamic nuclei	Reticular formation, substantia nigra, corpus striatum, premotor cortex, other thalamic nuclei	Influences activity of motor cortex
Ventral lateral	As in ventral anterior nucleus but also major input from cerebellum and minor input from red nucleus		Influences motor activity of motor cortex
Ventral posteromedial (VPM)	Trigeminal lemniscus, gustatory fibers	Primary somatic sensory (areas 3, 1, and 2) cortex	Relays common sensations to consciousness
Ventral posterolateral (VPL)	Medial and spinal lemnisci	Primary somatic sensory (areas 3, 1, and 2) cortex	Relays common sensations to consciousness
Intralaminar	Reticular formation, spinothalamic and trigeminothalamic tracts	To cerebral cortex via other thalamic nuclei, corpus striatum	Influences levels of consciousness and alertness
Midline	Reticular formation	Unknown	Unknown
Reticular	Cerebral cortex, reticular formation	Other thalamic nuclei	Cerebral cortex regulates thalamus
Medial geniculate body	Inferior colliculus, lateral lemniscus from both ears but predominantly the contralateral ear	Auditory radiation to superior temporal gyrus	Hearing
Lateral geniculate body	Optic tract	Optic radiation to visual cortex of occipital lobe	Visual information from opposite field of vision

FUNCTION

A practicing physician does not need to have a detailed knowledge of *all* the thalamic nuclei and their connections. Although an enormous amount of research has been devoted to this area, we still know very little about the functional significance of many of the nuclei.

However, the following basic principles *should* be committed to memory:

1. The thalamus is made up of complicated collections of nerve cells that are centrally placed in the brain and are interconnected.
2. A vast amount of sensory information of all types (except smell) converges on the thalamus and presumably is integrated through the interconnections between the nuclei. The resulting information pattern is distributed to other parts of the central nervous system. Olfactory information is probably first integrated at a lower level with taste and other sensations and is relayed to the thalamus from the amygdaloid complex and hippocampus through the mammillothalamic tract.
3. Anatomically and functionally, the thalamus and the cerebral cortex are closely linked. The fiber connections have been established, and, following removal of the cortex, the thalamus can appreciate crude sensations. However, the cerebral cortex is required for the interpretation of sensations based on past experiences. For example, if the sensory cortex is destroyed, one can still appreciate the presence of a hot object in the hand; however, appreciation of the shape, weight, and exact temperature of the object would be impaired.
4. The thalamus possesses certain very important nuclei whose connections have been clearly established. These include the ventral posteromedial nucleus, the ventral posterolateral nucleus, the medial geniculate body, and the lateral geniculate body. Their positions and connections should be learned.

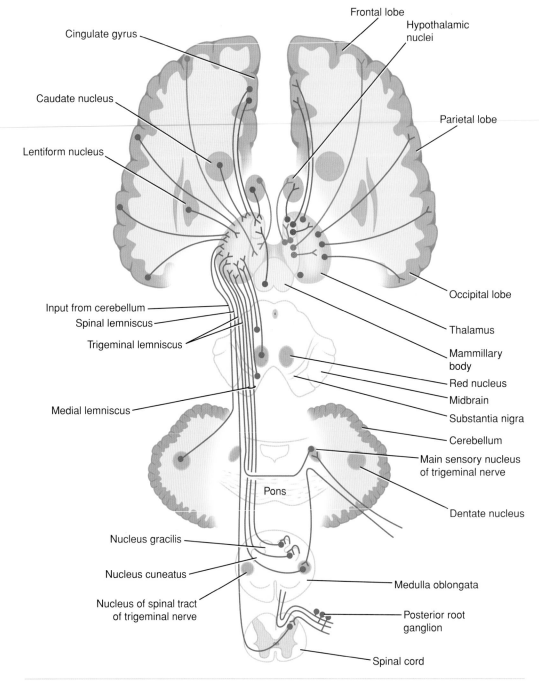

Figure 12-4 Main connections of the thalamus. Afferent fibers are shown on the left, and efferent fibers are shown on the right.

5. The ventroanterior and the ventrolateral nuclei of the thalamus form part of the basal nuclei circuit and thus are involved in the performance of voluntary movements. These nuclei receive input from the globus pallidus and send fibers to the prefrontal, supplemental, and premotor areas of the cerebral cortex.

6. The large dorsomedial nucleus has extensive connections with the frontal lobe cortex and hypothalamus. Considerable evidence suggests that this nucleus lies on the pathway that is concerned with subjective feeling states and the personality of the individual.

7. The intralaminar nuclei are closely connected with the activities of the reticular formation, and they receive much of their information from this source. Their strategic position enables them to control the level of overall activity of the cerebral cortex. The intralaminar nuclei are thus able to influence the levels of consciousness and alertness in an individual.

Clinical Notes

Lesions

Because the thalamus is such an important relay and integrative center, disease of this area of the central nervous system will have profound effects. The thalamus may be invaded by neoplasm, undergo degeneration following disease of its arterial supply, or be damaged by hemorrhage.

Sensory Loss

These lesions usually result from thrombosis or hemorrhage of one of the arteries supplying the thalamus. Damage to the ventral posteromedial nucleus and the ventral posterolateral nucleus will result in the loss of all forms of sensation, including light touch, tactile localization and discrimination, and muscle joint sense from the opposite side of the body.

The thalamus is centrally located among other important nervous structures. Usually, a thalamic lesion results in dysfunction of neighboring structures, producing symptoms and signs that overshadow those produced by the thalamic disease. For example, a vascular lesion of the thalamus may also involve the midbrain, with resulting coma, or a lateral extension of thalamic disease may involve the internal capsule and produce extensive motor and sensory deficits.

Surgical Relief of Pain by Thalamic Cauterization

The intralaminar nuclei of the thalamus are known to take part in the relay of pain to the cerebral cortex. Cauterization of these nuclei has been shown to relieve severe and intractable pain associated with terminal cancer.

Thalamic Pain

Thalamic pain may occur as the patient is recovering from a thalamic infarct. Spontaneous pain, which is often excessive (thalamic overreaction), occurs on the opposite side of the body. The painful sensation may be aroused by light touch or by cold and may fail to respond to powerful analgesic drugs.

ABNORMAL INVOLUNTARY MOVEMENTS

Choreoathetosis with ataxia may follow vascular lesions of the thalamus. Whether these signs in all cases are due to the loss of function of the thalamus or to involvement of the neighboring caudate and lentiform nuclei is not certain. The ataxia may arise as the result of the loss of appreciation of muscle and joint movement caused by a thalamic lesion.

THALAMIC HAND

The contralateral hand is held in an abnormal posture in some patients with thalamic lesions. The wrist is pronated and flexed, the metacarpophalangeal joints are flexed, and the interphalangeal joints are extended. The fingers can be moved actively, but the movements are slow. The condition is due to altered muscle tone in the different muscle groups.

Key Concepts

General Appearance

- The thalamus is a large egg-shaped mass that forms a major part of the diencephalon.
- It is located on either side of the third ventricle and attached by a band of gray matter called the interthalamic adhesion.
- The lateral thalamus contains the anterior thalamic nuclei, which are involved with the limbic system.
- The medial thalamus contains the large dorsomedial nucleus and two smaller nuclei, all of which are involved with somatic, visceral, and olfactory sensory information.
- The lateral thalamus is divided into dorsal and ventral tiers of nuclei.

- The dorsal tier includes the lateral dorsal nucleus, lateral posterior nucleus, and the pulvinar.
- The ventral tier includes the ventral anterior nucleus, ventral lateral nucleus, and the ventral posterior nuclei (posteromedial and posterolateral).

Functions

- A vast amount of sensory information converges on the thalamus and is distributed to other parts of the central nervous system.
- The thalamus is closely linked to the cortex but not for appreciation of sensation. For instance, upon removal of the cortex, the thalamus can still sense a hot object, but the interpretation of location, shape, weight, or temperature would be impaired.

Clinical Problem Solving

1. A 45-year-old man who has suddenly developed weakness of the left leg 12 hours previously is admitted to a medical ward. On examination, he is found to have paralysis of the left leg and weakness of the muscles of the left arm. The muscles of the affected limbs show increased tone, and tendon reflexes are exaggerated on the left side of the body. Also, considerable sensory loss on the left side of the body involves both the superficial and deep sensations. During the examination, the patient exhibits spontaneous jerking movements of the left leg. When asked to touch the tip of his nose with the left index finger, he demonstrates considerable intention tremor. The same test with the right arm shows nothing abnormal. Three days later, the patient starts to complain of agonizing pain down the left leg. The pain starts spontaneously or is initiated by the light touch of the bed sheet. What is your diagnosis? How can you explain the various signs and symptoms?

✓ Answers and Explanations to Clinical Problem Solving

1. This man had a thrombosis of the thalamogeniculate branch of the right posterior cerebral artery. This resulted in a degenerative lesion within the right thalamus, causing the impairment of superficial and deep sensations on the left side of the body. The contralateral hemiparesis, involving the left leg and left arm with increased muscle tone, was produced by edema in the nearby posterior limb of the right internal capsule, causing blocking of the corticospinal fibers. As the edema resolved, the paralysis and spasticity improved. The choreoathetoid movements of the left leg and the intention tremor of the left arm were probably due to damage to the right thalamus or to the right dentatothalamic nerve fibers. The agonizing pain felt down the left leg was due to the lesion in the right thalamus.

 Review Questions

Directions: Each of the numbered items in this section is followed by answers. Select the ONE lettered answer that is CORRECT.

1. The following statements concern the thalamus:
   (a) All types of sensory information, with the exception of smell, reach the thalamic nuclei via afferent fibers.
   (b) Very few afferent fibers reach the thalamic nuclei from the cerebral cortex.
   (c) The intralaminar nuclei of the thalamus are not connected to the reticular formation.
   (d) The intralaminar nuclei cannot influence the levels of consciousness and alertness.
   (e) The thalamus is covered on its inferior surface by a thin layer of white matter called the stratum zonale.

2. The following statements concern the thalamus:
   (a) The external medullary lamina is an area of gray matter lying on the lateral surface of the thalamus.
   (b) The Y-shaped external medullary lamina subdivides the thalamus into three main parts.
   (c) The ventral posteromedial nucleus receives the descending trigeminal and gustatory pathways.
   (d) The cerebellar–rubro–thalamic–cortical–ponto–cerebellar neuron pathway is important in voluntary movement.
   (e) The mammillary body–thalamus–amygdaloid nucleus–dentate gyrus neuron pathway is important in maintaining posture.

3. The following statements concern the thalamic nuclei:
   (a) The intralaminar nuclei lie outside the internal medullary lamina.
   (b) The ventral posterolateral nucleus receives the descending sensory tracts of the medial and spinal lemnisci.
   (c) The projections of the anterolateral nucleus ascend to the postcentral gyrus.
   (d) The reticular nucleus is part of the reticular formation.
   (e) The projections of the ventral posterolateral nucleus ascend to the postcentral gyrus through the posterior limb of the internal capsule.

4. The following statements concern the medial geniculate body:
   (a) The medial geniculate body receives auditory information from the superior colliculus and from the lateral lemniscus.
   (b) Efferent fibers from the medial geniculate body form the inferior brachium.
   (c) The medial geniculate body receives auditory information from both ears but predominantly from the opposite ear.
   (d) The medial geniculate body projects to the auditory cortex of the inferior temporal gyrus.
   (e) The medial geniculate body is a swelling on the anterior surface of the thalamus.
5. The following statements concern the lateral geniculate body:
   (a) The lateral geniculate body receives most of the fibers of the optic nerve.
   (b) Each lateral geniculate body receives visual information from the opposite field of vision.
   (c) The lateral geniculate body has a nucleus made up of 12 layers of nerve cells.
   (d) The lateral geniculate body is part of the midbrain at the level of the red nucleus.
   (e) The afferent fibers to the lateral geniculate body are the axons of the rods and cones of the retina.

Figure 12-5 CT scan of the brain showing a horizontal (axial) cut.

Directions: Each of the numbered incomplete statements in this section is followed by completions of the statement. Select the ONE lettered completion that is BEST in each case. For questions 6 through 13, study Figure 12-5, showing a computed tomography (CT) scan of the brain (horizontal cut [axial] section).

6. Structure number 1 is the:
   (a) falx cerebelli.
   (b) anterior cerebral artery.
   (c) crest of frontal bone.
   (d) sagittal suture.
   (e) longitudinal fissure.
7. Structure number 2 is the:
   (a) genu of corpus callosum.
   (b) lamina terminalis.
   (c) septum pellucidum.
   (d) anterior column of fornix.
   (e) interthalamic connection.
8. Structure number 3 is the:
   (a) lentiform nucleus.
   (b) internal capsule.
   (c) putamen.
   (d) head of caudate nucleus.
   (e) globus pallidus.
9. Structure number 4 is the:
   (a) pineal body.
   (b) falx cerebri.
   (c) third ventricle.
   (d) septum pellucidum.
   (e) great cerebral vein.

10. Structure number 5 is the:
    (a) medial geniculate body.
    (b) thalamus.
    (c) choroid plexus of lateral ventricle.
    (d) body of caudate nucleus.
    (e) third ventricle.
11. Structure number 6 is the:
    (a) thalamus.
    (b) head of caudate nucleus.
    (c) internal capsule.
    (d) claustrum.
    (e) lentiform nucleus.
12. Structure number 7 is the:
    (a) body of lateral ventricle.
    (b) tail of lateral ventricle.
    (c) anterior horn of lateral ventricle.
    (d) third ventricle.
    (e) fourth ventricle.
13. Structure number 8 is the:
    (a) septum pellucidum.
    (b) falx cerebri.
    (c) anterior cerebral artery.
    (d) lamina terminalis.
    (e) interthalamic adhesion.

Answers and Explanations to Review Questions

1. A is correct. All types of sensory information, with the exception of smell, reach the thalamic nuclei via afferent fibers. B. Large numbers of afferent fibers reach the thalamic nuclei from the cerebral cortex. C. The intralaminar nuclei of the thalamus are closely connected with the reticular formation. D. The intralaminar nuclei of the thalamus do influence the levels of consciousness and alertness. E. The thalamus is covered on its superior surface by a thin layer of white matter called the stratum zonale (see Fig. 12-1).

2. D is correct. The cerebellar–rubro–thalamic–cortical–ponto–cerebellar neuron pathway is important in voluntary movement. A. The external medullary lamina is an area of white matter lying on the lateral surface of the thalamus (see Fig. 12-1). B. The Y-shaped internal medullary lamina subdivides the thalamus into three main parts. C. The ventral posteromedial nucleus receives the ascending trigeminal and gustatory pathways. E. The mammillary body–thalamus–amygdaloid nucleus–dentate gyrus neuron pathway is not important in maintaining posture.

3. E is correct. The projections of the ventral posterolateral nucleus ascend to the postcentral gyrus through the posterior limb of the internal capsule. A. The intralaminar nuclei lie within the internal medullary lamina (see Fig. 12-3). B. The ventral posterolateral nucleus receives the ascending sensory tracts of the medial and spinal lemnisci. C. The projections of the posterolateral nucleus ascend to the postcentral gyrus. D. The reticular nucleus is not part of the reticular formation, although it receives afferent fibers from the formation.

4. C is correct. The medial geniculate body receives auditory information from both ears but predominantly from the opposite ear. A. The medial geniculate body receives auditory information from the inferior colliculus and from the lateral lemniscus. B. Afferent fibers from the medial geniculate body form the inferior brachium. D. The medial geniculate body projects to the auditory cortex of the superior temporal gyrus. E. The medial geniculate body is a swelling on the posterior surface of the thalamus (see Fig. 12-3).

5. B is correct. Each lateral geniculate body receives visual information from the opposite field of vision. A. The lateral geniculate body receives most of the fibers of the optic tract. C. The lateral geniculate body has a nucleus made up of six layers of nerve cells. D. The lateral geniculate body is a swelling on the undersurface of the pulvinar of the thalamus (see Fig. 12-3). E. The afferent fibers to the lateral geniculate body are the axons of the ganglion cells of the retina.

The answers for Figure 12-5, which shows a CT scan of the brain (horizontal cut [axial] section), are as follows:

6. E is correct. Structure number 1 is the longitudinal fissure.
7. A is correct. Structure number 2 is the genu of the corpus callosum.
8. D is correct. Structure number 3 is the head of the caudate nucleus.
9. C is correct. Structure number 4 is the third ventricle.
10. B is correct. Structure number 5 is the thalamus.
11. E is correct. Structure number 6 is the lentiform nucleus.
12. C is correct. Structure number 7 is the anterior horn of the lateral ventricle.
13. A is correct. Structure number 8 is the septum pellucidum.

13 Hypothalamus

CHAPTER OBJECTIVES

- To learn the location and boundaries of the hypothalamus and the various nuclei that make up this important area
- To review the main connections of the nuclei, especially the connections between

the hypothalamus and the pituitary gland

- To review some of the common clinical problems involving the hypothalamus

A 16-year-old girl is taken by her mother to a pediatrician because she is rapidly losing weight. The mother states that the weight loss started about 1 year ago. The child's eating habits changed from eating practically anything put before her to being a very choosy eater. Her personality is also changed, and she fears meeting strangers. Her relatives notice that she is impatient and irritable and cries a great deal. On being urged to eat more food, the girl countered by saying she was getting fat and must diet to improve her figure. Although she would not admit to having anything wrong with her, she admitted that menstruation had ceased 3 months previously.

On being questioned by the pediatrician, the girl admits to calorie counting, and sometimes, when she feels she has overeaten, will force herself to vomit by sticking her fingers down her throat. On physical examination, she shows obvious signs of weight loss with hollow facial features, prominent bones, and wasted buttocks. Apart from having cold extremities and a low blood pressure of 85/60 mm Hg, no further abnormalities are discovered.

The pediatrician makes the diagnosis of anorexia nervosa and admits her to the local hospital. Psychological treatment includes getting the confidence of the patient by using nursing personnel who understood the condition. The primary treatment is to restore the patient's weight by persuading the individual to eat adequate amounts of food.

Anorexia nervosa is a disorder of feeding and endocrine function that is normally controlled by the hypothalamus. However, strong evidence suggests that it is also of psychogenic origin.

The hypothalamus, although small (0.3% of the total brain), is a very important part of the central nervous system. It is essential for life. It controls the autonomic nervous system and the endocrine system and thus indirectly controls body homeostasis. The hypothalamus is well placed for this purpose, lying in the center of the limbic system. It is the site of numerous converging and diverging neuronal pathways, and through its adequate blood supply, it is able to sample the blood chemistry. The hypothalamus makes appropriate controlling responses following the integration of its nervous and chemical inputs.

HYPOTHALAMUS

The hypothalamus is the part of the diencephalon that extends from the region of the optic chiasma to the caudal border of the mammillary bodies. It lies below the thalamus and forms the floor and the inferior part of the lateral walls of the third ventricle (Fig. 13-1). Anterior to the hypothalamus is an area that, for functional reasons, is often included in the hypothalamus. Because it extends forward from the optic chiasma to the lamina terminalis and the anterior commissure, it is referred to as the **preoptic area**. Caudally, the hypothalamus merges into the tegmentum of the midbrain. The lateral boundary of the hypothalamus is formed by the internal capsule.

When observed from below (Fig. 13-2), the hypothalamus is seen to be related to the following structures, from anterior to posterior: (1) the optic chiasma, (2) the tuber cinereum and the infundibulum, and (3) the mammillary bodies.

This small area of the brain will be seen in the following paragraphs to control body homeostasis, through

Figure 13-1 Sagittal section of the brain showing the position of the hypothalamus.

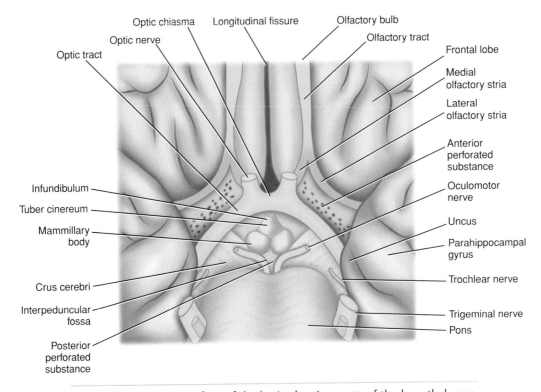

Figure 13-2 Inferior surface of the brain showing parts of the hypothalamus.

the autonomic nervous system and the neuroendocrine system, and to play a vital role in emotional behavior.

HYPOTHALAMIC NUCLEI

Microscopically, the hypothalamus is composed of small nerve cells that are arranged in groups or nuclei, many of which are not clearly segregated from one another. For functional reasons, the **preoptic area** is included as part of the hypothalamus. For purposes of description, the nuclei are divided by an imaginary parasagittal plane into medial and lateral zones (Fig. 13-3). Lying within the plane are the columns of the fornix and the mammillothalamic tract, which serve as markers (Fig. 13-4; also see Fig. 13-3).

Medial Zone

In the medial zone, the following hypothalamic nuclei can be recognized, from anterior to posterior: (1) part of the **preoptic nucleus**; (2) the **anterior nucleus**, which merges with the preoptic nucleus; (3) part of the **suprachiasmatic nucleus**; (4) the **paraventricular nucleus**;

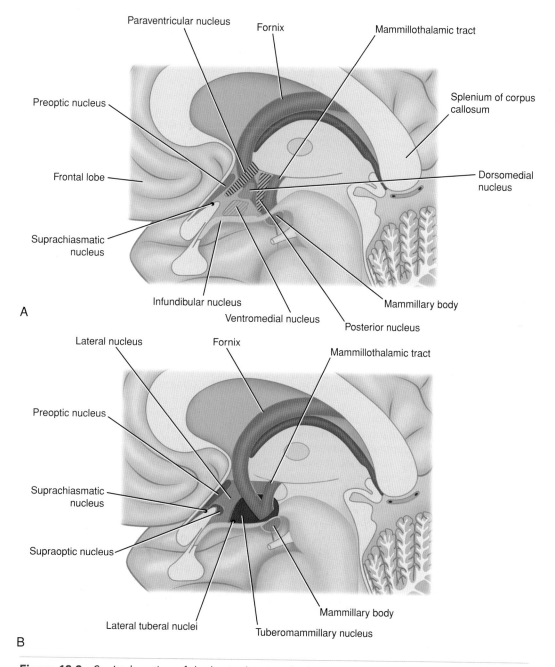

Figure 13-3 Sagittal section of the brain showing the hypothalamic nuclei. **A:** Medial zone nuclei lying medial to the plane of the fornix and the mammillothalamic tract. **B:** Lateral zone nuclei lying lateral to the plane of the fornix and the mammillothalamic tract.

Figure 13-4 Coronal section of the cerebral hemispheres showing the position of the hypothalamic nuclei.

(5) the **dorsomedial nucleus**; (6) the **ventromedial nucleus**; (7) the **infundibular (arcuate) nucleus**; and (8) the **posterior nucleus**.

Lateral Zone

In the lateral zone, the following hypothalamic nuclei can be recognized, from anterior to posterior: (1) part of the **preoptic nucleus**, (2) part of the **suprachiasmatic nucleus**, (3) the **supraoptic nucleus**, (4) the **lateral nucleus**, (5) the **tuberomammillary nucleus**, and (6) the **lateral tuberal nuclei**.

Some of the nuclei, such as the preoptic nucleus, the suprachiasmatic nucleus, and the mammillary nuclei, overlap both zones. It should be emphasized that most of the hypothalamic nuclei have ill-defined boundaries. With the use of modern technology, including histochemical, immunochemical, and anterograde and retrograde tracer studies, groups of neurons and their connections are being more precisely identified. Unfortunately, as new nuclear groups are discovered and given names, the reader has difficulty coming to terms with the old and new nomenclature. Only the major nuclear groups with well-established names and their connections are described in this account.

HYPOTHALAMIC LINES OF COMMUNICATION

The hypothalamus receives information from the rest of the body through (1) nervous connections, (2) the bloodstream, and (3) cerebrospinal fluid (CSF). The neurons of the hypothalamic nuclei respond and exert their control via the same routes. The CSF may serve as a conduit between the neurosecretory cells of the hypothalamus and distant sites of the brain.

Afferent Nervous Connections

The hypothalamus, which lies in the center of the limbic system, receives many afferent fibers from the viscera, the olfactory mucous membrane, the cerebral cortex, and the limbic system.

The afferent connections are numerous and complex; the main pathways (Fig. 13-5) are as follows:

1. **Somatic and visceral afferents.** General somatic sensation and gustatory and visceral sensations reach the hypothalamus through collateral branches of the lemniscal afferent fibers and the tractus solitarius and through the reticular formation.
2. **Visual afferents** leave the optic chiasma and pass to the suprachiasmatic nucleus.
3. **Olfaction** travels through the medial forebrain bundle.
4. **Auditory afferents** have not been identified, but since auditory stimuli can influence the activities of the hypothalamus, they must exist.
5. **Corticohypothalamic fibers** arise from the frontal lobe of the cerebral cortex and pass directly to the hypothalamus.
6. **Hippocampohypothalamic fibers** pass from the hippocampus through the fornix to the mammillary body. Many neurophysiologists regard the hypothalamus as the main output pathway of the limbic system.

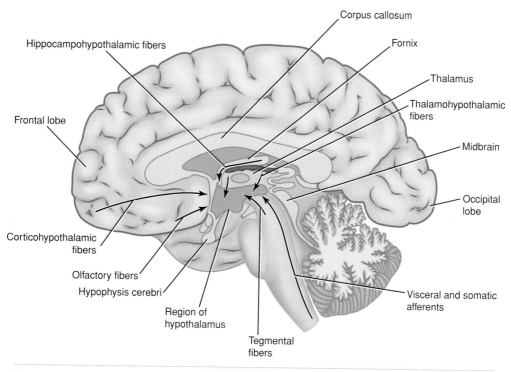

Figure 13-5 Sagittal section of the brain showing the main afferent pathways entering the hypothalamus.

7. **Amygdalohypothalamic fibers** pass from the amygdaloid complex to the hypothalamus through the stria terminalis and by a route that passes inferior to the lentiform nucleus.
8. **Thalamohypothalamic fibers** arise from the dorsomedial and midline thalamic nuclei.
9. **Tegmental fibers** arise from the midbrain.

The main afferent nervous connections of the hypothalamus are summarized in Table 13-1.

Efferent Nervous Connections

The efferent connections of the hypothalamus are also numerous and complex, and only the main pathways (Fig. 13-6) are described here:

1. **Descending fibers to the brainstem and spinal cord** influence the peripheral neurons of the autonomic nervous system. They descend through a series of neurons in the reticular formation. The hypothalamus is connected to the parasympathetic nuclei of the oculomotor, facial, glossopharyngeal, and vagus nerves in the brainstem. In a similar manner, the reticulospinal fibers connect the hypothalamus with sympathetic cells of origin in the lateral gray horns of the first thoracic segment to the second lumbar segment of the spinal cord and the sacral parasympathetic outflow at the level of the second, third, and fourth sacral segments of the spinal cord.
2. The **mammillothalamic tract** arises in the mammillary body and terminates in the anterior nucleus of the thalamus. Here, the pathway is relayed to the cingulate gyrus.

3. The **mammillotegmental tract** arises from the mammillary body and terminates in the cells of the reticular formation in the tegmentum of the midbrain.
4. Multiple pathways to the **limbic system**.

The main efferent nervous connections of the hypothalamus are summarized in Table 13-1.

Connections With the Hypophysis Cerebri

The hypothalamus is connected to the hypophysis cerebri (pituitary gland) by two pathways: (1) nerve fibers that travel from the supraoptic and paraventricular nuclei to the posterior lobe of the hypophysis and (2) long and short portal blood vessels that connect sinusoids in the median eminence and infundibulum with capillary plexuses in the anterior lobe of the hypophysis (Fig. 13-7). These pathways enable the hypothalamus to influence the activities of the endocrine glands.

Hypothalamohypophyseal Tract

The hormones **vasopressin** and **oxytocin** are synthesized in the nerve cells of the supraoptic and paraventricular nuclei. The hormones are passed along the axons together with carrier proteins called **neurophysins** and are released at the axon terminals (see Fig. 13-7). Here, the hormones are absorbed into the bloodstream in fenestrated capillaries of the posterior lobe of the hypophysis. The hormone vasopressin (antidiuretic hormone) is produced mainly in the nerve cells of the supraoptic nucleus. Its function is to cause **vasoconstriction**. It also has an important **antidiuretic function**, causing an increased absorption of water in

Table 13-1   Main Hypothalamic Afferent and Efferent Nervous Connections

Pathway	Origin	Destination
Afferent		
Medial and spinal lemnisci, tractus solitarius, reticular formation	Viscera and somatic structures	Hypothalamic nuclei
Visual fibers	Retina	Suprachiasmatic nucleus
Medial forebrain bundle	Olfactory mucous membrane	Hypothalamic nuclei
Auditory fibers	Inner ear	Hypothalamic nuclei
Corticohypothalamic fibers	Frontal lobe of cerebral cortex	Hypothalamic nuclei
Hippocampohypothalamic fibers; possibly main output pathway of limbic system	Hippocampus	Nuclei of mammillary body
Amygdalohypothalamic fibers	Amygdaloid complex	Hypothalamic nuclei
Thalamohypothalamic fibers	Dorsomedial and midline nuclei of thalamus	Hypothalamic nuclei
Tegmental fibers	Tegmentum of midbrain	Hypothalamic nuclei
Efferent		
Descending fibers in reticular formation to brainstem and spinal cord	Preoptic, anterior, posterior, and lateral nuclei of hypothalamus	Craniosacral parasympathetic and thoracolumbar sympathetic outflows
Mammillothalamic tract	Nuclei of mammillary body	Anterior nucleus of thalamus; relayed to cingulate gyrus
Mammillotegmental tract	Nuclei of mammillary body	Reticular formation in tegmentum of midbrain
Multiple pathways	Hypothalamic nuclei	Limbic system

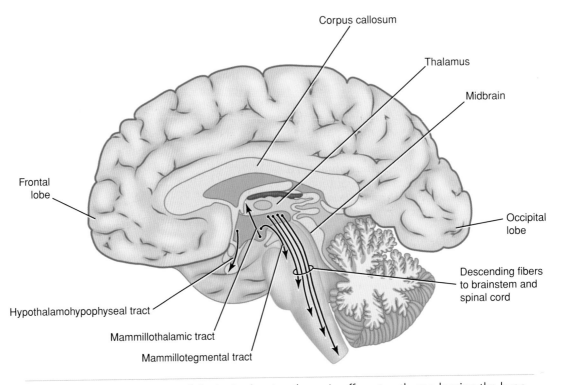

Figure 13-6 Sagittal section of the brain showing the main efferent pathways leaving the hypothalamus.

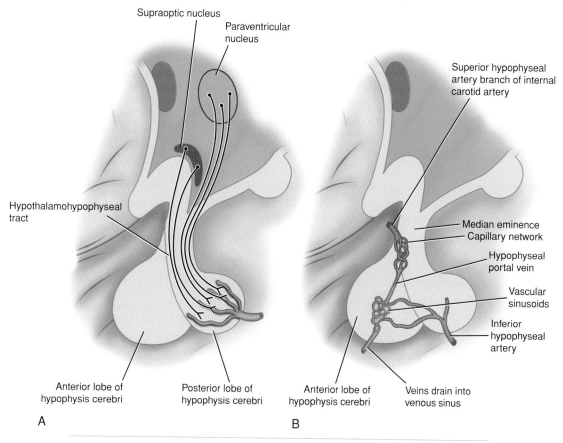

Figure 13-7 A: Hypothalamohypophyseal tract. **B:** Hypophyseal portal system.

the distal convoluted tubules and collecting tubules of the kidney. The other hormone is oxytocin, which is produced mainly in the paraventricular nucleus. Oxytocin stimulates the contraction of the smooth muscle of the uterus and causes contraction of the myoepithelial cells that surround the alveoli and ducts of the breast. Toward the end of pregnancy, oxytocin is produced in large amounts and stimulates labor contractions of the uterus. Later, when the baby suckles at the breast, a nervous reflex from the nipple stimulates the hypothalamus to produce more of the hormone. This promotes contraction of the myoepithelial cells and assists in the expression of the milk from the breasts.

The supraoptic nucleus, which produces vasopressin, acts as an **osmoreceptor**. Should the osmotic pressure of the blood circulating through the nucleus be too high, the nerve cells increase their production of vasopressin, and the antidiuretic effect of this hormone will increase the reabsorption of water from the kidney. By this means, the osmotic pressure of the blood will return to normal limits.

Hypophyseal Portal System

Neurosecretory cells situated mainly in the medial zone of the hypothalamus are responsible for the production of the **releasing hormones** and **release-inhibitory hormones.** The hormones are packaged into granules and

are transported along the axons of these cells into the median eminence and infundibulum. Here, the granules are released by exocytosis onto fenestrated capillaries at the upper end of the hypophyseal portal system.

The hypophyseal portal system is formed on each side from the superior hypophyseal artery, which is a branch of the internal carotid artery (see Fig. 13-7B). The artery enters the median eminence and divides into tufts of capillaries. These capillaries drain into long and short descending vessels that end in the anterior lobe of the hypophysis by dividing into vascular sinusoids that pass between the secretory cells of the anterior lobe.

The portal system carries the releasing hormones and the release-inhibiting hormones to the secretory cells of the anterior lobe of the hypophysis. The releasing hormones stimulate the production and release of **adrenocorticotropic hormone (ACTH)**, **follicle-stimulating hormone (FSH)**, **luteinizing hormone (LH)**, **thyrotropic hormone** or **thyroid-stimulating hormone (TSH)**, and **growth hormone (GH)**. The release of inhibiting hormones inhibits the release of the **melanocyte-stimulating hormone (MSH)** and **luteotropic hormone (LTH)**. LTH (also known as the **lactogenic hormone** or **prolactin**) stimulates the corpus luteum to secrete progesterone and the mammary gland to produce milk. The GH inhibitory hormone (somatostatin) inhibits the release of GH. A summary of the hypothalamic-releasing and inhibitory hormones and their effects

Table 13-2   Hypothalamic-Releasing and Inhibitory Hormones and Their Effects on Hypophysis (Pituitary) Anterior Lobe

Hypothalamic Regulatory Hormone	Anterior Pituitary Hormone	Functional Result
Growth hormone–releasing hormone (GHRH)	Growth hormone (GH)	Stimulates linear growth in epiphyseal cartilages
Growth hormone–inhibiting hormone (GHIH) or somatostatin	Growth hormone (reduced production)	Reduces linear growth in epiphyseal cartilages
Prolactin-releasing hormone (PRH)	Prolactin (luteotropic hormone, LTH)	Stimulates lactogenesis
Prolactin-inhibiting hormone (PIH), dopamine	Prolactin (luteotropic hormone, LTH) (reduced production)	Reduces lactogenesis
Corticotropin-releasing hormone (CRH)	Adrenocorticotropic hormone (ACTH)	Stimulates adrenal gland to produce corticosteroids and sex hormones
Thyrotropin-releasing hormone (TRH)	Thyroid-stimulating hormone (TSH)	Stimulates thyroid gland to produce thyroxine
Luteinizing hormone–releasing hormone (LHRH)	Luteinizing hormone (LH) and follicle-stimulating hormone (FSH)	Stimulates ovarian follicles and production of estrogen and progesterone

on the anterior lobe of the hypophysis are shown in Table 13-2.

The neurons of the hypothalamus that are responsible for the production of the releasing hormones and the release-inhibiting hormones are influenced by the afferent fibers passing to the hypothalamus. They also are influenced by the level of the hormone produced by the target organ controlled by the hypophysis. Should the level of thyroxine in the blood fall, for example, then the releasing factor for the thyrotropic hormone would be produced in increased quantities. Table 13-3 summarizes the presumed nuclear origin of the pituitary-releasing and inhibitory hormones in the hypothalamus.

FUNCTIONS

Table 13-4 summarizes the functions of the main hypothalamic nuclei.

Table 13-3   Nuclear Origin[a] of the Hypophysis (Pituitary)-Releasing and Inhibitory Hormones in the Hypothalamus

Hypothalamic Regulatory Hormone	Presumed Nuclear Origin
Growth hormone–releasing hormone (GHRH)	Infundibular or arcuate nucleus
Growth hormone–inhibiting hormone (GHIH) or somatostatin	Suprachiasmatic nucleus
Prolactin-releasing hormone (PRH)	?
Prolactin-inhibiting hormone (PIH)	?
Corticotropin-releasing hormone (CRH)	Paraventricular nuclei
Thyrotropin-releasing hormone (TRH)	Paraventricular and dorsomedial nuclei and adjacent areas
Luteinizing hormone–releasing hormone (LHRH)	Preoptic and anterior nuclei

[a]Origin is presumed.

Table 13-4   Main Hypothalamic Nuclei Functions

Hypothalamic Nucleus	Presumed Function
Supraoptic nucleus	Synthesizes vasopressin (antidiuretic hormone)
Paraventricular nucleus	Synthesizes oxytocin
Preoptic and anterior nuclei	Control parasympathetic system
Posterior and lateral nuclei	Control sympathetic system
Anterior hypothalamic nuclei	Regulate temperature (response to heat)
Posterior hypothalamic nuclei	Regulate temperature (response to cold)
Lateral hypothalamic nuclei	Initiate eating and increase food intake (hunger center)
Medial hypothalamic nuclei	Inhibit eating and reduce food intake (satiety center)
Lateral hypothalamic nuclei	Increase water intake (thirst center)
Suprachiasmatic nucleus	Controls circadian rhythms

Figure 13-8 Diagram depicting the hypothalamus as the chief center of the brain for controlling the internal milieu of the body.

Autonomic Control

The hypothalamus has a controlling influence on the autonomic nervous system and appears to integrate the autonomic and neuroendocrine systems, thus preserving body homeostasis. Essentially, the hypothalamus should be regarded as a higher nervous center for the control of lower autonomic centers in the brainstem and spinal cord (Fig. 13-8).

Electrical stimulation of the hypothalamus in animal experiments shows that the anterior hypothalamic area and the preoptic area influence parasympathetic responses; these include lowering of the blood pressure, slowing of the heart rate, contraction of the bladder, increased motility of the gastrointestinal tract, increased acidity of the gastric juice, salivation, and pupillary constriction.

Stimulation of the posterior and lateral nuclei causes sympathetic responses, which include elevation of blood pressure, acceleration of the heart rate, cessation of peristalsis in the gastrointestinal tract, pupillary dilation, and hyperglycemia. These responses would lead one to believe that in the hypothalamus, there exists areas that might be termed *parasympathetic and sympathetic centers*. However, it has been shown that considerable overlap of function occurs in these areas.

Endocrine Control

The nerve cells of the hypothalamic nuclei, by producing the releasing factors or release-inhibiting factors (see Table 13-2), control the hormone production of the anterior lobe of the hypophysis (pituitary gland). The anterior lobe hormones include GH, prolactin (LTH), ACTH, TSH, LH, and FSH. Some of these hormones act directly on body tissues, while others, such as ACTH, act through an endocrine organ, which in turn produces additional hormones that influence the activities of general body tissues. It should be pointed out that each stage is controlled by negative and positive feedback mechanisms.

Neurosecretion

The secretion of vasopressin and oxytocin by the supraoptic and paraventricular nuclei is discussed on page 377.

Temperature Regulation

The anterior portion of the hypothalamus controls those mechanisms that dissipate heat loss. Experimental stimulation of this area causes dilatation of skin blood vessels and sweating, which lower the body temperature. Stimulation of the posterior portion of the hypothalamus results in vasoconstriction of the skin blood vessels and inhibition of sweating; there also may be shivering, in which the skeletal muscles produce heat.

Normally, the hypothalamus sets the body temperature at 98.08° to 98.68°F when measured orally and 18°F higher when measured rectally. The temperature set can be altered in response to extremes, such as in environmental temperatures or in infection.

Regulation of Food and Water Intake

Stimulation of the lateral region of the hypothalamus initiates the feeling of hunger and results in an increase in food intake. This lateral region sometimes is referred to as the **hunger center**. Bilateral destruction of this center results in anorexia, with the consequent loss in body weight. Stimulation of the medial region of the hypothalamus inhibits eating and reduces food intake. This area is referred to as the **satiety center**. Bilateral destruction of the satiety center produces an uncontrolled voracious appetite, causing extreme obesity.

Experimental stimulation of other areas in the lateral region of the hypothalamus causes an immediate increase in the desire to drink water; this area is referred to as the **thirst center**. In addition, the supraoptic nucleus of the hypothalamus exerts a careful control on the osmolarity of the blood through the secretion of vasopressin (antidiuretic hormone) by the posterior lobe of the hypophysis. This hormone causes a great increase in the reabsorption of water in the distal convoluted tubules and collecting tubules of the kidneys.

Emotion and Behavior

Emotion and behavior are a function of the hypothalamus, the limbic system, and the prefrontal cortex. Some authorities believe that the hypothalamus is the integrator of afferent information received from other areas of the nervous system and brings about the physical expression of emotion; it can produce an increase in the heart rate, elevate the blood pressure, cause dryness of the mouth, flushing or pallor of the skin, and sweating. As well, it can often produce a massive peristaltic activity of the gastrointestinal tract.

Stimulation of the lateral hypothalamic nuclei may cause the symptoms and signs of rage, whereas lesions of these areas may lead to passivity. Stimulation of the ventromedial nucleus may cause passivity, whereas lesions of this nucleus may lead to rage.

Control of Circadian Rhythms

The hypothalamus controls many circadian rhythms, including body temperature, adrenocortical activity, eosinophil count, and renal secretion. Sleeping and wakefulness, although dependent on the activities of the thalamus, the limbic system, and the reticular activating system, are also controlled by the hypothalamus. Lesions of the anterior part of the hypothalamus seriously interfere with the rhythm of sleeping and waking. The suprachiasmatic nucleus, which receives afferent fibers from the retina, appears to play an important role in controlling the biologic rhythms. Nerve impulses generated in response to variations in the intensity of light are transmitted via this nucleus to influence the activities of many of the hypothalamic nuclei.

 Clinical Notes

General Considerations

In summary, the activities of the hypothalamus are modified by information received along numerous afferent pathways from different parts of the central nervous system (especially from the limbic system and the prefrontal cortex) and by the plasma levels of circulating hormones. It exerts its influence on bodily functions through the autonomic nervous system and the endocrine system.

Although small, the hypothalamus should not be interpreted as a structure of little importance. It is the chief center of the brain for maintaining the internal milieu of the body (see Fig. 13-8). Hardly any tissue in the body escapes its influence.

The connections of the hypothalamus are extremely complicated, and only the major pathways should be committed to memory for use in clinical work.

Clinical Disorders Associated With Hypothalamic Lesions

The hypothalamus may be the site of inflammation, neoplasm, or vascular disorder. Because of its deep-seated central position, it can be pressed on by tumors of the surrounding brain tissue or may be compressed as the result of the development of internal hydrocephalus. Its widespread influence on many homeostatic and behavioral functions means that a lesion of the hypothalamus will produce a large number of different syndromes. Importantly, an acute lesion is more likely to produce signs and symptoms than is a slowly growing tumor.

Obesity and Wasting

Severe obesity can occur as the result of hypothalamic lesions. It is generally associated with genital hypoplasia or atrophy.

Wasting is less common than obesity in hypothalamic disease. Severe cachexia is suggestive of damage to the hypophysis (pituitary gland).

Sexual Disorders

In children, sexual retardation and, rarely, sexual precocity may result from hypothalamic lesions. After puberty, the patient with hypothalamic disease may have impotence or amenorrhea.

Hyperthermia and Hypothermia

Hyperthermia can follow lesions of the hypothalamus caused by head injury or following surgical operations in the region of the hypothalamus. The patient with hyperthermia is otherwise normal and has no signs of malaise, which occurs with pyrexia secondary to infections. Hypothermia also can follow a lesion of the hypothalamus.

Diabetes Insipidus

Diabetes insipidus results from a lesion of the supraoptic nucleus or from the interruption of the nervous pathway to the posterior lobe of the hypophysis. Characteristically, the patient passes large volumes of urine of low specific gravity. As a result, the patient is extremely thirsty and drinks large quantities of fluids. The condition must be distinguished from diabetes mellitus, which is characterized by glucosuria.

Sleep Disturbance

The occurrence of either frequent short periods of sleep during the waking hours or insomnia has been observed in patients with hypothalamic lesions.

Emotional Disorders

Attacks of unexplained weeping or laughter, uncontrollable rage, depressive reactions, and even maniacal outbursts all have been observed in patients with hypothalamic lesions.

Key Concepts

Hypothalamus

- The hypothalamus controls body homeostasis through the autonomic nervous and endocrine systems and plays a vital role in emotional behavior.

Hypothalamic Nuclei

- The nerve cells in the hypothalamus are arranged in many small groups, or nuclei, which are not clearly segregated from one another. However, some nuclei such as the preoptic, suprachiasmatic, and mammillary nuclei are distinct and demonstrate functional significance.
- The hypothalamus not only receives information through nervous connections but also through the bloodstream and CSF.

Hypothalamic Connections With the Hypophysis Cerebri

- The hypothalamus is connected with the pituitary gland by two pathways: 1) nerve fibers from supraoptic and paraventricular nuclei to the posterior lobe of the hypophysis, and 2) long and short portal blood vessels that connect sinusoids in the median eminence and infundibulum with capillary plexuses in the anterior lobe of the hypophysis.

- The hypothalamohypophyseal tract: Vasopressin and oxytocin hormones are synthesized in the nerve cells of the supraoptic and paraventricular nuclei, released at axon terminals, and absorbed into the bloodstream via fenestrated capillaries of the posterior lobe of the hypophysis.
- Hypophyseal portal system: Neurosecretory cells in the hypothalamus produce releasing hormones and release-inhibitory hormones that are packaged into granules and released by exocytosis into fenestrated capillaries at the upper end of the portal system.
- The portal system carries the releasing hormone to the anterior lobe of the pituitary gland, which then stimulates production and release of hormones or inhibits the release of different hormones.

Hypothalamic Functions

- The hypothalamus shows influence and control over the autonomic nervous system, the endocrine system, temperature regulation, regulation of food and water intake, emotion and behavior, and circadian rhythms.

❓ Clinical Problem Solving

1. A 17-year-old boy is admitted into the medical ward for observation. The tentative diagnosis is Fröhlich syndrome. He has a 3-month history of severe headaches. More recently, he has attacks of vomiting, and 1 week ago he had noticed problems with his eyesight. The patient says that he has difficulty seeing objects on the lateral side of both eyes. His parents are concerned that he is putting on weight, as he has increased adiposity over the lower part of the trunk. On physical examination, the boy is found to be 6 ft 3 in tall; he has excessive trunk obesity. The testes and penis are small, and pubic and axillary hairs are absent. A lateral radiograph of the skull shows enlargement of the sella turcica with erosion of the dorsum sellae. An examination of the eye fields confirms that the patient has partial bitemporal hemianopia. Using your knowledge of neuroanatomy, explain the symptoms and signs of this patient.
2. A 40-year-old woman is involved in an automobile accident in which she sustains severe head injuries. Following a slow but uneventful recovery, she is released from the hospital without any residual signs or symptoms. Six months later, the patient starts to complain of frequency of micturition and is passing very large quantities of pale urine. She also says that she always seems thirsty and will often drink 10 glasses of water in one morning. Using your knowledge of neuroanatomy and neurophysiology, do you think a connection exists between the urinary symptoms and her automobile accident?
3. Do you think a patient with hydrocephalus could have a malfunctioning hypothalamus? If so, explain the connection.
4. Sherrington once stated in a scientific publication in 1947 that the hypothalamus should be regarded as the "head ganglion" of the autonomic nervous system (ANS). What is the relationship that exists between the hypothalamus and the ANS?
5. Explain what is meant by the terms *hypothalamohypophyseal tract* and *hypophyseal portal system*.

Answers and Explanations to Clinical Problem Solving

1. This boy was suffering from Fröhlich syndrome secondary to a chromophobe adenoma of the anterior lobe of the hypophysis. This space-occupying lesion had gradually eroded the sella turcica of the skull and had compressed the optic chiasma, producing bitemporal hemianopia. The size of the tumor was causing a raised intracranial pressure that was responsible for the headaches and attacks of vomiting. Pressure on the hypothalamus interfered with its function and resulted in the characteristic accumulation of fat in the trunk, especially the lower part of the abdomen. The hypogonadism and absence of secondary sex characteristics could have been due to pressure of the tumor on the hypothalamic nuclei and the consequent loss of control on the anterior lobe of the hypophysis, or it may have been due to the direct effect of the tumor pressing on the neighboring cells of the anterior lobe of the hypophysis.

2. Yes, the accident and the urinary symptoms are connected. This patient is suffering from diabetes insipidus caused by traumatic damage either to the posterior lobe of the hypophysis or to the supraoptic nucleus of the hypothalamus. In any event, production of vasopressin was inhibited. It should be pointed out that a lesion of the posterior lobe of the hypophysis is usually not followed by diabetes insipidus, since the vasopressin produced by the neurons of the supraoptic nucleus escapes directly into the bloodstream. The action of vasopressin on the distal convoluted tubules and collecting tubules of the kidney is fully explained on page 381.

3. Yes, it is possible. Hydrocephalus, caused by blockage of the three foramina in the roof of the fourth ventricle or by blockage of the cerebral aqueduct, will result in a rise in pressure in the third ventricle, with pressure on the hypothalamus. This pressure on the hypothalamus, which is situated in the floor and lower part of the lateral walls of the third ventricle, if great enough, could easily cause malfunctioning of the hypothalamus.

4. The hypothalamus is the main subcortical center regulating the parasympathetic and sympathetic parts of the autonomic system. It exerts its influence through descending pathways in the reticular formation.

5. The hypothalamohypophyseal tract is described on page 377, and the hypophyseal portal system is described on page 379. Remember that the hypothalamus exerts its control over metabolic and visceral functions through the hypophysis cerebri and the autonomic nervous system.

 Review Questions

Directions: Each of the numbered items in this section is followed by answers. Select the ONE lettered answer that is CORRECT.

1. The following statements concern the hypothalamus:
   (a) It lies below the thalamus in the tectum of the midbrain.
   (b) It is not related to the limbic system.
   (c) The nuclei of the hypothalamus are divided by an imaginary plane formed by the columns of the fornix and the mammillothalamic tract into medial and lateral groups.
   (d) The suprachiasmatic nucleus does not receive nerve fibers from the retina.
   (e) The lateral boundary of the hypothalamus is formed by the external capsule.

2. The following statements concern the hypothalamus:
   (a) When seen from the inferior aspect, the hypothalamus is related to the following structures, from anterior to posterior: (i) the olfactory stria, (ii) the anterior perforated substance, and (iii) the mammillary bodies.
   (b) The margins of the different nuclei can be clearly seen with the naked eye.
   (c) The mammillary body does not overlap the medial and lateral groups of hypothalamic nuclei.
   (d) The preoptic area of the hypothalamus is located between the septum pellucidum and the optic chiasma.
   (e) The blood–brain barrier is absent in the median eminence of the hypothalamus, thus permitting the neurons to sample the chemical content of the plasma directly.

3. The following statements concern the afferent fibers passing to the hypothalamus:
   (a) Fibers pass from the hippocampus to the mammillary bodies, bringing information from the auditory system.
   (b) Olfactory impulses reach the hypothalamus through the lateral forebrain bundle.
   (c) The hypothalamus receives many afferent fibers from the viscera via the reticular formation.
   (d) The dorsomedial nucleus receives axons from the posterior lobe of the pituitary.
   (e) The pineal gland sends fibers via the habenular commissure to the hypothalamus.

4. The following statements concern the hypothalamus:
   (a) Somatic efferent fibers leave the hypothalamic nuclei via the medial and spinal lemnisci.
   (b) It does not integrate the autonomic and neuroendocrine systems.
   (c) The posterior portion of the hypothalamus controls those mechanisms that dissipate heat loss.
   (d) The nerve cells of the hypothalamus produce releasing and release-inhibiting hormones that control the production of various hormones in the anterior lobe of the hypophysis.
   (e) The hunger center is probably located in the posterior hypothalamic nuclei.

5. The following statements concern the functional activities of the hypothalamus:
   (a) The hypothalamus brings about the physical changes associated with emotion, such as increased heart rate and flushing or pallor of the skin.
   (b) The medial hypothalamic nuclei are concerned with fluid intake.
   (c) The corticotropin-releasing hormone (CRH) is produced in the anterior nucleus of the hypothalamus.
   (d) The suprachiasmatic nucleus plays no part in controlling circadian rhythms.
   (e) The hypothalamus controls the lower autonomic centers by means of pathways through the tectospinal tract.

6. The following statements concern the hypothalamohypophyseal tract:
   (a) Oxytocin inhibits the contraction of the smooth muscle of the uterus.
   (b) The nerve cells of the supraoptic and paraventricular nuclei produce the hormones vasopressin and oxytocin.
   (c) The hormones travel in lymph vessels with protein carriers called neurophysins.
   (d) Vasopressin stimulates the proximal convoluted tubules of the kidney, causing increased absorption of water from the urine.
   (e) The hormones are absorbed into the bloodstream in the capillaries of the anterior lobe of the hypophysis.

7. The following statements concern the hypophyseal portal system:
   (a) It carries releasing hormones and release-inhibiting hormones to the secretory cells of the anterior lobe of the hypophysis.
   (b) The production of the releasing hormones and the release-inhibiting hormones cannot be influenced by the level of the hormone produced by the target organ controlled by the hypophysis.
   (c) The blood vessels commence superiorly in the median eminence and end inferiorly in the vascular sinusoids of the posterior lobe of the hypophysis cerebri.
   (d) Efferent nerve fibers leaving the hypothalamus influence the production of the releasing hormones by nerve cells.
   (e) The neuroglial cells of the hypothalamus are responsible for the production of the release-inhibiting hormones.

 Answers and Explanations to Review Questions

1. C is correct. The nuclei of the hypothalamus are divided by an imaginary plane formed by the columns of the fornix and the mammillothalamic tract into medial and lateral groups (see Fig. 13-3). A. The hypothalamus lies below the thalamus and not in the tectum of the midbrain (see Fig. 13-1). B. The hypothalamus lies in the center of the limbic system. D. The suprachiasmatic nucleus does receive nerve fibers from the retina. E. The lateral boundary of the hypothalamus is formed by the internal capsule.

2. E is correct. The blood–brain barrier is absent in the median eminence of the hypothalamus, thus permitting the neurons to sample the chemical content of the plasma directly. A. When seen from the inferior aspect, the hypothalamus is related to the following structures: (i) the optic chiasma, (ii) the tuber cinereum, and (iii) the mammillary bodies (see Fig. 13-2). B. The margins of the different hypothalamic nuclei are ill-defined and cannot be seen with the naked eye. C. The mammillary body overlaps both the medial and lateral groups of hypothalamic nuclei. D. The preoptic area of the hypothalamus is located between the lamina terminalis and the optic chiasma.

3. C is correct. The hypothalamus receives many afferent fibers from the viscera via the reticular formation. A. Fibers pass from the hippocampus to the mammillary bodies, bringing information from the limbic system. B. Olfactory impulses reach the hypothalamus through the medial forebrain bundle. D. The dorsomedial nucleus of the hypothalamus does not receive axons from the posterior lobe of the pituitary. E. The pineal gland does not send nerve fibers to the hypothalamus.

4. D is correct. The nerve cells of the hypothalamus produce releasing and release-inhibiting hormones that control the production of various hormones in the anterior lobe of the hypophysis. A. Somatic afferent fibers enter the hypothalamic nuclei via the medial and spinal lemnisci. B. The hypothalamus does integrate the autonomic and neuroendocrine systems, thus preserving homeostasis. C. The anterior portion of the hypothalamus controls those mechanisms that

dissipate heat loss. E. The hunger center is probably located in the lateral region of the hypothalamus.

5. A is correct. The hypothalamus probably brings about the physical changes associated with emotion, such as increased heart rate and flushing or pallor of the skin. B. The lateral hypothalamic nuclei are concerned with fluid intake. C. The CRH is produced in the paraventricular nuclei of the hypothalamus (see Table 13-3). D. The suprachiasmatic nucleus plays an important role in controlling circadian rhythms. E. The hypothalamus controls the lower autonomic centers by means of pathways through the reticular formation.

6. B is correct. The nerve cells of the supraoptic and paraventricular nuclei produce the hormones vasopressin and oxytocin. A. Oxytocin stimulates the contraction of the smooth muscle of the uterus. C. The hormones travel in the axons of the hypothalamohypophyseal tract with protein carriers called neurophysins. D. Vasopressin stimulates the distal convoluted tubules and collecting tubules of the kidney, causing increased absorption of water from the urine. E. The hormones leave the axons of the tract and are absorbed into the bloodstream in the capillaries of the posterior lobe of the hypophysis.

7. A is correct. The hypophyseal portal system carries releasing hormones and release-inhibiting hormones to the secretory cells of the anterior lobe of the hypophysis. B. The production of the releasing hormones and the release-inhibiting hormones can be influenced by the level of the hormone produced by the target organ controlled by the hypophysis. C. The blood vessels of the hypophyseal portal system commence superiorly in the median eminence and end inferiorly in the vascular sinusoids of the anterior lobe of the hypophysis cerebri. D. Afferent nerve fibers entering the hypothalamus influence the production of the releasing hormones by the nerve cells. E. The neuroglial cells of the hypothalamus are not responsible for the production of the release-inhibiting hormones.

14 Autonomic Nervous System

CHAPTER OBJECTIVES

- To understand the structure and physiology of the autonomic nervous system

- To understand the pharmacologic differences between the sympathetic and parasympathetic nervous systems

A 46-year-old man underwent a right-sided pneumonectomy for carcinoma of the bronchus and is seen by his thoracic surgeon for follow-up. The patient says that he feels surprisingly fit and is gaining some of the weight that he had lost prior to the operation. His wife comments that the upper lid of his right eye tends to droop slightly when he gets tired at the end of the day.

During a careful physical examination, the surgeon notices that in addition to the ptosis of the right eye, the patient's right pupil is constricted and that his face is slightly flushed on the right side. Further examination reveals that the skin on the right side of the face appears to be warmer and drier than normal. Palpation of the deep cervical group of lymph nodes reveals a large, hard, fixed node just above the right clavicle.

Based on his clinical findings, the surgeon makes the diagnosis of a right-sided Horner syndrome. These findings were not present before the operation. The presence of the enlarged right-sided deep cervical lymph node indicates that the bronchial carcinoma has metastasized to the lymph node in the neck and is spreading to involve the cervical part of the sympathetic trunk on the right side. This observation explains the abnormal eye and facial skin findings.

Knowledge of the sympathetic innervation of the structures of the head and neck enables the surgeon to make an accurate diagnosis in this patient.

The autonomic nervous system (ANS) and the endocrine system control the internal environment of the body. The ANS provides a fine discrete control over the functions of many organs and tissues, including heart muscle, smooth muscle, and the exocrine glands. The endocrine system, by means of its blood-borne hormones, exerts a slower more diffuse control.

The ANS, like the somatic nervous system, has afferent, connector, and efferent neurons. The afferent impulses originate in visceral receptors and travel via afferent pathways to the central nervous system (CNS), where they are integrated through connector neurons at different levels and then leave via efferent pathways to visceral effector organs. The majority of the activities of the autonomic system do not impinge on consciousness.

The efferent pathways of the autonomic system are made up of preganglionic and postganglionic neurons. The cell bodies of the preganglionic neurons are situated in the lateral gray column of the spinal cord and in the motor nuclei of the 3rd, 7th, 9th, and 10th cranial nerves. The axons of these cell bodies synapse on the cell bodies of the postganglionic neurons that are collected together to form **ganglia** outside the CNS.

The control exerted by the autonomic system is extremely rapid; it is also widespread, since one preganglionic axon may synapse with several postganglionic neurons. Large collections of afferent and efferent fibers and their associated ganglia form **autonomic plexuses** in the thorax, abdomen, and pelvis.

The visceral receptors include chemoreceptors, baroreceptors, and osmoreceptors. Pain receptors are present in viscera and certain types of stimuli, such as lack of oxygen or stretch, can cause extreme pain.

The information provided in this chapter is extensively used in clinical practice. The examples of autonomic innervations given are important and are commonly used by examiners to construct good questions.

ORGANIZATION

The ANS is distributed throughout the central and peripheral nervous systems. It is divided into two parts, the **sympathetic** and the **parasympathetic** and, as emphasized earlier, consists of both afferent and efferent fibers. This division between sympathetic and parasympathetic is made on the basis of anatomic differences, differences in the neurotransmitters, and differences in the physiologic effects.

Both the sympathetic and parasympathetic divisions produce opposite effects in most organs and are thus considered as physiologic antagonists. However, both divisions operate in conjunction with one another and the balance in the activities maintains a stable internal environment.

Sympathetic Part

The sympathetic system is the larger of the two parts of the autonomic system and is widely distributed throughout the body, innervating the heart and lungs, the muscle in the walls of many blood vessels, the hair follicles and the sweat glands, and many abdominopelvic viscera.

The function of the sympathetic system is to prepare the body for an emergency. The heart rate is increased, arterioles of the skin and intestine are constricted, arterioles of skeletal muscle are dilated, and the blood pressure is raised. Blood is redistributed; thus, it leaves the skin and gastrointestinal tract and passes to the brain, heart, and skeletal muscle. In addition, the sympathetic nerves dilate the pupils; inhibit smooth muscle of the bronchi, intestine, and bladder wall; and close the sphincters. The hair is made to stand on end, and sweating occurs.

The sympathetic system consists of the efferent outflow from the spinal cord, two ganglionated sympathetic trunks, important branches, plexuses, and regional ganglia.

Efferent Nerve Fibers (Sympathetic Outflow)

The lateral gray columns (horns) of the spinal cord from the first thoracic segment to the second lumbar segment (sometimes third lumbar segment) possess the cell bodies of the sympathetic connector neurons (Fig. 14-1). The myelinated axons of these cells leave the cord in the anterior nerve roots and pass via the **white rami communicantes** (the white rami are white because the nerve fibers are covered with white myelin) to the **paravertebral ganglia** of the **sympathetic trunk**. Once these fibers (preganglionic) reach the ganglia in the sympathetic trunk, they are distributed as follows:

1. They synapse with an excitor neuron in the ganglion. The gap between the two neurons is bridged by the neurotransmitter **acetylcholine (ACh)**. The postganglionic nonmyelinated axons leave the ganglion and pass to the thoracic spinal nerves as **gray rami communicantes** (the gray rami are gray because the nerve fibers are devoid of myelin). They are distributed in branches of the spinal nerves to smooth muscle in the blood vessel walls, sweat glands, and arrector pili muscle of the hairs of the skin.

2. They travel cephalad in the sympathetic trunk to synapse in ganglia in the cervical region (Fig. 14-2). The postganglionic nerve fibers pass via gray rami communicantes to join the cervical spinal nerves. Many of the preganglionic fibers entering the lower part of the sympathetic trunk from the lower thoracic and upper two lumbar segments of the spinal cord travel caudad to synapse in ganglia in the lower lumbar and sacral regions. Here again, the postganglionic nerve

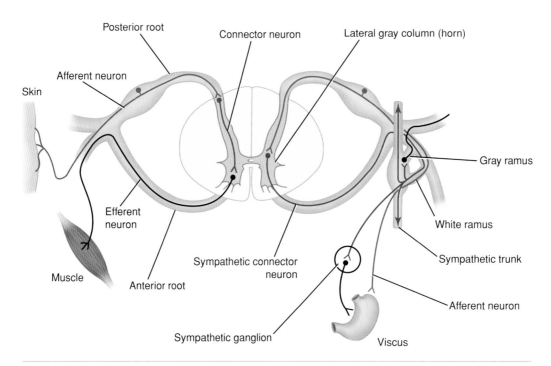

Figure 14-1 General arrangement of the somatic part of the nervous system (on **left**) compared with the autonomic part of the nervous system (on **right**).

Figure 14-2 Efferent part of the autonomic nervous system. Preganglionic parasympathetic fibers are shown in solid blue and postganglionic parasympathetic fibers are shown in interrupted blue. Preganglionic sympathetic fibers are shown in solid red and postganglionic sympathetic fibers are shown in interrupted red.

fibers pass via gray rami communicantes to join the lumbar, sacral, and coccygeal spinal nerves.

3. They may pass through the ganglia of the sympathetic trunk without synapsing. These myelinated fibers leave the sympathetic trunk as the **greater splanchnic**, **lesser splanchnic**, and **lowest** or **least splanchnic nerves**. The greater splanchnic nerve is formed from branches from the fifth to the ninth thoracic ganglia. It descends obliquely on the sides of the bodies of the thoracic vertebrae and pierces the crus of the diaphragm to synapse with excitor cells in the ganglia of the **celiac plexus**, the **renal plexus**, and the suprarenal medulla. The lesser splanchnic nerve is formed from branches of the 10th and 11th thoracic ganglia. It descends with the greater splanchnic

nerve and pierces the diaphragm to join excitor cells in ganglia in the lower part of the **celiac plexus.** The lowest splanchnic nerve (when present) arises from the 12th thoracic ganglion, pierces the diaphragm, and synapses with excitor neurons in the ganglia of the **renal plexus**. The splanchnic nerves, therefore, are formed of preganglionic fibers. The postganglionic fibers arise from the excitor cells in the peripheral plexuses and are distributed to the smooth muscle and glands of the viscera. A few preganglionic fibers, traveling in the greater splanchnic nerve, end directly on the cells of the **suprarenal medulla**. These medullary cells, which may be regarded as modified sympathetic excitor neurons, are responsible for the secretion of epinephrine and norepinephrine.

The ratio of preganglionic to postganglionic sympathetic fibers is about 1:10, permitting a wide control of involuntary structures.

Afferent Nerve Fibers

Afferent myelinated nerve fibers travel from the viscera through the sympathetic ganglia without synapsing. They pass to the spinal nerve via white rami communicantes and reach their cell bodies in the posterior root ganglion of the corresponding spinal nerve (see Fig. 14-1). The central axons then enter the spinal cord and may form the afferent component of a local reflex arc or ascend to higher centers, such as the hypothalamus.

Sympathetic Trunks

The sympathetic trunks are two ganglionated nerve trunks that extend the whole length of the vertebral column (see Fig. 14-2). In the neck, each trunk has 3 ganglia; in the thorax, 11 or 12; in the lumbar region, 4 or 5; and in the pelvis, 4 or 5. In the neck, the trunks lie anterior to the transverse processes of the cervical vertebrae; in the thorax, they are anterior to the heads of the ribs or lie on the sides of the vertebral bodies; in the abdomen, they are anterolateral to the sides of the bodies of the lumbar vertebrae; and in the pelvis, they are anterior to the sacrum. Below, the two trunks terminate by joining together to form a single ganglion, the **ganglion impar**.

Parasympathetic Part

The activities of the parasympathetic part of the autonomic system are directed toward conserving and restoring energy. The heart rate is slowed, pupils are constricted, peristalsis and glandular activity is increased, sphincters are opened, and the bladder wall is contracted.

Efferent Nerve Fibers (Craniosacral Outflow)

The connector nerve cells of the parasympathetic part of the ANS are located in the brainstem and the sacral segments of the spinal cord (see Fig. 14-2).

Those nerve cells located in the brainstem form nuclei in the following cranial nerves: the **oculomotor** (parasympathetic or Edinger–Westphal nucleus), the **facial** (superior salivatory nucleus and lacrimatory nucleus), the **glossopharyngeal** (inferior salivatory nucleus), and the **vagus** nerves (dorsal nucleus of the vagus). The axons of these connector nerve cells are myelinated and emerge from the brain within the cranial nerves.

The sacral connector nerve cells are found in the gray matter of the **second**, **third**, and **fourth sacral segments of the spinal cord**. These cells are not sufficiently numerous to form a lateral gray horn, as do the sympathetic connector neurons in the thoracolumbar region. The myelinated axons leave the spinal cord in the anterior nerve roots of the corresponding spinal nerves. They then leave the sacral nerves and form the **pelvic splanchnic nerves**.

The myelinated efferent fibers of the craniosacral outflow are preganglionic and synapse in peripheral ganglia located close to the viscera they innervate. Here again, acetylcholine is the neurotransmitter. The cranial parasympathetic ganglia are the **ciliary, pterygopalatine, submandibular**, and **otic**. In certain locations, the ganglion cells are placed in nerve plexuses, such as the **cardiac plexus, pulmonary plexus, myenteric plexus (Auerbach plexus)**, and **submucosal plexus (Meissner plexus)**; the last two plexuses are associated with the gastrointestinal tract. The pelvic splanchnic nerves synapse in ganglia in the **hypogastric plexuses**. Characteristically, the postganglionic parasympathetic fibers are nonmyelinated and of relatively short length compared with sympathetic postganglionic fibers.

The ratio of preganglionic to postganglionic fibers is about 1:3 or less, which is much more restricted than in the sympathetic part of the system.

Afferent Nerve Fibers

Afferent myelinated fibers span from the viscera to their cell bodies, located either in the sensory ganglia of the cranial nerves or in the posterior root ganglia of the sacrospinal nerves. The central axons then enter the CNS and take part in the formation of local reflex arcs or pass to higher centers of the ANS, such as the hypothalamus.

The afferent component of the autonomic system is identical to the afferent component of somatic nerves, and it forms part of the general afferent segment of the entire nervous system. The nerve endings in the autonomic afferent component may not be activated by such sensations as heat or touch but rather by stretch or lack of oxygen. Once the afferent fibers gain entrance to the spinal cord or brain, they are thought to travel alongside, or mixed with, the somatic afferent fibers.

LARGE AUTONOMIC PLEXUSES

Large collections of sympathetic and parasympathetic efferent nerve fibers and their associated ganglia, together with visceral afferent fibers, form **autonomic nerve plexuses** (a collection of nerve fibers that form a network, possibly containing nerve cells) in the thorax, abdomen, and pelvis. Branches from these plexuses innervate the viscera. The thorax contains the cardiac, pulmonary, and esophageal plexuses. In the abdomen, the plexuses are associated with the aorta and its branches, and subdivisions of these autonomic plexuses are named according to the branch of the aorta along which they are lying: celiac, superior mesenteric, inferior mesenteric, and aortic plexuses. The pelvis contains the superior and inferior hypogastric plexuses.

AUTONOMIC GANGLIA

The **autonomic ganglion** (a knotlike mass of nerve cells found outside the CNS) is the site where preganglionic

Figure 14-3 **A:** An autonomic ganglion as an integrator. Shows SIF cells. **B:** The liberation of acetylcholine (*ACh*) at an autonomic synapse.

nerve fibers synapse on postganglionic neurons (Fig. 14-3). Note that this term must be distinguished from the ganglion within the CNS consisting of nuclear groups (e.g., basal ganglia). Ganglia are situated along the course of efferent nerve fibers of the ANS. Sympathetic ganglia form part of the sympathetic trunk or are prevertebral in position (e.g., celiac and superior mesenteric ganglia). Parasympathetic ganglia, on the other hand, are situated close to or within the walls of the viscera.

An autonomic ganglion consists of a collection of multipolar neurons together with capsular or satellite cells and a connective tissue capsule. Nerve bundles are attached to each ganglion and consist of preganglionic nerve fibers that enter the ganglion, postganglionic nerve fibers that have arisen from neurons within the ganglion and are leaving the ganglion, and afferent and efferent nerve fibers that pass through the ganglion without synapsing. The preganglionic fibers are myelinated,

small, and relatively slow-conducting B fibers. The postganglionic fibers are unmyelinated, smaller, and slower-conducting C fibers.

The structure of synapses in autonomic ganglia shows the characteristic membrane thickening and small clear vesicles as well as some larger granular vesicles. The smaller vesicles contain ACh; the content of the granular vesicles is unknown.

Although an autonomic ganglion is the site where preganglionic fibers synapse on postganglionic neurons, the presence of small interneurons has been recognized. These cells exhibit catecholamine fluorescence and are referred to as **small intensely fluorescent (SIF)** cells. In some ganglia, these interneurons receive preganglionic cholinergic fibers and may modulate ganglionic transmission. In other ganglia, they receive collateral branches and may serve some integrative function. Many SIF cells contain **dopamine**, which is thought to be their transmitter.

PREGANGLIONIC TRANSMITTERS

As the preganglionic nerve fibers approach their termination, they wind around and between the dendritic processes of the postganglionic neuron, making multiple synaptic contacts. When the wave of excitation reaches the synaptic contacts, the synaptic transmitter is liberated, crosses the synaptic cleft to reach the receptor, and excites the postganglionic neuron (see Fig. 14-3B).

The synaptic transmitter that excites the postganglionic neurons in both sympathetic and parasympathetic ganglia is **ACh** (Fig. 14-4). The action of ACh in autonomic ganglia is quickly terminated by hydrolysis by **acetylcholinesterase (AChE)**.

Acetylcholine Receptors

ACh receptors are located on the outside of the cell membrane of postganglionic neurons. They are protein complexes that are bound to protein molecules that penetrate the cell membrane. Once the ACh molecule binds with the receptor, the structure of the protein molecule of the cell membrane changes and excitation or inhibition of the postganglionic neuron takes place. Two types of ACh receptors exist and are known as **nicotinic** and **muscarinic** receptors. These receptors are so named because nicotinic receptors respond specifically to nicotine (from tobacco), and muscarinic receptors respond specifically to muscarine (poison from toadstools). ACh is capable of binding to both of these receptors.

In both sympathetic and parasympathetic preganglionic neurons, the release of ACh binds predominantly with the nicotinic receptors on the postganglionic neurons.

FAST, SLOW, AND INHIBITORY SYNAPTIC POTENTIALS

ACh activation of the postsynaptic nicotinic receptors on the dendrites and cell bodies of the postganglionic neurons results in a depolarization of the membrane, an influx of Na^+ and Ca^{2+} ions, and the generation of the fast excitatory postsynaptic potential (fast **EPSP**). Usually, several presynaptic axon terminals must fire simultaneously and summation has to occur for transmission along the postsynaptic axon to take place. The fast EPSP reaches a maximum within about 15 msec.

ACh is also believed to activate small numbers of postsynaptic muscarinic receptors. This results in the development of the slow excitatory postsynaptic potential (slow **EPSP**), which lasts for 2 to 5 seconds. The underlying mechanism is complicated, and the slow potential occurs when the Na^+ and Ca^{2+} channels are open and M-type K^+ channels close; this leads to membrane depolarization. Late slow **EPSP** lasting as long as 1 to 2 minutes can also be produced by neuropeptide transmitters.

The activation of postsynaptic muscarinic receptors may also result in the development of the slow inhibitory postsynaptic potential (slow **IPSP**), which lasts about 10 seconds. The IPSP results from the opening of K^+ channels, permitting K^+ ions to flow out into the synaptic space, producing hyperpolarization.

The existence of these complex postsynaptic potentials in both sympathetic and parasympathetic ganglia (see Fig. 14-4) illustrates how the postsynaptic membrane potential can be altered and ganglionic transmission modulated.

GANGLION-STIMULATING AGENTS

Stimulating drugs, such as nicotine, lobeline, and dimethylphenylpiperazinium, stimulate sympathetic and parasympathetic ganglia by activating the nicotinic receptors on the postsynaptic membrane and producing a fast EPSP.

GANGLION-BLOCKING AGENTS

The two types of ganglion-blocking agents are depolarizing and nonpolarizing. **Nicotine** in high concentrations acts as a blocking agent by first stimulating the postganglionic neuron and causing depolarization and then by maintaining depolarization of the excitable membrane. During this latter phase, the postganglionic

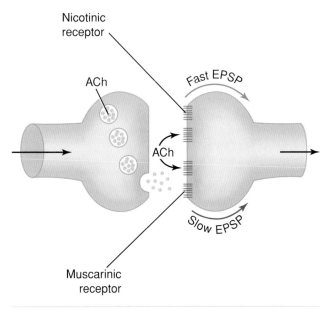

Figure 14-4 Example of the release of acetylcholine from a presynaptic terminal. A single presynaptic stimulus evokes a fast excitatory postsynaptic potential (fast **EPSP**) at a nicotinic receptor. Further stimulation may lead to a slow excitatory postsynaptic potential (slow **EPSP**) or a slow inhibitory postsynaptic potential (slow **IPSP**) at a muscarinic receptor. In preganglionic neurons, both sympathetic and parasympathetic, the release of acetylcholine binds predominantly with the nicotinic receptors on the postganglionic neurons.

neuron will fail to respond to the administration of any stimulant, regardless of the type of receptor it activates.

Hexamethonium and **tetraethylammonium** block ganglia by competing with ACh at the nicotinic receptor sites.

POSTGANGLIONIC NERVE ENDINGS

The postganglionic fibers terminate on the effector cells without special discrete endings. The axons run between the gland cells and the smooth and cardiac muscle fibers and lose their covering of Schwann cells. At sites where transmission occurs, clusters of vesicles are present within the axoplasm (see Fig. 3-35). The site on the axon may lie at some distance from the effector cell; thus, the transmission time may be slow at these endings. The diffusion of the transmitter through the large extracellular distance also permits a given nerve to have an action on a large number of effector cells.

POSTGANGLIONIC TRANSMITTERS

Parasympathetic postganglionic nerve endings liberate **ACh** as their transmitter substance (Fig. 14-5). All neurons that release ACh at their endings are called **cholinergic** (work like ACh). The ACh traverses the synaptic cleft and binds reversibly with the cholinergic

(**muscarinic**) receptor on the postsynaptic membrane. Within 2 to 3 msec, ACh is hydrolyzed into acetic acid and choline by the enzyme **AChE**, which is located on the surface of the nerve and receptor membranes. The choline is reabsorbed into the nerve ending and used again for synthesis of ACh.

Most sympathetic postganglionic nerve endings liberate **norepinephrine** as their transmitter substance. In addition, some sympathetic postganglionic nerve endings, particularly those that end on cells of sweat glands and the blood vessels in skeletal muscle, release **ACh**, which binds with muscarinic receptors on the postsynaptic membrane.

Sympathetic endings that use norepinephrine are called **adrenergic endings**. The two major kinds of receptors in the effector organs are called α and β **receptors**.

Two subgroups of α receptors (α_1 and α_2 receptors) and two subgroups of β receptors (β_1 and β_2 receptors) have been described. Norepinephrine has a greater effect on α receptors than on β receptors. **Phenylephrine** is a pure α stimulator. The bronchodilating drugs, such as **metaproterenol** and **albuterol**, mainly act on β_2 receptors. As a general rule, α receptor sites are associated with most of the excitatory functions of the sympathetic system (e.g., smooth muscle contraction, vasoconstriction, diaphoresis), whereas the β receptor sites are associated with most of the inhibitory functions (e.g., smooth muscle relaxation). β_2 Receptors are mainly in the lung, and stimulation results in

Figure 14-5 Efferent parts of the autonomic nervous system and the chemical transmitter substances released at the nerve endings. (ACh, acetylcholine; N. ep., norepinephrine.)

bronchodilation. β₁ Receptors are in the myocardium, where they are associated with excitation.

The action of norepinephrine on the receptor site of the effector cell is terminated by reuptake into the nerve terminal, where it is stored in presynaptic vesicles for reuse. Some of the norepinephrine escapes from the synaptic cleft into the general circulation and is subsequently metabolized in the liver.

OTHER POSTGANGLIONIC TRANSMITTERS

Sympathetic and parasympathetic postganglionic neurons have been shown to liberate substances other than ACh or norepinephrine at their endings; these include adenosine triphosphate (ATP), neuropeptide **Y**, and substance **P**. These substances may be released alone or from neurons that release ACh or norepinephrine; they have their own specific receptors. The function of these transmitters is probably to modulate the effects of the primary transmitter.

CHOLINERGIC RECEPTOR BLOCKADE

In the case of the parasympathetic and the sympathetic postganglionic nerve endings that liberate ACh as the transmitter substance, the receptors on the effector cells are **muscarinic**. This means that the action can be blocked by **atropine**. Atropine competitively antagonizes the muscarinic action by occupying the cholinergic receptor sites on the effector cells.

ADRENERGIC RECEPTOR BLOCKADE

The α-adrenergic receptors can be blocked by agents such as **phenoxybenzamine**, and the β-adrenergic receptors can be blocked by agents such as **propranolol**. The synthesis and storage of norepinephrine at sympathetic endings can be inhibited by **reserpine**.

HIGHER CONTROL

The hypothalamus has a controlling influence on the ANS and appears to integrate the autonomic and neuroendocrine systems, thus preserving body homeostasis (Fig. 14-6). Essentially, the hypothalamus should be regarded as a higher nervous center for the control of lower autonomic centers in the brainstem and spinal cord.

Stimulation of the anterior region of the hypothalamus can influence parasympathetic responses, whereas stimulation of the posterior part of the hypothalamus gives rise to sympathetic responses. In addition, lower brainstem centers such as **vasopressor**, **vasodilator**, **cardioaccelerator**, **cardiodecelerator**, and **respiratory centers** have been found in the reticular formation as the result of experimental stimulation in more primitive animals. The various levels of control are believed to be exerted as the result of interconnections of the different regions by ascending and descending pathways. The neurons of the thoracolumbar outflow of the sympathetic part of the system and the neurons of the craniosacral outflow of the parasympathetic part of the system receive their control through the descending tracts of the reticular formation.

Stimulation of different parts of the cerebral cortex and the limbic system produces autonomic effects, and this is presumably brought about through the hypothalamus. The ANS can be brought under voluntary control to some extent. This is seen, for example, in young individuals who may blush easily when embarrassed. As they mature, they are usually able to consciously train themselves to control this response. Also note that the higher centers of the brain can abnormally influence the activities of the ANS and induce diseases such as cardiac palpitations (arrhythmias) and even myocardial infarction.

ENTERIC NERVOUS SYSTEM

Two important plexuses of nerve cells and fibers extend continuously along and around the length of the gastrointestinal tract from the esophagus to the anal canal. The submucous or Meissner plexus lies between the mucous membrane and the circular muscle layer, and the myenteric or Auerbach plexus lies between the circular and longitudinal muscle layers. The submucous plexus is mainly concerned with the control of the glands of the mucous membrane, whereas the myenteric plexus controls the muscle and movements of the gut wall.

Different types of neurons have been recognized in the plexuses. Some neurons are bipolar or unipolar and are thought to be sensory and involved in local reflex activity; other neurons send axons to the celiac

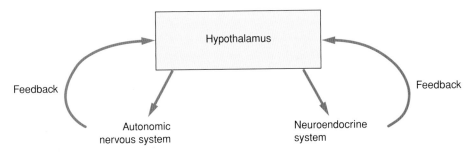

Figure 14-6 Hypothalamus as the control center for the autonomic nervous system and the neuroendocrine system.

and mesenteric plexuses. Preganglionic parasympathetic fibers synapse on nerve cells that give rise to postganglionic fibers that innervate the smooth muscle and glands. Postganglionic sympathetic fibers have been seen to terminate on parasympathetic nerve cells and probably exert an inhibitory role in parasympathetic activity. Internuncial neurons are also present. Interestingly, the nerve cells and their processes are surrounded by neuroglialike cells that closely resemble astrocytes in the CNS. It has been suggested that while the enteric plexuses can coordinate the activities of the gut wall, the parasympathetic and sympathetic inputs modulate these activities.

FUNCTIONS

The ANS, along with the endocrine system, maintains body homeostasis. The endocrine control is slower and exerts its influence by means of blood-borne hormones.

The ANS functions for the most part at the subconscious level. We are not aware, for example, that our pupils are dilating or that our arteries are constricting. The system should not be regarded as an isolated portion of the nervous system; it can play a role with somatic activity in expressing emotion and certain autonomic activities, such as micturition, can be brought under voluntary control. The various activities of the autonomic and endocrine systems are integrated within the hypothalamus.

The sympathetic and parasympathetic components of the ANS cooperate in maintaining the stability of the internal environment. The sympathetic part prepares and mobilizes the body in an emergency when sudden severe exercise, fear, or rage occurs. The parasympathetic part aims at conserving and storing energy, for example, in the promotion of digestion and the absorption of food by increasing the secretions of the glands of the gastrointestinal tract and stimulating peristalsis.

The sympathetic and parasympathetic parts of the ANS usually have antagonistic control over a viscus. For example, the sympathetic activity will increase the heart rate, whereas the parasympathetic activity will slow the heart rate. The sympathetic activity will make the bronchial smooth muscle relax, but the muscle is contracted by parasympathetic activity.

However, many viscera do not possess this fine dual control from the ANS. For example, the smooth muscle of the hair follicles (the arrector pili muscle) is made to contract by the sympathetic activity without parasympathetic control.

The activities of some viscera are kept under a constant state of inhibition by one or the other components of the ANS. The heart in a trained athlete is maintained at a slow rate by the activities of the parasympathetic system. This is of considerable importance because the heart is a more efficient pump when contracting slowly than when contracting very quickly, thus permitting adequate diastolic filling of the ventricles.

DIFFERENCES BETWEEN SYMPATHETIC AND PARASYMPATHETIC SYSTEMS

Important anatomic, physiologic, and pharmacologic differences between the sympathetic and parasympathetic parts of the ANS are shown in Table 14-1.

1. The sympathetic efferent nerve fibers originate (see Fig. 14-2) from nerve cells in the lateral gray column of the spinal cord between the first thoracic and second lumbar segments (the **thoracic outflow**). The parasympathetic efferent nerve fibers originate from nerve cells in the 3rd, 7th, 9th, and 10th cranial nerves and in the gray matter of the 2nd, 3rd, and 4th sacral segments of the cord (the **craniosacral outflow**).
2. The sympathetic ganglia are located either in the paravertebral sympathetic trunks or in the prevertebral ganglia, such as the celiac ganglion. The parasympathetic ganglion cells are located as small ganglia close to the viscera or within plexuses within the viscera.
3. The sympathetic part of the autonomic system has long postganglionic fibers, whereas the parasympathetic system has short fibers (see Fig. 14-5).
4. The sympathetic part of the system has a widespread action on the body as the result of the preganglionic fibers synapsing on many postganglionic neurons and the suprarenal medulla releasing the sympathetic transmitters epinephrine and norepinephrine, which are distributed throughout the body through the bloodstream. The parasympathetic part of the autonomic system has a more discrete control, since the preganglionic fibers synapse on only a few postganglionic neurons with no comparable organ to the suprarenal medulla.
5. The sympathetic postganglionic endings liberate norepinephrine at most endings and ACh at a few endings (e.g., sweat glands). The parasympathetic postganglionic endings liberate ACh.
6. The sympathetic part of the autonomic system prepares the body for emergencies and severe muscular activity, whereas the parasympathetic part conserves and stores energy.

To assist with the learning of the different actions of these two components of the autonomic system, imagine that sympathetic activity would be maximal in a man who finds himself suddenly alone in a field with a bull that is about to charge. His hair will stand on end with fear; his skin will be pale as the result of vasoconstriction, which causes a redistribution of blood away from the skin and viscera to the heart muscle and skeletal muscle. His upper eyelids will be raised and his pupils will be widely dilated so that he can see where to run. His heart rate will rise and the peripheral resistance of the arterioles will be increased, causing a rise in blood pressure. His bronchi will dilate to permit maximum respiratory flow of air. His peristaltic activity will be inhibited and his gut sphincters will be contracted. His vesical sphincter will also be contracted (this is certainly not the time to be thinking of defecation or

Table 14-1 Anatomic, Physiologic, and Pharmacologic Characteristics of Sympathetic Versus Parasympathetic Systems

	Sympathetic	Parasympathetic
Action	Prepares body for emergency	Conserves and restores energy
Outflow	T1–L2 (3)	Cranial nerves III, VII, IX, and X; S2–S4
Preganglionic fibers	Myelinated	Myelinated
Ganglia	Paravertebral (sympathetic trunks), prevertebral (e.g., celiac, superior mesenteric, inferior mesenteric)	Small ganglia close to viscera (e.g., otic, ciliary) or ganglion cells in plexuses (e.g., cardiac, pulmonary)
Neurotransmitter within ganglia	Acetylcholine	Acetylcholine
Ganglion-blocking agents	Hexamethonium and tetraethylammonium by competing with acetylcholine	Hexamethonium and tetraethylammonium by competing with acetylcholine
Postganglionic fibers	Long, nonmyelinated	Short, nonmyelinated
Characteristic activity	Widespread due to many postganglionic fibers and liberation of epinephrine and norepinephrine from suprarenal medulla	Discrete action with few postganglionic fibers
Neurotransmitter at postganglionic endings	Norepinephrine at most endings and acetylcholine at few endings (sweat glands)	Acetylcholine at all endings
Blocking agents on receptors of effector cells	α-Adrenergic receptors— phenoxybenzamine β-Adrenergic receptors— propranolol	Atropine, scopolamine
Agents inhibiting synthesis and storage of neurotransmitter at postganglionic endings	Reserpine	
Agents inhibiting hydrolysis of neurotransmitter at site of effector cells		Acetylcholinesterase blockers (e.g., neostigmine)
Drugs mimicking autonomic activity	Sympathomimetic drugs Phenylephrine: α receptors; Isoproterenol: β receptors	Parasympathomimetic drugs Pilocarpine Methacholine
Higher control	Hypothalamus	Hypothalamus

micturition). Glycogen will be converted into glucose for energy and he will sweat to lose body heat.

On the other hand, the parasympathetic activity will be great in a woman who has fallen asleep in an armchair after a satisfying meal. Her heart rate will be slow and her blood pressure will not be high. Her upper eyelids will droop or be closed and her pupils will be constricted. Her breathing will be noisy owing to bronchial constriction. Her abdomen may rumble owing to excessive peristaltic activity. She may feel the inclination to defecate or micturate.

AUTONOMIC INNERVATIONS

Some important ANS innervations are shown in Table 14-2.

Eye

Both sympathetic and parasympathetic nervous systems control involuntary function in the iris and lacrimal glands, whereas the eyelids are only affected by the sympathetic nervous system.

Upper Lid

The upper lid is raised by the levator palpebrae superioris muscle. The major part of this muscle is formed by skeletal muscle innervated by the oculomotor nerve. A small part is composed of smooth muscle fibers innervated by sympathetic postganglionic fibers from the superior cervical sympathetic ganglion (Fig. 14-7).

Iris

The smooth muscle fibers of the iris consist of circular and radiating fibers. The circular fibers form the sphincter pupillae and the radial fibers form the dilator pupillae.

The sphincter pupillae is supplied by parasympathetic fibers from the parasympathetic nucleus (Edinger–Westphal nucleus) of the oculomotor nerve.

Table 14-2   Autonomic Nervous System Effects on Body Organs

Organ		Sympathetic Action	Parasympathetic Action
Eye	Pupil	Dilates	Constricts
	Ciliary muscle	Relaxes	Contracts
Glands	Lacrimal, parotid, submandibular, sublingual, nasal	Reduce secretion by causing vasoconstriction of blood vessels	Increase secretion
	Sweat	Increases secretion	
Heart	Cardiac muscle	Increases force of contraction	Decreases force of contraction
	Coronary arteries (mainly controlled by local metabolic factors)	Dilates (β receptors), constricts (α receptors)	
Lung	Bronchial muscle	Relaxes (dilates bronchi)	Contracts (constricts bronchi)
	Bronchial secretion		Increases secretion
	Bronchial arteries	Constricts	Dilates
Gastrointestinal tract	Muscle in walls	Decreases peristalsis	Increases peristalsis
	Muscle in sphincters	Contracts	Relaxes
	Glands	Reduces secretion by vasoconstriction of blood vessels	Increases secretion
Liver		Breaks down glycogen into glucose	
Gallbladder		Relaxes	Contracts
Kidney		Decreases output due to constriction of arteries	
Urinary bladder	Bladder wall (detrusor)	Relaxes	Contracts
	Sphincter vesicae	Contracts	Relaxes
Erectile tissue of penis and clitoris			Relaxes, causes erection
Ejaculation		Contracts smooth muscle of vas deferens, seminal vesicles, and prostate	
Systemic arteries			
Skin		Constrict	
Abdominal		Constrict	
Muscle		Constrict (α receptors), dilate (β receptors), dilate (cholinergic)	
Arrector pili muscle		Contract	
Suprarenal			
Cortex		Stimulates	
Medulla		Liberates epinephrine and norepinephrine	

After synapsing in the **ciliary ganglion,** the postganglionic fibers pass forward to the eyeball in the **short ciliary nerves.** (The ciliary muscle of the eye is also supplied by the short ciliary nerves; see p. 406.)

The dilator pupillae is supplied by postganglionic fibers from the superior cervical sympathetic ganglion. The postganglionic fibers reach the orbit along the internal carotid and ophthalmic arteries. They pass uninterrupted through the ciliary ganglion and reach the eyeball in the **short ciliary nerves.** Other sympathetic fibers reach the eyeball in the **long ciliary nerves.**

Lacrimal Gland

The parasympathetic secretomotor nerve supply to the lacrimal gland originates in the **lacrimatory nucleus**

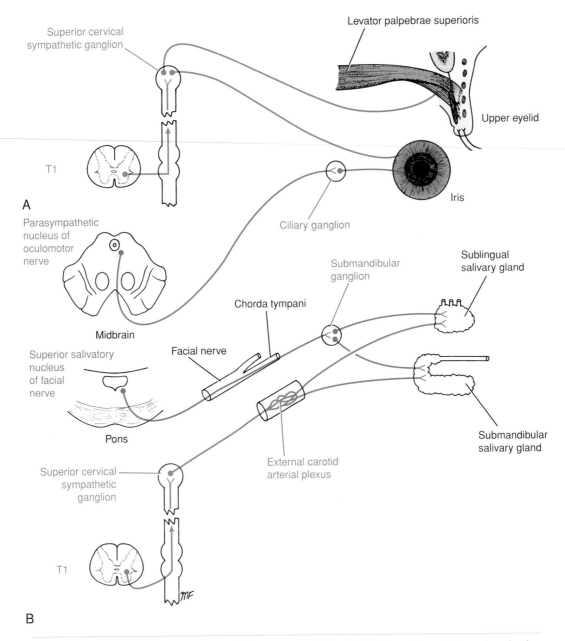

Figure 14-7 Autonomic innervation of the upper eyelid and iris (**A**) and the sublingual and submandibular salivary glands (**B**).

of the facial nerve (Fig. 14-8). The preganglionic fibers reach the **pterygopalatine ganglion** through the **nervus intermedius** and its **great petrosal branch** and through the **nerve of the pterygoid canal**. The postganglionic fibers leave the ganglion and join the maxillary nerve. They then pass into its **zygomatic branch** and the **zygomaticotemporal nerve.** They reach the lacrimal gland within the **lacrimal nerve**.

The sympathetic postganglionic fibers arise from the superior cervical sympathetic ganglion and travel in the plexus of nerves around the internal carotid artery. They join the **deep petrosal nerve, the nerve of the pterygoid canal, the maxillary nerve, the zygomatic nerve, zygomaticotemporal nerve,** and finally the lacrimal nerve. They function as vasoconstrictor fibers.

Salivary Glands

The involuntary action of the salivary glands is controlled by the ANS. These three, paired glands have similar sympathetic nerve origination but have unique parasympathetic origins.

Submandibular and Sublingual Glands

The parasympathetic secretomotor supply originates in the **superior salivatory nucleus** of the facial nerve (see Fig. 14-7). The preganglionic fibers pass to the **submandibular ganglion** and other small ganglia close to the duct through the **chorda tympani nerve** and the **lingual nerve.** Postganglionic fibers reach the submandibular gland either directly or along the duct. Postganglionic

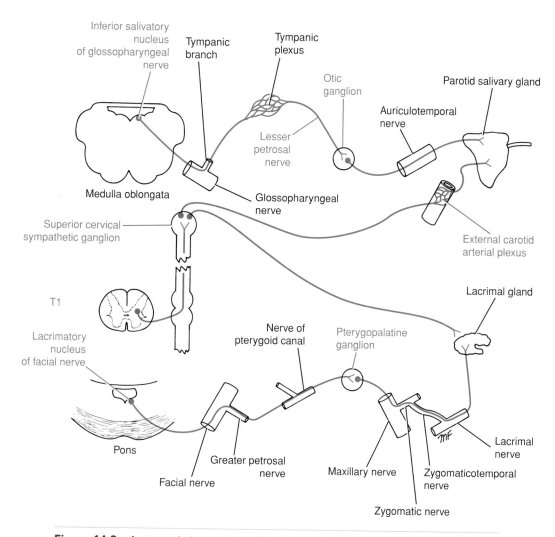

Figure 14-8 Autonomic innervation of the parotid salivary gland and lacrimal gland.

fibers to the sublingual gland travel through the lingual nerve.

Sympathetic postganglionic fibers arise from the superior cervical sympathetic ganglion and reach the glands as a plexus of nerves around the external carotid, facial, and lingual arteries. They function as vasoconstrictor fibers.

Parotid Gland

Parasympathetic secretomotor fibers from the **inferior salivatory nucleus** of the glossopharyngeal nerve supply the gland (see Fig. 14-8). The preganglionic nerve fibers pass to the otic ganglion through the **tympanic branch of the glossopharyngeal nerve** and the **lesser petrosal nerve**. Postganglionic fibers reach the gland through the auriculotemporal nerve.

Sympathetic postganglionic fibers arise from the superior cervical sympathetic ganglion and reach the gland as a plexus of nerves around the external carotid artery. They function as vasoconstrictor fibers.

Heart

The sympathetic postganglionic fibers arise from the cervical and upper thoracic portions of the sympathetic

trunks (Fig. 14-9). Postganglionic fibers reach the heart by way of the **superior**, **middle**, and **inferior cardiac branches** of the cervical portion of the sympathetic trunk and a number of **cardiac branches** from the thoracic portion of the sympathetic trunk. The fibers pass through the **cardiac plexuses** and terminate on the **sinoatrial** and **atrioventricular nodes**, on cardiac muscle fibers, and on coronary arteries. Activation of these nerves results in cardiac acceleration, increased force of contraction of the cardiac muscle, and dilatation of the coronary arteries. The coronary dilatation is mainly produced in response to local metabolic needs rather than by direct nerve stimulation of the coronary arteries.

The parasympathetic preganglionic fibers originate in the **dorsal nucleus of the vagus nerve** and descend into the thorax in the vagus nerves. The fibers terminate by synapsing with postganglionic neurons in the **cardiac plexuses**. Postganglionic fibers terminate on the **sinoatrial** and **atrioventricular nodes** and on the coronary arteries. Activation of these nerves results in a reduction in the rate and force of contraction of the myocardium and a constriction of the coronary arteries. Here again, the coronary constriction is mainly produced by the reduction in local metabolic needs rather than by neural effects.

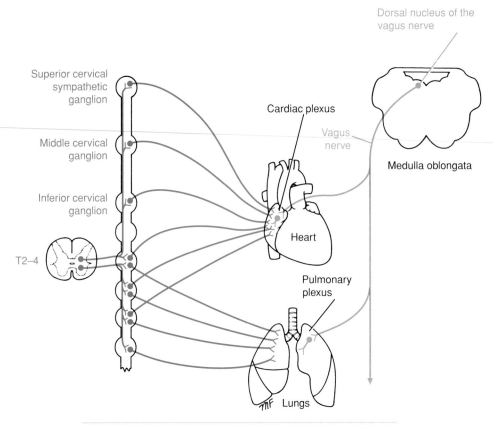

Figure 14-9   Autonomic innervation of the heart and lungs.

Lungs

The sympathetic postganglionic fibers arise from the second to the fifth thoracic ganglia of the sympathetic trunk (see Fig. 14-9). The fibers pass through the pulmonary plexuses and enter the lung, where they form networks around the bronchi and blood vessels. The sympathetic fibers produce bronchodilation and slight vasoconstriction.

The parasympathetic preganglionic fibers arise from the **dorsal nucleus of the vagus** and descend to the thorax within the vagus nerves. The fibers terminate by synapsing with postganglionic neurons in the pulmonary plexuses. The postganglionic fibers enter the lung, where they form networks around the bronchi and blood vessels. The parasympathetic fibers produce bronchoconstriction and slight vasodilation and increase glandular secretion.

Gastrointestinal Tract

Stomach and Intestine (to Splenic Flexure)

Preganglionic parasympathetic fibers enter the abdomen in the **anterior (left)** and **posterior (right) vagal trunks** (Fig. 14-10). The fibers are distributed to many abdominal viscera and to the gastrointestinal tract from the stomach to the splenic flexure of the colon. The fibers that pass to the gastrointestinal tract terminate on postganglionic neurons in the **myenteric (Auerbach)**

and **submucosal (Meissner) plexuses**. The postganglionic fibers supply the smooth muscle and glands. The parasympathetic nerves stimulate peristalsis and relax the sphincters; they also stimulate secretion.

Sympathetic preganglionic nerve fibers pass through the thoracic part of the sympathetic trunk and enter the **greater** and **lesser splanchnic nerves**. These descend into the abdomen and synapse with postganglionic neurons in the **celiac** and **superior mesenteric ganglia**. The postganglionic nerve fibers are distributed to the stomach and intestine as nerve plexuses around the branches of the celiac and superior mesenteric arteries. The sympathetic nerves inhibit peristalsis and cause contraction of the sphincters; they also inhibit secretion (see the enteric nervous system, p. 394).

Descending Colon, Pelvic Colon, and Rectum

The preganglionic parasympathetic fibers originate in the gray matter of the spinal cord from the second to the fourth sacral segments (see Fig. 14-10). The fibers pass through the **pelvic splanchnic nerves** and the nerve plexuses around the branches of the inferior mesenteric artery. They terminate on postganglionic neurons in the myenteric (Auerbach) and submucosal (Meissner) plexuses. The postganglionic fibers supply the smooth muscle and glands. The parasympathetic nerves stimulate peristalsis and secretion.

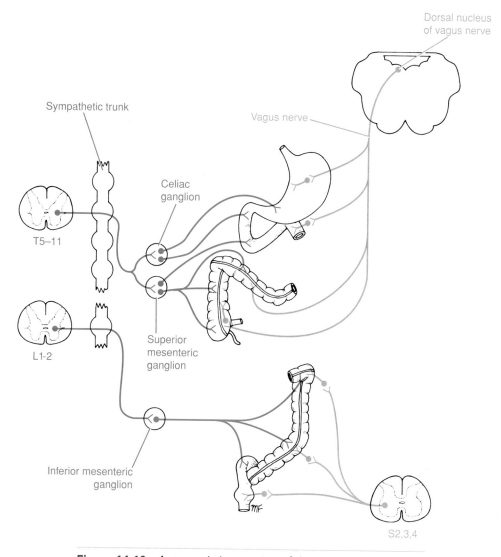

Figure 14-10   Autonomic innervation of the gastrointestinal tract.

The sympathetic preganglionic nerve fibers pass through the lumbar part of the sympathetic trunk and synapse with postganglionic neurons in the **inferior mesenteric plexus**. Postganglionic fibers are distributed to the bowel as nerve plexuses around the branches of the inferior mesenteric arteries. The sympathetic nerves inhibit peristalsis and secretion.

Gallbladder and Biliary Ducts

The gallbladder and biliary ducts receive postganglionic parasympathetic and sympathetic fibers from the hepatic plexus. Parasympathetic fibers derived from the vagus are thought to be motor fibers to the smooth muscle of the gallbladder and bile ducts and inhibitory to the sphincter of Oddi.

Autonomic afferent fibers are also present. Some of the fibers are believed to leave the hepatic plexus and join the right phrenic nerve, thus partially explaining the phenomenon of referred shoulder pain in the presence of gallbladder disease (see p. 410).

Kidney

Preganglionic sympathetic fibers pass through the lower thoracic part of the sympathetic trunk and the lowest thoracic splanchnic nerve to join the **renal plexus** around the renal artery (Fig. 14-11). The preganglionic fibers synapse with postganglionic neurons in the renal plexus. The postganglionic fibers are distributed to the branches of the renal artery. The sympathetic nerves are vasoconstrictor in action to the renal arteries within the kidney.

Preganglionic parasympathetic fibers enter the renal plexus from the vagus. Here, they synapse with postganglionic neurons whose fibers are distributed to the kidney along the branches of the renal artery. The parasympathetic nerves are thought to be vasodilator in action.

Suprarenal Gland Medulla

Preganglionic sympathetic fibers descend to the gland in the **greater splanchnic nerve**, a branch of the thoracic

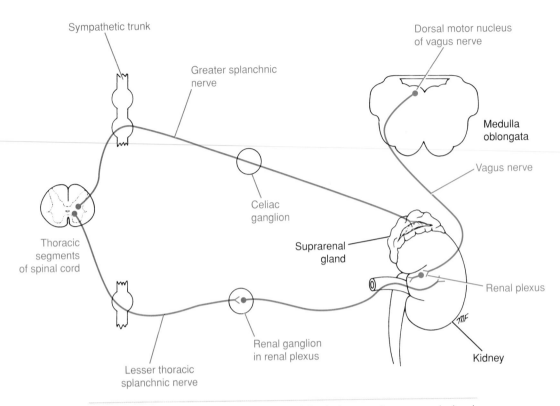

Figure 14-11 Autonomic innervation of the kidney and suprarenal gland.

part of the sympathetic trunk (see Fig. 14-11). The nerve fibers terminate on the secretory cells of the medulla, which are comparable to postganglionic neurons. ACh is the transmitter substance between the nerve endings and the secretory cells, as at any other preganglionic endings. The sympathetic nerves stimulate the secretory cells of the medulla to increase the output of epinephrine and norepinephrine. The medulla of the suprarenal gland lacks parasympathetic innervation.

Anal Canal Involuntary Internal Sphincter

The circular smooth muscle coat is thickened at the upper end of the anal canal to form the involuntary internal sphincter. The sphincter is innervated by postganglionic sympathetic fibers from the **hypogastric plexuses** (Fig. 14-12). Each hypogastric plexus receives sympathetic fibers from the **aortic plexus** and from the lumbar and pelvic parts of the sympathetic trunks. The sympathetic nerves cause the internal anal sphincter to contract.

Urinary Bladder

The muscular coat of the bladder is composed of smooth muscle, which at the bladder neck is thickened to form the **sphincter vesicae**. The nerve supply of the smooth muscle is from the hypogastric plexuses (see Fig. 14-12). The sympathetic postganglionic fibers originate in the first and second lumbar ganglia of the sympathetic trunk and travel to the hypogastric plexuses.

The parasympathetic preganglionic fibers arise as the pelvic splanchnic nerves from the second, third, and fourth sacral nerves; they pass through the hypogastric plexuses to reach the bladder wall, where they synapse with postganglionic neurons.

The sympathetic nerves to the detrusor muscle have little or no action on the smooth muscle of the bladder wall and are distributed mainly to the blood vessels. The sympathetic nerves to the sphincter vesicae play only a minor role in causing contraction of the sphincter in maintaining urinary continence. However, in the male, the sympathetic innervation of the sphincter causes active contraction of the bladder neck during ejaculation (brought about by sympathetic action), thus preventing seminal fluid from entering the bladder. The parasympathetic nerves stimulate the contraction of the smooth muscle of the bladder wall and, in some way, inhibit the contraction of the sphincter vesicae.

Penile and Clitoral Erection

In erection, the genital **erectile tissue** becomes engorged with blood. The initial vascular engorgement is controlled by the parasympathetic part of the ANS. The parasympathetic preganglionic fibers originate in the gray matter of the second, third, and fourth sacral segments of the spinal cord (Fig. 14-13). The fibers enter the hypogastric plexuses and synapse on the postganglionic neurons. The postganglionic fibers join the internal pudendal arteries and are distributed along their branches, which enter the erectile tissue. The parasympathetic nerves

Figure 14-12 Autonomic innervation of the sphincters of the anal canal and urinary bladder.

cause vasodilatation of the arteries and greatly increase the blood flow to the erectile tissue.

Ejaculation

During the increasing sexual excitement that occurs during sex play, the external urinary meatus of the glans penis becomes moist as a result of the secretions of the bulbourethral glands. Friction on the glans penis, reinforced by other afferent nervous impulses, results in a discharge along the sympathetic nerve fibers to the smooth muscle of the duct of the epididymis and the vas deferens on each side, the seminal vesicles, and the prostate. The smooth muscle contracts and the spermatozoa, together with the secretions of the seminal vesicles and prostate, are discharged into the prostatic urethra. The fluid now joins the secretions of the bulbourethral glands and penile urethral glands and is then ejected from the penile urethra as a result of the rhythmic contractions of the bulbospongiosus muscles, which compress the urethra. Meanwhile, the sphincter of the bladder contracts and prevents a reflux of the spermatozoa into the bladder. The spermatozoa and the secretions of the several accessory glands constitute the **seminal fluid**, or **semen**. At the climax of male sexual excitement, a mass discharge of nervous impulses takes place in the CNS. Impulses pass down the spinal cord to the sympathetic outflow (T1–L2). The nervous impulses that pass to the

genital organs are thought to leave the cord at the first and second lumbar segments in the preganglionic sympathetic fibers (see Fig. 14-13). Many of these fibers synapse with postganglionic neurons in the first and second lumbar ganglia. Other fibers may synapse in ganglia in the lower lumbar or pelvic parts of the sympathetic trunks. The postganglionic fibers are then distributed to the **vas deferens**, the **seminal vesicles**, and the **prostate** through the **hypogastric plexuses**. The sympathetic nerves stimulate the contractions of the smooth muscle in the walls of these structures and cause the spermatozoa, together with the secretions of the seminal vesicles and prostate, to be discharged into the urethra.

Uterus

Preganglionic sympathetic nerve fibers leave the spinal cord at segmental levels T12 and L1 and are believed to synapse with ganglion cells in the sympathetic trunk or possibly in the inferior hypogastric plexuses (Fig. 14-14). The postganglionic fibers supply the smooth muscle of the uterus. Parasympathetic preganglionic fibers leave the spinal cord at levels S2–S4 and synapse with ganglion cells in the inferior hypogastric plexuses. Although the uterine muscle is largely under hormonal control, sympathetic innervation may cause uterine contraction and vasoconstriction, whereas parasympathetic fibers have the opposite effect.

Figure 14-13 Autonomic innervation of the male reproductive tract.

Figure 14-14 Autonomic innervation of the uterus; the pathway taken by the afferent sensory fibers is shown as well.

Afferent pain fibers from the fundus and the body of the uterus ascend to the spinal cord through the hypogastric plexuses, entering it through the posterior roots of the 10th, 11th, and 12th thoracic spinal nerves. Fibers from the cervix run in the pelvic splanchnic nerves and enter the spinal cord through the posterior roots of the second, third, and fourth sacral nerves.

Upper Limb Arteries

The arteries of the upper limb are innervated by sympathetic nerves. The preganglionic fibers originate from cell bodies in the second to the eighth thoracic segments of the spinal cord (Fig. 14-15). They pass to the sympathetic trunk through white rami and ascend in the trunk to synapse in the middle cervical, inferior cervical, first thoracic, or stellate ganglia. The postganglionic fibers join the nerves that form the brachial plexus and are distributed to the arteries within the branches of the plexus. The sympathetic nerves cause vasoconstriction of cutaneous arteries and vasodilatation of arteries that supply skeletal muscle.

Lower Limb Arteries

The arteries of the lower limb are also innervated by sympathetic nerves (see Fig. 14-15). The preganglionic fibers originate from cell bodies in the lower three thoracic and upper two or three lumbar segments of the spinal cord. The preganglionic fibers pass to the lower thoracic and upper lumbar ganglia of the sympathetic trunk through white rami. The fibers synapse in the lumbar and sacral ganglia and the postganglionic fibers reach the arteries through branches of the lumbar and sacral plexuses.

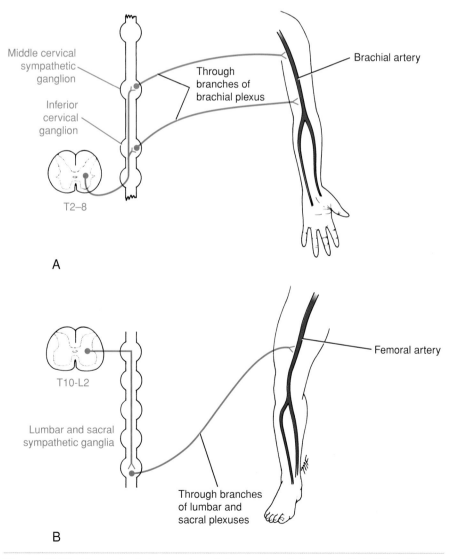

Figure 14-15 Sympathetic innervation of the arteries of the upper limb (**A**) and lower limb (**B**).

ANS PHYSIOLOGIC REFLEXES

The ANS is involved in important visual and cardiovascular reflexes.

Direct and Consensual Light Reflexes

Afferent nervous impulses travel from the retina through the optic nerve, optic chiasma, and optic tract (see Fig. 11-3). A small number of fibers leave the optic tract and synapse on nerve cells in the **pretectal nucleus**, which lies close to the superior colliculus. The impulses are passed by axons of the pretectal nerve cells to the parasympathetic nuclei (Edinger–Westphal nuclei) of the oculomotor nerve on both sides. Here, the fibers synapse and the parasympathetic nerves travel through the oculomotor nerve to the **ciliary ganglion** in the orbit. Finally, postganglionic parasympathetic fibers pass through the **short ciliary nerves** to the eyeball and to the constrictor pupillae muscle of the iris. Both pupils constrict in the consensual light reflex because the pretectal nucleus sends fibers to the parasympathetic nuclei on both sides of the midbrain.

Accommodation Reflex

When the eyes are directed from a distant to a near object, contraction of the medial recti brings about convergence of the ocular axes, the lenses thicken to increase their refractive power by contraction of the ciliary muscle, and the pupils constrict to restrict the light waves to the thickest central part of the lenses. The afferent impulses travel through the optic nerve, the optic chiasma, the optic tract, the lateral geniculate body, and the optic radiation to the visual cortex (see Fig. 11-3). The visual cortex is connected to the eye field of the frontal cortex. From here, cortical fibers descend through the internal capsule to the oculomotor nuclei in the midbrain. The oculomotor nerve travels to the medial recti muscles. Some of the descending cortical fibers synapse with the parasympathetic nuclei (Edinger–Westphal nuclei) of the oculomotor nerve on both sides. The parasympathetic preganglionic fibers

then travel through the oculomotor nerve to the **ciliary ganglion** in the orbit where they synapse. Finally, postganglionic parasympathetic fibers pass through the **short ciliary nerves** to the ciliary muscle and the constrictor pupillae muscle of the iris.

Carotid Sinus and Aortic Arch Reflexes

The carotid sinus, located in the bifurcation of the common carotid artery, and the aortic arch serve as baroreceptors. As the blood pressure rises, nerve endings situated in the walls of these vessels are stimulated. The afferent fibers from the carotid sinus ascend in the glossopharyngeal nerve and terminate in the **nucleus solitarius** (see Figs. 11-16 and 11-17). The afferent fibers from the aortic arch ascend in the vagus nerve. Connector neurons in the medulla oblongata activate the parasympathetic nucleus (dorsal nucleus) of the vagus, which slows the heart rate. At the same time, reticulospinal fibers descend to the spinal cord and inhibit the preganglionic sympathetic outflow to the heart and cutaneous arterioles. The combined effect of stimulation of the parasympathetic action on the heart and inhibition of the sympathetic action on the heart and peripheral blood vessels reduces the rate and force of contraction of the heart and reduces the peripheral resistance of the blood vessels. Consequently, the blood pressure falls. The blood pressure of the individual is thus modified by the afferent information received from the baroreceptors. The modulator of the ANS, namely, the hypothalamus, in turn, can be influenced by other, higher centers in the CNS.

Bainbridge Right Atrial Reflex

This reflex is initiated when the nerve endings in the wall of the right atrium and in the walls of the venae cavae are stimulated by a rise of venous pressure. The afferent fibers ascend in the vagus to the medulla oblongata and terminate on the **nucleus of the tractus solitarius** (see Fig. 11-18). Connector neurons inhibit the parasympathetic nucleus (dorsal) of the vagus, and reticulospinal fibers stimulate the thoracic sympathetic outflow to the heart, resulting in cardiac acceleration.

 Clinical Notes

General Considerations

Clearly, the ANS is not an isolated part of the nervous system. It should be regarded as the part of the nervous system that, with the endocrine system, is particularly involved in maintaining the stability of the internal environment of the body. Its activities are modified by the hypothalamus, whose function is to integrate vast amounts of afferent information received from other areas of the nervous system and to translate changing hormonal levels of the bloodstream into appropriate nervous and hormonal activities.

Because the ANS is so important in maintaining normal body homeostasis, not surprisingly, the system is subject to many pharmacologic interventions. Propranolol and atenolol,

for example, are β-adrenergic antagonists that can be used in the treatment of hypertension and ischemic heart disease.

Autonomic Nervous System Injury

Trauma to the ANS is usually limited to either sympathetic or parasympathetic components, rarely both at the same time, due to their relative locations in the thorax or cranial cavity, respectively.

Sympathetic Injuries

The sympathetic trunk in the neck can be injured by stab and bullet wounds. Traction injuries to the first thoracic root of the brachial plexus can damage sympathetic nerves destined for the stellate ganglion. All these conditions can produce a preganglionic type of Horner syndrome. Injuries to the spinal cord or cauda equina can disrupt the sympathetic control of the bladder (see p. 402).

Parasympathetic Injuries

The oculomotor nerve is vulnerable in head injuries (herniated uncus) and can be damaged by compression by aneurysms in the junction between the posterior cerebral artery and posterior communicating artery. The preganglionic parasympathetic fibers traveling in this nerve are situated in the periphery of the nerve and can be damaged. Surface aneurysmal compression characteristically causes dilation of the pupil and loss of the visual light reflexes.

The autonomic fibers in the facial nerve can be damaged by fractures of the skull involving the temporal bone. The vestibulocochlear nerve is closely related to the facial nerve in the internal acoustic meatus, so clinical findings involving both nerves are common. Involvement of the parasympathetic fibers in the facial nerve may produce impaired lacrimation in addition to paralysis of the facial muscles.

The glossopharyngeal and vagus nerves are at risk in stab and bullet wounds of the neck. The parasympathetic secretomotor fibers to the parotid salivary gland leave the glossopharyngeal nerve just below the skull; therefore, they are rarely damaged.

The parasympathetic outflow in the sacral region of the spinal cord (S2–S4) may be damaged by spinal cord and cauda equina injuries, leading to disruption of bladder, rectal, and sexual functions.

Degeneration and Regeneration of Autonomic Nerves

The structural changes are identical to those found in other areas of the peripheral and central parts of the nervous system. Functional recoveries following sympathectomy operations can be explained only by the assumption either that the operative procedure was inadequate and nerve fibers were left intact or regenerated or that alternative nervous pathways existed and were left undisturbed.

The denervation of viscera supplied by autonomic nerves is followed by their increased sensitivity to the agent that was previously the transmitter substance. One explanation is that following nerve section, there may be an increase in the number of receptor sites on the post-synaptic membrane. Another possibility, which applies to endings where norepinephrine is the transmitter, is that the reuptake of the transmitter by the nerve terminal is interfered with in some way.

Urinary Bladder Dysfunction

Injuries to the spinal cord are followed by disruption of the nervous control of micturition. The normal bladder is innervated as follows:

Sympathetic innervation is from the first and second lumbar segments of the spinal cord.

Parasympathetic innervation is from the second, third, and fourth sacral segments of the spinal cord.

Sensory nerve fibers enter the spinal cord at the above segments.

The **atonic bladder** occurs during the phase of spinal shock immediately following the injury and may last from a few days to several weeks. The bladder wall muscle is relaxed, the sphincter vesicae is tightly contracted (loss of inhibition from higher levels), and the sphincter urethrae is relaxed. The bladder becomes greatly distended and finally overflows. Depending on the level of the cord injury, the patient may or may not be aware that the bladder is full but has no voluntary control.

The **automatic reflex bladder** occurs after the patient has recovered from spinal shock, provided that the cord lesion lies above the level of the parasympathetic outflow (S2–S4). This is the type of bladder normally found in infancy. The descending fibers in the spinal cord are sectioned, so voluntary control is not possible. The bladder fills and empties reflexly. Stretch receptors in the bladder wall are stimulated as the bladder fills and the afferent impulses pass to the spinal cord (S2–S4). Efferent impulses pass down to the bladder muscle, which contracts; the sphincter vesicae and the urethral sphincter both relax. This simple reflex occurs every 1 to 4 hours.

The **autonomous bladder** is the condition that occurs if the sacral segment of the spinal cord is destroyed or if the cauda equina is severed. The bladder has no reflex control or voluntary control. The bladder wall is flaccid and the capacity of the bladder is greatly increased. It fills to capacity and overflows, which results in continual dribbling. The bladder may be partially emptied by manual compression of the lower part of the anterior abdominal wall, but infection of the urine and back pressure effects on the ureters and kidneys are inevitable.

Defecation

The act of defecation involves a coordinated reflex that results in the emptying of the descending colon, pelvic colon, rectum, and anal canal. It is assisted by a rise in the intra-abdominal pressure brought about by contraction of the muscles of the anterior abdominal wall. The involuntary internal sphincter of the anal canal normally is innervated by postganglionic sympathetic fibers from the hypogastric plexuses, and the voluntary external sphincter of the anal canal is innervated by the inferior rectal nerve. The desire to defecate is initiated by stimulation of the stretch receptors in the wall of the rectum.

Following severe spinal cord injuries (or cauda equina injuries), the patient is not aware of rectal distention. Moreover, the parasympathetic influence on the peristaltic activity of the descending colon, sigmoid colon, and rectum is lost. In addition, control over the abdominal musculature and sphincters of the anal canal may be severely impaired. The rectum, now an isolated structure, responds by contracting when the pressure within its lumen rises. This local reflex response is much more efficient if the sacral segments of the spinal cord and the cauda equina are intact. At best, however, the force of the contractions of the rectal wall is small and constipation and impaction are the usual outcome. The treatment of patients with spinal cord injuries is to empty the rectum with biweekly enemas; the use of suppositories also may be helpful.

Erection and Ejaculation

As described previously, erection of the penis or clitoris is controlled by the parasympathetic nerves that originate from the second, third, and fourth sacral segments of the spinal cord. Bilateral damage to the reticulospinal tracts in the spinal cord above the second sacral segment of the spinal cord will result in loss of erection. Later, when the effects of spinal shock have disappeared, spontaneous or reflex erection may occur if the sacral segments of the spinal cord are intact.

Ejaculation is controlled by sympathetic nerves that originate in the first and second lumbar segments of the spinal cord. Ejaculation brings about a flow of seminal fluid into the prostatic urethra. The final ejection of the fluid from the penis is the result of the rhythmic contractions of the bulbospongiosus muscles, which compress the urethra. The bulbospongiosus muscles are innervated by the pudendal nerve (S2–S4). Discharge of the seminal fluid into the bladder is prevented by the contraction of the sphincter vesicae, which is innervated by the sympathetic nerves (L1–L2). As in the case of erection, severe bilateral damage to the spinal cord results in loss of ejaculation. Later, reflex ejaculation may be possible in patients with spinal cord transections in the thoracic or cervical regions. Some individuals have a normal ejaculation without external emission, and the seminal fluid passes into the bladder owing to paralysis of the sphincter vesicae.

Diseases Involving the Autonomic Nervous System

The ANS can be affected by a variety of diseases that compromise the integrity of peripheral nerves containing sympathetic and parasympathetic fibers.

Diabetes Mellitus

Diabetes mellitus is a common cause of peripheral nerve neuropathy. This involves sensory and motor dysfunction and may also include autonomic dysfunction. The clinical features of autonomic dysfunction include postural hypotension, peripheral edema, pupillary abnormalities, and impaired sweating. The cause is probably associated with chronic hyperglycemia.

Horner Syndrome

Horner syndrome consists of (1) constriction of the pupil (miosis), (2) slight drooping of the eyelid (ptosis), (3) enophthalmos (which, although apparent, is not real and is caused by the ptosis; however, the orbitalis muscle is paralyzed, and involvement may be responsible), (4) vasodilation of skin arterioles, and (5) loss of sweating (anhydrosis). All these symptoms result from an interruption of the sympathetic nerve supply to the head and neck. Pathologic causes include lesions in the brainstem or cervical part of the spinal cord that interrupt the reticulospinal tracts descending from the hypothalamus to the sympathetic outflow in the lateral gray column of the first thoracic segment of the spinal cord. Such lesions include **multiple sclerosis** and **syringomyelia**. Traction on the stellate ganglion due to a **cervical rib** or involvement of the ganglion in a metastatic lesion may interrupt the peripheral part of the sympathetic pathway.

All patients with Horner syndrome have miosis and ptosis. However, a distinction should be made between lesions occurring at the first neuron (the descending reticulospinal fibers within the CNS), the second neuron (the preganglionic fibers), and the third neuron (postganglionic fibers). For example, the clinical signs suggestive of a first-neuron defect (central Horner syndrome) could include contralateral hyperesthesia of the body and loss of sweating of the entire half of the body. Signs suggesting a second-neuron involvement (preganglionic Horner syndrome) include loss of sweating limited to the face and neck and the presence of flushing or blanching of the face and neck. Signs suggesting third-neuron involvement (postganglionic Horner syndrome) include facial pain or ear, nose, or throat disease.

The presence or absence of other localizing signs and symptoms may assist in differentiating the three types of Horner syndrome.

Argyll Robertson Pupil

Argyll Robertson pupil is characterized by a small pupil, which is of fixed size and does not react to light but does contract with accommodation. It is usually caused by a neurosyphilitic lesion interrupting the fibers that run from the pretectal nucleus to the parasympathetic nuclei (Edinger–Westphal nuclei) of the oculomotor nerve on both sides. The fact that the pupil constricts with accommodation implies that the connections between the parasympathetic nuclei and the constrictor pupillae muscle of the iris are intact.

Adie Tonic Pupil Syndrome

In Adie tonic pupil syndrome, the pupil has a decreased or absent light reflex, a slow or delayed contraction to near vision, and a slow or delayed dilatation in the dark. This benign syndrome, which probably results from a disorder of the parasympathetic innervation of the constrictor pupillae muscle, must be distinguished from the Argyll Robertson pupil (see above), which is caused by neurosyphilis. Adie syndrome can be confirmed by looking for hypersensitivity to cholinergic agents. Drops commonly used for this test are 2.5% methacholine (Mecholyl) or 0.1% pilocarpine. The Adie tonic pupil should constrict when these drops are put in the eye. These cholinergic agents do not cause pupillary constriction in mydriasis caused by oculomotor lesion or in drug-related mydriasis.

Frey Syndrome

Frey syndrome is an interesting complication that sometimes follows penetrating wounds of the parotid gland. During the process of healing, the postganglionic parasympathetic secretomotor fibers traveling in the auriculotemporal nerve grow out and join the distal end of the great auricular nerve, which supplies the sweat glands of the overlying facial skin. By this means, a stimulus intended for saliva production instead produces sweat secretion.

A similar syndrome may follow injury to the facial nerve. During the process of regeneration, parasympathetic fibers normally destined for the submandibular and sublingual salivary glands are diverted to the lacrimal gland. This produces watering of the eyes associated with salivation, the so-called **crocodile tears**.

Hirschsprung Disease

Hirschsprung disease (megacolon) is a congenital condition in which the myenteric plexus (Auerbach plexus) fails to develop in the distal part of the colon. The involved part of the colon possesses no parasympathetic ganglion cells and peristalsis is absent. This effectively blocks the passage of feces and the proximal part of the colon becomes enormously distended.

Disease Caused by Botulinum Toxin

A very small amount of botulinum toxin binds irreversibly to the nerve plasma membranes and prevents the release of ACh at cholinergic synapses and neuromuscular junctions, producing an atropinelike syndrome with skeletal muscle weakness.

Disease Caused by Black Widow Spider Venom

The venom of a black widow spider causes a brief release of ACh at the nerve endings followed by a permanent blockade.

Disease Caused by Anticholinesterase Agents

AChE, which is responsible for hydrolyzing and limiting the action of ACh at nerve endings, can be blocked by certain drugs. Physostigmine, neostigmine, pyridostigmine, and carbamate and organophosphate insecticides are effective AChE inhibitors. Their use results in an excessive stimulation of the cholinergic receptors, producing the "SLUDG syndrome"—salivation, lacrimation, urination, defecation, and gastrointestinal distress.

Sympathectomy

Sympathectomy, or surgical removal of a sympathetic nerve ganglion, can be used to treat arterial disease.

Raynaud Disease

Raynaud disease is a vasospastic disorder involving the digital arteries of the upper limb. The disorder is usually bilateral and an attack is provoked by exposure to cold. Pallor or cyanosis of the fingers is seen as well as severe pain. Gangrene of the tips of the fingers may occur.

In mild cases of Raynaud disease, the treatment is the avoidance of cold and no smoking (smoking causes vasoconstriction). In more severe cases, drugs that inhibit sympathetic activity, such as reserpine, bring about arterial vasodilatation with consequent increase in blood flow to the fingers. Cervicothoracic preganglionic sympathectomy has been used, but the long-term results are disappointing.

Intermittent Claudication

Intermittent claudication, which is common in men, is due to arterial occlusive disease of the leg. Ischemia of the muscles produces a cramplike pain on exercise. Lumbar preganglionic sympathectomy may be advocated as a form of treatment in order to bring about vasodilatation and an increase in blood flow through the collateral circulation. Preganglionic sympathectomy is performed by removing the upper three lumbar ganglia and the intervening parts of the sympathetic trunk.

Hypertension

In the past, severe essential hypertension was treated by bilateral thoracolumbar sympathectomy to reduce the vasomotor control over the peripheral resistance and thus lower the blood pressure. Today, chemical blocking agents of the sympathetic system are widely used with great success and the resulting reduction in the force of myocardial contraction reduces the arterial blood pressure.

Referred Visceral Pain

Most viscera are innervated only by autonomic nerves. Therefore, it follows that visceral pain is conducted along afferent autonomic nerves. Visceral pain is diffuse and poorly localized, whereas somatic pain is intense and discretely localized. Visceral pain frequently is referred to skin areas that are innervated by the same segments of the spinal cord as the painful viscus (Fig. 14-16). The explanation for referred pain is not known. One theory is that the nerve fibers from the viscus and the dermatome ascend in the CNS along a common pathway and the cerebral cortex is incapable of distinguishing between the sites of origin. Another theory is that under normal conditions, the viscus does not give rise to painful stimuli, whereas the skin area

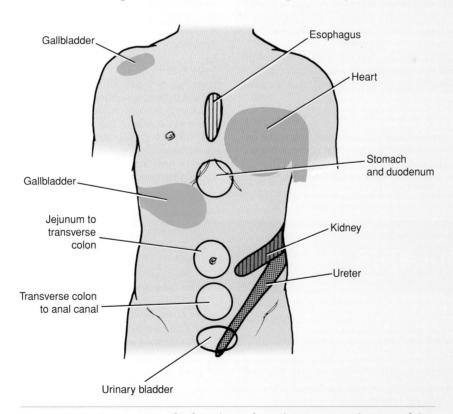

Gallbladder

Esophagus

Heart

Gallbladder

Stomach and duodenum

Jejunum to transverse colon

Kidney

Ureter

Transverse colon to anal canal

Urinary bladder

Figure 14-16 Some areas of referred pain from the viscera. In the case of the heart, the pain is usually referred to the left side of the thorax; occasionally, it is referred to both sides.

repeatedly receives noxious stimuli. Because both afferent fibers enter the spinal cord at the same segment, the brain interprets the information as coming from the skin rather than from the viscus. Pain arising from the gastrointestinal tract is referred to the midline. This can probably be explained by the fact that the tract arises embryologically as a midline structure and receives a bilateral nerve supply.

Cardiac Pain

Pain originating in the heart as the result of acute myocardial ischemia is assumed to be caused by oxygen deficiency and the accumulation of metabolites, which stimulate the sensory nerve endings in the myocardium. The afferent nerve fibers ascend to the CNS through the cardiac branches of the sympathetic trunk and enter the spinal cord through the posterior roots of the upper four thoracic nerves. The nature of the pain varies considerably, from a severe crushing pain to nothing more than a mild discomfort.

The pain is not felt in the heart but is referred to the skin areas supplied by the corresponding spinal nerves. The skin areas supplied by the upper four intercostal nerves and by the intercostobrachial nerve (T2) are therefore affected. The intercostobrachial nerve communicates with the medial cutaneous nerve of the arm and is distributed to skin on the medial side of the upper part of the arm. A certain amount of spread of nervous information must occur within the CNS, as the pain is sometimes felt in the neck and the jaw.

Myocardial infarction involving the inferior wall or diaphragmatic surface of the heart often gives rise to discomfort in the epigastrium, just below the sternum. One must assume that the afferent pain fibers from the heart ascend in the sympathetic nerves and enter the spinal cord in the posterior roots of the seventh, eighth, and ninth thoracic spinal nerves and give rise to referred pain in the T7–T9 thoracic dermatomes in the epigastrium.

Because the heart and the thoracic part of the esophagus probably have similar afferent pain pathways, pain from **acute esophagitis** can mimic the pain of myocardial infarction.

Stomach Pain

Referred pain from the stomach is commonly felt in the epigastrium. The afferent pain fibers from the stomach ascend in company with the sympathetic nerves and pass through the celiac plexus and the greater splanchnic nerves. The sensory fibers enter the spinal cord at segments T5–T9 and give rise to referred pain in the dermatomes T5–T9 on the lower chest and abdominal walls.

Appendicular Pain

Visceral pain from the appendix is produced by distention of its lumen or spasm of its muscle. It travels in nerve fibers that accompany sympathetic nerves through the superior mesenteric plexus and the lesser splanchnic nerve to the spinal cord (T10 segment). The vague referred pain is felt in the region of the umbilicus, which is innervated by the 10th intercostal nerve (T10 dermatome). Later, when the inflammatory process involves the parietal peritoneum in the right iliac fossa, which is innervated by the 12th thoracic and 1st lumbar spinal nerves, the now somatic pain becomes severe and dominates the clinical picture. The somatic pain is localized precisely to the right lower quadrant of the anterior abdominal wall (T12–L1 dermatomes).

Gallbladder Pain

Visceral pain impulses from the gallbladder (acute cholecystitis, gallstone colic) travel in nerve fibers that accompany sympathetic fibers through the celiac plexus and the greater splanchnic nerves to the spinal cord (segments T5–T9). The vague referred pain is felt in the dermatomes (T5–T9) on the lower chest and upper abdominal walls. Should the inflammatory process spread to involve the parietal peritoneum of the anterior abdominal wall or peripheral diaphragm, the now severe somatic pain will be felt in the right upper quadrant of the anterior abdominal wall and through to the back below the inferior angle of the scapula. Involvement of the central diaphragmatic parietal peritoneum, which is innervated by the phrenic nerve (C3–C5), may give rise to referred pain to the tip of the shoulder, since the skin in this area is innervated by the supraclavicular nerves (C3–C4).

Causalgia

Causalgia is a painful condition of the arm or leg accompanied by trophic changes in the affected skin and nails. It commonly follows crushing or partial division of the median nerve in the arm or the tibial nerve in the leg. It is thought that the descending impulses in the sympathetic postganglionic fibers in some way evoke ascending impulses in the afferent pain fibers at the site of injury. In many instances, sympathectomy has relieved the pain of causalgia.

Key Concepts

Organization

- The ANS is divided into two parts, sympathetic and parasympathetic.
- The function of the sympathetic system is to prepare the body for emergency by increasing heart rate, constricting peripheral blood vessels, increasing blood supply to muscles, and increasing blood pressure. Thus, it redistributes blood to organs that need high performance in emergency situations.

- Efferent fibers of the sympathetic system originate in the lateral gray columns of the spinal cord. Myelinated axons leave the cord in the anterior root and pass via the white rami communicantes to the paravertebral ganglia of the sympathetic trunk.

- Once these presynaptic fibers reach the sympathetic trunks, they are distributed as follows:

  - Synapse with a postsynaptic sympathetic neuron in the ganglion.

- Travel superiorly or inferiorly to synapse at a different level of the sympathetic trunk. For instance, T1 fibers must travel superiorly to the superior cervical ganglion.
- Pass through the ganglia without synapsing, as the greater, lesser, or least splanchnic nerve, to synapse in a prevertebral sympathetic ganglion.
- Afferent information from the viscera travels through the sympathetic ganglia without synapsing and ascends to higher centers.
- The function of the parasympathetic system is to conserve and restore energy. The heart rate is slowed, pupils are constricted, peristalsis and glandular activity is increased, and the bladder walls are contracted.
- Efferent fibers of the parasympathetic system originate in the parasympathetic nuclei of cranial nerves III, VII, IX, and X and the sacral spinal cord segments S2–S4.
- Presynaptic parasympathetic fibers of cranial nerves II, VII, and IX synapse in the parasympathetic ganglia of the head—specifically—ciliary, otic, pterygopalatine, and submandibular.
- Afferent fibers from viscera travel with the cranial nerves and the pelvic splanchnic nerves.
- The sympathetic system has long postganglionic fibers, whereas the parasympathetic has short fibers.

Neurotransmitters

- The preganglionic fibers in both the sympathetic and parasympathetic systems are cholinergic, meaning they synthesize and release ACh at the synapse.

- The postganglionic fibers in the parasympathetic are also cholinergic.
- Most postganglionic sympathetic neurons release norepinephrine; however, fibers to sweat glands and blood vessels are cholinergic.

Important Autonomic Innervations

- The skin of the upper eyelid receives sympathetic innervation from the superior cervical ganglion.
- The pupil of the iris is constricted by parasympathetic from cranial nerve III and dilated by sympathetic fibers from the superior cervical ganglion.
- The lacrimal gland receives parasympathetic fibers from cranial nerve VII and sympathetic vasoconstrictor fibers from the superior cervical ganglion.
- Submandibular and sublingual glands receive parasympathetic innervation from cranial nerve VII and sympathetic fibers from the superior cervical ganglion.
- The parotid gland receives parasympathetic fibers from cranial nerve IX and sympathetic fibers from the superior cervical ganglion.
- The gastrointestinal tract, up to the splenic flexure, receives parasympathetic innervation from cranial nerve X and sympathetic fibers from the greater and lesser splanchnic nerves.
- The descending colon, sigmoid colon, and rectum receive parasympathetic innervation from the pelvic splanchnic nerves and sympathetic fibers from the lumbar part of the sympathetic trunk.

? Clinical Problem Solving

1. A 35-year-old man is getting off the back of a truck when it starts to move. With his feet on the ground, he grabs a rail on the truck with his right hand and holds on. The truck continues along the road for one block before it stops. In the meantime, the man is dragged along the road as he holds onto the truck. He is seen in the emergency department in a state of shock, with cuts and abrasions to his legs. On careful examination of his right arm, the following muscles are found to be paralyzed: the flexor carpi ulnaris, flexor digitorum profundus, palmar and dorsal interossei, and the thenar and hypothenar muscles. Loss of sensation occurs on the medial side of the arm, forearm, and hand. The deep tendon reflex for the biceps brachii is present, but the triceps reflex is absent. The pupil of the right eye is constricted and the right upper eyelid droops. The right eyeball seems to be less prominent than the left. The skin of the right cheek feels warmer and drier and is redder in color than the left cheek. Using your knowledge of neuroanatomy, explain the clinical findings.

2. A 3-year-old boy with a history since infancy of chronic constipation and abdominal distention is taken to a pediatrician. The child's mother says that the constipation is getting progressively worse. It is not responding to laxatives and she is finding it necessary to give her son an enema once a week to relieve his abdominal distention. On physical examination, the child's abdomen is obviously distended and a doughlike mass is palpated along the course of the descending colon in the left iliac fossa.

Examination of the rectum shows it to be empty and not dilated. Following an enema and repeated colonic irrigation with saline solution, the patient is given a barium enema for a radiographic examination. The radiograph shows a grossly distended descending colon and an abrupt change in lumen diameter where the descending colon joined the sigmoid colon. Notably, the child fails to empty the colon of the barium. Using your knowledge of the autonomic nerve supply to the colon, what is the diagnosis? How would you treat this patient?

3. A nervous 25-year-old woman attends her physician because she is experiencing attacks of painful discoloration of the fourth and fifth fingers of both hands. She says that her symptoms started 2 years previously, during the winter, and affects her right hand first and, in subsequent attacks, her left hand as well. Her fingers turn white on exposure to cold and then become deep blue. The color change is confined to the distal half of each finger and is accompanied by an aching pain. Holding her hands over a hot stove or going into a hot room is the only treatment that relieves the pain. As the pain disappears, she says her fingers become red and swollen. She tells her physician that she notices that her fingers are moist with sweat during some of the attacks. Using your knowledge of neuroanatomy, make the diagnosis. What is the autonomic nerve supply to the blood vessels of the upper limb? How would you treat this patient?

4. An obese 45-year-old mother of six children is examined by her physician because her symptoms are suggestive of gallbladder disease. She complains of having severe attacks of colicky pain beneath the right costal margin, which radiate through to the back beneath the right scapula. The physician turns to a medical student and says, "Note that the patient complains of referred pain to the back." What does he mean by that statement? Explain the phenomenon of referred pain to the back and sometimes the right shoulder in gallbladder disease.

5. Examination of a patient with neurosyphilis indicates that the pupil of her left eye is small and fixed and does not react to light but contracts when she is asked to look at a near object. What is the innervation of the iris? Using your knowledge of neuroanatomy, state where you believe the neurologic lesion would be situated to account for these defects.

6. A 36-year-old man is admitted to the emergency department following a gunshot wound to the lower back. Radiographic examination reveals that the bullet is lodged in the vertebral canal at the level of the third lumbar vertebra. A complete neurologic examination reveals the symptoms and signs that indicate a complete lesion of the cauda equina. What is the autonomic nerve supply to the bladder? Is this patient going to have any interference with bladder function?

7. On routine medical examination, a 40-year-old black man is found to have essential hypertension. His blood pressure readings are 180 systolic and 100 diastolic (mm Hg). How would you treat this patient medically? What is the action of the various types of drugs that are commonly used in the treatment of hypertension?

8. What transmitter substances are liberated at the following nerve endings: (a) preganglionic sympathetic, (b) preganglionic parasympathetic, (c) postganglionic parasympathetic, (d) postganglionic sympathetic fibers to the heart muscle, and (e) postganglionic sympathetic fibers to the sweat glands of the hand?

 Answers and Explanations to Clinical Problem Solving

1. As a result of holding onto the moving truck with the right hand, this man has sustained a severe traction injury of the eighth cervical and first thoracic roots of the brachial plexus. The various paralyzed forearm and hand muscles together with the sensory loss were characteristic of Klumpke paralysis. In this case, the pull on the first thoracic nerve was so severe that the white ramus communicans to the inferior cervical sympathetic ganglion was torn. This effectively cut off the preganglionic sympathetic fibers to the right side of the head and neck, causing a right-sided Horner syndrome (preganglionic type). This was exemplified by (a) constriction of the pupil, (b) drooping of the upper lid, and (c) enophthalmos. The arteriolar vasodilatation due to loss of sympathetic vasoconstrictor fibers was responsible for the red, hot cheek on the right side. The dryness of the skin of the right cheek also was due to the loss of the sympathetic secretomotor supply to the sweat glands.

2. This 3-year-old boy has Hirschsprung disease, a congenital condition in which the myenteric plexus (Auerbach plexus) fails to develop in the distal part of the colon. The proximal part of the colon is normal but becomes greatly distended due to the accumulation of feces. In this patient, the lower sigmoid colon, later at operation, was shown to have no parasympathetic ganglion cells. Thus, this segment of the bowel had no peristalsis and effectively blocked the passage of feces. Once the diagnosis had been confirmed by performing a biopsy of the distal segment of the bowel, the treatment was to remove the aganglionic segment of the bowel by surgical resection.

3. This patient has given a classic history of Raynaud disease. The disease is much more common in women than in men, especially those who have a nervous disposition. The initial pallor of the fingers is due to spasm of the digital arterioles. The cyanosis that follows is due to local capillary dilatation

due to accumulation of metabolites. Because blood flow through the capillaries is absent, deoxygenated hemoglobin accumulates within them. During this period of prolonged cyanosis, the patient experiences severe, aching pain. On exposing the fingers to warmth, the vasospasm disappears and oxygenated blood flows back into the very dilated capillaries. Reactive hyperemia results, as well as increased tissue fluid responsible for the swelling of the affected fingers. The sweating of the fingers during the attack probably is due to the excessive sympathetic activity, which may be responsible in part for the arteriolar vasospasm.

The arteries of the upper limb are innervated by sympathetic nerves. The preganglionic fibers originate from the cell bodies in the second to the eighth thoracic segments of the spinal cord. They ascend in the sympathetic trunk to synapse in the middle cervical, inferior cervical, and first thoracic or stellate ganglia. The postganglionic fibers join the nerves that form the brachial plexus and are distributed to the digital arteries within the branches of the brachial plexus.

In this patient, the attacks were relatively mild. The patient should be reassured and told to keep her hands warm as much as possible. However, should the condition worsen, the patient should be treated with drugs, such as reserpine, that inhibit sympathetic activity. This would result in arterial vasodilatation with consequent increase in blood flow to the fingers.

4. The patient was suffering from gallstone colic. The visceral pain originated from the cystic duct or bile duct and was due to stretching or spasm of the smooth muscle in its wall. The pain afferent fibers pass through the celiac ganglia and ascend in the greater splanchnic nerve to enter the fifth to the ninth thoracic segments of the spinal cord. The pain was referred to the fifth through the ninth thoracic dermatomes on the right side—that is, to the skin over and inferior to the right scapula.

Referred pain to the right shoulder in gallbladder disease is discussed on page 410.

5. This patient has an Argyll Robertson pupil, which is a small fixed pupil that does not react to light but contracts with accommodation. The condition usually is due to a syphilitic lesion. The innervation of the iris is described on page 396. The neurologic lesion in this patient interrupted the fibers running from the pretectal nucleus to the parasympathetic nuclei of the oculomotor nerve on both sides.

6. The urinary bladder is innervated by sympathetic fibers from the first and second lumbar segments of the spinal cord and by parasympathetic fibers from the second, third, and fourth sacral segments of the spinal cord. In this patient, the cauda equina was sectioned at the level of the third lumbar vertebra. This meant that the preganglionic sympathetic fibers that descend in the anterior roots of the first and second lumbar nerves were left intact, since they leave the vertebral canal to form the appropriate spinal nerves above the level of the bullet. The preganglionic parasympathetic fibers were, however, sectioned as they descended in the vertebral canal within the anterior roots of the second, third, and fourth sacral nerves. The patient would therefore have an autonomous bladder and would be without any external reflex control. The bladder would fill to capacity and then overflow. Micturition could be activated by powerful contraction of the abdominal muscles by the patient, assisted by manual pressure on his anterior abdominal wall in the suprapubic region.

7. The precise cause of essential hypertension is unknown. Nevertheless, the objective of the treatment is to lower the blood pressure and keep it, if possible, within normal limits before the complications of cerebral hemorrhage, renal failure, or heart failure develop. The best way to accomplish this in patients with mild hypertension is to reduce the plasma fluid volume by the use of diuretics. β-Receptor–blocking agents are now extensively used. These reduce the rate and force of contraction of the cardiac muscle and lower the cardiac output.

8. (a) Acetylcholine, (b) acetylcholine, (c) acetylcholine, (d) norepinephrine, and (e) acetylcholine.

 Review Questions

Directions: Each of the numbered items in this section is followed by answers. Select the ONE lettered answer that is CORRECT.

1. The following statements concern the autonomic nervous system (ANS):
   (a) The enteric nervous system is made up of the submucous plexus of Meissner and the myenteric plexus of Auerbach.
   (b) The nerve fibers of the enteric nervous system are naked axons.
   (c) The activities of the parasympathetic part of the ANS are used in an emergency.
   (d) The parasympathetic part of the autonomic system contains only efferent nerve fibers.
   (e) The pretectal nucleus is concerned with the auditory reflexes.

2. The following statements concern the autonomic nervous system:
    (a) An Argyll Robertson pupil indicates that the accommodation reflex for near vision is normal but that the light reflex is lost.
    (b) White rami communicantes are limited to the thoracic part of the sympathetic trunk.
    (c) White rami communicantes contain postganglionic sympathetic fibers.
    (d) The greater splanchnic nerves are formed of nonmyelinated axons.
    (e) The lesser splanchnic nerves arise from the eighth and ninth ganglia of the thoracic part of the sympathetic trunks.

3. The following general statements concern the autonomic nervous system (ANS):
    (a) The hypothalamus has little control over the ANS.
    (b) The cerebral cortex has no control over the ANS.
    (c) A patient with Adie tonic pupil syndrome has an increased light reflex and a fast pupillary contraction to near vision and a fast dilatation in the dark.
    (d) Pain arising in the gastrointestinal tract is referred to the midline.
    (e) Visceral pain frequently is referred to skin areas that are innervated by different segments of the spinal cord as the painful viscus.

4. The following statements concern Horner syndrome:
    (a) The pupil is dilated.
    (b) The upper eyelid is retracted.
    (c) The patient has vasodilation of the facial skin arterioles.
    (d) The patient has excessive facial sweating.
    (e) The patient has exophthalmos.

Directions: Each of the numbered items or incomplete statements in this section is followed by answers or completions of the statement. Select the ONE lettered answer or completion that is BEST in each case.

5. The sympathetic outflow:
    (a) arises from nerve cells that are situated in the posterior gray column (horn) of the spinal cord.
    (b) has preganglionic nerve fibers that leave the spinal cord in the posterior roots of the spinal nerves.
    (c) is restricted to the T1–L2 segments of the spinal cord.
    (d) receives descending fibers from supraspinal levels that pass down the spinal cord in the posterior white column.
    (e) has many preganglionic nerve fibers that synapse in the posterior root ganglia of the spinal nerves.

6. Norepinephrine is secreted at the endings of the:
    (a) preganglionic sympathetic fibers.
    (b) preganglionic parasympathetic fibers.
    (c) postganglionic parasympathetic fibers.
    (d) postganglionic sympathetic fibers.
    (e) preganglionic fibers to the suprarenal medulla.

7. The parasympathetic innervation controlling the parotid salivary gland arises from the:
    (a) facial nerve.
    (b) oculomotor nerve.
    (c) vagus nerve.
    (d) carotid plexus.
    (e) glossopharyngeal nerve.

8. Which of the following statements best describes the parasympathetic part of the autonomic nervous system (ANS)?
    (a) It is associated with the thoracolumbar part of the spinal cord.
    (b) Effects are local and discrete due to preganglionic neurons synapsing with few postganglionic neurons.
    (c) It has short preganglionic axons.
    (d) It is active during an emotional crisis.
    (e) Its activity mobilizes glucose from glycogen.

9. Anticholinesterase drugs act at synapses by:
    (a) mimicking the action of acetylcholine at its receptor sites.
    (b) preventing the release of acetylcholine.
    (c) increasing the secretion of acetylcholine.
    (d) blocking the breakdown of acetylcholine.
    (e) preventing the uptake of acetylcholine by the nerve ending.

10. Atropine has the following effect on the autonomic nervous system:
    (a) It is an anticholinesterase drug.
    (b) It increases the activity of norepinephrine.
    (c) It blocks the action of acetylcholine on effector sites in the parasympathetic system.
    (d) It blocks norepinephrine reuptake by presynaptic terminals in the sympathetic system.
    (e) It blocks norepinephrine receptor sites.

11. The parasympathetic outflow in the spinal cord occurs at levels:
    (a) S1–S2
    (b) S3–S5
    (c) S1–S3
    (d) S2–S4
    (e) L1–L2

Directions: Each of the numbered items in this section is followed by answers. Select the ONE lettered answer that is CORRECT.

12. The following statements concern autonomic innervation of the urinary bladder:
    (a) The parasympathetic part brings about relaxation of the bladder wall muscle and contraction of the sphincter vesicae.
    (b) The sympathetic part in the male causes relaxation of the sphincter vesicae and does not prevent reflux of semen into the bladder during ejaculation.
    (c) The afferent fibers from the bladder reach the spinal cord at the first and second lumbar segments and the second, third, and fourth sacral segments.
    (d) The sympathetic part causes contraction of the sphincter urethrae.
    (e) The parasympathetic part innervates the blood vessels supplying the bladder wall.

13. The following statements concern the autonomic innervation of the heart:
    (a) The parasympathetic part causes dilation of the coronary arteries.
    (b) The postganglionic fibers do not terminate on the sinoatrial and atrioventricular nodes.
    (c) The sympathetic postganglionic fibers liberate acetylcholine at their nerve endings.
    (d) The sympathetic nerves cause cardiac acceleration and increased force of contraction of the heart.
    (e) The neural control of dilatation of the coronary arteries is more important than the chemical control exerted by the products of cardiac muscle metabolism.

Matching Questions. Directions: Match the numbered glands with the most appropriate lettered autonomic ganglion listed below. Each lettered option may be selected once, more than once, or not at all.

14. Submandibular gland   (a) Otic ganglion
15. Lacrimal gland   (b) Submandibular ganglion
16. Nasal glands   (c) Pterygopalatine ganglion
17. Parotid gland   (d) Ciliary ganglion
18. Sublingual gland   (e) None of the above

Match the numbered autonomic ganglia with the most appropriate lettered viscus or muscle listed below. Each lettered option may be selected once, more than once, or not at all.

19. Superior cervical ganglion   (a) Levator palpebrae superioris (smooth muscle only)
20. Ciliary ganglion
21. Celiac ganglion   (b) Vermiform appendix
22. Inferior mesenteric ganglion   (c) Constrictor pupillae
23. Superior mesenteric ganglion   (d) Descending colon
   (e) None of the above

Match the numbered cranial nerves with the appropriate lettered nuclei listed below. Each lettered option may be selected once, more than once, or not at all.

24. Facial nerve   (a) Inferior salivatory nucleus
25. Oculomotor nerve   (b) Edinger–Westphal nucleus
26. Glossopharyngeal nerve   (c) Lacrimatory nucleus
27. Hypoglossal nerve   (d) None of the above

The following questions apply to Figure 14-17. Match the numbered areas of referred pain with the appropriate lettered viscus originating the pain listed below. Each lettered option may be selected once, more than once, or not at all.

28. Number 1   (a) Heart
29. Number 2   (b) Appendix
30. Number 3   (c) Gallbladder
31. Number 4   (d) Stomach
   (e) None of the above

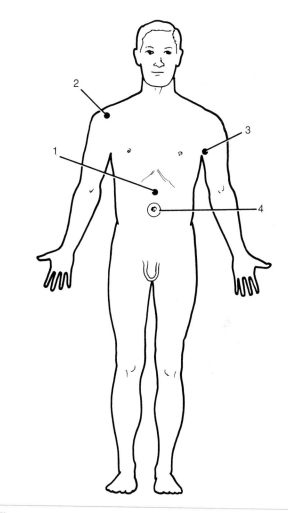

Figure 14-17 Areas of referred pain.

Answers and Explanations to Review Questions

1. A is correct. The enteric nervous system is made up of the submucous plexus of Meissner and the myenteric plexus of Auerbach. B. The nerve cells and the nerve fibers in the enteric nervous system are surrounded by neuroglialike cells that closely resemble astrocytes. C. The activities of the parasympathetic part of the ANS aim at conserving and restoring energy. D. The parasympathetic part of the autonomic system contains both afferent and efferent nerve fibers. E. The pretectal nucleus is concerned with the light reflex.

2. A is correct. An Argyll Robertson pupil indicates that the accommodation reflex for near vision is normal but that the light reflex is lost. B. White rami communicantes are found in the thoracic and first and second lumbar parts of the sympathetic trunk. C. Gray rami communicantes contain postganglionic sympathetic fibers. D. The greater splanchnic nerves are formed of myelinated axons. E. The lesser splanchnic nerves arise from the 10th and 11th ganglia of the thoracic part of the sympathetic trunks.

3. D is correct. Pain arising in the gastrointestinal tract is referred to the midline. A. The hypothalamus has great control over the ANS. B. The cerebral cortex can influence the ANS. C. A patient with Adie tonic pupil syndrome has a decreased or absent light reflex and a slow or delayed pupillary contraction to near vision and a slow or delayed dilatation in the dark. E. Visceral pain frequently is referred to skin areas that are innervated by the same segment of the spinal cord as the painful viscus.

4. C is correct. In Horner syndrome, the patient has vasodilation of the facial skin arterioles. A. The pupil is constricted. B. Ptosis of the upper eyelid occurs. D. Facial sweating is absent. E. Enophthalmos occurs.

5. C is correct. The sympathetic outflow is restricted to T1–L2 segments of the spinal cord (see Fig. 14-2).

6. D is correct. Norepinephrine is secreted at the endings of most postganglionic sympathetic fibers.

7. E is correct. The parasympathetic innervation controlling the parotid salivary gland is the glossopharyngeal nerve.

8. B is correct. The parasympathetic part of the ANS produces effects that are local and discrete due to preganglionic neurons synapsing with few postganglionic neurons.

9. D is correct. Anticholinesterase drugs act at synapses by blocking the breakdown of acetylcholine.

10. C is correct. Atropine blocks the action of acetylcholine on the effector sites in the parasympathetic part of the autonomic system.

11. D is correct. The parasympathetic outflow in the spinal cord occurs at the level of S2–S4 (see Fig. 14-2).

12. C is correct. The afferent sensory fibers from the bladder reach the spinal cord at the first and second lumbar segments and the second, third, and fourth sacral segments. A. The parasympathetic innervation of the bladder brings about contraction of the bladder wall muscle and relaxation of the sphincter vesicae. B. The sympathetic innervation of the bladder in the male causes contraction of the sphincter vesicae and prevents the reflux of semen into the bladder during ejaculation. D. The sphincter urethrae is not under the control of the autonomic nervous system; it is made to contract voluntarily by the internal pudendal nerve. E. The sympathetic nerves innervate the blood vessels supplying the bladder wall.

13. D is correct. The sympathetic nerves supplying the heart cause cardiac acceleration and increased force of contraction of the cardiac muscle. A. The parasympathetic part of the autonomic system brings about constriction of the coronary arteries. B. The postganglionic autonomic nerves to the heart do terminate on the sinoatrial and atrioventricular nodes. C. The sympathetic postganglionic fibers supplying the heart liberate norepinephrine at their endings. E. The local metabolic needs of the cardiac muscle exert a greater control over the degree of dilation of the coronary arteries than the neural control of the arteries.

14. B is correct. The submandibular salivary gland receives secretomotor parasympathetic nerves through the submandibular ganglion.

15. C is correct. The lacrimal gland receives secretomotor parasympathetic nerves through the pterygopalatine ganglion.

16. C is correct. The nasal glands receive secretomotor parasympathetic nerves through the pterygopalatine ganglion.

17. A is correct. The parotid salivary gland receives secretomotor parasympathetic nerves through the otic ganglion.

18. B is correct. The sublingual salivary gland receives secretomotor parasympathetic nerves through the submandibular salivary ganglion.

19. A is correct. The levator palpebrae superioris (smooth muscle only) is innervated by sympathetic fibers from the superior cervical sympathetic ganglion.

20. C is correct. The constrictor pupillae is innervated by parasympathetic nerves from the ciliary ganglion.

21. E is correct. The celiac ganglion gives rise to nerves that supply the smooth muscle of the gut from the gastroesophageal junction down to the middle of the second part of the duodenum; it also supplies the liver, the pancreas, and the spleen.

22. D is correct. The descending colon receives sympathetic nerves from the inferior mesenteric ganglion.

23. B is correct. The vermiform appendix receives sympathetic nerves from the superior mesenteric ganglion.

24. C is correct. Parasympathetic nerve fibers from the lacrimatory nucleus travel in the facial nerve and

its branches to the pterygopalatine ganglion, synapse, and then pass to the lacrimal gland.

25. B is correct. Parasympathetic nerve fibers from the Edinger–Westphal nucleus travel in the oculomotor nerve to the ciliary ganglion, synapse, and then pass to the constrictor pupillae and the ciliary muscle.

26. A is correct. Parasympathetic nerve fibers from the inferior salivatory nucleus travel in the glossopharyngeal nerve and its branches to the otic ganglion, synapse, and then pass to the parotid salivary gland.

27. D is correct. The hypoglossal nerve supplies the muscles of the tongue.

28. D is correct.

29. C is correct.

30. A is correct.

31. B is correct.

15 Meninges

CHAPTER OBJECTIVES

- To learn the structure and function of the three meninges that surround the brain and spinal cord

- To understand the venous sinuses within the skull and see how the meninges contribute to their walls

- To appreciate the relationship of the meninges to the different forms of cerebral hemorrhage

A 44-year-old woman is seen by a neurologist because she is experiencing intense pain in the right eye. On physical examination, she is found to have a slight medial strabismus of the right eye, and the right pupil is smaller than normal. Further examination reveals numbness over the right cheek. A computed tomography (CT) scan shows the presence of an aneurysm of the right internal carotid artery within the cavernous sinus. The aneurysm is about the size of a pea.

The location of the carotid aneurysm within the cavernous sinus explains the ocular pain; pressure on the right abducens nerve is responsible for the paralysis of the lateral rectus muscle producing the medial strabismus. The small pupil of the right eye is caused by the aneurysm pressing on the sympathetic plexus surrounding the carotid artery and producing paralysis of the dilator pupillae muscle. The numbness over the right cheek is due to pressure of the aneurysm on the right maxillary division of the trigeminal nerve as it passes forward through the lateral wall of the sinus.

This patient illustrates the necessity of knowing the relationships between the structures within the skull, especially in regions like the cavernous sinus, where so many important neural structures lie close to one another.

BRAIN MENINGES

The brain in the skull is surrounded by three protective membranes or meninges: the dura mater, the arachnoid mater, and the pia mater.

Dura Mater

The dura mater of the brain is conventionally described as two layers: the endosteal layer and the meningeal layer (Fig. 15-1). These are closely united except along certain lines where they separate to form **venous sinuses**.

The **endosteal layer** is nothing more than the periosteum covering the inner surface of the skull bones. At the foramen magnum, it does not become continuous with the dura mater of the spinal cord. Around the margins of all the foramina in the skull, it becomes continuous with the **periosteum** on the outside of the skull bones. At the sutures, it is continuous with the **sutural ligaments**. It is most strongly adherent to the bones over the base of the skull.

The **meningeal layer** is the dura mater proper. It is a dense, strong fibrous membrane covering the brain (Figs. 15-2 and 15-3) and is continuous through the foramen magnum with the dura mater of the spinal cord. It provides tubular sheaths for the cranial nerves as the latter pass through the foramina in the skull. Outside the skull, the sheaths fuse with the epineurium of the nerves (see Fig. 15-2B).

The meningeal layer sends inward four septa—the falx cerebri, falx cerebelli, tentorium cerebelli, and diaphragma sellae—which divide the cranial cavity into freely communicating spaces that lodge the subdivisions of the brain (see Figs. 15-1 and 15-3). The function of these septa is to restrict the displacement of the brain associated with acceleration and deceleration when the head is moved.

The **falx cerebri** is a sickle-shaped fold of dura mater that lies in the midline between the two cerebral hemispheres. Its narrow anterior end is attached to the internal frontal crest and the crista galli. Its broad posterior part blends in the midline with the upper surface of the

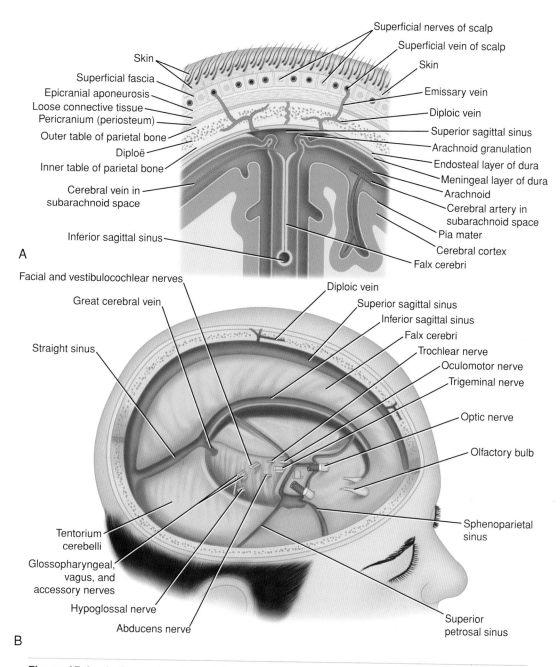

Figure 15-1 **A:** Coronal section of the upper part of the head showing the layers of the scalp, sagittal suture of the skull, falx cerebri, venous sinuses, arachnoid granulations, emissary veins, and relation of the cerebral blood vessels to the subarachnoid space. **B:** Interior of the skull showing the dura mater and its contained venous sinuses.

tentorium cerebelli. The **superior sagittal sinus** runs in its upper fixed margin, the **inferior sagittal sinus** runs in its lower concave free margin, and the **straight sinus** runs along its attachment to the tentorium cerebelli.

The **tentorium cerebelli** is a crescent-shaped fold of dura mater that roofs over the posterior cranial fossa (Fig. 15-1; also see Fig. 15-4). It covers the upper surface of the cerebellum and supports the occipital lobes of the cerebral hemispheres. In the anterior edge, a gap, the **tentorial notch**, allows passage of the midbrain,

which produces an inner free border and an outer attached or fixed border. The fixed border is attached to the posterior clinoid processes, the superior borders of the petrous bones, and the margins of the grooves for the transverse sinuses on the occipital bone. The free border runs forward at its two ends, crosses the attached border, and is affixed to the anterior clinoid process on each side. At the point where the two borders cross, the third and fourth cranial nerves pass forward to enter the lateral wall of the cavernous sinus.

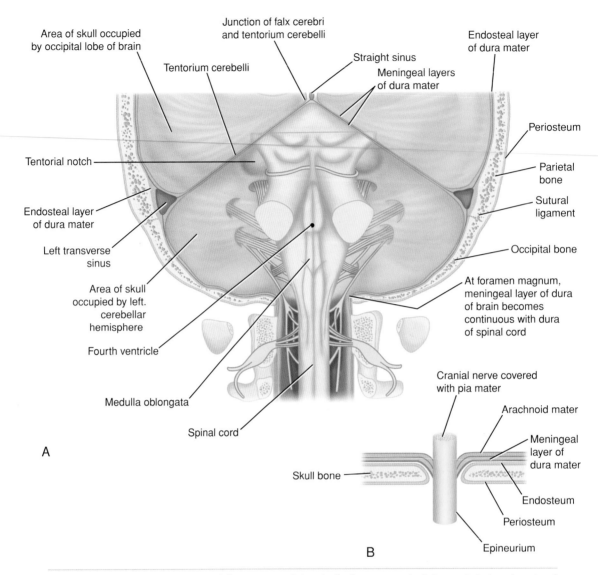

Area of skull occupied by occipital lobe of brain

Junction of falx cerebri and tentorium cerebelli

Tentorium cerebelli

Straight sinus

Meningeal layers of dura mater

Endosteal layer of dura mater

Periosteum

Tentorial notch

Parietal bone

Endosteal layer of dura mater

Sutural ligament

Left transverse sinus

Occipital bone

Area of skull occupied by left. cerebellar hemisphere

At foramen magnum, meningeal layer of dura of brain becomes continuous with dura of spinal cord

Fourth ventricle

Cranial nerve covered with pia mater

Medulla oblongata

Arachnoid mater

Meningeal layer of dura mater

Spinal cord

Skull bone

Endosteum

A

Periosteum

Epineurium

B

Figure 15-2 A: Posterior view of the interior of the skull after removal of the occipital and parietal bones showing the arrangement of the endosteal and meningeal layers of the dura mater. The brainstem has been left in situ. **B:** The arrangement of the meninges as a cranial nerve passes through a foramen in the skull.

Close to the apex of the petrous part of the temporal bone, the lower layer of the tentorium is pouched forward beneath the superior petrosal sinus to form a recess for the trigeminal nerve and the trigeminal ganglion.

The falx cerebri and the falx cerebelli are attached to the upper and lower surfaces of the tentorium, respectively. The straight sinus runs along its attachment to the falx cerebri, the superior petrosal sinus runs along its attachment to the petrous bone, and the **transverse sinus** runs along its attachment to the occipital bone (see Figs. 15-1 and 15-4).

The **falx cerebelli,** a small, sickle-shaped fold of dura mater attached to the internal occipital crest projects forward between the two cerebellar hemispheres. Its posterior fixed margin contains the **occipital sinus.**

The **diaphragma sellae** is a small, circular fold of dura mater that forms the roof for the sella turcica (Fig. 15-5). A small opening in its center allows passage of the stalk of the **hypophysis cerebri.**

Dural Nerve Supply

Branches of the trigeminal, vagus, and the first three cervical spinal nerves and branches from the sympathetic trunk pass to the dura.

The dura possesses numerous sensory endings that are sensitive to stretching, which produces the sensation of headache. Stimulation of the sensory endings of the trigeminal nerve above the level of the tentorium cerebelli produces referred pain to an area of skin on the same side of the head. Stimulation of the dural endings below the level of the tentorium produces pain referred

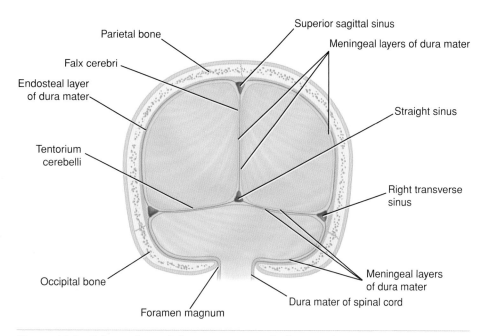

Figure 15-3 Falx cerebri and the tentorium cerebelli. Note the continuity between the meningeal layer of dura mater within the skull and the dura mater of the spinal cord at the foramen magnum.

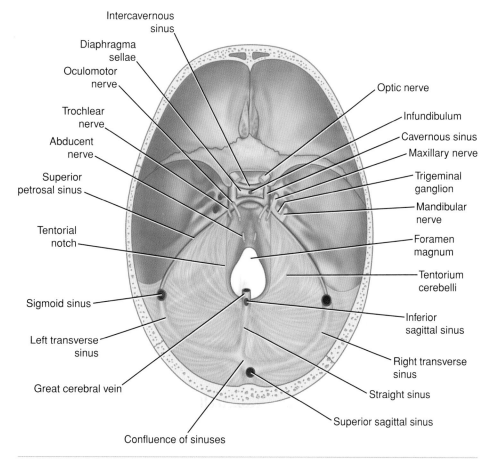

Figure 15-4 Superior view of the diaphragma sellae and tentorium cerebelli. Note the position of the cranial nerves and venous sinuses.

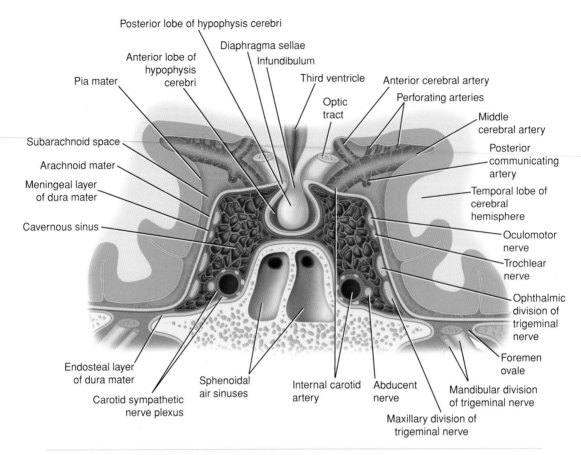

Figure 15-5 Coronal section through the body of the sphenoid bone showing the hypophysis cerebri and cavernous sinuses. Note the position of the internal carotid artery and the cranial nerves.

to the back of the neck and the back of the scalp along the distribution of the greater occipital nerve.

Dural Arterial Supply

Numerous arteries supply the dura mater from the **internal carotid, maxillary, ascending pharyngeal, occipital,** and **vertebral arteries**. From the clinical standpoint, the most important is the **middle meningeal artery**, which can be damaged in head injuries (Fig. 15-6).

The **middle meningeal artery** arises from the maxillary artery in the infratemporal fossa. It enters the cranial cavity through the **foramen spinosum** and then lies between the meningeal and endosteal layers of dura. The artery then runs forward and laterally in a groove on the upper surface of the squamous part of the temporal bone. The anterior branch deeply grooves or tunnels the anterior-inferior angle of the parietal bone, and its course corresponds roughly to the line of the underlying precentral gyrus of the brain. The posterior branch curves backward and supplies the posterior part of the dura mater (Fig. 15-7).

The **meningeal veins** lie in the endosteal layer of dura (see Fig. 15-6). The middle meningeal vein follows the branches of the middle meningeal artery and drains into the pterygoid venous plexus or the sphenoparietal sinus. The veins lie lateral to the arteries.

Dural Venous Sinuses

The venous sinuses of the cranial cavity are situated between the layers of the dura mater (see Figs. 15-3 to 15-5 and 15-7). Their main function is to receive blood from the brain through the cerebral veins and the cerebrospinal fluid (CSF) from the subarachnoid space through the **arachnoid villi** (see Fig. 16-18). The blood in the dural sinuses ultimately drains into the internal jugular veins in the neck. The dural sinuses are lined by endothelium, and their walls are thick but devoid of muscular tissue. They have no valves. **Emissary veins,** which are also valveless, connect the dural venous sinuses with the **diploic veins** of the skull and with the veins of the scalp (see Fig. 15-1).

The **superior sagittal sinus** occupies the upper fixed border of the falx cerebri (see Figs. 15-1 and 15-4). It begins anteriorly at the foramen cecum, where it occasionally receives a vein from the nasal cavity. It runs posteriorly, grooving the vault of the skull; at the internal occipital protuberance, it deviates to one or the other side (usually the right) and becomes continuous with the corresponding **transverse sinus.** The sinus

Underlying precentral gyrus
of cerebral cortex

Region of anterior inferior
portion of parietal bone

Meningeal layer
of dura mater

Endosteal layer

Anterior branches
of middle meningeal
vessels (arteries
and veins)

Posterior branches of
middle meningeal vessels

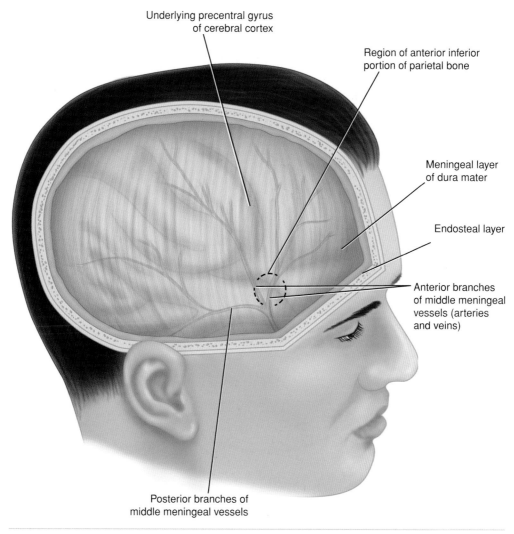

Figure 15-6   Right side of the head showing the relation of the middle meningeal vessels to the layers of the dura mater and the skull.

communicates through small openings with two or three irregularly shaped **venous lacunae** on each side (see Fig. 15-7). Numerous arachnoid villi and granulations project into the lacunae, which also receive the diploic and meningeal veins (see Fig. 15-1).

The superior sagittal sinus in its course receives the **superior cerebral veins** (Fig. 15-1; see Fig. 17-5). At the internal occipital protuberance, it is dilated to form the **confluence of the sinuses** (see Fig. 15-4). Here, the superior sagittal sinus usually becomes continuous with the right transverse sinus; it is connected to the opposite transverse sinus and receives the **occipital sinus**. The **inferior sagittal sinus** occupies the free lower margin of the falx cerebri (see Fig. 15-1). It runs backward and joins the **great cerebral vein** at the free margin of the tentorium cerebelli to form the straight sinus (see Figs. 15-1 and 15-4). It receives a few cerebral veins from the medial surface of the cerebral hemispheres.

The **straight sinus** occupies the line of junction of the falx cerebri with the tentorium cerebelli. It is formed by the union of the **inferior sagittal sinus** with the **great**

cerebral vein. It ends by turning to the left (sometimes to the right) to form the **transverse sinus**.

The **transverse sinuses** are paired structures that begin at the internal occipital protuberance (see Figs. 15-3 and 15-4). The right sinus is usually continuous with the superior sagittal sinus, and the left is continuous with the straight sinus. Each sinus occupies the attached margin of the tentorium cerebelli, grooving the occipital bone and the posteroinferior angle of the parietal bone. The transverse sinuses receive the **superior petrosal sinuses**, the **inferior cerebral** and **cerebellar veins**, and the **diploic veins**. They end by turning downward as the **sigmoid sinuses** (see Fig. 15-4).

The **sigmoid sinuses** are a direct continuation of the transverse sinuses. Each sinus turns downward and medially and grooves the mastoid part of the temporal bone. Here, the sinus lies posterior to the mastoid antrum. The sinus then turns forward and then inferiorly through the posterior part of the jugular foramen to become continuous with the **superior bulb** of the **internal jugular vein**.

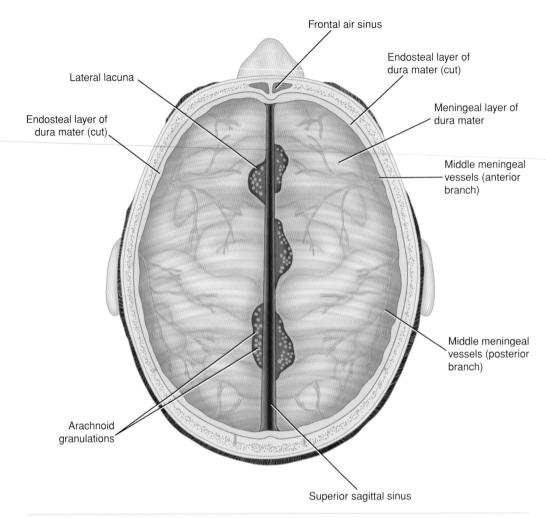

Frontal air sinus

Endosteal layer of
dura mater (cut)

Lateral lacuna

Meningeal layer of
dura mater

Endosteal layer of
dura mater (cut)

Middle meningeal
vessels (anterior
branch)

Middle meningeal
vessels (posterior
branch)

Arachnoid
granulations

Superior sagittal sinus

Figure 15-7 Superior view of the head with the calvarium removed. The greater part of the endosteal layer of dura mater has been removed, exposing the underlying meningeal layer of dura and the interior of the superior sagittal venous sinus.

The **occipital sinus** is a small sinus occupying the attached margin of the falx cerebelli. It commences near the foramen magnum where it communicates with the **vertebral veins** and drains into the **confluence of sinuses**.

The **cavernous sinuses** are situated in the middle cranial fossa on each side of the body of the sphenoid bone (see Fig. 15-5). Numerous trabeculae cross their interior, giving them a spongy appearance, hence the name. Each sinus extends from the superior orbital fissure in front to the apex of the petrous part of the temporal bone behind.

The **internal carotid artery**, surrounded by its **sympathetic nerve plexus**, runs forward through the sinus. The **abducens nerve** also passes through the sinus. The internal carotid artery and the nerves are separated from the blood by an endothelial covering.

The **third** and **fourth cranial nerves** and the **ophthalmic** and **maxillary divisions of the trigeminal nerve** run forward in the lateral wall of the sinus. They lie between the endothelial lining and the dura mater.

The tributaries are the **superior** and **inferior ophthalmic veins**, the **inferior cerebral veins**, the **sphenoparietal sinus**, and the **central vein of the retina**.

The sinus drains posteriorly into the **superior** and **inferior petrosal sinuses** and inferiorly into the **pterygoid venous plexus**.

The two sinuses communicate with each other by means of the **anterior** and **posterior intercavernous sinuses**, which run in the diaphragma sellae anterior and posterior to the stalk of the hypophysis cerebri (see Fig. 15-4). Each sinus has an important communication with the facial vein through the superior ophthalmic vein. (This is a route by which infection can travel from the facial skin to the cavernous sinus.)

The **superior** and **inferior petrosal sinuses** are small sinuses situated on the superior and inferior borders of the petrous part of the temporal bone on each side of the skull. Each superior sinus drains the cavernous sinus into the transverse sinus, and each inferior sinus drains the cavernous sinus into the internal jugular vein.

Arachnoid Mater

The arachnoid mater is a delicate, impermeable membrane covering the brain and lying between the pia mater internally and the dura mater externally (see Fig. 15-1). It is separated from the dura by a potential space, the **subdural space**, filled by a film of fluid; it is separated from the pia by the **subarachnoid space**, which is filled with **CSF**. The outer and inner surfaces of the arachnoid are covered with flattened mesothelial cells.

The arachnoid bridges over the sulci on the surface of the brain, and in certain situations, the arachnoid and pia are widely separated to form the **subarachnoid cisternae**. The **cisterna cerebellomedullaris** lies between the inferior surface of the cerebellum and the roof of the fourth ventricle. The **cisterna interpeduncularis** lies between the two cerebral peduncles. All the cisternae are in free communication with one another and with the remainder of the subarachnoid space.

In certain areas, the arachnoid projects into the venous sinuses to form **arachnoid villi.** The arachnoid villi are most numerous along the superior sagittal sinus. Aggregations of arachnoid villi are referred to as **arachnoid granulations** (see Fig. 15-7). Arachnoid villi serve as sites where the CSF diffuses into the bloodstream.

The arachnoid is connected to the pia mater across the fluid-filled subarachnoid space by delicate strands of fibrous tissue.

Structures passing to and from the brain to the skull or its foramina must pass through the subarachnoid space. All the cerebral arteries and veins lie in the space, as do the cranial nerves (see Figs. 15-1 and 15-5). The arachnoid fuses with the epineurium of the nerves at their point of exit from the skull (see Fig. 15-2B). In the case of the **optic nerve**, the arachnoid forms a sheath for the nerve, which extends into the orbital cavity through the optic canal and fuses with the sclera of the eyeball (Fig. 15-8). Thus, the subarachnoid space extends around the optic nerve as far as the eyeball.

The **CSF** is produced by the **choroid plexuses** within the lateral, third, and fourth ventricles of the brain. It escapes from the ventricular system of the brain through the three foramina in the roof of the fourth ventricle and so enters the subarachnoid space. It now circulates both upward over the surfaces of the cerebral hemispheres and downward around the spinal cord. The spinal subarachnoid space extends down as far as the **second sacral vertebra** (see pp. 426-427). Eventually, the fluid enters the bloodstream by passing into the arachnoid villi and diffusing through their walls.

In addition to removing waste products associated with neuronal activity, the CSF provides a fluid medium in which the brain floats. This mechanism effectively protects the brain from trauma. In addition, the fluid is now believed to play a role in hormonal transport.

Pia Mater

The pia mater is a vascular membrane covered by flattened mesothelial cells. It closely invests the brain, covering the gyri and descending into the deepest sulci (see Fig. 15-1). It extends out over the cranial nerves and fuses with their epineurium. The cerebral arteries entering the substance of the brain carry a sheath of pia with them.

The pia mater forms the **tela choroidea** of the roof of the third and fourth ventricles of the brain, and it fuses with the ependyma to form the choroid plexuses in the lateral, third, and fourth ventricles of the brain.

SPINAL CORD MENINGES

Like the brain, the spinal cord in the vertebral column is also protected by three layers of meninges.

Dura Mater

The dura mater is a dense, strong, fibrous membrane that encloses the spinal cord and the cauda equina

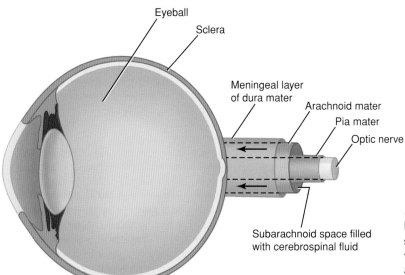

Eyeball

Sclera

Meningeal layer of dura mater

Arachnoid mater

Pia mater

Optic nerve

Subarachnoid space filled with cerebrospinal fluid

Figure 15-8 Sagittal section of the eyeball showing the attachment of the meninges to the sclera. Note the extension of the subarachnoid space around the optic nerve to the eyeball.

Figure 15-9 This silver stain of a cat spinal cord shows the spinal cord and its meninges: dura mater (DM), arachnoid mater (A) with its subarachnoid space (SS), and pia mater (PM). W, white matter; G, gray matter; DH, dorsal horn; VH, ventral horn; Gc, gray commissure; CC, central canal; VR, ventral roots; DR, dorsal roots. (From Gartner, L. P. (2018). *Color atlas and text of histology* (7th ed.). Baltimore, MD: Wolters Kluwer.)

(Figs. 15-9 to 15-11). It is continuous above through the foramen magnum with the meningeal layer of dura covering the brain. Inferiorly, it ends on the filum terminale at the level of the lower border of the second sacral vertebra. The dural sheath lies loosely in the vertebral canal and is separated from the wall of the canal by the **extradural space**. This contains loose areolar tissue and the **internal vertebral venous plexus**. The dura mater extends along each nerve root and becomes continuous with the connective tissue surrounding each spinal nerve (epineurium). The inner surface of the dura mater is in contact with the arachnoid mater (see Fig. 4-5).

Arachnoid Mater

The arachnoid mater is a delicate impermeable membrane that covers the spinal cord and lies between the pia mater internally and dura mater externally. It is separated from the pia mater by a wide space, the **subarachnoid space**, which is filled with **CSF**. The

subarachnoid space is crossed by a number of fine strands of connective tissue. The arachnoid mater is continuous above through the foramen magnum with the arachnoid covering the brain. Inferiorly, it ends on the filum terminale at the level of the lower border of the second sacral vertebra (see Figs. 15-10 and 15-11). The arachnoid mater continues along the spinal nerve roots, forming small lateral extensions of the subarachnoid space.

Pia Mater

The pia mater, a vascular membrane that closely covers the spinal cord (see Fig. 15-9B), is thickened on either side between the nerve roots to form the **ligamentum denticulatum**, which passes laterally to adhere to the arachnoid and dura. By this means, the spinal cord is suspended in the middle of the dural sheath. The pia mater extends along each nerve root and becomes continuous with the connective tissue surrounding each spinal nerve.

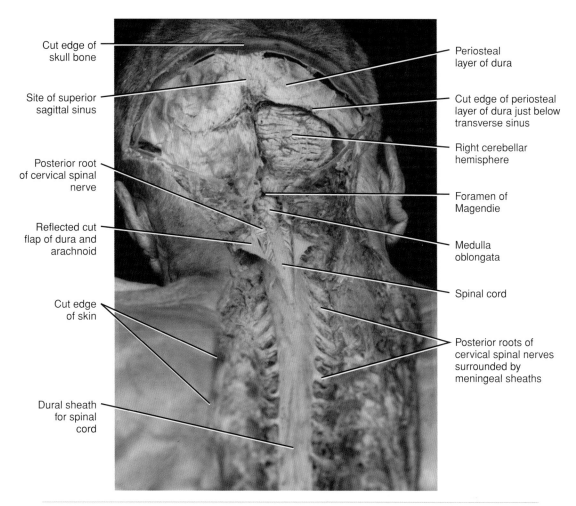

Cut edge of
skull bone

Site of superior
sagittal sinus

Posterior root
of cervical spinal
nerve

Reflected cut
flap of dura and
arachnoid

Cut edge
of skin

Dural sheath
for spinal
cord

Periosteal
layer of dura

Cut edge of periosteal
layer of dura just below
transverse sinus

Right cerebellar
hemisphere

Foramen of
Magendie

Medulla
oblongata

Spinal cord

Posterior roots of
cervical spinal nerves
surrounded by
meningeal sheaths

Figure 15-10 Dissection of the back of the head and neck. The greater part of the occipital bone has been removed, exposing the periosteal layer of dura. On the right side, a window has been made in the dura below the transverse venous sinus to expose the cerebellum and the medulla oblongata in the posterior cranial fossa. In the neck, the dura and arachnoid have been incised in the midline to expose the spinal cord and rootlets of the cervical spinal nerves. Note the cervical spinal nerves leaving the vertebral canal enveloped in a meningeal sheath.

Reflected cut
edge of dura
and arachnoid

Spinal cord

Conus
medullaris

Anterior and
posterior nerve
roots of
cauda equina

Lower end of
spinal cord

Filum
terminale

Cut lamina
of sacrum

Lower end of
subarachnoid
space

Filum
terminale

Figure 15-11 Dissection of the lower part of the back, including a complete laminectomy of the lumbar and sacral regions of the vertebral column. The meningeal sheath has been incised and reflected laterally, exposing the subarachnoid space, the lower end of the spinal cord, and the cauda equina. Note the filum terminale surrounded by the anterior and posterior nerve roots of the lumbar and sacral spinal nerves forming the cauda equina.

Clinical Notes

Functional Significance

The meninges of the brain and spinal cord form three concentric membranous coverings. The outermost covering, the dura mater, by virtue of its toughness, serves to protect the underlying nervous tissue. The dura protects the cranial nerves by forming a sheath that covers each cranial nerve for a short distance as it passes through foramina in the skull. The dura mater also provides each spinal nerve root with a protective sheath.

In the skull, the falx cerebri, which is a vertical sheet of dura between the cerebral hemispheres, and the tentorium cerebelli, which is a horizontal sheet that projects forward between the cerebrum and cerebellum, serve to limit excessive movements of the brain within the skull.

The arachnoid mater is a much thinner impermeable membrane that loosely covers the brain. The interval between the arachnoid and pia mater, the subarachnoid space, is filled with CSF. The CSF gives buoyancy to the brain and protects the nervous tissue from mechanical forces applied to the skull.

The pia mater is a vascular membrane that closely invests and supports the brain and spinal cord.

Excessive Brain Movement

When a moving patient's head is suddenly halted, the momentum of the brain causes it to travel onward until its movement is resisted by the skull or the strong septa of the dura mater. In lateral movements, the lateral surface of one hemisphere hits the side of the skull and the medial surface of the opposite hemisphere hits the side of the falx cerebri. In superior movements, the superior surfaces of the cerebral hemispheres hit the vault of the skull, and the superior surface of the corpus callosum hits the sharp free edge of the falx cerebri; the superior surface of the cerebellum presses against the inferior surface of the tentorium cerebelli.

Movements of the brain relative to the skull and dural septa may seriously injure the cranial nerves that are tethered as they pass through the various foramina. Furthermore, the fragile cortical veins that drain into the dural sinuses may be torn, resulting in severe **subdural** or **subarachnoid hemorrhage**. The tortuous arteries, with their strong walls, are rarely damaged.

Intracranial Hemorrhage

Excessive brain movement or other cranial trauma can put significant traction on the cranial vessels, leading to rupture and hemorrhage. Intracranial hemorrhage is described based on its relationship to the adjacent layers of the meninges: epidural, subdural, and subarachnoid.

Epidural Hemorrhage

Epidural hemorrhage results from injuries to the meningeal arteries or veins. The most common artery to be damaged is the **anterior division of the middle meningeal artery**. A comparatively minor blow to the side of the head, resulting in fracture of the skull in the region of the anterior-inferior portion of the parietal bone, may sever the artery. Arterial or venous injury is especially liable to occur if the vessels enter a bony canal in this region. Bleeding occurs and strips up the meningeal layer of dura from the internal surface of the skull. The intracranial pressure rises and the enlarging blood clot exerts local pressure on the underlying motor area in the precentral gyrus. Blood also passes laterally through the fracture line to form a soft swelling under the temporalis muscle.

To stop the hemorrhage, the torn artery or vein must be ligated or plugged. The burr hole through the skull wall should be placed about 1½ in (4 cm) above the midpoint of the zygomatic arch.

Subdural Hemorrhage

Subdural hemorrhage results from tearing of the **superior cerebral veins** at their point of entrance into the superior sagittal sinus. The cause is usually a blow on the front or the back of the head, causing excessive anteroposterior displacement of the brain within the skull. Acute and chronic forms of the condition occur.

Computed Tomography Scans

The different appearances of the blood clots in these two conditions as seen on CT scans are related to the anatomy of the area (Fig. 15-12). In an epidural hemorrhage, the blood strips up the meningeal layer of the dura from the endosteal layer of dura (periosteum of the skull), producing a **lens-shaped** hyperdense collection of blood that compresses the brain and displaces the midline structures to the opposite side. The shape of the blood clot is determined by the adherence of the meningeal layer of dura to the periosteal layer of dura.

In patients with subdural hematoma, the blood accumulates in the extensive potential space between the meningeal layer of dura and the arachnoid, producing a long **crescent-shaped,** hyperdense rim of blood that extends from anterior to posterior along the inner surface of the skull. With a large hematoma, the brain sulci are obliterated and the midline structures are displaced to the opposite side.

Subarachnoid and Cerebral Hemorrhages

Subarachnoid and cerebral hemorrhages are described on page 474.

Intracranial Hemorrhage in the Infant

Intracranial hemorrhage may occur during birth and may result from excessive molding of the head. Bleeding may occur from the cerebral veins or the venous sinuses. Excessive anteroposterior compression of the head often tears the anterior attachment of the falx cerebri from the tentorium cerebelli. Bleeding then takes place from the great cerebral veins, the straight sinus, or the inferior sagittal sinus.

The shaken baby syndrome is described on page 22.

Headache

The brain itself is insensitive to pain; therefore, headaches are due to the stimulation of receptors outside the brain.

Meningeal Headaches

The dura mater receives its sensory nerve supply from the trigeminal and the first three cervical nerves. The dura above the tentorium is innervated by the trigeminal nerve, and the headache is referred to the forehead and face. The dura below the tentorium is innervated by the cervical nerves, and the headache is referred to the back of the head and neck. **Meningitis**, or inflammation of the meninges, causes severe headache over the entire head and back of the neck.

Headaches Caused by Cerebral Tumors

An expanding tumor with its associated raised intracranial pressure produces severe, continuous, and progressive headache caused by the irritation and stretching of the dura. A tumor above the tentorium tends to produce a headache referred to the front of the head, while a tumor below the tentorium produces a headache referred to the back of the head.

Migraine Headache

Migraine is a common form of headache, which may be unilateral or bilateral, recurring at intervals and associated with prodromal visual disturbances. The prodromal visual disturbances are thought to be due to sympathetic vasoconstriction of the cerebral arteries supplying the visual cortex. The headache is chiefly due to the dilation and stretching of other cerebral arteries and branches of the external carotid artery. The disease therefore appears to affect arteries both inside and outside the skull, and its cause is unknown, although genetic, hormonal, and biochemical factors may initiate an attack. β-blockers bring relief to some patients due to the reduction in cerebral vasodilation.

Alcoholic Headache

Alcoholic headache is due to the direct toxic effect of alcohol on the meninges.

Headaches Due to Diseases of the Teeth, Paranasal Sinuses, and Eyes

Dental infection and sinusitis are common causes of headache. The pain is referred to the skin of the face and the forehead along the branches of the trigeminal nerve. Tonic spasm of the ciliary muscle of the eye, when attempting to focus on an object for prolonged periods (e.g., reading small print), may cause severe orbital headache. This commonly occurs in individuals who need lenses for the correction of presbyopia.

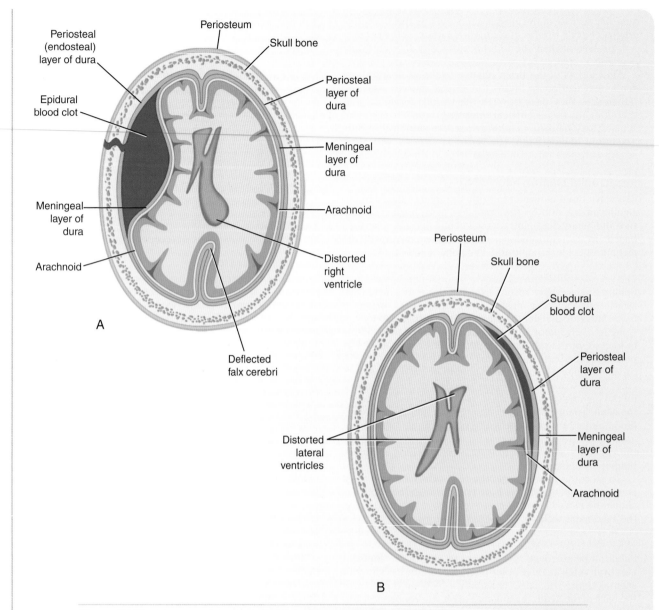

Figure 15-12 Diagrammatic representation of an epidural hemorrhage and a subdural hemorrhage. **A:** Epidural hemorrhage from the middle meningeal artery or vein on the left side. The hematoma is lens shaped and occupies the space between the endosteal layer of dura (periosteum of the skull) and the meningeal layer of dura (true dura, hence the name *epidural*). **B:** Subdural hemorrhage from the cerebral veins at the site of entrance into the venous sinus on the right side. The hematoma is crescent shaped and occupies the space between the meningeal layer of dura and the arachnoid (i.e., beneath the dura).

Key Concepts

Brain Meninges

- The brain in the skull and the spinal cord in the vertebral canal are surrounded by three protective membranes or meninges: dura mater, arachnoid mater, and pia mater.

Dura Mater

- In the skull, the dura mater has two layers, an endosteal layer and a meningeal layer. The endosteal layer is essentially the periosteum of the skull and therefore not present in the vertebral canal.

- The meningeal layer or dura mater proper is a dense, strong fibrous membrane that forms four inward septa, which divide the cranial cavity into freely communicating spaces.

- The falx cerebri is the largest dural fold and separates the two cerebral hemispheres at midline.

- The tentorium cerebelli is continuous with the falx cerebri and separates the cerebrum from the cerebellum.

- The falx cerebelli separates the two cerebellar hemispheres.

- The diaphragma sellae forms the roof over the sella turcica, which houses the pituitary gland.

DURAL NERVE SUPPLY

- Branches of the trigeminal, vagus, and the first three cervical spinal nerves innervate the cranial dura.

DURAL ARTERIAL SUPPLY

- Multiple arteries supply the dura but from the clinical standpoint, the middle meningeal artery is the most important as it is the only arterial vessel found between the meningeal and endosteal layers of dura.

DURAL VENOUS SINUSES

- The venous sinuses are found between the two layers of dura.

- The superior and inferior sagittal sinuses are located within the falx cerebri.

- The inferior sagittal sinus joins the straight sinus which is located at the junction of the falx cerebri and tentorium cerebelli.

- The occipital sinus is located within the falx cerebelli.

- The superior sagittal sinus, straight sinus, and occipital sinus come together at the confluence of sinuses, which then drains laterally into two transverse sinuses.

- The sigmoid sinuses are a direct continuation of the transverse sinuses and eventually exit the cranial cavity through the jugular foramen, at this point becoming the internal jugular vein.

Arachnoid Mater

- A delicate impermeable membrane lying between the dura mater and pia mater.

- It is separated from the pia mater by the subarachnoid space, which is filled with CSF.

- In certain areas, the arachnoid protrudes into the dural venous sinuses as arachnoid villi, which serve as sites where CSF diffuses into the bloodstream.

- The vasculature for the central nervous system is located in the subarachnoid space.

Pia Mater

- The pia mater is a vascular membrane that closely invests the brain, covering the gyri and descending into the deepest sulci.

- The cerebral arteries entering the substance carry a sheath of pia with them.

Spinal Cord Meninges

- The dura mater of the spinal cord is continuous with the meningeal layer of the cranial dura.

- The arachnoid mater is continuous with cranial arachnoid mater and maintains the same meningeal relationships in the vertebral canal as the cranial cavity.

- The pia mater closely covers the spinal cord and has multiple thickenings on either side, called denticulate ligaments, that form a means of suspension for the spinal cord in the dural sheath.

? Clinical Problem Solving

1. In a head trauma accident, which structures within the skull limit damage to the cerebral hemispheres and other parts of the brain? Which blood vessels are damaged more commonly, the cerebral arteries or the cerebral veins? Are cranial nerves likely to be damaged in head injuries? If so, which ones are damaged most commonly and what is the reason for their increased susceptibility?

2. While performing an autopsy on a patient who had died of a meningioma, the pathologist explains to a group of students that these tumors arise from the arachnoid mater. She explains that they occur in those areas in which the arachnoid pierces the dura to form the arachnoid villi that project into the dural venous sinuses. She then asks the students where they would expect to find meningiomas. How would you answer that question?

3. A 10-year-old girl is admitted to hospital for surgical correction of medial strabismus of the right eye. Twenty-four hours after successful completion of the operation, her right eyeball is noted to project forward excessively (proptosis) and the conjunctiva of the right eye is inflamed. A watery, purulent discharge is expressed from beneath the eyelids. The ophthalmologist is greatly concerned because he does not want the complication of cavernous sinus thrombosis to occur. What is the connection between infection of the eye and cavernous sinus thrombosis? Is cavernous sinus thrombosis a serious condition?

4. On examination, a 41-year-old man is found to have paralysis of the lateral rectus muscle of his left eye; the left pupil is dilated but reacts slowly to light, and anesthesia of the skin over the left side of the forehead is noted. A carotid arteriogram reveals the presence of an aneurysm of the right internal carotid artery situated in the cavernous sinus. Using your knowledge of anatomy, explain the clinical findings on physical examination.

5. On ophthalmoscopic examination, a 45-year-old woman is found to have edema of both optic discs (*bilateral papilledema*) and congestion of the retinal veins. The cause of the condition is found to be a rapidly growing intracranial tumor. Using your knowledge of anatomy, explain the papilledema. Why does the patient exhibit bilateral papilledema?

6. A pediatrician is observing a 6-year-old boy playing with his toys. He notes that the child has perfectly normal use of his arms but that his legs are stiff; and when he walks, he tends to cross his legs and has a scissorlike gait. A diagnosis of cerebral diplegia secondary to birth injuries is made. (Note that congenital cerebral diplegia is believed by some authorities to occur early in fetal life and to be caused by a viral infection that arrests cerebral development.) Apparently, the child was born prematurely and he was a breech presentation. Using your knowledge of anatomy, explain what happens to the fetal skull bones during delivery. Why are the dural venous sinuses likely to be damaged at birth? Why is cerebral hemorrhage more likely to occur in a premature baby with a malpresentation?

7. A 25-year-old woman is admitted to the emergency department unconscious after being hit on the side of the head by a car while crossing the road. Within an hour, her state of unconsciousness deepens. On examination, she is found to have a large, doughlike swelling over the right temporalis muscle. She also has the signs of right-sided hemiplegia. Later, a right-sided, fixed, dilated pupil develops. A lateral radiograph of the skull shows a fracture line across the groove for the anterior division of the right middle meningeal artery. Her coma deepens and she dies 4 hours after the accident. Using your knowledge of neuroanatomy, make a diagnosis in this case. Explain the clinical findings. How could you account for the homolateral hemiplegia?

8. A 50-year-old woman complaining of a severe headache of 3 days' duration visits her physician. She says that the headache had started getting very severe about 1 hour after she hit her head on the mantelpiece after bending down to poke the fire. She is admitted to the hospital for observation. Three hours later, she becomes confused and also develops a right-sided hemiplegia on the side of the body opposite to the head injury. She has exaggeration of the deep reflexes and a positive Babinski response on the right side. Examination of the cerebrospinal fluid with a lumbar puncture shows raised pressure and the presence of blood in the fluid. Radiographic examination shows no fracture of the skull. A CT scan reveals the presence of a subdural hematoma. What exactly is a subdural hematoma?

Answers and Explanations to Clinical Problem Solving

1. The meninges and the cerebrospinal fluid afford a remarkable degree of protection to the delicate brain. The dural partitions, especially the falx cerebri and the tentorium cerebelli, limit the extent of brain movement within the skull.

   The thin-walled cerebral veins are liable to be damaged during excessive movements of the brain relative to the skull, especially at the point where the veins join the dural venous sinuses. The thick-walled cerebral arteries are rarely damaged.

   The small-diameter cranial nerves of long length are particularly prone to damage during head injuries. The trochlear, abducens, and oculomotor nerves are commonly injured.

2. Meningiomas arise from the arachnoid villi found along the dural venous sinuses. They are therefore most commonly found along the superior sagittal sinus and the sphenoparietal sinuses. They are rare below the tentorium cerebelli.

3. The anterior facial vein, the ophthalmic veins, and the cavernous sinus are in direct communication with one another. Infection of the skin of the face alongside the nose, ethmoidal sinusitis, and infection of the orbital contents can lead to thrombosis of the veins and ultimately cavernous sinus thrombosis. If untreated with antibiotics, this condition can be fatal, since the cavernous sinus drains many cerebral veins from the inferior surface of the brain.

4. The internal carotid artery passes forward on the lateral surface of the body of the sphenoid within the cavernous sinus. An aneurysm of the artery may press on the abducens nerve and cause paralysis of the lateral rectus muscle. Further expansion of the aneurysm may cause compression of the oculomotor nerve and the ophthalmic division of the trigeminal nerve as they lie in the lateral wall of the cavernous sinus. This patient had left lateral rectus paralysis and paralysis of the left pupillary constrictor muscle owing to involvement of the abducens and oculomotor nerves, respectively. The slight anesthesia of the skin over the left side of the forehead was due to pressure on the ophthalmic division of the left trigeminal nerve.

5. The optic nerves are surrounded by sheaths derived from the pia mater, arachnoid mater, and dura mater. The intracranial subarachnoid space extends forward around the optic nerve to the back of the eyeball. A rise in cerebrospinal fluid pressure due to an intracranial tumor will compress the thin walls of the retinal vein as it crosses the extension of the subarachnoid space in the orbital cavity. This will result in congestion of the retinal vein and bulging of the optic disc involving both eyes.

6. During the descent of the fetal head through the birth canal during labor, the bones of the calvarium overlap, a process known as molding. If this process is excessive or takes place too rapidly, as in malpresentations or in premature deliveries (when a small fetus is birthed rapidly), an abnormal strain is put on the falx cerebri. This stress involves the superior sagittal sinus, especially if the anteroposterior compression is excessive, and the sinus may tear where it joins the transverse sinus. The great cerebral vein may tear as well. The result is either a subarachnoid or subdural hemorrhage with accompanying brain damage.

7. The initial loss of consciousness was due to concussion or cerebral trauma. The swelling over the right temporalis and the radiographic finding of a fracture over the right middle meningeal artery were due to hemorrhage from the artery into the overlying muscle and soft tissue. This patient had an extradural hemorrhage. The right homolateral hemiplegia was due to the compression of the left cerebral peduncle against the edge of the tentorium cerebelli. This is unusual. A left hemiplegia due to pressure on the right precentral gyrus is more common. The right-sided, fixed, dilated pupil was due to the pressure on the right oculomotor nerve by the hippocampal gyrus, which had herniated through the tentorial notch.

8. A subdural hematoma is an accumulation of blood in the interval between the meningeal layer of dura and the arachnoid mater. It results from tearing of the superior cerebral veins at their point of entrance into the superior sagittal sinus. The cause is usually a blow on the front or the back of the head, causing excessive anteroposterior displacement of the brain within the skull. A subdural hematoma can be easily identified by CT as a dense rim of blood extending along the inner table of the skull, obliterating the cerebral fissures and displacing the cerebral structures to the opposite side.

Review Questions

Directions: Each of the numbered items in this section is followed by answers. Select the ONE lettered answer that is CORRECT.

1. The following statements concern the meninges of the brain:
   (a) Both layers of the dura mater covering the brain are continuous through the foramen magnum with the dura covering the spinal cord.
   (b) The periosteal layer of dura mater is not continuous with the sutural ligaments of the skull.
   (c) As each cranial nerve passes through a foramen in the skull, it is surrounded by a tubular sheath of arachnoid mater only.
   (d) The cranial venous sinuses run between the meningeal and endosteal layers of dura mater.
   (e) The meninges extend anteriorly through the optic canal and fuse with the periosteum of the orbital cavity.

2. The following general statements concern the meninges:
   (a) The cisterna cerebellomedullaris lies between the inferior surface of the cerebellum and the roof of the fourth ventricle and contains lymph.
   (b) The arachnoid mater is permeable to cerebrospinal fluid (CSF).
   (c) The CSF in the arachnoid villi is able to drain into the venous sinuses through small tubules lined with endothelial cells.
   (d) The arachnoid mater surrounding the spinal cord ends inferiorly on the filum terminale at the level of the lower border of the first sacral vertebra.
   (e) The extradural space that separates the dural sheath of the spinal cord and the walls of the vertebral canal contains the external vertebral venous plexus.

3. The following statements concern the tentorium cerebelli:
   (a) The free border is attached anteriorly to the posterior clinoid processes.
   (b) It is formed from the meningeal layer of the dura mater.
   (c) It separates the cerebellum from the temporal lobes of the brain.
   (d) The sigmoid sinus lies within its attached border to the occipital bone.
   (e) The anterior edge houses the occipital venous sinus.

4. The following statements concern headache:
   (a) Brain tissue is insensitive to pain.
   (b) Intracranial pain arises from receptors situated in the pia mater.
   (c) An expanding cerebral tumor located in the posterior cranial fossa would produce pain referred to the face.
   (d) Migraine headache is believed to be due to dilation of the cerebral veins.
   (e) Headaches associated with presbyopia are due to tonic spasm of the frontalis muscles of the forehead.

5. The following statements concern the subarachnoid space:
   (a) It is filled with cerebrospinal fluid (CSF).
   (b) It extends inferiorly as far as the fourth sacral vertebra.
   (c) The cerebral arteries and veins are not located in the subarachnoid space.
   (d) The cranial nerves lie outside the subarachnoid space in sheaths derived from the dura mater.
   (e) The arachnoid villi project into the venous sinuses as large outpouchings of the subarachnoid space.

6. The following statements concern the cavernous sinus:
   (a) The external carotid artery passes through it.
   (b) Its medial wall contains the oculomotor, trochlear, and ophthalmic divisions of the trigeminal nerve.
   (c) It drains directly posteriorly into the straight sinus.
   (d) It does not communicate with the facial vein.
   (e) It is related medially to the pituitary gland and the sphenoid air sinus.

7. The following structure limits rotatory movements of the brain within the skull:
   (a) Tentorium cerebelli
   (b) Diaphragma sellae
   (c) Falx cerebri
   (d) Dorsum sellae
   (e) Squamous part of the temporal bone

8. The following nerves are sensory to the dura mater:
   (a) Oculomotor nerve
   (b) Trochlear nerve
   (c) Sixth cervical spinal nerve
   (d) Trigeminal nerve
   (e) Hypoglossal nerve

Answers and Explanations to Review Questions

1. D is correct. The cranial venous sinuses run between the meningeal and endosteal layers of dura mater (see Fig. 15-3). A. The periosteal (endosteal) layer of dura covering the brain is continuous through the foramen magnum with the periosteum outside the skull; only the meningeal layer of dura covering the brain is continuous through the foramen magnum with the dura covering the spinal cord (see Fig. 15-3). B. The periosteal layer of dura mater is continuous with the sutural ligaments of the skull. C. As each cranial nerve passes through a foramen in the skull, the cranial nerve is surrounded by a tubular sheath of pia, arachnoid, and dura mater (see Fig. 15-2). E. The meninges within the skull extend anteriorly through the optic canal and fuse with the sclera of the eyeball (see Fig. 15-8).

2. C is correct. The CSF in the arachnoid villi is able to drain into the venous sinuses through small tubules lined with endothelial cells (see Fig. 16-18). A. The cisterna cerebellomedullaris is filled with CSF and lies between the inferior surface of the cerebellum and the roof of the fourth ventricle. B. The arachnoid mater is not permeable to CSF. D. The arachnoid mater surrounding the spinal cord ends inferiorly on the filum terminale at the level of the lower border of the second sacral vertebra (see Fig. 15-9). E. The extradural space that separates the dural sheath of the spinal cord and the walls of the vertebral canal is filled with loose areolar tissue and contains the internal vertebral venous plexus (see Fig. 1-3).

3. B is correct. The tentorium cerebelli is formed from the meningeal layer of the dura mater (see Fig. 15-3). A. The free border of the tentorium cerebelli is attached anteriorly to the anterior clinoid processes of the sphenoid bone. C. The tentorium cerebelli separates the cerebellum from the occipital lobes of the brain. D. The sigmoid sinus does not lie within the free border of the tentorium cerebelli. E. In the anterior edge of the tentorium cerebelli is the tentorial notch (see Fig. 15-4).

4. A is correct. Brain tissue is insensitive to pain. B. Intracranial pain arises from receptors situated in the dura mater. C. An expanding cerebral tumor located in the posterior cranial fossa would produce pain referred to the back of the neck. D. Migraine headache is believed to be due to dilation of cerebral arteries and branches of the external carotid artery. E. Headaches associated with presbyopia are due to tonic spasm of the ciliary muscles of the eyes.

5. A is correct. The subarachnoid space is filled with CSF. B. The subarachnoid space extends inferiorly as far as the second sacral vertebra (see Fig. 15-9). C. The subarachnoid space contains the cerebral arteries and veins. D. The cranial nerves lie inside the subarachnoid space. E. The arachnoid villi project into the venous sinuses as minute outpouchings of the subarachnoid space.

6. E is correct. The cavernous sinus is related medially to the pituitary gland and the sphenoid air sinus (see Fig. 15-5). A. The cavernous sinus has the internal carotid artery and the abducens nerve passing through it (see Fig. 15-5). B. The cavernous sinus has the oculomotor, trochlear, and ophthalmic divisions of the trigeminal nerve in its lateral wall (see Fig. 15-5). C. The cavernous sinus drains posteriorly into the superior and inferior petrosal sinuses (see Fig. 15-1). D. The cavernous sinus has an important clinical communication anteriorly via the superior ophthalmic vein with the facial vein.

7. C is correct. The falx cerebri limits rotatory movements of the brain within the skull.

8. D is correct. The trigeminal nerve is an important sensory nerve to the dura mater within the skull.

16 Ventricular System and Cerebrospinal Fluid

CHAPTER OBJECTIVES

- To learn the locations, functions, origins, and fate of cerebrospinal fluid

- To understand the structure and function of the blood–brain and blood–cerebrospinal fluid barriers

- To learn how certain parts of the brain are protected from potentially toxic drugs or other exogenous materials

A 26-year-old woman involved in an automobile accident is admitted to the emergency department. Her mother, who is also involved in the accident, told the physician that at the time of impact, her daughter's head was thrown forward against the windshield.

On examination, the patient is unconscious and shows evidence of a severe head injury on the left side. After a thorough physical examination, the physician decides to perform a spinal tap. The cerebrospinal fluid (CSF) pressure is 160 mm of water, and two samples of the fluid are collected. The specimens show red blood cells at the bottom of the tubes, and the supernatant fluid is blood stained. After standing for an hour, the supernatant fluid in both tubes becomes colorless.

The physician makes the diagnosis of subarachnoid hemorrhage secondary to the head injury. The blood could be originating from a severe fracture of the skull, damage to one of the cerebral blood vessels, or a tear involving the brain or meninges. The physician is confident that the blood in the CSF specimens did not originate from an accidental puncture of a vertebral vein during the spinal tap procedure. He eliminates this possibility by drawing two specimens of the fluid. If a local vein is accidentally punctured by the first needle, the first specimen will be blood stained, however, the second specimen most probably will be clear. With this patient, both specimens are uniformly blood stained, so the blood is in the subarachnoid space.

The management of this patient in the emergency department and the evaluation of the spinal tap specimen depends on knowledge of the CSF system and the anatomy involved in the spinal tap procedure.

VENTRICULAR SYSTEM

The ventricles are four fluid-filled cavities located within the brain; these are the two lateral ventricles, the third ventricle, and the fourth ventricle (Fig. 16-1; see also Atlas Plates 3, 4, 7, and 8). The two **lateral ventricles** communicate through the **interventricular foramina** (of Monro) with the **third ventricle**. The third ventricle is connected to the **fourth ventricle** by the narrow **cerebral aqueduct** (**aqueduct of Sylvius**). The fourth ventricle, in turn, is continuous with the narrow **central canal** of the spinal cord and, through the three foramina in its roof, with the subarachnoid space. The central canal in the spinal cord has a small dilatation at its inferior end, referred to as the **terminal ventricle**.

The ventricles are lined throughout with **ependyma** and are filled with **CSF**. The ventricles are developmentally derived from the cavity of the neural tube.

Lateral Ventricles

One of each of the two large lateral ventricles is present in each cerebral hemisphere (Fig. 16-2). The ventricle is a roughly C-shaped cavity and may be divided into a **body** which occupies the parietal lobe and from which **anterior**, **posterior**, and **inferior horns** extend into the frontal, occipital, and temporal lobes, respectively. The lateral ventricle communicates with the cavity of the third ventricle through the **interventricular foramen** (Figs. 16-3 and 16-4; also see Fig. 16-2). This opening, which lies in the anterior part of the medial wall of the ventricle, is bounded anteriorly by the anterior column of the fornix and posteriorly by the anterior end of the thalamus.

The **body of the lateral ventricle** extends from the interventricular foramen posteriorly as far as the posterior end of the thalamus. Here, it becomes continuous

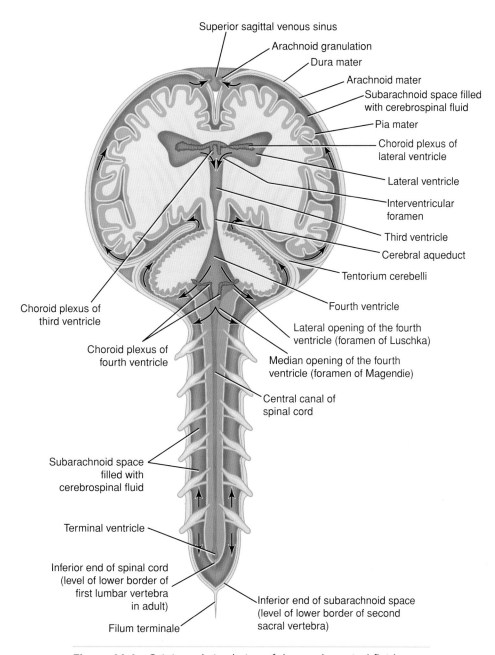

Superior sagittal venous sinus

Arachnoid granulation

Dura mater

Arachnoid mater

Subarachnoid space filled
with cerebrospinal fluid

Pia mater

Choroid plexus of
lateral ventricle

Lateral ventricle

Interventricular
foramen

Third ventricle

Cerebral aqueduct

Tentorium cerebelli

Fourth ventricle

Lateral opening of the fourth
ventricle (foramen of Luschka)

Median opening of the fourth
ventricle (foramen of Magendie)

Central canal of
spinal cord

Choroid plexus of
third ventricle

Choroid plexus of
fourth ventricle

Subarachnoid space
filled with
cerebrospinal fluid

Terminal ventricle

Inferior end of spinal cord
(level of lower border of
first lumbar vertebra
in adult)

Filum terminale

Inferior end of subarachnoid space
(level of lower border of second
sacral vertebra)

Figure 16-1   Origin and circulation of the cerebrospinal fluid.

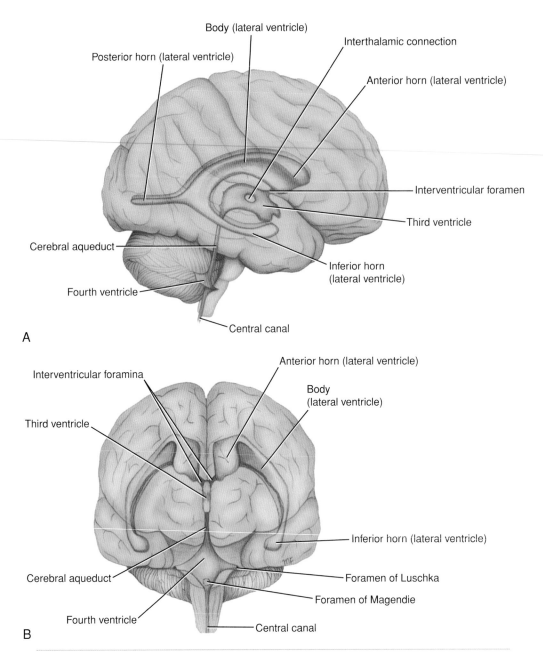

Figure 16-2 Cast of the ventricular cavities of the brain. **A:** Lateral view. **B:** Anterior view.

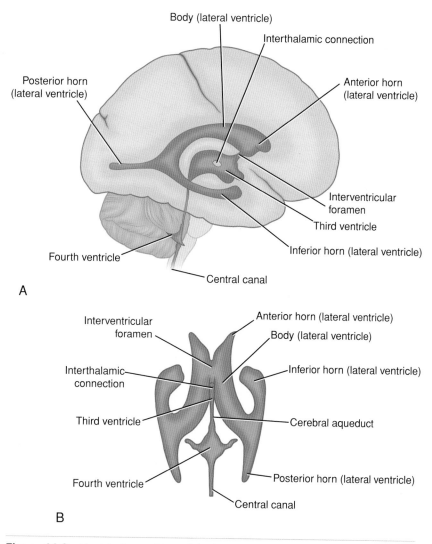

Figure 16-3   Ventricular cavities of the brain. **A:** Lateral view. **B:** Superior view.

with the posterior and the inferior horns. The body of the lateral ventricle has a roof, a floor, and a medial wall (Fig. 16-5).

The **roof** is formed by the undersurface of the **corpus callosum**. The **floor** is formed by the body of the **caudate nucleus** and the lateral margin of the thalamus. The superior surface of the thalamus is obscured in its medial part by the **body of the fornix**. The **choroid plexus** of the ventricle projects into the body of the ventricle through the slitlike gap between the body of the fornix and the superior surface of the thalamus. This slitlike gap is known as the **choroidal fissure**; through it, the blood vessels of the plexus invaginate the pia mater of the tela choroidea and the ependyma of the lateral ventricle. The **medial wall** is formed by the **septum pellucidum** anteriorly; posteriorly, the roof and the floor come together on the medial wall.

The **anterior horn of the lateral ventricle** extends forward into the frontal lobe (see Figs. 16-2 and 16-3). It is continuous posteriorly with the body of the ventricle at the interventricular foramen. The anterior horn has

a roof, a floor, and a medial wall. The **roof** is formed by the undersurface of the anterior part of the **corpus callosum**; the **genu of the corpus callosum** limits the anterior horn anteriorly (see Fig. 16-5A). The **floor** is formed by the rounded **head of the caudate nucleus**; medially, a small portion is formed by the superior surface of the **rostrum of the corpus callosum**. The **medial wall** is formed by the **septum pellucidum** and the **anterior column of the fornix**.

The **posterior horn of the lateral ventricle** extends posteriorly into the occipital lobe (see Figs. 16-2 and 16-3). The **roof** and **lateral wall** are formed by the fibers of the **tapetum of the corpus callosum**. Lateral to the tapetum are the fibers of the **optic radiation** (see Fig. 16-5C). The **medial wall** of the posterior horn has two elevations. The superior swelling is caused by the splenial fibers of the corpus callosum, called the **forceps major**, passing posteriorly into the occipital lobe; this superior swelling is referred to as the **bulb of the posterior horn**. The inferior swelling is produced by the **calcarine sulcus** and is called the **calcar avis**.

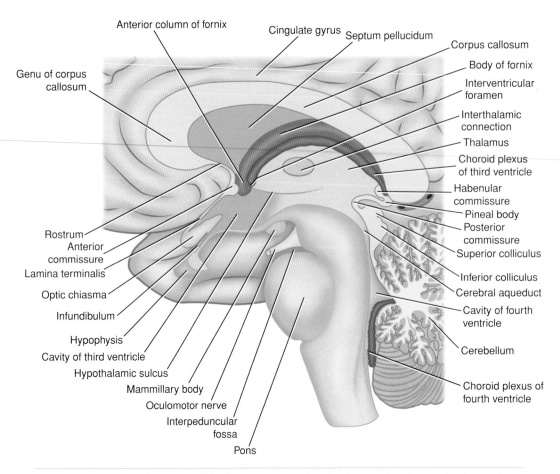

Figure 16-4 Sagittal section of the brain showing the third ventricle, the cerebral aqueduct, and the fourth ventricle.

The **inferior horn of the lateral ventricle** extends anteriorly into the temporal lobe (see Figs. 16-2 and 16-3). The inferior horn has a roof and a floor (see Fig. 16-5B).

The **roof** is formed by the inferior surface of the **tapetum of the corpus callosum** and by the **tail of the caudate nucleus** (see Fig. 9-5). The latter passes anteriorly to end in the **amygdaloid nucleus**. Medial to the tail of the caudate nucleus is the **stria terminalis**, which also ends anteriorly in the amygdaloid nucleus.

The **floor** is formed laterally by the **collateral eminence**, produced by the **collateral fissure**, and medially by the hippocampus (see Figs. 9-3 and 9-4). The anterior end of the hippocampus is expanded and slightly furrowed to form the **pes hippocampus**. The hippocampus is composed of gray matter; however, the ventricular surface of the hippocampus is covered by a thin layer of white matter called the **alveus**, which is formed from the axons of the cells of the hippocampus. These axons converge on the medial border of the hippocampus to form a bundle known as the **fimbria**. The fimbria of the hippocampus becomes continuous posteriorly with the **posterior column of the fornix**.

In the interval between the stria terminalis and the fimbria is the temporal part of the choroidal fissure. Here, the lower part of the **choroid plexus** of the lateral ventricle invaginates the ependyma from the medial side and closes the fissure (Fig. 16-6).

Choroid Plexus

The **choroid plexus** projects into the ventricle on its medial aspect and is a vascular fringe composed of pia mater covered with the ependymal lining of the ventricular cavity (Fig. 16-7). The choroid plexus is, in fact, the irregular lateral edge of the tela choroidea, which is a two-layered fold of pia mater situated between the fornix superiorly and the upper surface of the thalamus (see Fig. 16-6A). At the junction of the body of the lateral ventricle and the inferior horn, the choroid plexus is continued into the inferior horn and projects through the choroidal fissure. The function of the choroid plexus is to produce CSF.

Third Ventricle

The third ventricle is a slitlike cleft between the two thalami. It communicates anteriorly with the lateral ventricles through the interventricular foramina (of Monro) and posteriorly with the fourth ventricle through the cerebral aqueduct (of Sylvius) (see Fig. 16-4). The walls of the third ventricle are described on page 363.

Figure 16-5 Coronal sections of the brain passing through the anterior horn of the lateral ventricle (**A**), the body of the lateral ventricle (**B**), and the posterior horn of the lateral ventricle (**C**).

Choroid Plexuses

The choroid plexuses are formed from the tela choroidea situated above the roof of the ventricle (see Fig. 16-7). The vascular tela choroidea projects downward on each side of the midline, invaginating the ependymal roof of the ventricle. The two vascular ridges or fringes that hang from the roof of the third ventricle form the choroid plexuses. The function of the choroid plexuses is to produce CSF.

The blood supply of the tela choroidea and, therefore, also of the choroid plexuses of the third and lateral ventricles is derived from the **choroidal branches of the internal carotid and basilar arteries**. The venous blood drains into the internal cerebral veins, which

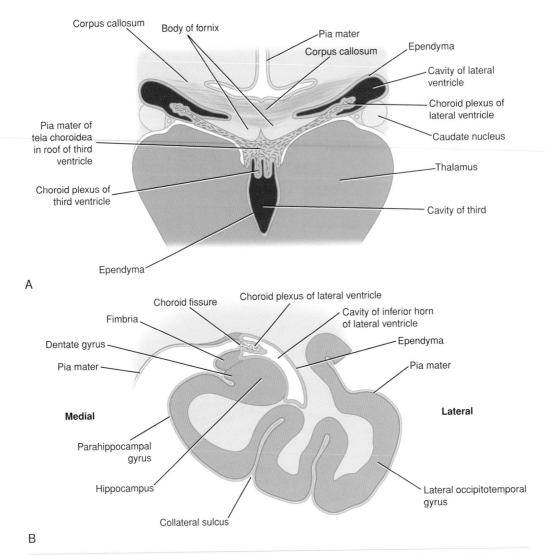

A

B

Figure 16-6 Coronal section of the cavities of the third and lateral ventricles (**A**) and the cavity of the inferior horn of the lateral ventricle (**B**).

Figure 16-7 Sagittal section of the fourth ventricle showing the origin and circulation of the cerebrospinal fluid. Note the position of the foramen of Magendie.

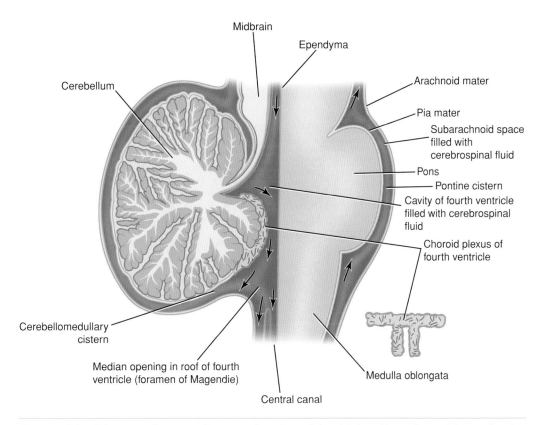

Midbrain

Ependyma

Cerebellum

Arachnoid mater

Pia mater

Subarachnoid space filled with cerebrospinal fluid

Pons

Pontine cistern

Cavity of fourth ventricle filled with cerebrospinal fluid

Choroid plexus of fourth ventricle

Cerebellomedullary cistern

Median opening in roof of fourth ventricle (foramen of Magendie)

Medulla oblongata

Central canal

Figure 16-8   Schematic diagram of a coronal section of the third and lateral ventricles at the site of the interventricular foramina showing the structure of the tela choroidea and its relationship with the ependyma and pia mater.

unite to form the great cerebral vein. The great cerebral vein joins the inferior sagittal sinus to form the straight sinus.

Cerebral Aqueduct

The cerebral aqueduct (aqueduct of Sylvius), a narrow channel about 3/4 of an inch (1.8 cm) long, connects the third ventricle with the fourth ventricle (see Figs. 16-2 and 16-3). It is lined with ependyma and is surrounded by a layer of gray matter called the **central gray**. The direction of CSF flow is from the third to the fourth ventricle. The cerebral aqueduct does not have a choroid plexus.

Fourth Ventricle

The fourth ventricle is a tent-shaped cavity filled with CSF. It is situated anterior to the cerebellum and posterior to the pons and the superior half of the medulla oblongata (Figs. 16-8 and 16-9; also see Fig. 16-4). It is lined with ependyma and is continuous above with the cerebral aqueduct of the midbrain and below with the central canal of the medulla oblongata and the spinal cord (Fig. 16-3). The fourth ventricle possesses lateral boundaries, a roof, and a rhomboid-shaped floor.

Lateral Boundaries

The caudal part of each lateral boundary is formed by the inferior cerebellar peduncle (Fig. 16-10). The cranial part of each lateral boundary is formed by the superior cerebellar peduncle.

Posterior Wall (Roof)

The tent-shaped roof projects into the cerebellum (see Figs. 16-8 and 16-9). The superior part is formed by the medial borders of the two superior cerebellar peduncles and a connecting sheet of white matter called the **superior medullary velum** (Fig. 16-11). The inferior part of the roof is formed by the **inferior medullary velum**, which consists of a thin sheet devoid of nervous tissue and formed by the ventricular ependyma and its posterior covering of pia mater (Fig. 16-12). This part of the roof is pierced in the midline by a large aperture, the **median aperture** or **foramen of Magendie**. Lateral recesses extend laterally around the sides of the medulla and open anteriorly as the **lateral openings of the fourth ventricle**, or the **foramina of Luschka** (Fig. 16-13). Thus, the cavity of the fourth ventricle communicates with the subarachnoid space through a single median opening and two lateral apertures. These important openings permit CSF flow from the ventricular system into the subarachnoid space.

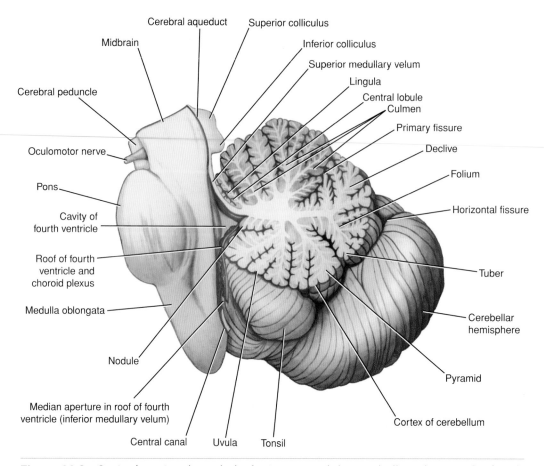

Figure 16-9 Sagittal section through the brainstem and the cerebellum showing the fourth ventricle.

Figure 16-10 Posterior surface of the brainstem showing the floor of the fourth ventricle. The cerebellum has been removed.

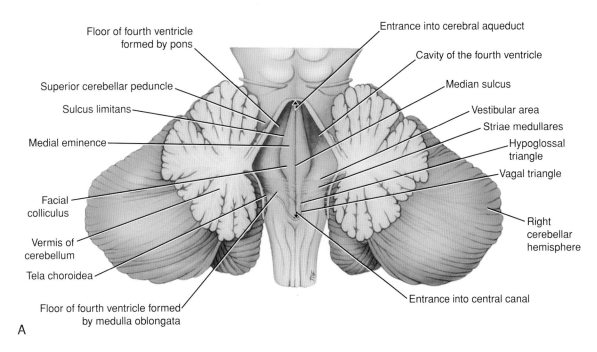

Floor of fourth ventricle formed by pons

Superior cerebellar peduncle

Sulcus limitans

Medial eminence

Facial colliculus

Vermis of cerebellum

Tela choroidea

Floor of fourth ventricle formed by medulla oblongata

Entrance into cerebral aqueduct

Cavity of the fourth ventricle

Median sulcus

Vestibular area

Striae medullares

Hypoglossal triangle

Vagal triangle

Right cerebellar hemisphere

Entrance into central canal

A

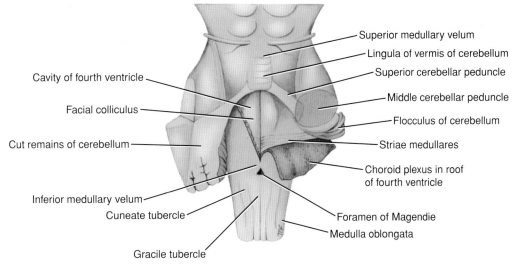

Cavity of fourth ventricle

Facial colliculus

Cut remains of cerebellum

Inferior medullary velum

Cuneate tubercle

Gracile tubercle

Superior medullary velum

Lingula of vermis of cerebellum

Superior cerebellar peduncle

Middle cerebellar peduncle

Flocculus of cerebellum

Striae medullares

Choroid plexus in roof of fourth ventricle

Foramen of Magendie

Medulla oblongata

B

Figure 16-11   Posterior view of the cavity of the fourth ventricle. **A:** The vermis of the cerebellum has been divided in the midline and the cerebellar hemispheres have been displaced laterally. **B:** The greater part of the cerebellum has been removed, leaving the superior and inferior medullary vela. Note that the right half of the inferior medullary velum has been reflected inferiorly to reveal the choroid plexus.

Rhomboid Fossa (Floor)

The diamond-shaped floor is formed by the posterior surface of the pons and the cranial half of the medulla oblongata (see Fig. 16-10). The floor is divided into symmetrical halves by the **median sulcus**. On each side of this sulcus, an elevation, the **medial eminence**, is bounded laterally by another sulcus, the **sulcus limitans**. Lateral to the sulcus limitans is an area known as the **vestibular area** (see Figs. 16-10 and 16-11). The vestibular nuclei lie beneath the vestibular area.

The **facial colliculus** is a slight swelling at the inferior end of the medial eminence that is produced by the fibers from the motor nucleus of the facial nerve looping over the abducens nucleus (Fig. 16-14). At the superior end of the sulcus limitans, a bluish gray area is produced by a cluster of nerve cells containing melanin pigment; the cluster of cells is called the **substantia ferruginea**. Strands of nerve fibers, the **stria medullaris**, derived from the arcuate nuclei, emerge from the median sulcus and pass laterally over the

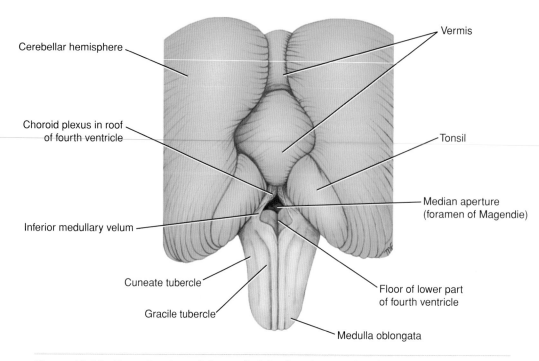

Figure 16-12 Posterior view of the roof of the fourth ventricle. The cerebellum has been displaced superiorly to show the large median aperture (foramen of Magendie).

medial eminence and the vestibular area and enter the inferior cerebellar peduncle to reach the cerebellum (see Fig. 16-10).

Inferior to the stria medullaris, the following features should be recognized in the floor of the ventricle. The most medial is the **hypoglossal triangle**, which indicates the position of the underlying **hypoglossal**

nucleus (see Fig. 16-11). Lateral to this is the **vagal triangle**, beneath which lies the dorsal motor nucleus of the vagus. The **area postrema** is a narrow area between the vagal triangle and the lateral margin of the ventricle, just rostral to the opening into the central canal. The inferior part of the vestibular area also lies lateral to the vagal triangle.

Figure 16-13 Posterior view of the roof of the fourth ventricle after removal of the greater part of the cerebellum. Shows the lateral recess and aperture (foramina of Luschka).

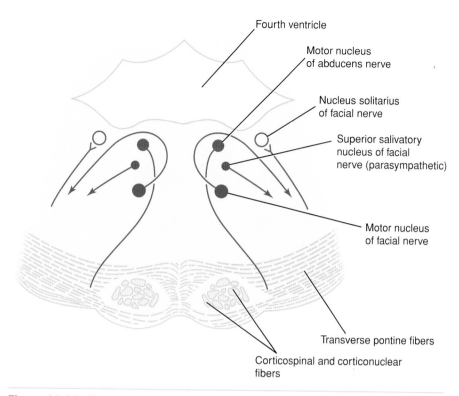

Figure 16-14   Transverse section through the fourth ventricle and the pons showing the nuclei of the facial nerve and their relationship to the nucleus of the abducens nerve.

Choroid Plexus

The choroid plexus has a T shape; the vertical part of the T is double (see Fig. 16-8). It is suspended from the inferior half of the roof of the ventricle and is formed from the highly vascular tela choroidea. The tela choroidea is a two-layered fold of pia mater that projects through the roof of the ventricle and is covered by ependyma. The blood supply to the plexus is from the **posterior inferior cerebellar arteries**. The function of the choroid plexus is to produce CSF.

Central Canal

The central canal opens superiorly into the fourth ventricle. Inferiorly, it extends through the inferior half of the medulla oblongata and through the entire length of the spinal cord. In the conus medullaris of the spinal cord, it expands to form the **terminal ventricle** (see Fig. 16-1). The central canal is closed at its lower end, is filled with CSF, and is lined with ependyma. The central canal is surrounded by gray matter, the **gray commissure**. The central canal does not have a choroid plexus.

SUBARACHNOID SPACE

The subarachnoid space is the interval between the arachnoid mater and pia mater and, therefore, is present where these meninges envelop the brain and spinal cord (see Fig. 16-1). The space is filled with CSF and contains the large blood vessels of the brain (Fig. 16-15). This space is traversed by a network of fine trabeculae, formed of delicate connective tissue. The subarachnoid space completely surrounds the brain and extends along the olfactory nerves to the mucoperiosteum of the nose. The subarachnoid space also extends along the cerebral blood vessels as they enter and leave the substance of the brain and stops where the vessels become an arteriole or a venule.

In certain situations around the base of the brain, the arachnoid does not closely follow the surface of the brain. In such a case, the subarachnoid space expands to form **subarachnoid cisterns**. The descriptions of the **cerebellomedullary cistern**, the **pontine cistern**, and the **interpeduncular cistern**, which are the largest cisterns, are on page 449.

Inferiorly, the subarachnoid space extends beyond the lower end of the spinal cord and invests the **cauda equina** (see Fig. 1-15). The subarachnoid space ends below at the level of the interval between the second and third sacral vertebrae.

The subarachnoid space surrounds the cranial and spinal nerves and follows them to the point where they leave the skull and vertebral canal. Here, the arachnoid mater and pia mater fuse with the perineurium of each nerve.

Meningeal layer of dura mater

Arachnoid mater

Fine connective tissue trabeculae

Covering of cerebral blood vessel derived from arachnoid

Cerebral blood vessel

Pia mater

Cerebral cortex

Perivascular space

Figure 16-15   Diagram of the subarachnoid space around the cerebral hemisphere showing the relationship of the cerebral blood vessel to the meninges and cerebral cortex.

CEREBROSPINAL FLUID

The CSF is found in the ventricles of the brain and in the subarachnoid space around the brain and spinal cord. It has a volume of about 150 mL. It is a clear, colorless fluid and possesses, in solution, inorganic salts similar to those in the blood plasma. The glucose content is about half that of blood, with only a trace of protein. Only a few cells are present, and these are lymphocytes. The normal lymphocyte count is 0 to 3 cells per cubic millimeter. CSF pressure is **kept remarkably constant**. In the lateral recumbent position, the pressure, as measured by spinal tap, is about 60 to 150 mm of water. This pressure may be raised by straining, coughing, or compressing the internal jugular veins in the neck (see p. 256). Table 16-1 summarizes CSF physical characteristics and composition.

Functions

CSF, which bathes the external and internal surfaces of the brain and spinal cord, serves as a cushion between the central nervous system (CNS) and the surrounding bones, thus protecting it against mechanical trauma. Because the density of the brain is only slightly greater than that of the CSF, the CSF provides mechanical buoyancy and support for the brain. The close relationship of the fluid to the nervous tissue and the blood enables it to serve as a reservoir and assist in the regulation of the contents of the skull. For example, if the brain volume or the blood volume increases, CSF volume decreases. Because the CSF is an ideal physiologic substrate, it probably plays an active part in the nourishment of the nervous tissue; it almost certainly assists

in the removal of products of neuronal metabolism. Secretions of the pineal gland possibly influence the activities of the pituitary gland by circulating through the CSF in the third ventricle (see p. 253).

Table 16-2 summarizes CSF functions.

Formation

CSF is formed mainly in the choroid plexuses of the lateral, third, and fourth ventricles; some originates from the ependymal cells lining the ventricles and from the brain substance through the perivascular spaces.

Table 16-1	Cerebrospinal Fluid Physical Characteristics and Composition
Appearance	Clear and colorless
Volume	c. 150 mL
Rate of production	0.5 mL/min
Pressure (spinal tap with patient in lateral recumbent position)	60–150 mm of water
Composition	
Protein	15–45 mg/100 mL
Glucose	50–85 mg/100 mL
Chloride	720–750 mg/100 mL
Number of cells	0–3 lymphocytes/mm^3

Table 16-2   Cerebrospinal Fluid Functions

1. Cushions and protects the central nervous system from trauma
2. Provides mechanical buoyancy and support for the brain
3. Serves as a reservoir and assists in the regulation of the contents of the skull
4. Nourishes the central nervous system
5. Removes metabolites from the central nervous system
6. Serves as a pathway for pineal secretions to reach the pituitary gland

The choroid plexuses have a much-folded surface, and each fold consists of a core of vascular connective tissue covered with cuboidal epithelium of the ependyma (Fig. 16-16). Electron-microscopic examination of the epithelial cells shows that their free surfaces are covered with microvilli. The blood of the capillaries is separated from the ventricular lumen by endothelium, a basement membrane, and the surface epithelium. The epithelial cells are fenestrated and permeable to large molecules.

The choroid plexuses **actively secrete** CSF and this creates a small pressure gradient. At the same time, they actively transport nervous system metabolites from the CSF into the blood. Active transport also explains why concentrations of potassium, calcium, magnesium, bicarbonate, and glucose are lower in CSF than in blood plasma.

The CSF is produced continuously at a rate of about 0.5 mL/min and with a total volume of about 150 mL; this corresponds to a turnover time of about 5 hours.

Importantly, CSF production is not pressure regulated (as in the case of blood pressure) and it continues to be produced even if the reabsorption mechanisms are obstructed.

Circulation

The circulation begins with its secretion from the choroid plexuses in the ventricles (and a small amount from the brain surface). The fluid passes from the lateral ventricles into the third ventricle through the interventricular foramina (Fig. 16-17; also see Fig. 16-1). It then passes into the fourth ventricle through the narrow cerebral aqueduct. The circulation is aided by the arterial pulsations of the choroid plexuses and by the cilia on the ependymal cells lining the ventricles.

From the fourth ventricle, CSF passes slowly through the median aperture and the lateral foramina of the lateral recesses of the fourth ventricle and enters the subarachnoid space. It then moves through the cerebellomedullary cistern and pontine cisterns and flows superiorly through the tentorial notch of the tentorium

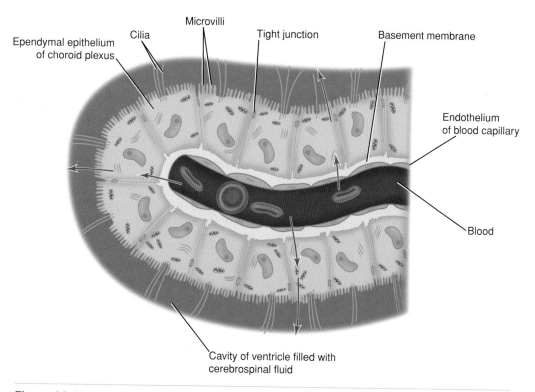

Figure 16-16 Microscopic structure of the choroid plexus showing the path taken by fluids in the formation of cerebrospinal fluid.

Figure 16-17 Circulation of the cerebrospinal fluid. The *dashed line* indicates the course taken by fluid within the cavities of the central nervous system.

cerebelli to reach the inferior surface of the cerebrum. It then moves superiorly over the lateral aspect of each cerebral hemisphere, assisted by the pulsations of the cerebral arteries. Some moves inferiorly in the subarachnoid space around the spinal cord and cauda equina. Here, it reaches a dead end and its further circulation relies on the pulsations of the spinal arteries and the movements of the vertebral column, respiration, coughing, and the changing of the positions of the body.

CSF not only bathes the ependymal and pial surfaces of the brain and spinal cord but also penetrates the nervous tissue along the blood vessels.

Absorption

The main sites for CSF absorption are the **arachnoid villi** that project into the dural venous sinuses, especially the **superior sagittal sinus** (Fig. 16-18). The arachnoid villi tend to be grouped together to form elevations known as **arachnoid granulations**. Structurally, each arachnoid villus is a diverticulum of the subarachnoid space that pierces the dura mater. The arachnoid diverticulum is capped by a thin cellular layer, which, in turn, is covered by the endothelium of the venous sinus. The arachnoid granulations increase in number and size with age and tend to become calcified with advanced age.

CSF absorption into the venous sinuses occurs when CSF pressure exceeds the venous pressure in the sinus. Electron-microscopic studies of the arachnoid villi indicate that fine tubules lined with endothelium permit a direct flow of fluid from the subarachnoid space into the lumen of the venous sinuses. Should the venous pressure rise and exceed CSF pressure, compression of the tips of the villi closes the tubules and prevents the reflux of blood into the subarachnoid space. The arachnoid villi thus serve as valves.

Some CSF probably is absorbed directly into the veins in the subarachnoid space and some possibly escapes through the perineural lymph vessels of the cranial and spinal nerves.

Because CSF production from the choroid plexuses is constant, the rate of CSF absorption through the arachnoid villi controls CSF pressure.

Subarachnoid Space Extensions

A sleeve of the subarachnoid space extends around the optic nerve to the back of the eyeball (Fig. 16-19). Here, the arachnoid mater and pia mater fuse with the sclera. The central artery and vein of the retina cross this extension of the subarachnoid space to enter the optic nerve, and they may be compressed in patients with raised CSF pressure.

Small extensions of the subarachnoid space also occur around the other cranial and spinal nerves. Here, some communication may occur between the subarachnoid space and the perineural lymph vessels.

The subarachnoid space also extends around the arteries and veins of the brain and spinal cord at points where they penetrate the nervous tissue (see Fig. 16-15). The pia mater, however, quickly fuses with the outer coat of the blood vessel below the surface of the brain and spinal cord, thus closing off the subarachnoid space.

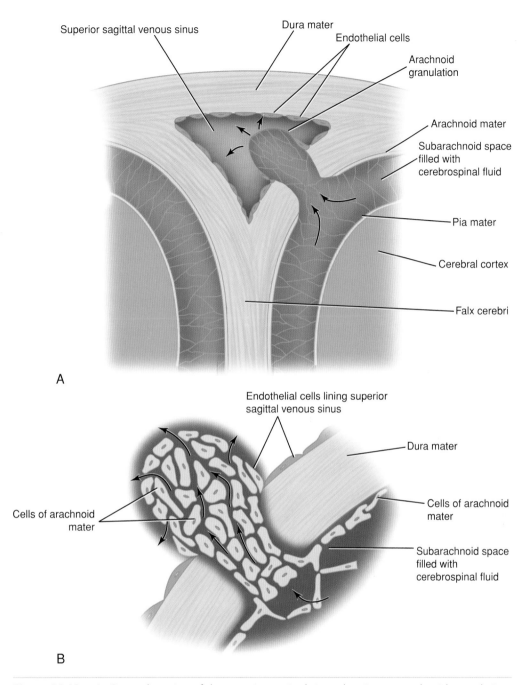

Figure 16-18 **A:** Coronal section of the superior sagittal sinus showing an arachnoid granulation. **B:** Magnified view of an arachnoid granulation showing the path taken by the cerebrospinal fluid into the venous system.

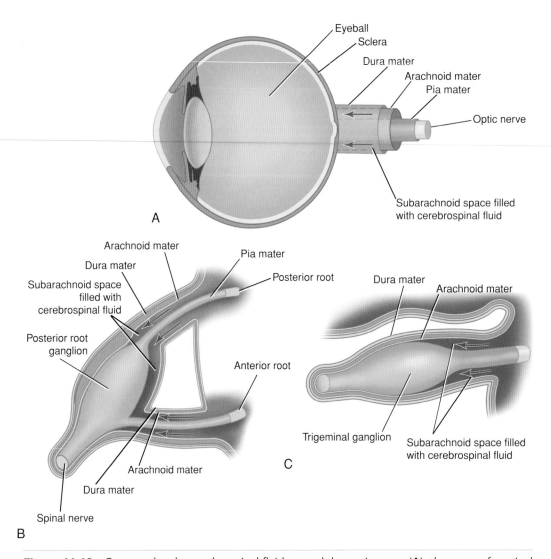

Figure 16-19 Course taken by cerebrospinal fluid around the optic nerve (**A**), the roots of a spinal nerve (**B**), and the trigeminal nerve (**C**).

BLOOD–BRAIN AND BLOOD–CEREBROSPINAL FLUID BARRIERS

The CNS requires a very stable environment in order to function normally. This stability is provided by isolating the nervous system from the blood by the existence of the so-called blood–brain barrier (BBB) and the blood–cerebrospinal fluid barrier.

Blood–Brain Barrier

The experiments of Paul Ehrlich in 1882 showed that living animals injected intravascularly with vital dyes, such as trypan blue, demonstrated staining of all the tissues of the body except the brain and spinal cord. Later, researchers demonstrated that although most of the brain is not stained after the intravenous injection of trypan blue, the following areas do become stained: the pineal gland, the posterior lobe of the pituitary, the tuber cinereum, the wall of the optic recess, and

the vascular area postrema (area of the medulla on the floor of the fourth ventricle just rostral to the opening into the central canal). These observations led to the concept of a BBB (for which blood–brain–spinal cord barrier would be a more accurate name).

BBB permeability is inversely related to the size of the molecules and directly related to their lipid solubility. Gases and water pass readily through the barrier, whereas glucose and electrolytes pass more slowly. The barrier is almost impermeable to plasma proteins and other large organic molecules. Compounds with molecular weights of about 60,000 and higher remain within the blood circulatory system. This would explain why in the early experiments with trypan blue, which quickly binds to the plasma protein albumin, the dye did not pass into the neural tissue in the greater part of the brain.

Structure

Examination of a CNS electron micrograph shows that the lumen of a blood capillary is separated from the

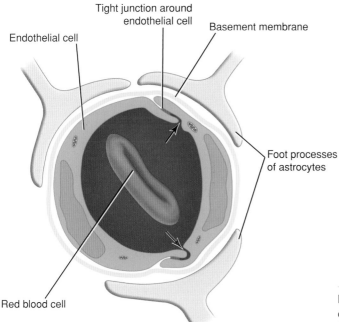

Endothelial cell

Tight junction around
endothelial cell

Basement membrane

Foot processes
of astrocytes

Red blood cell

Figure 16-20 Cross section of a blood capillary of the central nervous system in the area where the blood–brain barrier exists.

extracellular spaces around the neurons and neuroglia by the following structures: (1) the endothelial cells in the wall of the capillary, (2) a continuous basement membrane surrounding the capillary outside the endothelial cells, and (3) the foot processes of the astrocytes that adhere to the outer surface of the capillary wall (Fig. 16-20).

The use of electron-dense markers such as lanthanum and horseradish peroxidase has shown that these substances do not penetrate between the endothelial cells of the capillaries because of the presence of tight junctions that form belts around the cells. When the dense markers are introduced into the extracellular spaces of the neuropil, they pass between the perivascular foot processes of the astrocytes as far as the endothelial lining of the capillary. This evidence demonstrates that the tight junctions between the endothelial

cells of the blood capillaries are responsible for the BBB. (Peripheral nerves are isolated from the blood in the same manner as those of the CNS. The endothelial cells of the blood capillaries in the endoneurium have tight junctions; thus, there is a blood–nerve barrier.) In molecular terms, the BBB is thus a continuous lipid bilayer that encircles the endothelial cells and isolates the brain tissue from the blood. This explains how lipophilic molecules can readily diffuse through the barrier, whereas hydrophilic molecules are excluded.

Although a BBB exists in the newborn, it is likely more permeable to certain substances than it is in the adult.

BBB structure is not identical in all CNS regions: In those areas where it appears to be absent, the capillary endothelium contains fenestrations across which proteins and small organic molecules may pass from the blood to the nervous tissue (Fig. 16-21). The area

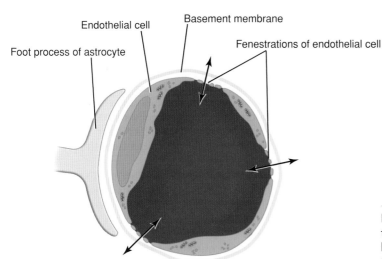

Figure 16-21 Cross section of a blood capillary of the central nervous system where the blood–brain barrier appears to be absent. Note the presence of fenestrations in the endothelial cells.

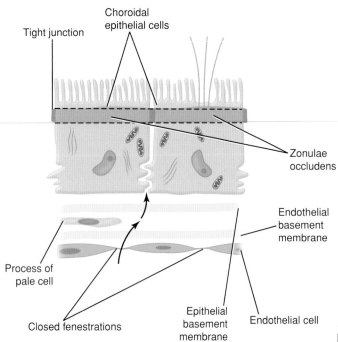

Figure 16-22 Section of villus of choroid plexus.

postrema of the floor of the fourth ventricle and the hypothalamus may serve as sites at which neuronal receptors may sample the chemical content of the plasma directly. The hypothalamus, which is involved in the regulation of the metabolic activity of the body, might bring about appropriate modifications of activity, thereby protecting the nervous tissue.

Blood–Cerebrospinal Fluid Barrier

Water, gases, and lipid-soluble substances pass freely from the blood to the CSF. Macromolecules such as proteins and most hexoses other than glucose are unable to enter the CSF. A barrier similar to the BBB may exist in the choroid plexuses.

Structure

Electron-microscopic examination of a villus of a choroid plexus shows that the lumen of a blood capillary is separated from the lumen of the ventricle by the following structures: (1) the endothelial cells, which are fenestrated and have very thin walls (the fenestrations are not true perforations but are filled by a thin diaphragm); (2) a continuous basement membrane surrounding the capillary outside the endothelial cells; (3) scattered pale cells with flattened processes; and (4) a continuous basement membrane, on which rest (5) the choroidal epithelial cells (Fig. 16-22). The use of electron-dense markers has not been entirely successful in localizing the barrier precisely. Horseradish peroxidase injected intravenously appears as a coating on the luminal surface of the endothelial cells and in many areas

examined, it did pass between the endothelial cells. Tight junctions between the choroidal epithelial cells probably serve as the barrier.

Cerebrospinal Fluid–Brain Interface

Although vital dyes given by intravenous injection do not gain access to most brain tissues, if the dyes are injected into the subarachnoid space or into the ventricles, they soon enter the extracellular spaces around the neurons and glial cells. Thus, a comparable physiologic barrier between CSF and the CNS extracellular compartment does not exist. However, three structures separate CSF from nervous tissue: (1) the pia-covered surface of the brain and spinal cord, (2) the perivascular extensions of the subarachnoid space into the nervous tissue, and (3) the ependymal surface of the ventricles (Fig. 16-23).

The pia-covered surface of the brain consists of a loosely arranged layer of pial cells resting on a basement membrane. Beneath the basement membrane are the astrocyte foot processes. No intercellular junctions exist between adjacent pial cells or between adjacent astrocytes; therefore, the extracellular spaces of the nervous tissue are in almost direct continuity with the subarachnoid space.

The prolongation of the subarachnoid space into the central nervous tissue quickly ends below the surface of the brain, where the fusion of the outer covering of the blood vessel with the pial covering of the nervous tissue occurs.

The ventricular surface of the brain is covered with columnar ependymal cells with localized tight junctions.

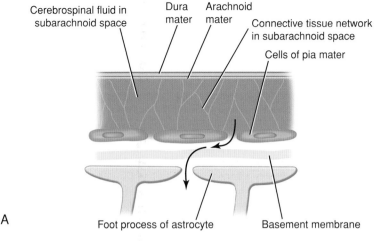

Cerebrospinal fluid in subarachnoid space

Dura mater

Arachnoid mater

Connective tissue network in subarachnoid space

Cells of pia mater

Foot process of astrocyte

Basement membrane

A

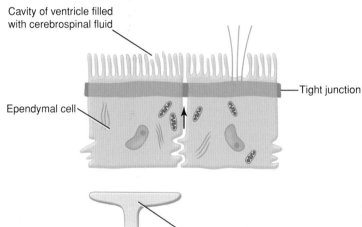

Cavity of ventricle filled with cerebrospinal fluid

Tight junction

Ependymal cell

Processes of astrocytes and other glial cells

B

Figure 16-23 Section of the cerebrospinal fluid–brain interface. **A:** Outer surface of the brain. **B:** Ventricular surface of the brain.

Intercellular channels permit free communication between the ventricular cavity and the extracellular neuronal space. The ependyma does not have a basement membrane, and specialized astrocytic foot processes are absent because the neuroglia cells are loosely arranged.

Functional Significance of the Barriers

In normal conditions, the BBB and blood–cerebrospinal fluid barrier are two important semipermeable barriers that protect the brain and spinal cord from potentially harmful substances while permitting gases and nutrients to enter the nervous tissue.

 Clinical Notes

Optic Nerve and Papilledema

The optic nerves are surrounded by sheaths derived from the pia mater, arachnoid mater, and dura mater. The intracranial subarachnoid space extends forward around the optic nerve to the back of the eyeball (see Fig. 16-19A). A rise of CSF pressure caused by an intracranial tumor will compress the thin walls of the retinal vein as it crosses the extension of the subarachnoid space to enter the optic nerve. This will result in congestion of the retinal vein, bulging forward of the optic disc, and edema of the disc; the last condition is referred to as **papilledema**. As both subarachnoid extensions are continuous with the intracranial subarachnoid

space, both eyes will exhibit papilledema. Persistent papilledema leads to optic atrophy and blindness.

Hydrocephalus

Hydrocephalus is an abnormal increase in CSF volume within the skull. If the hydrocephalus is accompanied by raised CSF pressure, then it is due to one of the following: (1) abnormal increase in CSF formation, (2) blockage of CSF circulation, or (3) diminished CSF absorption. Rarely, hydrocephalus occurs with normal CSF pressure; these patients exhibit compensatory hypoplasia or atrophy of the brain substance.

Two varieties of hydrocephalus are described: In **noncommunicating hydrocephalus**, the raised CSF pressure is due to blockage at some point between its formation at the choroid plexuses and its exit through the foramina in the roof of the fourth ventricle. In **communicating hydrocephalus**, no obstruction exists within or to the outflow from the ventricular system; the CSF freely reaches the subarachnoid space and is found to be under increased pressure.

Excessive Cerebrospinal Fluid Formation

Excessive CSF formation is a rare condition that may occur with a tumor of the choroid plexuses.

Blockage of Cerebrospinal Fluid Circulation

An obstruction of the interventricular foramen by a tumor will block the drainage of the lateral ventricle on that side. Continued CSF production by the choroid plexus of that ventricle will cause distention of that ventricle and atrophy of the surrounding neural tissue.

An obstruction in the cerebral aqueduct may be congenital or may result from inflammation or pressure from a tumor. This causes a symmetrical distention of both lateral ventricles and distention of the third ventricle.

Obstruction of the median aperture (foramen of Magendie) in the roof of the fourth ventricle and the two lateral apertures (foramina of Luschka) in the lateral recesses of the fourth ventricle by inflammatory exudate or by tumor growth will produce symmetrical dilatation of both lateral ventricles and the third and fourth ventricles.

Sometimes, inflammatory exudate secondary to meningitis will block the subarachnoid space and obstruct CSF flow over the outer surface of the cerebral hemispheres. Here again, the entire ventricular system of the brain will become distended.

Diminished Cerebrospinal Fluid Absorption

Interference with CSF at the arachnoid granulations may be caused by inflammatory exudate, venous thrombosis or pressure on the venous sinuses, or obstruction of the internal jugular vein.

Clinical Investigation of the Cerebral Ventricles

The size of the cerebral ventricles may be investigated clinically by the use of (1) computed tomography (CT) and magnetic resonance imaging (MRI) and, if necessary, (2) intracranial pneumography.

CT and **MRI** are safe and easy to perform. The outline of the ventricles may be demonstrated by using these methods (see Figs. 1-24 and 1-25). Apart from ventricular distention or distortion, the cerebral tumor causing the condition also may be demonstrated.

Intracranial pneumography is essentially the replacement of CSF within the ventricles and subarachnoid space with air or oxygen. Because the air or gas is less dense than CSF or neural tissue, the ventricles and cerebral gyri can be visualized. In an **encephalogram**, the air or oxygen is introduced through a spinal tap and radiographs of the skull are then made. In a **ventriculogram**, the air or oxygen is introduced into the lateral ventricle through a needle inserted through a hole in the skull (in a young child, the needle may be inserted through a suture) and skull radiographs are made. In ventriculography, only the ventricles are visualized.

Cerebrospinal Fluid Pressure and Composition in Disease

CSF examination can be of great assistance in making a neurologic diagnosis.

Clinical measurement of CSF pressure by means of a spinal tap is described on page 19. An increase in pressure is usually due to meningitis or an increase in volume of the brain produced by edema, tumor formation, a cerebral abscess, or the presence of a hematoma.

The gross appearance of a specimen of CSF is of great value. Normally, it is clear and colorless. Cloudiness usually indicates the presence of polymorphonuclear leukocytes or an excessive quantity of protein. An increase in the white cells would suggest inflammation of the meninges or encephalitis. An increase in protein content implies a change in the vascular permeability, and protein escapes into the CSF. Raised protein content is seen in tuberculous meningitis and poliomyelitis. In multiple sclerosis, the gamma globulin is elevated due to production of immunoglobulins in the brain and spinal cord.

Normal CSF does not contain red blood cells. Gross blood in the CSF is usually caused by contamination brought about by puncture of a vertebral vein by the spinal tap needle. Uniform blood staining is found in subarachnoid hemorrhage. Yellow coloration or **xanthochromia** is caused by the presence of oxyhemoglobin in the fluid some hours after subarachnoid hemorrhage.

Normal CSF contains fewer than four white cells. In bacterial infections, many thousands of cells may be present per cubic millimeter. In viral infections of the nervous system, a moderate lymphocyte reaction may occur. A slight rise in lymphocyte count may also occur in cerebral tumors, cerebral infarction, and multiple sclerosis.

The glucose level in the CSF may disappear completely in acute bacterial meningitis but remains normal in viral infections.

Normal CSF physical characteristics and composition are summarized in Table 16-1.

Subarachnoid Space Blockage

A block of the subarachnoid space in the vertebral canal may be caused by a tumor of the spinal cord or the meninges. Performing a spinal tap is of great value in making a diagnosis. The normal pressure of CSF with the patient lying quietly on his or her side and breathing through the mouth is between 60 and 150 mm of water. If CSF flow in the subarachnoid space is blocked, the normal variations in pressure corresponding to the pulse and respiration are reduced or absent. Compression of the internal jugular veins in the neck raises the cerebral venous pressure and inhibits CSF absorption in the arachnoid villi and granulations, thus producing a rise in the manometric reading of CSF pressure. If this fails to occur, the subarachnoid space is blocked and the patient is exhibiting a positive **Queckenstedt sign**. Should the tumor completely occupy the vertebral canal in the region of the cauda equina, no CSF can flow out of the spinal tap needle.

Normally, CSF is clear. In the presence of a tumor, it may be yellow and clot spontaneously owing to the rise in protein content.

Fourth Ventricle Tumors

Tumors may arise in the vermis of the cerebellum or in the pons and invade the fourth ventricle. **Ependymomas** arising from the ependymal cells lining the ventricle also occur. Tumors in this region may invade the cerebellum and produce the symptoms and signs of cerebellar deficiency, or they may press on the vital nuclear centers situated beneath the floor of the ventricle; the hypoglossal and vagal nuclei, for example, control movements of the tongue, swallowing, respiration, heart rate, and blood pressure.

Blood–Brain Barrier in the Fetus and Newborn

In the fetus, newborn child, and premature infant, the BBB is not fully developed, and toxic substances such as bilirubin can readily enter the CNS and produce yellowing of the brain and kernicterus. This is not possible in the adult.

Brain Trauma and the Blood–Brain Barrier

Any injury to the brain, whether it be due to direct trauma or to inflammatory or chemical toxins, causes a breakdown of the BBB, allowing free diffusion of large molecules into the nervous tissue. This is believed to be brought about by actual destruction of the vascular endothelial cells or disruption of their tight junctions.

Drugs and the Blood–Brain Barrier

The systemic administration of **penicillin** results in only a small amount entering the CNS. This is fortunate because penicillin in high concentrations is toxic to nervous tissue. In the presence of meningitis, however, the meninges become more permeable locally at the site of inflammation, thus permitting sufficient antibiotic to reach the infection. **Chloramphenicol** and the **tetracyclines** readily cross the BBB and enter the nervous tissue. The **sulfonamide** drugs also easily pass through the BBB.

Lipid-soluble substances such as the anesthetic agent **thiopental** rapidly enter the brain after intravenous injection. On the other hand, water-soluble substances such as exogenous **norepinephrine** cannot cross the BBB. **Phenylbutazone** is a drug that becomes bound to plasma protein, and the large drug protein molecule is unable to cross the barrier. Most tertiary amines such as **atropine** are lipid soluble and quickly enter the brain, whereas the quaternary compounds such as **atropine methyl nitrate** do not.

In Parkinson disease, the neurotransmitter dopamine is deficient in the corpus striatum. Unfortunately, dopamine cannot be used in the treatment, as it will not cross the BBB. L-Dopa readily crosses the barrier and has been used with great success.

Tumors and the Blood–Brain Barrier

Brain tumors frequently possess blood vessels that have no BBB. Anaplastic malignant astrocytomas, glioblastomas, and secondary metastatic tumors lack the normal barriers. However, slow-growing tumors often have normal vascular barriers.

Key Concepts

Ventricular System

- The ventricles are fluid-filled cavities located within the brain.
- The ventricles are lined throughout with ependyma and are filled with CSF.
- Lateral ventricles are the largest ventricles and are described as having a body, and anterior, posterior, and lateral horns.
- The lateral ventricles communicate with a singular, medially located third ventricle via the interventricular foramen.
- The third ventricle is found between the two thalami.
- The cerebral aqueduct of the midbrain communicates CSF between the third and fourth ventricles.
- The fourth ventricle is located between the pons/medulla and the cerebellum.
- CSF exits the fourth ventricle through the singular median opening (foramen of Magendie) and two lateral openings (foramina of Luschka).
- The choroid plexus is found within the lateral ventricles and produces CSF.
- Blood–Brain and Blood–Cerebrospinal Fluid Barriers
- The BBB freely allows gases and water, slowly allows glucose and electrolytes, but restricts passage of plasma proteins and other large organic molecules.
- The structure of the BBB is formed by the endothelial capillary walls, a continuous basement membrane around the vessels, and the foot processes of astrocytes that adhere to the capillary wall.
- Tight junctions between endothelial cells are responsible for the restriction of large molecules but yet allow lipophilic molecules to cross the barrier.
- Water, gases, and lipid-soluble substances pass freely from the blood to the CSF but macromolecules are restricted, suggesting a similar barrier exists in the choroid plexus.

? Clinical Problem Solving

1. A 55-year-old man is being investigated for signs and symptoms that suggest the presence of a cerebral tumor. Examination of the CT scan shows gross enlargement and distortion of the left lateral ventricle. What other investigation might be carried out in this patient to display the ventricles of the brain? Using your knowledge of neuroanatomy, determine the location of the tumor in this patient.

2. A 3-year-old child is referred to the children's hospital because the circumference of his head greatly exceeds the normal limit for his age. After a careful history is taken and a detailed physical examination is performed, a diagnosis of hydrocephalus is made. What is your definition of hydrocephalus? Name three common causes of hydrocephalus in young children.

3. A 50-year-old man is found on ophthalmoscopic examination to have edema of both optic discs (bilateral papilledema) and congestion of the retinal veins. The cause of the condition is found to be a rapidly growing intracranial tumor. Using your knowledge of neuroanatomy, explain the papilledema. Why does the patient exhibit bilateral papilledema?

4. A 38-year-old man is admitted to the neurosurgery ward with symptoms of persistent headache and vomiting and some unsteadiness in walking. The headache started 6 weeks previously and became progressively worse. On examination, he cannot sit up in bed unsupported. The limbs on the right side of the body show some loss of tone. Examination of the patient when he is standing up shows a marked loss of equilibrium. Examination of the cranial nerves shows central deafness of the right ear. Ophthalmoscopic examination shows severe bilateral papilledema. Using your knowledge of neuroanatomy, explain the symptoms and signs experienced by this patient and try to make a diagnosis.

5. A 4-year-old girl is found to have tuberculous meningitis. She is immediately admitted to the hospital and administration of streptomycin and isoniazid is commenced. As soon as this therapy is started, she is also administered steroid hormones to reduce the incidence of adhesions. She recovers fully with no complications. Using your knowledge of neuroanatomy, explain why preventing adhesion formation in the subarachnoid space is important.

6. A 5-year-old girl with symptoms of headache, general malaise, and vomiting is admitted to the children's hospital. On examination, the body temperature is found to be 104°F and the pulse rate is rapid. Attempts to flex the neck produce pain and result in the patient flexing her hip and knee joints. A spinal tap is performed; the cerebrospinal fluid (CSF) is seen to be cloudy and the pressure is raised to 190 mm of water. Microscopic examination of the fluid shows a large number of polymorphonuclear leukocytes. A diagnosis of meningitis is made. Subsequent culture reveals the infection to be a meningococcal meningitis. The resident vaguely remembers reading in a textbook the importance of the blood–brain barrier (BBB) in the use of antibiotics for the treatment of meningitis. What is the BBB? Does the presence of the BBB influence your choice and dose of antibiotics to be used in this patient?

7. During a ward round in the children's hospital, the pediatrician informs the students that a 4-day-old baby with jaundice has a serum indirect bilirubin level of 45 mg/100 mL and that by now the bile pigment is staining the brain a yellow color (kernicterus). The neuronal damage is revealed clinically by lethargy and poor feeding habits and by occasional muscle spasms. She says the prognosis is very poor. One of the students observes that he cannot understand why the bile pigment is having such a dramatic effect on the baby. Recently, he examined a patient who was dying of inoperable carcinoma of the head of the pancreas with total obstruction of the common bile duct. In that patient, the skin was a deep yellow, but apart from complaints of the intense skin irritation owing to the high concentration of bile salts in the blood and loss of weight, the patient had no symptoms and no neurologic abnormalities. Explain why the baby had neuronal damage and the adult did not.

8. Name five areas of the brain where the blood–brain barrier (BBB) appears to be absent. What do you think is the significance of the fact that in a few areas of the brain, the barrier is absent?

Answers and Explanations to Clinical Problem Solving

1. An MRI shows the outline of the ventricles very well. Occasionally, when these methods show insufficient detail, a ventriculogram can be obtained. This procedure consists of the introduction of air or oxygen into the lateral ventricle through a needle inserted through a burr hole in the skull. Since the left lateral ventricle was the only part of the ventricular system that showed distention and distortion, one can assume that the tumor had closed off the left interventricular foramen and, therefore, was in the vicinity of that foramen. This was confirmed on the CT scan.

2. Hydrocephalus is an abnormal increase in the volume of cerebrospinal fluid within the skull. Congenital atresia of the cerebral aqueduct, meningitis, tumors, and blockage of the arachnoid granulations by subarachnoid bleeding or inflammatory exudate are common causes of this condition in young children.

3. The intracranial subarachnoid space extends forward around the optic nerve to the back of the eyeball. A rise in cerebrospinal fluid pressure caused by an intracranial tumor will compress the thin walls of the retinal vein as it crosses the extension of the subarachnoid space to enter the optic nerve. This will result in congestion of the retinal vein, bulging of the optic disc, and edema of the disc. Since both subarachnoid extensions are continuous with the intracranial subarachnoid space, both eyes will exhibit papilledema.

4. This man was operated on and was found to have a large astrocytoma of the vermis of the cerebellum. The tumor had severely encroached on the cavity of the fourth ventricle, producing internal hydrocephalus and pressure on the floor of the ventricle. The symptoms of headache and persistent vomiting were produced by a raised intracranial pressure caused by the enlarging tumor. The tumor also blocked off the median and lateral apertures in the roof of the fourth ventricle, causing an internal hydrocephalus, which further raised the intracranial pressure. The bilateral papilledema was secondary to the raised intracranial pressure. The inability to sit up in bed (truncal ataxia) and the loss of equilibrium on standing were due to the tumor involvement of the vermis of the cerebellum. The loss of tone of the muscles of the right limbs indicated spread of the tumor to involve the right cerebellar hemisphere. Central deafness on the right side was due to involvement of the right eighth cranial nerve nuclei by the tumor mass. The patient died 6 months after neurosurgical exploration.

5. Steroid hormones (e.g., prednisone) inhibit the normal inflammatory reaction and thereby reduce the incidence of fibrous adhesions. Preventing adhesion formation is important, as it can block the openings in the roof of the fourth ventricle thus preventing the escape of cerebrospinal fluid (CSF) into the subarachnoid space from within the ventricular system. Adhesions also can prevent the flow of CSF over the cerebral hemispheres or reduce the absorption of the fluid into the arachnoid granulations. Thus, adhesions of the meninges may result in hydrocephalus.

6. The BBB is a semipermeable barrier that exists between the blood and the extracellular spaces of the nervous tissue of the brain. It permits the passage of water, gases, glucose, electrolytes, and amino acids, but it is impermeable to substances with a large molecular weight. Yes, the presence of the BBB does affect the choice and dose of antibiotics. The antibiotic penicillin, when injected intramuscularly into a normal individual, is found in much lower concentrations in the CSF than in the blood; this is due to the existence of the BBB and the blood–cerebrospinal fluid barrier. Inflammation of the meninges results in an increased permeability of the meningeal blood vessels, and consequently, the concentration of penicillin rises in the CSF. However, for treatment to be effective in patients with meningitis, very large doses of penicillin must be given intravenously. By contrast, chloramphenicol and the sulfonamides rapidly cross the blood–brain and blood–cerebrospinal fluid barriers; therefore, an adequate concentration in the CSF can easily be maintained.

7. The blood–brain barrier in the newborn child is not fully developed and is more permeable than that in the adult. Indirect bilirubin readily crosses the barrier in the newborn but does not do so in the adult. Once the bile pigment reaches the extracellular spaces of the brain tissue in the newborn, it passes into the neurons and neuroglia cells. This results in abnormal cell function and eventually neuronal death.

8. The pineal gland, the posterior lobe of the pituitary, the tuber cinereum, the wall of the optic recess, and the vascular area postrema at the inferior end of the fourth ventricle are parts of the brain where the capillary endothelium contains open fenestrations across which proteins and small organic molecules may pass. In these areas, a BBB appears to be absent. The significance of the absence of the barrier in the pineal gland is not understood. To function normally, pinealocytes possibly require a close relationship with the blood plasma in order to sample the concentrations of hormones. The absence of the BBB in the region of the hypothalamus may allow this area of the brain to sample the chemical content of the plasma, so appropriate modifications of metabolic activity may take place, thus protecting the nervous tissue as a whole.

? Review Questions

Directions: Each of the numbered items in this section is followed by answers. Select the ONE lettered answer that is CORRECT.

1. The following statements concern the ventricular system:
   (a) The cerebral aqueduct connects the third ventricle with the fourth ventricle.
   (b) The two lateral ventricles communicate directly with one another through the foramen of Monro.
   (c) The ventricles are developed from the embryonic endoderm.
   (d) It is lined throughout with squamous epithelium.
   (e) Choroid plexuses are found only in the lateral ventricles.

2. The following statements concern the ventricular system:
   (a) The fourth ventricle has a rectangular-shaped floor.
   (b) The pineal body is suspended from the roof of the fourth ventricle.
   (c) The nerve centers controlling the heart rate and blood pressure lie beneath the floor of the third ventricle.
   (d) The choroid plexus of the lateral ventricle projects into the cavity on its medial side through the choroidal fissure.
   (e) The foramen of Magendie is an aperture in the roof of the third ventricle.

3. The following statements concern the blood–brain barrier (BBB):
   (a) It protects the brain from toxic compounds of low molecular weight.
   (b) It is present in the pineal gland.
   (c) The endothelial cells of the blood capillaries are nonfenestrated.
   (d) The endothelial cells of the blood capillaries are held together by localized tight junctions.
   (e) L-Dopa has difficulty passing through it in the treatment of Parkinson disease.

4. The following statements concern the blood–brain barrier (BBB):
   (a) Chloramphenicol and the tetracyclines cannot cross the barrier.
   (b) In the newborn child, the BBB is not fully developed.
   (c) Cerebral trauma or inflammation has little effect on BBB integrity.
   (d) Gases and water pass with difficulty through the barrier.
   (e) Glucose and electrolytes pass quickly through the barrier.

5. The following statements concern the blood–cerebrospinal fluid barrier:
   (a) The beltlike tight junctions between the choroidal ependymal cells form the barrier.
   (b) The proteins and most hexoses, other than glucose, are able to cross the barrier.
   (c) Gases and water cannot pass through the barrier.
   (d) Lipid-soluble substances have difficulty passing through the barrier.
   (e) The basement membrane of the endothelial cells plays a vital part in the formation of the barrier.

6. The following structures are associated with the roof of the fourth ventricle:
   (a) Tectum of the midbrain
   (b) Choroid plexus
   (c) Pineal gland
   (d) Corpus callosum
   (e) Temporal lobes of the cerebral hemispheres

7. The following statements concern the cerebrospinal fluid (CSF) in the fourth ventricle:
   (a) It is produced mainly by the choroid plexus of the cerebral aqueduct.
   (b) It leaves the midbrain through the interventricular foramina.
   (c) It enters the spinal cord through the foramen of Luschka.
   (d) It is dark yellow in color.
   (e) It escapes into the subarachnoid space through the apertures in the roof of the fourth ventricle.

8. The lateral boundaries of the fourth ventricle are formed by:
   (a) the tentorium cerebelli.
   (b) the sulcus limitans.
   (c) the cerebellar peduncles.
   (d) the cerebral peduncles.
   (e) the striae medullares.

9. The following important nuclei lie beneath the floor of the fourth ventricle:
   (a) Oculomotor nucleus
   (b) Trochlear nucleus
   (c) Trigeminal nucleus
   (d) Hypoglossal nucleus
   (e) Olfactory nucleus

10. The following statements concern the third ventricle:
    (a) It is situated between the two thalami.
    (b) It communicates with the lateral ventricles through the cerebral aqueduct.
    (c) It is continuous with the fourth ventricle through the interventricular foramen.
    (d) The choroid plexus is located on the floor.
    (e) The choroid plexus receives its arterial supply through the posterior cerebral arteries.

11. The following statements concern the subarachnoid space:
    (a) It contains cerebrospinal fluid (CSF) and the cerebral arteries but not the cerebral veins.
    (b) It does not communicate with the cisterns.
    (c) The fourth ventricle drains into it through a single foramen.
    (d) The space does not surround the cranial and spinal nerves where they leave the skull and the vertebral canal.
    (e) It is the interval between the arachnoid mater and the pia mater.

12. The following statements concern cerebrospinal fluid (CSF) formation:
    (a) None of the fluid originates from the brain substance.
    (b) It is largely formed by the choroid plexuses.
    (c) It is passively secreted by the ependymal cells covering the choroid plexuses.
    (d) It is produced continuously at a rate of about 5 mL/min.
    (e) It is drained into the subarachnoid space from the lymphatic vessels of the brain and spinal cord.

13. The following statements concern the cerebrospinal fluid (CSF):
    (a) Its circulation through the ventricles is not aided by the pulsations of the choroid plexuses.
    (b) It extends inferiorly in the subarachnoid space to the level of the fifth sacral vertebra.
    (c) The CSF pressure in the subarachnoid space rises if the internal jugular veins in the neck are compressed.
    (d) It exits from the ventricular system through the ventricular foramina.
    (e) Its circulation in the subarachnoid space is aided by the pulsations of the cerebral and spinal veins.

14. The following statements concern cerebrospinal fluid (CSF) absorption:
    (a) The fluid is passed into the blood by active transport through the cells forming the arachnoid villi.
    (b) The major sites for its absorption are into the veins in the subarachnoid space and the perineural lymph vessels.
    (c) Arachnoid villi play an important role in its absorption.
    (d) Fine tubules found within the arachnoid villi play a minor role in CSF flow into the venous sinuses.
    (e) In communicating hydrocephalus, flow is obstructed within the ventricular system and to the outflow from the ventricular system to the subarachnoid space.

Matching Questions. Directions: The following questions apply to Figure 16-24. Match the numbers listed on the left with the appropriate lettered structures listed on the right. Each lettered option may be selected once, more than once, or not at all.

Figure 16-24   Lateral view of the brain showing an outline of ventricular cavities.

15. Number 1   (a) Cerebral aqueduct
16. Number 2   (b) Body of lateral ventricle
17. Number 3   (c) Third ventricle
18. Number 4   (d) Fourth ventricle
                    (e) None of the above

Directions: Each case history is followed by questions. Read the case history, then select the ONE BEST lettered answer.

A 24-year-old woman complaining of recent onset of severe headaches and several attacks of morning vomiting was seen by a neurologist. A thorough physical examination revealed findings suggesting that she might have an intracranial tumor involving the cerebellum. The physician ordered an MRI of the patient's brain with particular reference to the contents of the posterior cranial fossa.

19. Figure 16-25 is a coronal MRI (contrast enhanced) through the fourth ventricle. The radiologist made the following correct observations in his report except:
    (a) The bones of the skull showed nothing abnormal. The cerebral cortex appeared to be normal.
    (b) The midline structures were not deflected to one or the other side.
    (c) The cavity of the fourth ventricle was distorted and larger than normal.
    (d) The body of the lateral ventricle had a normal appearance.

A 21-year-old pregnant woman was invited to a reunion party and during the course of the evening, she drank several gin and tonics. The party was followed by several others extending over a 3-week period during which she drank heavily. Six months later, she gave birth to a boy who was diagnosed as having congenital hydrocephalus.

Figure 16-25 A coronal MRI (contrast enhanced) through the hindbrain showing the fourth ventricle and the surrounding neural and bony structures.

20. The pediatric neurologist carefully questioned the mother and came to the following correct conclusions except:
    (a) The consumption of a large amount of alcohol during pregnancy usually has no adverse effects on the developing fetus.
    (b) The high alcoholic intake coincided with the first trimester.
    (c) The alcohol had crossed the placental barrier and entered the fetal circulation.
    (d) The alcohol had probably also crossed the fetal blood–brain barrier (BBB) and entered the brain.
    (e) The neurologist was of the opinion that the toxic effect of alcohol was probably responsible for the hydrocephalus.

 Answers and Explanations to Review Questions

1. A is correct. The cerebral aqueduct connects the third ventricle with the fourth ventricle (see Fig. 16-4). B. The two lateral ventricles do not communicate directly with one another through the interventricular foramen (foramen of Monro) (see Fig. 16-2). C. The ventricles are developed from the neural tube in the embryo. D. The ventricular system is lined throughout with ependyma, which is a single layer of cuboidal or columnar cells. E. The choroid plexuses are found in the lateral ventricles and the third and the fourth ventricles.

2. D is correct. The choroid plexus of the lateral ventricle projects into the cavity on its medial side through the choroidal fissure (see Fig. 16-7). A. The fourth ventricle has a diamond-shaped floor called the rhomboid fossa (see Fig. 16-11).

B. The pineal body is not suspended from the roof of the fourth ventricle (see Fig. 16-4). C. The nerve centers controlling the heart rate and blood pressure lie beneath the floor of the fourth ventricle (see Fig. 16-11). E. The foramen of Magendie is an aperture in the roof of the fourth ventricle (see Fig. 16-12).

3. C is correct. The endothelial cells of the blood capillaries in the BBB are nonfenestrated. A. The BBB protects the brain from toxic compounds of high molecular weight. B. The BBB is not present in the pineal gland. D. The endothelial cells of the blood capillaries of the BBB are not held together by localized tight junctions; they pass around the endothelial cells. E. L-Dopa readily passes through the BBB in the treatment of Parkinson disease.

4. B is correct. In the newborn child, the BBB is not fully developed. A. Chloramphenicol and the tetracyclines can cross the BBB. C. Cerebral trauma and inflammation may have a great effect on the integrity of the BBB. D. Gases and water pass readily through the BBB. E. Glucose and electrolytes pass slowly through the BBB.

5. A is correct. In the blood–cerebrospinal fluid barrier, the beltlike tight junctions between the choroidal ependymal cells form the barrier. B. The proteins and most hexoses, other than glucose, are unable to cross the blood–cerebrospinal fluid barrier. C. Gases and water pass readily through the barrier. D. Lipid-soluble substances have no difficulty passing through the barrier. E. The basement membrane of the endothelial cells plays no part in the formation of the barrier.

6. B is correct. The choroid plexus is present in the roof of the fourth ventricle (see Fig. 16-8).

7. E is correct. The CSF in the fourth ventricle escapes into the subarachnoid space through apertures in the roof of the ventricle (see Fig. 16-13). A. The CSF in the fourth ventricle is produced mainly in the choroid plexuses of the lateral, third, and fourth ventricles. B. It leaves the midbrain through the cerebral aqueduct (Fig. 16-17). C. The CSF in the fourth ventricle enters the spinal cord through the central canal (see Fig. 16-7). D. The CSF is clear and colorless.

8. C is correct. The lateral boundaries of the fourth ventricle are formed by the cerebellar peduncles (see Fig. 16-10).

9. D is correct. The hypoglossal nucleus lies beneath the floor of the fourth ventricle (see hypoglossal triangle in Fig. 16-11).

10. A is correct. The third ventricle lies between the thalami (see Fig. 16-5). B. The third ventricle communicates with the lateral ventricles through the interventricular foramina (see Fig. 16-2). C. The third ventricle is continuous with the fourth ventricle through the cerebral aqueduct (see Fig. 16-3). D. The choroid plexus of the third ventricle is situated in the roof (see Fig. 16-6). E. The choroid plexus of the third ventricle receives its arterial supply from the internal carotid and basilar arteries.

11. E is correct. The subarachnoid space is the interval between the arachnoid mater and the pia mater (see Fig. 16-1). A. The subarachnoid space contains CSF, the cerebral arteries, and the cerebral veins. B. The subarachnoid space is in free communication with the cisterns. C. The fourth ventricle drains into the subarachnoid space through three openings in its roof (see Fig. 16-1). D. The subarachnoid space surrounds the cranial and spinal nerves to the point where they leave the skull and the vertebral canal.

12. B is correct. The CSF is largely formed by the choroid plexuses. A. Some of the fluid originates from the brain substance. C. The CSF is actively secreted by the ependymal cells covering the choroid plexuses. D. The CSF is produced continuously at a rate of 0.5 mL/min. E. The brain and spinal cord have no lymphatic vessels.

13. C is correct. The CSF pressure in the subarachnoid space rises if the internal jugular veins in the neck are compressed. A. The circulation of the CSF through the ventricles is aided by the pulsations of the arteries in the choroid plexuses. B. The CSF extends inferiorly in the subarachnoid space in the vertebral column to the level of the lower border of the second sacral vertebra (see Fig. 16-1). D. The CSF exits from the ventricular system of the brain through the foramina of Luschka and Magendie (see Fig. 16-1). E. The circulation of the CSF in the subarachnoid space is aided by the pulsations of the cerebral and spinal arteries.

14. C is correct. The arachnoid villi play an important role in the absorption of CSF into the cranial venous sinuses. A. The CSF does not pass into the blood by active transport through the cells forming the arachnoid villi. B. The veins in the subarachnoid space and the perineural lymph vessels are minor sites for the absorption of CSF. D. The fine tubules found within the arachnoid villi play a major role in the flow of the CSF into the venous sinuses. E. In communicating hydrocephalus, flow of the CSF is not obstructed within the ventricular system or to the outflow from the ventricular system to the subarachnoid space.

For answers to Questions 15 to 18, study Figure 16-21.

15. B is correct; 1 is body of the lateral ventricle.

16. A is correct; 2 is cerebral aqueduct.

17. D is correct; 3 is fourth ventricle.

18. C is correct; 4 is third ventricle.

19. C is correct. The size and the shape of the cavity of the fourth ventricle were within normal limits.

20. A is correct. Many chemical substances when consumed are toxic to the central nervous system (CNS), and alcohol in large quantities is one of the worst offenders. During the first trimester, alcohol can readily access the brain at a time when it is particularly vulnerable. Before a physician prescribes a therapeutic drug, he or she must know whether the drug will cross the BBB and what effect, if any, that drug will have on the CNS.

CHAPTER OBJECTIVES

- To review the main arteries and veins supplying the brain and spinal cord

- To learn the areas of the cerebral cortex and spinal cord supplied by a particular artery and to

understand the dysfunction that would result if the artery were blocked

- To review the circle of Willis as well as the blood supply to the internal capsule

A 61-year-old woman collapsed in the supermarket and was in a coma when admitted to the emergency department of the local hospital. Twenty-four hours later, she recovered consciousness and was found to have paralysis on the left side of her body, mainly involving the lower limb. There was also some sensory loss of the left leg and foot. She was able to swallow normally and did not appear to have difficulty with her speech. The left-sided hemiplegia and hemianesthesia strongly suggested a cerebrovascular accident involving the right cerebral hemisphere. The limitation of the paralysis and anesthesia to the leg and foot indicated that the right anterior cerebral artery or one of its branches was blocked by a thrombus or embolus.

The diagnosis was confirmed by positron emission tomography (PET), which showed an absence of blood flow through the leg area on the medial surface of the right cerebral hemisphere.

Cerebrovascular accidents (stroke) remain the third leading cause of morbidity and death in the United States. Consequently, clinicians must know the areas of the cerebral cortex and spinal cord supplied by a particular artery and to understand the dysfunction that would result if the artery were blocked. The internal capsule that contains the major ascending and descending pathways to the cerebral cortex is commonly disrupted by arterial hemorrhage or thrombosis.

ARTERIES OF THE BRAIN

The brain is supplied by the two internal carotid and the two vertebral arteries. The four arteries lie within the subarachnoid space, and their branches anastomose on the inferior surface of the brain to form the circle of Willis.

Internal Carotid Artery

The internal carotid artery begins at the bifurcation of the common carotid artery (Fig. 17-1), where it usually possesses a localized dilatation, called the **carotid sinus**. It ascends the neck and perforates the base of the skull by passing through the carotid canal of the temporal bone. The artery then runs horizontally forward through the cavernous sinus and emerges on the medial side of the anterior clinoid process by perforating the dura mater. It now enters the subarachnoid space by piercing the arachnoid mater and turns posteriorly to the region of the medial end of the lateral cerebral

sulcus. Here, it divides into the **anterior** and **middle cerebral arteries** (Fig. 17-2; also see Fig. 17-1).

Cerebral Portion Branches

1. The **ophthalmic artery** arises as the internal carotid artery emerges from the cavernous sinus. It enters the orbit through the optic canal below and lateral to the optic nerve. It supplies the eye and other orbital structures, and its terminal branches supply the frontal area of the scalp, the ethmoid and frontal sinuses, and the dorsum of the nose.

2. The **posterior communicating artery** is a small vessel that originates from the internal carotid artery close to its terminal bifurcation. The posterior communicating artery runs posteriorly above the oculomotor nerve to join the posterior cerebral artery, thus forming part of the **circle of Willis**.

3. The **choroidal artery**, a small branch, also originates from the internal carotid artery close to its terminal

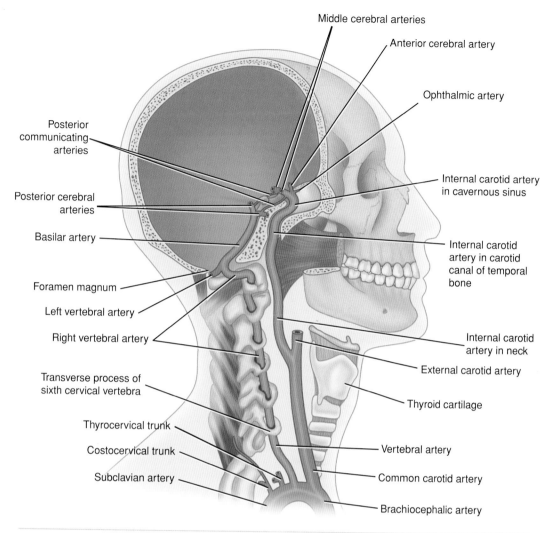

Middle cerebral arteries

Anterior cerebral artery

Ophthalmic artery

Posterior communicating arteries

Posterior cerebral arteries

Basilar artery

Internal carotid artery in cavernous sinus

Internal carotid artery in carotid canal of temporal bone

Foramen magnum

Left vertebral artery

Right vertebral artery

Internal carotid artery in neck

External carotid artery

Transverse process of sixth cervical vertebra

Thyroid cartilage

Thyrocervical trunk

Costocervical trunk

Vertebral artery

Subclavian artery

Common carotid artery

Brachiocephalic artery

Figure 17-1 Origin and courses of the internal carotid and vertebral arteries as they ascend the neck to enter the skull.

bifurcation. The choroidal artery passes posteriorly close to the optic tract, enters the inferior horn of the lateral ventricle, and ends in the choroid plexus. It gives off numerous small branches to surrounding structures, including the crus cerebri, the lateral geniculate body, the optic tract, and the internal capsule.

4. The **anterior cerebral artery** is the smaller terminal branch of the internal carotid artery. It runs forward and medially superior to the optic nerve and enters the longitudinal fissure of the cerebrum. Here, it is joined to the anterior cerebral artery of the opposite side by the **anterior communicating artery**. It curves backward over the corpus callosum and, finally, anastomoses with the posterior cerebral artery (Fig. 17-3; also see Fig. 17-8). The **cortical branches** supply the entire medial surface of the cerebral cortex as far back as the parieto-occipital sulcus. They also supply a strip of cortex about 1 in

(2.5 cm) wide on the adjoining lateral surface. The anterior cerebral artery thus supplies the "leg area" of the precentral gyrus. A group of **central branches** pierces the anterior perforated substance and helps to supply parts of the lentiform and caudate nuclei and the internal capsule.

5. The **middle cerebral artery,** the largest branch of the internal carotid, runs laterally in the lateral cerebral sulcus (see Fig. 17-2). **Cortical branches** supply the entire lateral surface of the hemisphere except for the narrow strip supplied by the anterior cerebral artery, the occipital pole, and the inferolateral surface of the hemisphere, which are supplied by the posterior cerebral artery (see Fig. 17-3). This artery thus supplies the entire motor area except the "leg area." **Central branches** enter the anterior perforated substance and supply the lentiform and caudate nuclei and the internal capsule (Fig. 17-4).

Figure 17-2   Arteries of the inferior surface of the brain. Note the formation of the circle of Willis. Part of the right temporal lobe has been removed to show the course of the middle cerebral artery.

Vertebral Artery

The vertebral artery, a branch of the first part of the subclavian artery, ascends the neck by passing through the foramina in the transverse processes of the upper six cervical vertebrae (see Fig. 17-1). It enters the skull through the foramen magnum and pierces the dura mater and arachnoid to enter the subarachnoid space. It then passes upward, forward, and medially on the medulla oblongata (see Fig. 17-2). At the lower border of the pons, it joins the vessel of the opposite side to form the **basilar artery**.

Branches of the Cranial Portion

1. The **meningeal branches** are small and supply the bone and dura in the posterior cranial fossa.
2. The **posterior spinal artery** may arise from the vertebral artery or the posterior inferior cerebellar artery. It descends on the posterior surface of the spinal cord close to the posterior roots of the spinal

nerves. The branches are reinforced by radicular arteries that enter the vertebral canal through the intervertebral foramina. For the detailed distribution of this artery, see page 471.
3. The **anterior spinal artery** is formed from a contributory branch from each vertebral artery near its termination (see Fig. 17-2). The single artery descends on the anterior surface of the medulla oblongata and spinal cord and is embedded in the pia mater along the anterior median fissure. The artery is reinforced by radicular arteries that enter the vertebral canal through the intervertebral foramina. For the detailed distribution of this artery, see page 472.
4. The **posterior inferior cerebellar artery**, the largest branch of the vertebral artery, passes on an irregular course between the medulla and the cerebellum (see Fig. 17-2; also see Figs. 17-12 and 17-14). It supplies the inferior surface of the vermis, the central nuclei of the cerebellum, and the undersurface of the cerebellar hemisphere; it also supplies the medulla oblongata and the choroid plexus of the fourth ventricle.

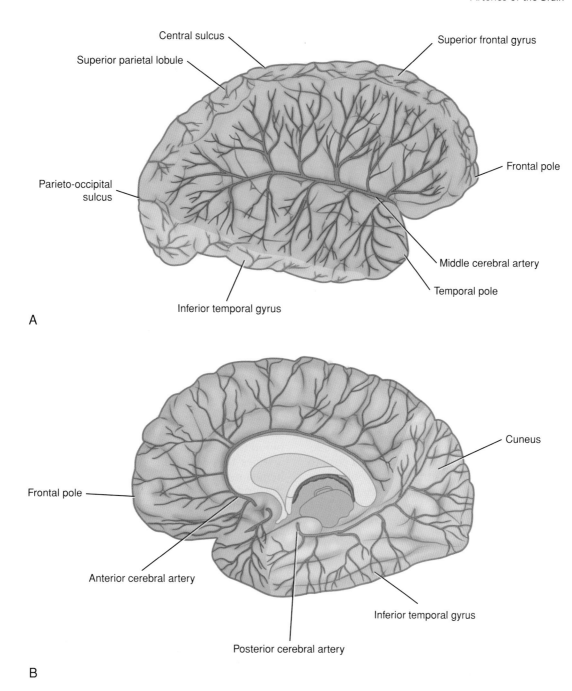

Figure 17-3   Areas supplied by the cerebral arteries. **A:** The lateral surface of the right cerebral hemisphere. **B:** The medial surface of the right cerebral hemisphere. The area supplied by the anterior cerebral artery is colored blue, the area supplied by the middle cerebral artery is pink, and the area supplied by the posterior cerebral artery is brown.

5. The **medullary arteries** are very small branches that are distributed to the medulla oblongata.

Basilar Artery

The basilar artery, formed by the union of the two vertebral arteries (see Fig. 17-1), ascends in a groove on the anterior surface of the pons (see Fig. 17-2; also see Figs. 17-13 and 17-14). At the upper border of the pons, it divides into the two posterior cerebral arteries.

Branches

1. The **pontine arteries** are numerous small vessels that enter the substance of the pons.
2. The **labyrinthine artery** is a long, narrow artery that accompanies the facial and the vestibulocochlear nerves into the internal acoustic meatus and supplies the internal ear. It often arises as a branch of the anterior inferior cerebellar artery.

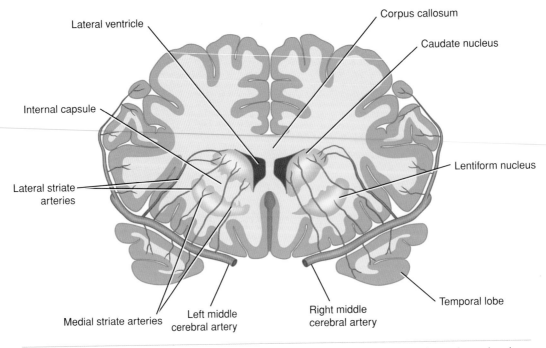

Figure 17-4 Coronal section of the cerebral hemispheres showing the arterial supply to the deep cerebral structures from the middle cerebral artery.

3. The **anterior inferior cerebellar artery** passes posteriorly and laterally and supplies the anterior and inferior parts of the cerebellum. A few branches pass to the pons and the upper part of the medulla oblongata.
4. The **superior cerebellar artery** arises close to the termination of the basilar artery (see Fig. 17-2; also see Figs. 17-11 to 17-14). It winds around the cerebral peduncle and supplies the superior surface of the cerebellum. It also supplies the pons, the pineal gland, and the superior medullary velum.
5. The **posterior cerebral artery** curves laterally and backward around the midbrain and is joined by the posterior communicating branch of the internal carotid artery (see Figs. 17-1 and 17-2; also see Figs. 17-11 to 17-14). **Cortical branches** supply the inferolateral and medial surfaces of the temporal lobe and the lateral and medial surfaces of the occipital lobe (see Fig. 17-3). Thus, the posterior cerebral artery supplies the visual cortex. **Central branches** pierce the brain substance and supply parts of the thalamus and the lentiform nucleus as well as the midbrain, the pineal, and the medial geniculate bodies. A **choroidal branch** enters the inferior horn of the lateral ventricle and supplies the choroid plexus; it also supplies the choroid plexus of the third ventricle.

Circle of Willis

The circle of Willis lies in the interpeduncular fossa at the base of the brain. It is formed by the anastomosis between the two internal carotid arteries and the two vertebral arteries (see Fig. 17-2). The anterior communicating, anterior cerebral, internal carotid, posterior communicating, posterior cerebral, and basilar arteries

all contribute to the circle. The circle of Willis allows blood that enters by either internal carotid or vertebral arteries to be distributed to any part of both cerebral hemispheres. Cortical and central branches arise from the circle and supply the brain substance.

Variations in the sizes of the arteries forming the circle are common, and the absence of one or both posterior communicating arteries has been reported.

Arteries to Specific Brain Areas

The **corpus striatum** and the **internal capsule** are supplied mainly by the medial and lateral striate central branches of the middle cerebral artery (see Fig. 17-4); the central branches of the anterior cerebral artery supply the remainder of these structures.

The **thalamus** is supplied mainly by branches of the posterior communicating, basilar, and posterior cerebral arteries.

The **midbrain** is supplied by the posterior cerebral, superior cerebellar, and basilar arteries.

The **pons** is supplied by the basilar and the anterior, inferior, and superior cerebellar arteries.

The **medulla oblongata** is supplied by the vertebral, anterior and posterior spinal, posterior inferior cerebellar, and basilar arteries.

The **cerebellum** is supplied by the superior cerebellar, anterior inferior cerebellar, and posterior inferior cerebellar arteries.

Nerve Supply of Cerebral Arteries

The cerebral arteries receive a rich supply of sympathetic postganglionic nerve fibers. These fibers are derived from the superior cervical sympathetic ganglion. Stimulation of these nerves causes vasoconstriction of the cerebral arteries. However, under normal conditions, the local blood flow is mainly controlled by the concentrations of carbon dioxide, hydrogen ions, and oxygen present in the nervous tissue; a rise in the carbon dioxide and hydrogen ion concentrations and a lowering of the oxygen tension bring about a vasodilatation.

VEINS OF THE BRAIN

The veins of the brain have no muscular tissue in their very thin walls, and they possess no valves. They emerge from the brain and lie in the subarachnoid space. They pierce the arachnoid mater and the meningeal layer of the dura and drain into the cranial venous sinuses (Fig. 17-5).

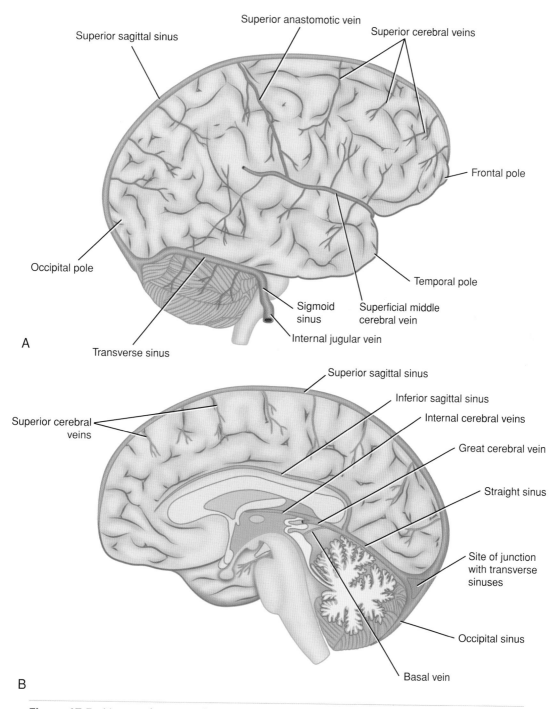

Figure 17-5 Venous drainage of the right cerebral hemisphere. **A:** Lateral surface. **B:** Medial surface.

External Cerebral Veins

The **superior cerebral veins** pass upward over the lateral surface of the cerebral hemisphere and empty into the superior sagittal sinus.

The **superficial middle cerebral vein** drains the lateral surface of the cerebral hemisphere. It runs inferiorly in the lateral sulcus and empties into the cavernous sinus.

The **deep middle cerebral vein** drains the insula and is joined by the **anterior cerebral** and **striate veins** to form the **basal vein**. The basal vein ultimately joins the great cerebral vein, which in turn drains into the straight sinus.

Internal Cerebral Veins

The two internal cerebral veins are formed by the union of the **thalamostriate vein** and the **choroid vein** at the interventricular foramen. The two veins run posteriorly in the tela choroidea of the third ventricle and unite beneath the splenium of the corpus callosum to form the great cerebral vein, which empties into the straight sinus.

Veins of Specific Brain Areas

The **midbrain** is drained by veins that open into the basal or great cerebral veins.

The **pons** is drained by veins that open into the basal vein, cerebellar veins, or neighboring venous sinuses.

The **medulla oblongata** is drained by veins that open into the spinal veins and neighboring venous sinuses.

The **cerebellum** is drained by veins that empty into the great cerebral vein or adjacent venous sinuses.

BRAIN CAPILLARIES

The capillary blood supply to the brain is greater in the gray matter than in the white matter. This is to be expected, since the metabolic activity in the neuronal cell bodies in the gray matter is much greater than in the nerve processes in the white matter. The blood–brain barrier isolates the brain tissue from the rest of the body and is formed by the tight junctions that exist between the endothelial cells in the capillary beds (see pp. 452-453).

CEREBRAL CIRCULATION

The blood flow to the brain must deliver oxygen, glucose, and other nutrients to the nervous tissue and remove carbon dioxide, lactic acid, and other metabolic by-products. The brain has been shown to be supplied with arterial blood from the two internal carotid arteries and the two vertebral arteries. The blood supply to half of the brain is provided by the internal carotid and vertebral arteries on that side, and their respective streams come together in the posterior communicating artery at a point where the pressure of the two is equal and they do not mix (Fig. 17-6). If, however, the internal carotid or vertebral artery is occluded, the blood passes forward or backward across that point to compensate for the reduction in blood flow. The arterial circle also permits the blood to flow across the midline, as shown when the internal carotid or vertebral artery on one side is occluded. It also has been shown that the two streams of blood from the vertebral arteries remain separate and on the same side of the lumen of the basilar artery and do not mix.

Although the cerebral arteries anastomose with one another at the circle of Willis and by means of branches on the surface of the cerebral hemispheres, once they enter the brain substance, no further anastomoses occur.

The most important factor in forcing the blood through the brain is the arterial blood pressure. This is opposed by such factors as a raised intracranial pressure, increased blood viscosity, and narrowing of the vascular diameter. Cerebral blood flow remains

■ Right internal carotid

■ Left internal carotid

■ Right vertebraa

■ Left vertebral

Figure 17-6 Circle of Willis showing the distribution of blood from the four main arteries.

remarkably constant despite changes in the general blood pressure. This autoregulation of the circulation is accomplished by a compensatory lowering of the cerebral vascular resistance when the arterial pressure is decreased and a rising of the vascular resistance when the arterial pressure is increased. Needless to say, this autoregulation does not maintain an adequate blood flow when the arterial blood pressure falls to a very low level.

The diameter of the cerebral blood vessels is the main factor contributing to the cerebrovascular resistance. While cerebral blood vessels are innervated by sympathetic postganglionic nerve fibers and respond to norepinephrine, they apparently play little or no part in the control of cerebrovascular resistance in normal human beings. The most powerful vasodilator influence on cerebral blood vessels is an increase in carbon dioxide or hydrogen ion concentration; a reduction in oxygen concentration also causes vasodilatation. It has been shown, using PET, that an increase in neuronal activity in different parts of the brain causes a local increase in blood flow. For example, viewing an object will increase the oxygen and glucose consumption in the visual cortex of the occipital lobes. This results in an increase in the local concentrations of carbon dioxide and hydrogen ions and brings about a local increase in blood flow.

The cerebral blood flow in patients can be measured by the intracarotid injection or inhalation of radioactive krypton or xenon. Normal cerebral blood flow, per minute, is around 50 to 60 mL/100g of brain tissue.

SPINAL CORD ARTERIES

The spinal cord receives its arterial supply from three small arteries: the two posterior spinal arteries and the anterior spinal artery. These longitudinally running arteries are reinforced by small segmentally arranged arteries that arise from arteries outside the vertebral column and enter the vertebral canal through the intervertebral foramina. These vessels anastomose on the surface of the cord and send branches into the substance of the white and gray matter. Considerable variation exists as to the size and segmental levels at which the reinforcing arteries occur.

Posterior Spinal Arteries

The posterior spinal arteries arise either directly from the vertebral arteries inside the skull or indirectly from the posterior inferior cerebellar arteries. Each artery descends on the posterior surface of the spinal cord close to the posterior nerve roots and gives off branches that enter the substance of the cord (Fig. 17-7). The posterior spinal arteries supply the posterior third of the spinal cord.

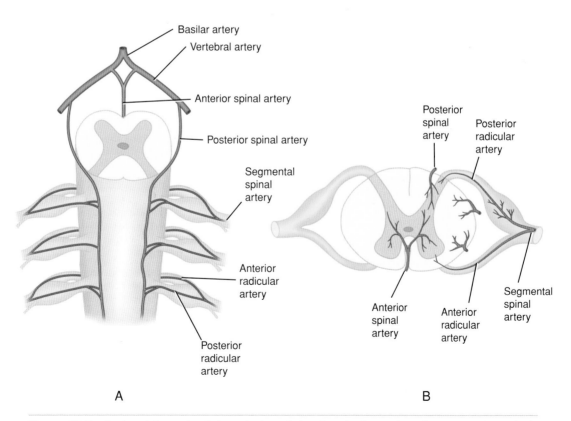

A

B

Figure 17-7   A: Arterial supply of the spinal cord showing the formation of two posterior spinal arteries and one anterior spinal artery. **B:** Transverse section of the spinal cord showing the segmental spinal arteries and the radicular arteries.

The posterior spinal arteries are small in the upper thoracic region, and the first three thoracic segments of the spinal cord are particularly vulnerable to ischemia should the segmental or radicular arteries in this region be occluded.

Anterior Spinal Artery

The anterior spinal artery is formed by the union of two arteries, each of which arises from the vertebral artery inside the skull. The anterior spinal artery then descends on the anterior surface of the spinal cord within the anterior median fissure. Branches from the anterior spinal artery enter the substance of the cord and supply the anterior two-thirds of the spinal cord.

In the upper and lower thoracic segments of the spinal cord, the anterior spinal artery may be extremely small. Should the segmental or radicular arteries be occluded in these regions, the fourth thoracic and the first lumbar segments of the spinal cord would be particularly liable to ischemic necrosis.

Segmental Spinal Arteries

At each intervertebral foramen, the longitudinally running posterior and anterior spinal arteries are reinforced by small segmental arteries on both sides. The arteries are branches of arteries outside the vertebral column (deep cervical, intercostal, and lumbar arteries). Having entered the vertebral canal, each segmental spinal artery gives rise to **anterior** and **posterior radicular arteries** that accompany the anterior and posterior nerve roots to the spinal cord.

Additional **feeder arteries** enter the vertebral canal and anastomose with the anterior and posterior spinal arteries; however, the number and size of these arteries vary considerably from one individual to another. One large and important feeder artery, the **great anterior medullary artery of Adamkiewicz**, arises from the aorta in the lower thoracic or upper lumbar vertebral levels; it is unilateral and, in the majority of persons, enters the spinal cord from the left side. The importance of this artery lies in the fact that it may be the major source of blood to the lower two-thirds of the spinal cord.

SPINAL CORD VEINS

The veins of the spinal cord drain into six tortuous longitudinal channels that communicate superiorly within the skull with the veins of the brain and the venous sinuses. They drain mainly into the internal vertebral venous plexus.

 # Clinical Notes

The brain receives about 15% of the resting cardiac output. The arterial blood reaches the brain through the two internal carotid and the two vertebral arteries; the internal carotid arteries are the major supply of arterial blood.

The distributing arteries—the anterior, middle, and posterior cerebral arteries—that arise from the circle of Willis pass over the outer surface of the brain and anastomose with one another. They give rise to branches that penetrate the brain at right angles. In the brain substance, further branching occurs, but no further anastomoses take place. Anastomoses on the brain surface provide the vital collateral circulation should one of the arteries be occluded by disease.

Despite the recent decrease in cerebrovascular disease, which has been brought about by the treatment of high blood cholesterol and the aggressive treatment of hypertension, cerebrovascular disease is still responsible for about 50% of all adult neurologic hospital admissions.

Cerebral Ischemia

Unconsciousness occurs in 5 to 10 seconds if the blood flow to the brain is completely cut off. Irreversible brain damage with death of nervous tissue rapidly follows complete arrest of cerebral blood flow. Neuronal function is estimated to cease after about 1 minute, and irreversible changes start to occur after about 4 minutes, although this time may be longer if the patient's body has been cooled. (However, brain damage might be reversed if the blood flow can be restored even after 5 minutes.) Cardiac arrest due to coronary thrombosis is the most common cause of this condition.

Cerebral Circulation Interruption

Vascular lesions of the brain are extremely common and the resulting neurologic defect will depend on the size of the artery occluded, the state of the collateral circulation, and the area of the brain involved.

CEREBRAL ARTERY SYNDROMES

Clinical studies and the examination of postmortem material have focused attention on the high frequency of lesions in the common carotid, internal carotid, and vertebral arteries in the neck.

ANTERIOR CEREBRAL ARTERY OCCLUSION

If the occlusion of the anterior cerebral artery is proximal to the anterior communicating artery, the collateral circulation is usually adequate to preserve the circulation. Occlusion distal to the communicating artery may produce the following signs and symptoms:

1. Contralateral hemiparesis and hemisensory loss involving mainly the leg and foot (paracentral lobule of cortex)
2. Inability to identify objects correctly, apathy, and personality changes (frontal and parietal lobes)

MIDDLE CEREBRAL ARTERY OCCLUSION

Occlusion of the middle cerebral artery may produce the following signs and symptoms, but the clinical picture will vary according to the site of occlusion and the degree of collateral anastomoses:

1. Contralateral hemiparesis and hemisensory loss involving mainly the face and arm (precentral and postcentral gyri)

2. Aphasia if the left hemisphere is affected (rarely if the right hemisphere is affected)
3. Contralateral homonymous hemianopia (damage to the optic radiation)
4. Anosognosia if the right hemisphere is affected (rarely if the left hemisphere is affected)

POSTERIOR CEREBRAL ARTERY OCCLUSION

Occlusion of the posterior cerebral artery may produce the following signs and symptoms, but the clinical picture will vary according to the site of the occlusion and the availability of collateral anastomoses:

1. Contralateral homonymous hemianopia with some degree of macular sparing (damage to the calcarine cortex, macular sparing due to the occipital pole receiving collateral blood supply from the middle cerebral artery)
2. Visual agnosia (ischemia of the left occipital lobe)
3. Impairment of memory (possible damage to the medial aspect of the temporal lobe)

INTERNAL CAROTID ARTERY OCCLUSION

Occlusion of the internal carotid artery can occur without causing symptoms or signs or can cause massive cerebral ischemia depending on the degree of collateral anastomoses.

1. The symptoms and signs are those of middle cerebral artery occlusion, including contralateral hemiparesis and hemianesthesia.
2. Partial or complete loss of sight occurs on the same side, but permanent loss is rare (emboli dislodged from the internal carotid artery reach the retina through the ophthalmic artery).

VERTEBROBASILAR ARTERY OCCLUSION

The vertebral and basilar arteries supply all the parts of the central nervous system in the posterior cranial fossa, and through the posterior cerebral arteries, they supply the visual cortex on both sides. The clinical signs and symptoms are extremely varied and may include the following:

1. Ipsilateral pain and temperature sensory loss of the face and contralateral pain and temperature sensory loss of the body
2. Attacks of hemianopia or complete cortical blindness
3. Ipsilateral loss of the gag reflex, dysphagia, and hoarseness as the result of lesions of the nuclei of the glossopharyngeal and vagus nerves
4. Vertigo, nystagmus, nausea, and vomiting
5. Ipsilateral Horner syndrome
6. Ipsilateral ataxia and other cerebellar signs
7. Unilateral or bilateral hemiparesis
8. Coma

Cerebral Blood Flow Impairment

Impairment of cerebral blood flow can be caused by a large number of conditions, and the more important conditions can be considered under the following headings: (1) diseases that produce alteration in blood pressure, (2) diseases of arterial walls, and (3) diseases that result in blockage of the arterial lumen.

POSTURAL HYPOTENSION

Patients who get up after being confined to bed for several days, soldiers who stand at attention for long periods on a hot day, and worshipers kneeling in church may experience the accumulation of venous blood in the limbs or impaired venous return to the heart, with a consequent fall in the cardiac output and a lowered arterial blood pressure. The general arterial pressure has to be lowered considerably before the cerebral blood flow is diminished.

PHYSICAL AND PSYCHOLOGIC SHOCK

The profound and prolonged fall in blood pressure that may follow physical trauma, such as an automobile accident or extensive surgery, especially in older adults in whom the cerebral arteries are already narrowed by disease, may cause the patient to lose consciousness. Hyperventilation in anxiety states may reduce the cerebral blood flow by lowering the carbon dioxide content of the blood.

BLOOD VISCOSITY CHANGES

In polycythemia vera, the cerebral blood flow is considerably reduced as the result of an increase in the viscosity of the blood.

CAROTID SINUS SYNDROME

The carotid sinus, situated at the proximal end of the internal carotid artery, is extremely sensitive to changes in arterial blood pressure. Distention of the arterial wall causes a reflex slowing of the heart rate and a fall in blood pressure. This occurs as the result of an increased number of nervous impulses passing up the sinus nerve, a branch of the glossopharyngeal nerve, which connects with the cardioinhibitory and vasomotor centers. Hypersensitivity of the reflex or external pressure may cause the blood pressure to fall suddenly and produce cerebral ischemia and loss of consciousness.

HEART DISEASE

Any severe cardiac disease, such as coronary thrombosis, auricular fibrillation, or heart block, that results in a marked fall in cardiac output will result in a severe fall in general arterial blood pressure and reduction in cerebral blood flow.

ARTERIAL WALL DISEASE

The most common cause of narrowing of the lumen of the arteries that supply the brain is atheroma. This disease may affect the main arteries supplying the brain in their course through the neck as well as their course within the skull. Moreover, the impairment of the cerebral circulation may be worsened by an attack of coronary thrombosis with its associated hypotension, shock due to surgical procedures, severe anemia, or even rotation of the head with external pressure on the carotid arteries.

Atheromatous degeneration of the cerebral arteries occurs most commonly in middle or old age and often complicates diabetes and hypertension. When actual blockage of an artery occurs, the effect will depend on the size and location of the vessel. The nerve cells and their fibers will degenerate in the avascular area, and the surrounding neuroglia will proliferate and invade the area. In patients with generalized narrowing of the cerebral arteries without blockage of a single artery, the brain will undergo a diffuse atrophy. It should be remembered that a very narrow atheromatous artery may be blocked by a thrombus, thus totally closing the lumen.

DISEASES CAUSING ARTERIAL LUMEN BLOCKAGE

Embolism of a cerebral artery can occur in two forms: (1) a thrombus (by far the most common) and (2) fat globules. The thrombus may develop anywhere on the endothelial lining from the left side of the heart to the parent vessels of the cerebral arteries. A common site of origin is an atheromatous plaque on the internal carotid, common carotid, or vertebral artery. Another area is the site of endocarditis on the mitral or aortic valve or the endocardial lining of a myocardial infarction following a coronary thrombosis. In women, cerebral thrombosis is more common among those taking oral contraceptives, especially those taking a high-dose estrogen–progesterone combination.

Fat embolism usually follows severe fractures of one of the long bones. Fat globules from the macerated yellow marrow enter the nutrient veins, pass through the pulmonary circulation, and end up blocking multiple small cerebral end arteries.

Cerebral Aneurysms

Congenital aneurysms occur most commonly at the site where two arteries join in the formation of the circle of Willis. At this point, the tunica media has a deficiency and this is complicated by the development of atheroma, which so weakens the arterial wall that a local dilatation occurs. The aneurysm may press on neighboring structures, such as the optic nerve or the third, fourth, or sixth cranial nerve, and produce signs or symptoms or may suddenly rupture into the subarachnoid space. In the latter case, a severe pain in the head suddenly develops, followed by mental confusion. Death may quickly occur, or the patient may survive the first bleeding only to die a few days or weeks later. Clipping or ligating the neck of the aneurysm offers the best chance of recovery.

Other than congenital aneurysms, aneurysms are rare and include those due to softening of the arterial wall following the lodging of an infected embolus; those due to damage of the internal carotid artery as it lies within the cavernous sinus following a fracture of the skull; and those that are associated with disease of the arterial wall, such as atheroma.

Intracranial Hemorrhage

Intracranial hemorrhage can result from trauma or cerebral vascular lesions. Four varieties are considered: (1) epidural, (2) subdural, (3) subarachnoid, and (4) cerebral. Epidural and subdural hemorrhages are described on pp. 429-430.

Subarachnoid Hemorrhage

Subarachnoid hemorrhage usually results from leakage or rupture of a congenital aneurysm on the cerebral arterial circle or, less commonly, from an angioma or contusion and laceration of the brain and meninges. The symptoms, which are sudden in onset, will include severe headache, stiffness of the neck, and loss of consciousness. The diagnosis is established by the use of computed tomography (CT). The dense areas of the blood in the subarachnoid space can be identified. The withdrawal of heavily blood-stained cerebrospinal fluid through a lumbar puncture is also diagnostic, but this method has been replaced by the use of CT.

Cerebral Hemorrhage

Cerebral hemorrhage generally is due to rupture of an atheromatous artery and is most common in patients with hypertension. It usually occurs in individuals of middle age and often involves a rupture of the thin-walled lenticulostriate artery, a branch of the middle cerebral artery. The important corticonuclear and corticospinal fibers in the internal capsule are damaged, producing hemiplegia on the opposite side of the body. The patient immediately loses consciousness, and the paralysis is evident when consciousness is regained. In some cases, the hemorrhage bursts into the lateral ventricle, resulting in deeper unconsciousness and corticospinal lesions on both sides of the body. Hemorrhage may also occur into the pons and cerebellum.

Computed Tomography, Magnetic Resonance Imaging, and Positron Emission Tomography

CT, magnetic resonance imaging (MRI), and PET are techniques that are indispensable in making the diagnosis of different forms of cerebrovascular disease. The diagnosis can usually be made with speed, accuracy, and safety. An intracranial blood clot can be recognized by its density. These techniques have largely replaced cerebral angiography (see below).

Cerebral Angiography

The technique of cerebral angiography is used for the detection of abnormalities of the blood vessels; the detection and localization of space-occupying lesions such as tumors, hematomas, or abscesses; or the determination of the vascular pattern of tumors to aid in the diagnosis of their pathology. With the patient under general anesthesia and in the supine position, the head is centered on a radiographic apparatus that will take repeated radiographs at 2-second intervals. Both anteroposterior and lateral projections are obtained. A radiopaque medium is injected rapidly into the lumen of the common carotid or vertebral artery or is indirectly introduced into one of these arteries through a catheter inserted into the radial or femoral artery. As the radiopaque material is rapidly introduced, a series of films is exposed. By this means, the cerebral arteries, the capillary flush, and the veins may be demonstrated. Examples of normal-appearing carotid and vertebral angiograms are shown in Figures 17-8 to 17-15.

Cerebral angiography is an invasive technique that unfortunately has a morbidity of 0.5% to 2.5%. CT and MRI should therefore be used whenever possible. PET is now also used extensively.

Spinal Cord Ischemia

The blood supply to the spinal cord is surprisingly meager considering the importance of this nervous tissue. The posterior and anterior spinal arteries are of small and variable diameter, and the reinforcing segmental arteries vary in number and size.

The posterior third of the spinal cord receives its arterial supply from the posterior spinal arteries. The anterior two-thirds of the spinal cord are supplied by the small, tenuous anterior spinal artery. This latter artery therefore supplies the anterior white column, the anterior gray horns, and the anterior part of the lateral white columns and the root of the posterior horns.

Occlusion of the anterior spinal artery may produce the following signs and symptoms (Fig. 17-16).

1. Loss of motor function (paraplegia) below the level of the lesion occurs due to bilateral damage to the corticospinal tracts.
2. Bilateral thermoanesthesia and analgesia occur below the level of the lesion due to bilateral damage to the spinothalamic tracts.
3. Weakness of the limb muscles may occur due to damage of the anterior gray horns in the cervical or lumbar regions of the cord.
4. Loss of bladder and bowel control occurs due to damage of the descending autonomic tracts.

Figure 17-8 Lateral internal carotid arteriogram. Male aged 20 years.

Middle cerebral artery

Opexrculofrontal branch

Callosomarginal trunk

Cortical (frontal) branches

Pericallosal artery

Anterior cerebral artery

Frontopolar artery

Ophthalmic artery

Internal carotid artery
in cavernous sinus

Superficial temporal artery

Maxillary artery

Ascending palatine artery

Facial artery

Lingual artery   Superior thyroid artery

Posterior parietal artery
Cortical (parietal) branches

Angular artery

Posterior temporal artery

Posterior cerebral artery

Posterior auricular artery

Occipital artery

External carotid artery

Internal carotid artery in neck

Bifurcation of common carotid artery

Common carotid artery

C1
C2
C3
C4

X-rays

Cassette

Figure 17-9 Main features seen in radiograph in Figure 17-8.

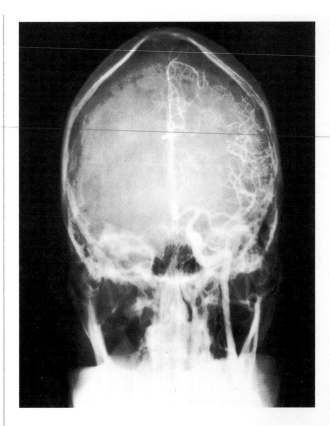

Figure 17-10 Anteroposterior internal carotid arteriogram. Male aged 20 years.

Figure 17-11 Main features seen in the radiograph in Figure 17-10.

Figure 17-12 Lateral vertebral arteriogram. Male aged 20 years.

Coronal suture

Anterior cerebral arteries

Posterior cerebral arteries

Internal occipital artery

Posterior temporal artery

Posterior communicating artery

Superior cerebellar artery

Basal artery

Posterior inferior cerebellar artery

Vertebral artery passing through foramen magnum of skull

Anterior arch of atlas

Meningeal branches

Posterior arch of atlas

Spinal branches

Muscular branches

Vertebral artery passing through foramina transversaria of first through sixth cervical vertebrae

X-rays

Cassette

Figure 17-13 Main features shown in the radiograph in Figure 17-12.

Figure 17-14 Anteroposterior (angled) vertebral arteriogram. Woman aged 35 years.

Figure 17-15 Main features shown in the radiograph in Figure 17-14.

Figure 17-16 Anterior spinal artery occlusion. Pink area denotes region of spinal cord affected.

5. Position sense, vibration, and light touch are normal due to preservation of the posterior white columns that are supplied by the posterior spinal arteries.

Ischemia of the spinal cord can easily follow minor damage to the arterial supply as the result of nerve block procedures, aortic surgery, or any operation in which severe hypotension occurs. The fourth thoracic and first lumbar segments of the cord are particularly prone to ischemia.

Spinal Cord Ischemia and Thoracic Aortic Dissection

The thoracic region of the spinal cord receives its segmental arteries from the posterior intercostal arteries, which arise directly from the thoracic aorta. In thoracic aortic dissection, the expanding blood clot in the aortic wall can block the origins of the posterior intercostal arteries, causing ischemia of the spinal cord.

Spinal Cord Ischemia as a Complication of a Leaking Abdominal Aortic Aneurysm

The lumbar region of the spinal cord receives its segmental arteries from the lumbar arteries, which are branches of the abdominal aorta. The effect of direct pressure on the lumbar arteries by a leaking aneurysm can interfere with the blood supply to the spinal cord.

Key Concepts

Blood Supply of the Brain

- The brain is supplied by the two internal carotid and the two vertebral arteries that lie within cerebrospinal fluid of the subarachnoid space.
- The internal carotid begins at the bifurcation of the common carotid in the neck, where it possesses a local dilation called the carotid sinus.
- The internal carotid enters the cranial cavity through the carotid canal of the temporal bone.
- The internal carotid terminates as the anterior and middle cerebral arteries after giving off ophthalmic and posterior communicating arteries.
- The two vertebral arteries enter the cranial cavity through the foramen magnum after ascending through the transverse foramina of the cervical vertebrae.
- The cranial portion of the vertebral artery gives off the posterior spinal, anterior spinal, posterior inferior cerebellar, medullary, and meningeal arteries.

- The vertebral arteries merge to form the basilar artery on the anterior surface of the pons.
- The basilar artery branches into pontine, labyrinthine, anterior inferior cerebellar, superior cerebellar, and posterior cerebral arteries.
- The circle of Willis is formed by the anastomosis between the two internal carotid and vertebral blood supplies by communication of the anterior cerebral and anterior communicating arteries, internal carotid arteries, posterior communicating and posterior cerebral arteries, and the basilar artery.
- The corpus striatum and internal capsule are supplied by the medial and lateral striate branches of the middle cerebral artery.
- The thalamus is supplied by branches of the posterior communicating, basilar, and posterior cerebral arteries.
- The midbrain is supplied by the posterior cerebral, superior cerebellar, and basilar arteries.

- The pons is supplied by the basilar, anterior inferior, and superior cerebellar arteries.
- The medulla oblongata is supplied by the vertebral, anterior and posterior spinal, posterior inferior cerebellar, and basilar arteries.
- The cerebellum is supplied by the superior cerebellar, anterior inferior cerebellar, and posterior inferior cerebellar arteries.

Blood Supply of the Spinal Cord

- The spinal cord receives its arterial supply from three small arteries: two posterior spinal arteries and the anterior spinal artery.
- These longitudinally running arteries are reinforced by small segmentally arranged arteries that enter the vertebral column through the intervertebral foramina of the vertebral column.

 Clinical Problem Solving

1. A distinguished neurosurgeon, while giving a lecture on cerebrovascular accidents, made the following statement: "It is generally agreed that there are no anastomoses of clinical importance between the terminal end arteries within the brain substance, but there are many important anastomoses between the large arteries, both within and outside the skull, and these may play a major role in determining the extent of brain damage in cerebral vascular disease." Comment on this statement, and name the sites at which important arterial anastomoses take place.
2. During examination of a carotid angiogram, the contrast medium had filled the anterior and middle cerebral arteries but had failed to fill the posterior cerebral artery. Careful following of the contrast medium showed it to enter the posterior communicating artery but to extend no farther. Explain this phenomenon in a normal person.
3. A 45-year-old man was admitted to the hospital after collapsing in his home 3 days previously. He was in a partial state of unconsciousness on the floor and was found by a friend. On physical examination, he had right-sided homonymous hemianopia, although careful examination of the fields of vision showed that the macular regions were normal. Right-sided hemianesthesia and hemianalgesia also were present, although the patient complained of severe burning pain in the right leg. During the first 24 hours in the hospital, the patient demonstrated mild right-sided hemiparesis of the flaccid type, which disappeared within 2 days. What is your diagnosis? Be specific in describing the branches of the artery that are involved.
4. During the course of an autopsy on a patient who had recently died of cerebrovascular disease, the pathologist made the comment that in atherosclerosis of the cerebral arteries, the atheromatous plaques tend to occur where the main arteries divide or where the arteries suddenly curve. At these sites, pressure flow changes may be a factor

in the causation of the disease process. Using your knowledge of anatomy, name as many sites as you can where the main cerebral arteries divide or undergo abrupt change in their course.
5. Having carefully examined a male patient with cerebrovascular disease, the physician met with the family to discuss the nature of the illness, the course of treatment, and the prognosis. The daughter asked the physician what was meant by the term *stroke* as well as its common causes. He was also asked why the clinical findings vary so much from patient to patient. Using your knowledge of the anatomy and physiology of cerebral blood flow, explain why patients with cerebrovascular disease present such a variety of syndromes.
6. The classic sign of cerebrovascular disease is hemiplegia, yet we know that most patients also exhibit sensory deficits of different types. Using your knowledge of the anatomical distribution of the cerebral arteries, discuss the main types of sensory loss that you may find in such patients.
7. During the discussion of the symptoms and signs of a 70-year-old woman who had been admitted to the hospital for treatment of cerebrovascular disease, a fourth-year medical student made the comment that she was surprised to find that many of the signs and symptoms were bilateral in this patient. She said that the three previous patients she had examined had displayed only unilateral signs and symptoms. Using your knowledge of neuroanatomy, explain why some patients exhibit bilateral signs and symptoms, while in others the syndrome is clearly unilateral.
8. Neurologists speak frequently of the dominant hemisphere and if cerebrovascular disease should involve that hemisphere, one would expect the patient possibly to have global or total sensorimotor aphasia. Explain this phenomenon.
9. Explain why patients with a thrombosis of the middle cerebral artery often present with homonymous hemianopia as well as hemiplegia and hemianesthesia.

10. During the neurobiology course, the professor of neuroanatomy emphasized the importance of knowing the structure and blood supply of the internal capsule. He explained the arrangement of the ascending and descending tracts within the capsule and showed how they were concentrated into a small area between the thalamus and caudate nucleus medially and the lentiform nucleus laterally. Clearly, an interruption of the blood supply to this vital area would produce widespread neurologic defects. What is the blood supply to the internal capsule?

11. A 36-year-old man visited his physician with a complaint that on three occasions during the past 6 months, he had fainted at work. During careful questioning, the patient stated that on each occasion, he had fainted while sitting at his desk and while interviewing office personnel; he added that the person being interviewed sat in a chair immediately to the right of the desk. He said that before each fainting attack he felt dizzy; then, he lost consciousness only to recover within a few moments. The previous evening, he had a similar dizzy spell when he turned his head quickly to the right to talk to a friend in the street. The physician noted that the patient wore a stiff collar that was rather close fitting. When the physician commented on this, the patient stated that he always wore this type of collar to work. No abnormal physical signs were found. Using your knowledge of anatomy and physiology, what diagnosis would you make?

12. A 45-year-old man, a company director, rose to give his annual after-dinner speech to the board when he suddenly experienced an "agonizing, crushing" pain over the sternum. Feeling giddy and weak, he fell back in his chair. A few moments later, he lapsed into unconsciousness. An attendant at the dinner, who had received some training in cardiopulmonary resuscitation while a member of the armed forces, ran forward and noted that the patient had stopped breathing. He quickly started mouth-to-mouth resuscitation and cardiac compression and kept going until ambulance personnel arrived to take the patient to the hospital. The physician in the intensive care unit at the hospital later told the patient that his life had been saved by the alertness and competence of the attendant at the dinner. Using your knowledge of neurophysiology, state how long brain tissue can survive with complete cardiac arrest and when breathing has ceased.

13. A 62-year-old man with a history of hypertension visited his physician because the day before, he had temporarily lost the sight in his right eye. He explained that the sight loss was partial and lasted about half an hour. On close questioning, the patient admitted that he had had similar episodes of blindness in the same eye during the previous 6 months, but they had lasted only a few minutes. The patient also mentioned that there were days when he could not remember the names of people and things. He also had recently experienced severe right-sided

headaches. When asked about his activities, he said that he could not walk as well as he used to and his left leg sometimes felt weak and numb. While performing a careful physical examination, the physician heard with his stethoscope a distinct systolic bruit over the right side of the neck. Given that the patient has vascular disease of the brain, which artery is likely to be involved in the disease process? What special clinical investigations could you perform to confirm the diagnosis?

14. A 39-year-old man was admitted to the hospital with a history of a sudden excruciating, generalized headache while gardening. This was followed, 10 minutes later, by the patient collapsing to the ground in a state of unconsciousness. After being carried indoors and placed on a settee, the patient regained consciousness but appeared confused. He complained of a severe headache and a stiff neck. Physical examination revealed some rigidity of the neck but nothing further. A careful neurologic examination 3 days later revealed some loss of tone in the muscles of the left leg. Using your knowledge of anatomy, make the diagnosis. What is the reason for the neck rigidity?

15. A 26-year-old man, on leaving a bar after a few drinks, stepped into the road at 1:00 AM and was struck by a passing car. Fortunately, the car was traveling slowly and struck the patient's head a glancing blow. One hour later, a policeman found the patient unconscious on the sidewalk. Physical examination at the local hospital found that the patient had recovered consciousness for a few minutes but then had quickly relapsed into an unconscious state. The right pupil was dilated, and the muscle tone of the left leg was found to be less than normal. A positive Babinski sign was obtained on the left side. Examination of the scalp showed a severe bruise over the right temple, and a lateral radiograph of the skull showed a fracture of the anterior inferior angle of the parietal bone. A CT scan showed a dense area extending from anterior to posterior along the inner table of the right parietal bone. What is the diagnosis? Let us suppose that the equipment for performing a CT scan was unavailable and that it was decided to perform a lumbar puncture; this test revealed a raised cerebrospinal fluid pressure, and the fluid was very slightly blood stained. Explain these additional findings.

16. A 50-year-old woman complaining of headaches, drowsiness, and mental confusion visited her physician. On close questioning, the patient distinctly remembered striking her head against a closet door when bending down 3 weeks previously. A CT scan revealed the presence of a large space-occupying lesion over the right frontal lobe of the brain. What is the possible diagnosis?

17. A 55-year-old man with a history of hypertension collapsed in the street while walking to work. He complained of a sudden severe headache. After 5 minutes, his face began to sag on the right side

and his speech became slurred. On admission to the hospital, his right arm and leg were found to be weaker than the left, and the muscles were hypotonic. The eyes were deviated to the left. Later, the right arm and leg showed complete paralysis and were insensitive to pinprick. A positive Babinski sign was present on the right side. Two hours later, the patient relapsed into a deep coma with bilateral dilated fixed pupils. Later, the respirations became deep and irregular, and the patient died 6 hours later. Using your knowledge of neuroanatomy, make the diagnosis.

18. What is the blood supply to the spinal cord? Which areas of the spinal cord are supplied by the anterior spinal artery? Which regions of the spinal cord are most susceptible to ischemia?

 Answers and Explanations to Clinical Problem Solving

1. Once the terminal branches of the cerebral arteries enter the brain substance, no further anastomoses occur. Blockage of such end arteries by disease is quickly followed by neuronal death and necrosis. The surrounding neuroglia then usually proliferates and invades the area, producing a neuroglial scar or forming a cystic cavity. The following important anastomoses exist between the cerebral arteries: (a) the circle of Willis; (b) anastomoses between the branches of the cerebral arteries on the surface of the cerebral hemispheres and the cerebellar hemispheres; and (c) anastomoses between the branches of the internal and external carotid arteries: (i) at their origin at the common carotid artery, (ii) at the anastomosis between the branches of the ophthalmic artery within the orbit and the facial and maxillary arteries, and (iii) between the meningeal branches of the internal carotid artery and the middle meningeal artery.

2. The work of McDonald and Potter in 1951 showed that the posterior communicating artery is the site at which the streams of blood from the internal carotid and vertebral arteries on the same side come together, and since their pressures at this point are equal, they do not mix. Nevertheless, in clinical practice, good filling of the posterior cerebral artery with radiopaque material as shown by carotid angiography occurs in about 25% of patients. Slight filling also may be seen in other normal individuals. The variable results can be explained on the basis that the size of the arteries making up the arterial circle is subject to considerable variation, and consequently, the blood flow in different individuals may vary.

3. Occlusion of the cortical branches of the left posterior cerebral artery will give rise to right-sided homonymous hemianopia because of ischemia of the primary visual area in the calcarine fissure. The escape of the macular region could be accounted for by the overlapping of the arterial supply of this area of the occipital lobe by the left posterior and left middle cerebral arteries. The right-sided hemianesthesia and the severe burning pain in the right leg are referred to clinically as the thalamic syndrome and are due to occlusion of one of the central branches of the left posterior cerebral artery that supplies the sensory nuclei of the left thalamus.

The presence of a mild fleeting right-sided hemiparesis could be explained by a temporary occlusion of a branch of the left posterior cerebral artery to the left cerebral peduncle.

4. Atheromatous plaques tend to occur at the following sites: (a) carotid sinus of the internal carotid artery at or just beyond the bifurcation of the common carotid artery, (b) the first main bifurcation of the middle cerebral artery, (c) where the vertebral arteries join to form the basilar artery, (d) where the anterior cerebral artery curves superiorly and posteriorly over the genu of the corpus callosum, and (e) where the posterior cerebral artery passes around the lateral side of the cerebral peduncle.

5. A stroke may be defined as a sudden development of a neurologic defect, usually associated with the development of some degree of hemiplegia and sometimes accompanied by unconsciousness; it is usually caused by a cerebrovascular accident. The symptoms and signs will depend on the cause of the interruption of cerebral blood flow and the size of the artery involved. For example, cerebral embolism or cerebral hemorrhage is a sudden event, whereas the development of atherosclerosis in a patient with hypertension is a slow process that suddenly may become worse when thrombosis occurs at the site of the atheromatous plaque. Hemiplegia is the most common sign, but many additional sensory defects may develop, depending on the artery blocked. Examples are hemianesthesia, hemianopia, dysphasia, and dysarthria.

6. Occlusion of the middle cerebral artery or its branches can produce, in addition to paralysis of the muscles of the opposite side of the body, contralateral hemianesthesia owing to ischemia of the postcentral gyrus and homonymous hemianopia owing to ischemia of the optic radiation. Occlusion of the anterior cerebral artery or its branches may produce contralateral sensory loss in the leg, foot, and toes owing to ischemia of the leg area of the cerebral cortex. Occlusion of the posterior cerebral artery or its branches may produce contralateral homonymous hemianopia owing to ischemia of the primary visual area in the region of the calcarine fissure. If the branches to the thalamus also are blocked, there will also be contralateral hemianesthesia and possibly the development of severe pain in the same areas.

These sensory deficits are the main ones seen. The degree of sensory involvement will depend on the size and number of branches of the artery occluded.

7. The internal carotid and the basilar arteries are equally affected by disease. The internal carotid artery supplies predominantly one cerebral hemisphere through the anterior cerebral and middle cerebral branches; therefore, occlusion of the internal carotid artery will produce contralateral hemiplegia, hemianesthesia, hemianopia, and aphasia and agnosia, depending on whether the dominant hemisphere is involved. On the other hand, the basilar artery contributes to the blood supply of both sides of the brain through the two posterior cerebral arteries and the many branches to both sides of the brainstem. Consequently, occlusion of the basilar artery will result in bilateral motor and sensory losses and involvement of the cranial nerves and cerebellum on both sides of the body.

8. The dominant hemisphere possesses the language function. In right-handed individuals (and in some left-handed persons), language is a function of the left hemisphere. A cerebrovascular accident involving the middle cerebral artery on the left side will therefore be more serious than one on the right side, since it will involve the cortical speech area and cause a total sensory motor aphasia. In persons who have a dominant right hemisphere, the reverse occurs.

9. The middle cerebral artery, in addition to giving off cortical branches, gives off central branches that supply part of the posterior limb of the internal capsule and the optic radiation. Occlusion of these branches will cause contralateral homonymous hemianopia.

10. Since so many important ascending and descending tracts travel in the internal capsule, an occlusion of its blood supply would produce a widespread neurologic deficit. The internal capsule is supplied by the medial and lateral striate central branches of the middle cerebral artery and by the central branches of the anterior cerebral artery.

11. This patient has the symptoms of the carotid sinus syndrome. For a full description of this syndrome, see page 473.

12. It has been estimated that irreversible changes start to occur in the cerebral nervous tissue about 4 minutes following the complete arrest of cerebral blood flow. (This figure may be higher if the patient's body has been cooled.)

13. The impairment of vision of the right eye with motor symptoms in the left leg strongly suggests partial occlusion of the right internal carotid artery. When these are coupled with impairment of memory and a systolic bruit over the right internal carotid artery, the diagnosis is almost certain. The right-sided headaches are also common symptoms in this condition. A right-sided carotid angiogram can confirm the presence of extreme narrowing of the internal carotid artery at its origin. Ophthalmodynamometric measurements can show diminished retinal arterial pressure on the right side owing to diminished pressure in the right ophthalmic artery.

14. This patient had a congenital aneurysm of the anterior communicating artery. The sudden onset of a severe headache, which is often so dramatic that the patient feels as though he or she has been hit on the head, is characteristic of rupture of a congenital aneurysm into the subarachnoid space. The stiff or rigid neck is due to meningeal irritation caused by the presence of blood in the subarachnoid space. This patient had no evidence of previous pressure on the optic nerve leading to unilateral visual defect, which sometimes occurs when the aneurysm is situated on the anterior part of the circle of Willis. The loss of tone in the left leg muscles is difficult to explain, although it may be due to the sudden hemorrhage into the subarachnoid space causing damage to the right cerebral hemisphere.

15. This patient had a right-sided extradural hemorrhage due to a fracture of the anterior part of the parietal bone, which tore the anterior division of the right middle meningeal artery. The history of the patient being found unconscious and then regaining consciousness for a period only to relapse into unconsciousness is a characteristic finding. The initial trauma usually is responsible for the initial loss of consciousness. The relapse into an unconscious state is due to the accumulation of a large blood clot under arterial pressure outside the meningeal layer of dura. This is responsible for the dilated pupil on the right side due to indirect pressure on the right oculomotor nerve. The pressure on the right precentral gyrus causes the hemiplegia and weakness of the left leg; it also causes the positive Babinski sign on the left side. The presence of a large blood clot in the intracranial cavity was easily recognized on a CT scan. The presence of the clot was also responsible for the raised cerebrospinal fluid pressure. The slight blood staining of the fluid obtained from a spinal tap was due to a small leakage of blood from the extradural space into the subarachnoid space at the fracture site.

16. This patient had a chronic subdural hematoma following trauma to the head 3 weeks previously. This resulted from one of the superior cerebral veins tearing at its point of entrance into the superior sagittal sinus. The blood accumulated under low pressure between the dura and the arachnoid. The headaches, drowsiness, and mental confusion were due to the raised intracranial pressure. The blood clot could be seen easily on the CT scan. The blood clot was successfully removed through a burr hole in the skull, and the patient had no further symptoms.

17. The history of hypertension, sudden onset of severe headache, slurring of speech, right lower facial weakness, right-sided hemiplegia, right positive Babinski sign, right-sided hemianesthesia, and deviation of the eyes to the left side are all diagnostic of a cerebrovascular accident involving the left cerebral hemisphere. The perforating central branches of the left middle cerebral artery were found at autopsy to be extensively affected by atherosclerosis. One of these arteries had ruptured, resulting in

a large hemorrhage into the left lentiform nucleus and left internal capsule. The combination of hypertension and atherosclerotic degeneration of the artery was responsible for the fatal hemorrhage. The dilated fixed pupils, the irregularity in breathing, and, finally, death were due to the raised pressure within the hemisphere causing downward pressure effects within the brainstem.

18. The blood supply to the spinal cord is fully described on pages 471-472. The anterior spinal artery supplies the anterior two-thirds of the spinal cord. The upper and lower thoracic segments of the spinal cord have a relatively poor supply of blood because the anterior spinal artery in this region may be extremely small; therefore, they are more susceptible to ischemia.

? Review Questions

Directions: Each of the numbered items in this section is followed by answers. Select the ONE lettered answer that is CORRECT.

1. The following statements concern the blood supply to the brain:
   (a) The brain receives its blood supply directly from the two external carotid arteries.
   (b) The circle of Willis is formed by the anterior cerebral, the internal carotid, the posterior cerebral, the basilar, and the anterior and posterior communicating arteries.
   (c) The cerebral arteries do not anastomose on the surface of the brain.
   (d) Numerous anastomoses occur between the branches of the cerebral arteries once they have entered the substance of the brain.
   (e) The main blood supply to the internal capsule is from the central branches of the anterior cerebral artery.

2. The areas of the cerebral cortex listed below receive their arterial supply as indicated:
   (a) The precentral gyrus (face area) is supplied by the middle cerebral artery.
   (b) The postcentral gyrus (face area) is supplied by the anterior cerebral artery.
   (c) The cuneus is supplied by the anterior cerebral artery.
   (d) The inferior temporal gyrus is supplied by the middle cerebral artery.
   (e) The Wernicke area is supplied by the posterior cerebral artery.

3. The arteries listed below arise from the main stem arteries as indicated:
   (a) The ophthalmic artery is a branch of the middle cerebral artery.
   (b) The pontine arteries are branches of the internal carotid artery.
   (c) The posterior communicating artery is a branch of the middle cerebral artery.
   (d) The posterior spinal artery arises from the vertebral artery.
   (e) The posterior inferior cerebellar artery is a branch of the basilar artery.

4. The veins listed below drain into the venous sinuses indicated:
   (a) The superior cerebral veins drain into the inferior sagittal sinus.
   (b) The great cerebral vein drains into the superior sagittal sinus.
   (c) The superior cerebellar veins drain only into the straight sinus.
   (d) The spinal veins drain into the external vertebral venous plexus.
   (e) The inferior sagittal sinus drains into the straight sinus.

5. The following statements concern the cerebral blood flow:
   (a) The sympathetic postganglionic fibers exert great control over the diameter of the cerebral blood vessels.
   (b) It varies greatly with changes in the general blood pressure.
   (c) Oxygen tension in the cerebral blood has no effect on the diameter of the cerebral blood vessels.
   (d) One of the most powerful vasodilators of cerebral blood vessels is carbon dioxide.
   (e) The blood flow for a particular area of nervous tissue following occlusion of a cerebral artery does not depend on the collateral circulation.

6. The following statements concern cerebral ischemia:
   (a) Atheromatous degeneration of a cerebral artery does not cause degeneration of the nerve cells in the avascular area due to the presence of cerebrospinal fluid.
   (b) Neuronal function ceases after the blood flow has stopped for about 10 seconds.
   (c) Irreversible cerebral damage starts to occur after the blood flow has ceased for about 4 minutes.
   (d) Shock occurring as the result of severe physical trauma does not result in cerebral ischemia.
   (e) Cooling of the patient's body following a cerebrovascular accident speeds up cerebral degeneration.

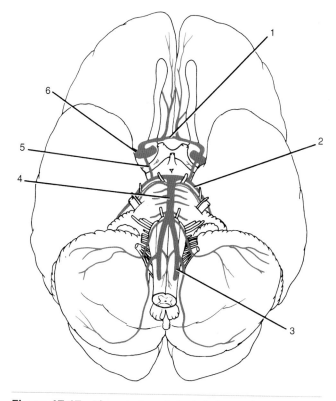

Figure 17-17   The arteries of the inferior surface of the brain.

Matching Questions. Directions: The following questions apply to Figure 17-17. Match the numbered arteries listed below with the appropriate lettered arteries. Each lettered option may be selected once, more than once, or not at all.

7. Number 1
8. Number 2
9. Number 3
10. Number 4
11. Number 5
12. Number 6

(a) Middle cerebral artery
(b) Anterior communicating artery
(c) Posterior cerebral artery
(d) Basilar artery
(e) None of the above

Directions: In the next item, select the ONE lettered answer that is CORRECT.

13. The following statements concern the blood supply to the spinal cord:
    (a) The posterior spinal arteries supply the posterior third of the spinal cord.
    (b) The veins do not communicate with the veins of the brain and the venous sinuses.
    (c) The arteria radicularis magna (artery of Adamkiewicz) arises in the lower thoracic region from the arch of the aorta.
    (d) The anterior spinal artery is double but usually arises from one vertebral artery.
    (e) The spinal arteries are not reinforced by branches of local arteries.

Directions: Each case history is followed by questions. Read the case history, then select the ONE BEST lettered answer.

A 58-year-old man, while eating his evening meal, suddenly complained of a severe headache. Moments later, he slumped forward and lost consciousness.

14. On being admitted to the hospital, the examining physician could have found the following physical signs **except:**
    (a) He was in a deep coma, and his breathing was deep and slow.
    (b) The patient's head was turned to the left.
    (c) The right side of his face was flattened, and saliva was drooling out of the right corner of his mouth.
    (d) The muscle tone of the limbs was less on the right side than on the left.
    (e) The right abdominal reflexes were absent, and there was a positive Babinski response on the left side.

15. Three days later, the patient regained consciousness, and the following additional signs could have become apparent **except:**
    (a) The right arm and, to a lesser extent, the right leg were paralyzed.
    (b) Movements of the left arm and leg and the left side of the face were normal.
    (c) The upper and lower parts of the right side of his face were paralyzed.
    (d) The patient had difficulty in swallowing.
    (e) The patient was unable to speak.

16. During the next 2 weeks, the following signs could have developed **except:**
    (a) The muscles of the limbs on the right side became hypertonic.
    (b) The tendon reflexes on the right side became hyperactive.
    (c) The patient had some sensory loss on the right side.
    (d) The patient was suffering from urinary incontinence.
    (e) The muscles on the left side exhibited hypotonia.

17. The neurologist in charge of this patient interpreted the findings as follows. All his interpretations were likely to be correct **except:**
    (a) The sudden onset of a severe headache followed by loss of consciousness is a common finding in patients with a blockage of a cerebral artery.
    (b) The depth of coma is unrelated to the extent of the arterial blockage.
    (c) Paralysis of the face on the right side indicated the presence of a lesion on the left side of the brain.
    (d) The patient's head and eyes were turned to the left (i.e., to the side of the lesion).
    (e) The loss of right-sided abdominal reflexes indicated the presence of a lesion on the left side of the brain.

18. The following physical signs and known anatomical data strongly suggested the involvement of the left middle cerebral artery **except:**
    (a) Paralysis of the right side of the face and the right arm was more severe than that of the right leg.
    (b) The presence of aphasia.
    (c) The central branches of the middle cerebral artery do not supply the lentiform nucleus, the caudate nucleus, and the internal capsule.
    (d) The left middle cerebral artery supplies the entire lateral surface of the cerebral hemisphere except for the narrow strip supplied by the anterior cerebral artery.
    (e) The left posterior cerebral artery supplies the occipital pole and the inferolateral surface of the cerebral hemisphere.

A 60-year-old man was admitted to the emergency department, complaining of the sudden onset of excruciating, sharp, tearing pain localized to the back of the chest and the back. After a thorough physical and radiologic examination, a diagnosis of dissection of the descending thoracic aorta was made. Within a few hours, the patient started to experience "girdle" pain involving the fourth thoracic dermatome on both sides. Later, he was found to have bilateral thermoanesthesia and analgesia below the level of the fourth thoracic dermatome. Position sense, vibration, and light touch remained normal. Complete spastic paralysis of both legs quickly developed.

19. The sudden onset of "girdle" pain in this patient was **most likely caused by:**
    (a) Pressure on the fourth thoracic spinal nerves
    (b) Blockage of the origins of the posterior intercostal arteries that give rise to the segmental spinal arteries by the aortic dissection
    (c) Discomfort caused by the expanding aneurysm
    (d) Osteoarthritis of the vertebral column
20. The development of bilateral thermoanesthesia and analgesia below the level of the fourth thoracic segment of the cord and the later development of paraplegia **could be caused by:**
    (a) Absent circulation in the posterior spinal arteries
    (b) Cerebral hemorrhage
    (c) Absent circulation in the anterior spinal artery
    (d) Collapse of the fourth thoracic vertebral body

 Answers and Explanations to Review Questions

1. B is correct. The circle of Willis is formed by the anterior cerebral, the internal carotid, the posterior cerebral, the basilar, and the anterior and posterior communicating arteries (see Fig. 17-6). A. The brain receives its blood supply directly and indirectly from the two internal carotid and the two vertebral arteries that lie within the subarachnoid space. C. The cerebral arteries anastomose on the surface of the brain. D. No anastomoses exist between the branches of the cerebral arteries once they have entered the substance of the brain. E. The main blood supply to the internal capsule is from the central branches of the middle cerebral artery.
2. A is correct. The precentral gyrus (face area) is supplied by the middle cerebral artery (see Figs. 8-5 and 17-3). B. The face area of the postcentral gyrus is supplied by the middle cerebral artery. C. The cuneus is supplied by the posterior cerebral artery (see Fig. 17-3). D. The inferior temporal gyrus is supplied by the posterior cerebral artery (see Fig. 17-3). E. The Wernicke area is supplied by the middle cerebral artery.
3. D is correct. The posterior spinal artery arises from the vertebral artery (see Fig. 17-7). A. The ophthalmic artery is a branch of the cerebral portion of the internal carotid artery. B. The pontine arteries are branches of the basilar artery (see Fig. 17-2). C. The posterior communicating artery is a branch of the internal carotid artery (see Fig. 17-2). E. The posterior inferior cerebellar artery is a branch of the vertebral artery (see Fig. 17-2).

4. E is correct. The inferior sagittal sinus drains into the straight sinus (see Fig. 17-5). A. The superior cerebral veins drain into the superior sagittal sinus (see Fig. 17-5). B. The great cerebral vein drains into the straight sinus (see Fig. 17-5). C. The superior cerebellar veins drain into the straight sinus, the transverse sinus, and the occipital sinus (see Fig. 17-5). D. The spinal veins drain into the internal vertebral venous plexus.
5. D is correct. One of the most powerful vasodilators of cerebral blood vessels is carbon dioxide. A. The sympathetic postganglionic fibers exert very little control over the diameter of the cerebral blood vessels. B. The cerebral blood flow varies only slightly with changes in the general blood pressure. C. Low oxygen tension in the cerebral blood causes vasodilation of the cerebral blood vessels. E. The blood flow for a particular area of nervous tissue following occlusion of a cerebral artery depends on the adequacy of the collateral circulation.
6. C is correct. Irreversible cerebral damage starts to occur after blood flow has ceased for about 4 minutes. A. Atheromatous degeneration of a cerebral artery may cause degeneration of the nerve cells in the avascular area and proliferation of the microglial cells in the surrounding area. B. Neuronal function ceases after blood flow has stopped for about 1 minute. D. Shock occurring as the result of severe physical trauma can result in cerebral ischemia. E. Cooling of the patient's body following a cerebrovascular accident slows down cerebral degeneration.

For answers to Questions 7 to 12, study Figure 17-17 which shows the arteries of the inferior surface of the brain.

7. B is correct; 1 is the anterior communicating artery.
8. C is correct; 2 is the posterior cerebral artery.
9. E is correct; 3 is the left vertebral artery.
10. D is correct; 4 is the basilar artery.
11. E is correct; 5 is the (right) posterior communicating artery.
12. A is correct; 6 is the (right) middle cerebral artery.
13. A is correct. The posterior spinal arteries supply the posterior third of the spinal cord (see p. 471). B. The spinal cord veins communicate with the veins of the brain and the venous sinuses. C. The arteria radicularis magna (artery of Adamkiewicz) arises from the aorta in the lower thoracic or upper lumbar vertebral levels. D. The anterior spinal artery is single but usually arises from both vertebral arteries. E. The spinal arteries are reinforced by radicular arteries, which are branches of local arteries.
14. E is the exception. A positive Babinski sign was present on the right side.
15. C is the exception. The muscles of the upper part of the face on the right side are not affected by a lesion involving the upper motor neurons on the left side of the brain. This is due to the fact that the part of the facial nucleus of the seventh cranial nerve that controls the muscles of the upper part of the face receives corticonuclear fibers from both cerebral hemispheres.
16. E is the exception. The cerebral lesion was on the left side of the brain, and the muscles of the left leg were completely unaffected by the vascular accident.

17. B is the exception. The depth of coma is related to the extent of the arterial blockage.
18. C is the exception. The central branches of the right middle cerebral artery do supply the right lentiform and caudate nuclei and the right internal capsule.
19. B is correct. In the thoracic region, the posterior intercostal arteries arise directly from the thoracic aorta and can be blocked by a blood clot as the aortic dissection progresses. The segmental spinal arteries, which are branches of the posterior intercostal arteries, give origin to the radicular arteries that supply the spinal nerves and their roots. If these arteries are compromised, severe pain is experienced in the distribution of the spinal nerves involved and, hence, the "girdle" pain.
20. C is correct. The blood supply to the spinal cord is meager and if the segmental arteries that reinforce the anterior and posterior spinal arteries are compromised, ischemia of the spinal cord could follow. In this patient, the circulation in the anterior spinal artery ceased and the blood supply to the anterior two-thirds of the spinal cord was cut off. This would explain the sudden development of bilateral thermoanesthesia and analgesia (spinothalamic tracts in both lateral white columns) and the paraplegia (corticospinal tracts in both lateral white columns). The sparing of the sensations of position, vibration, and light touch, which travel in the fasciculus gracilis and fasciculus cuneatus, can be explained by the fact that the posterior white columns are supplied by the posterior spinal arteries in which the circulation is adequate.

18 Nervous System Development

CHAPTER OBJECTIVES

- To review the development of the nervous system
- To visualize the relationship of different parts of the nervous system to one another
- To understand how the different nerve tracts insinuate themselves between the central masses of gray matter
- To review common congenital anomalies of the nervous system

A pediatrician examines a newborn baby boy after a difficult delivery and finds a soft, fluctuant swelling over the vertebral column in the lumbosacral region. The swelling measures about 3 in (7.5 cm) in diameter and is covered with a thin layer of intact skin. Transillumination of the sac reveals what appears to be solid nervous tissue. Any neurologic deficit is carefully looked for, and the baby is noted to move both legs normally and appears to respond normally to painful stimulation of the leg skin. Examination of the anal sphincter shows normal tone.

Careful examination for other congenital anomalies, especially hydrocephalus, is also made, but nothing abnormal is detected.

A diagnosis of meningomyelocele is made. In this condition, vertebral arches fail to develop, with herniation of the meninges and nervous tissue through the defect. The child must be operated on; the lower end of the spinal cord and the cauda equina are returned to the vertebral canal, and the vertebral defect is repaired. The child will make an uneventful recovery.

In Chapter 1, the early development of the nervous system was considered to give the reader some insight into how the brain and spinal cord came into existence (see p. 14). In this chapter, the process of development continues, and the different parts of the nervous system followed as they evolve. An embryologic explanation for some of the more common congenital anomalies will be discussed.

SPINAL CORD

In early development, the neural tube is seen to dilate at the cephalic end into the **forebrain vesicle**, the **midbrain vesicle**, and the **hindbrain vesicle** (see Fig. 1-18A). The rest of the tube elongates and remains smaller in diameter; it will form the **spinal cord**.

The wall of the neural tube consists of a single layer of pseudostratified columnar epithelial cells, called the **matrix cells**. This thick zone of epithelium, which extends from the cavity of the tube to the exterior, is referred to as the **ventricular zone**. The nuclei of these cells move in toward the cavity of the tube to divide, and out toward the periphery during the intermitotic phases of the cell cycle (see Fig. 1-18C). Repeated division of the matrix cells results in an increase in length and diameter of the neural tube. Eventually, the early **neuroblasts** are formed and are incapable of further division. These cells migrate peripherally to form the **intermediate zone**. The intermediate zone will form the **gray matter** of the spinal cord. The neuroblasts now give rise to nerve fibers that grow peripherally and form a layer external to the intermediate zone called the **marginal zone**. The nerve fibers in the marginal zone become myelinated and form the **white matter** of the spinal cord.

While the neuroblasts are being formed, the matrix cells also give rise to the **astrocytes** and the **oligodendrocytes** of the neuroglia. Later, the **microglial cells**, which are derived from the surrounding mesenchyme, migrate into the developing spinal cord along with blood vessels. The **ependymal cells** are formed from the matrix cells that line the neural tube.

The cavity of the neural tube now becomes narrowed to form a dorsiventral cleft with thick lateral walls and thin **floor** and **roof plates** (Fig. 18-1A). The intermediate zone of the lateral wall of the tube forms a large anterior thickening known as the **basal plate** and a smaller

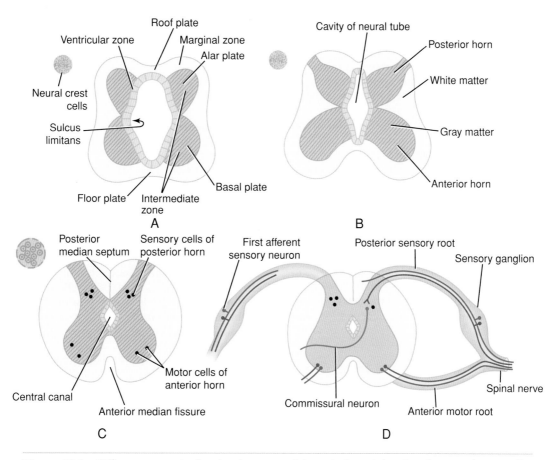

Figure 18-1 Different stages in the development of the spinal cord showing the neural crest cells, which will form the first afferent neurons in the sensory pathway.

posterior thickening known as the **alar plate**. The neuroblasts in the basal plate will form the motor cells of the anterior column (horn), while the neuroblasts in the alar plate will become the sensory cells of the posterior column. The motor basal plate and the sensory alar plate are separated on each side by the **sulcus limitans**. The roof and floor plates remain thin, and the cells contribute to the ependyma.

Continued growth of the basal plates on each side of the midline forms a deep longitudinal groove called the **anterior median fissure** (see Fig. 18-1C). The alar plates also increase in size and extend medially, compressing the posterior part of the lumen of the neural tube. Ultimately, the walls of the posterior portion of the tube fuse, forming the **posterior median septum**. The lumen of the neural tube becomes the **central canal**.

Further Development of the Motor Neurons

The medial group of motor neurons forms large multipolar cells whose axons will leave the anterior surface of the spinal cord to supply the musculature of the body. Currently occupying the minds of researchers is how the axons from a developing neuron are guided from their points of origin to a specific target. The growing end of the axon is believed to possess numerous receptors that respond to chemical cues along the way.

The lateral group of neurons gives rise to axons that will leave the anterior surface of the spinal cord as autonomic preganglionic fibers. Between the first thoracic and second or third lumbar segments of the mature spinal cord, the lateral group of neurons will form the **lateral gray column (horn)**, that is, the **sympathetic outflow**. Collectively, the axons leaving the anterior surface of the spinal cord will form the **anterior roots of the spinal nerves** (see Fig. 18-1D).

Afferent Neuron Development in the Sensory Pathway

The first neurons in the sensory pathway have their cell bodies situated outside the spinal cord and are derived from the neural crest (see Figs. 1-16 and 18-1D). The neural crest cells migrate to a posterolateral position on either side of the developing spinal cord and become segmented into cell clusters. Some of the cells in each cluster now differentiate into neuroblasts. Each neuroblast develops two processes: a peripheral process and a central process. The peripheral processes grow out laterally to become typical axons of sensory nerve fibers. The central processes, also axons, grow into the posterior part of the developing spinal cord and either end in the posterior gray column or ascend through the marginal zone (white matter) to one of the higher brain centers. These central processes are referred to collectively as the **posterior root of the spinal nerve** (see Fig. 18-1D). The peripheral processes join the anterior root to form the **spinal nerve**.

Some of the neural crest cells form the **capsular** or **satellite cells**, which surround the unipolar nerve cell bodies in a ganglion. Each **posterior root ganglion** is thus formed of the unipolar neurons and the capsular cells.

Further Development of Posterior Gray Column Sensory Neurons

The neuroblasts that have entered the alar plates now develop processes that enter the marginal zone (white matter) of the cord on the same side and either ascend or descend to a higher or lower level. Other nerve cells send processes to the opposite side of the cord through the floor plate, where they ascend or descend for variable distances (see Fig. 18-1A).

Development of the Meninges and Spinal Cord Relationship to Vertebral Column

The **pia mater**, **arachnoid mater**, and **dura mater** are formed from the mesenchyme (sclerotome) that surrounds the neural tube. The **subarachnoid space** develops as a cavity in the mesenchyme, which becomes filled with **cerebrospinal fluid (CSF)**. The **ligamentum denticulatum** is formed from areas of condensation of the mesenchyme.

During the first 2 months of intrauterine life, the spinal cord is the same length as the vertebral column. Thereafter, the developing vertebral column grows more rapidly than the spinal cord; thus, at birth, the coccygeal end of the cord lies at the level of the third lumbar vertebra. In the adult, the lower end of the spinal cord lies at the level of the lower border of the body of the first lumbar vertebra. As a result of this disproportion in the rate of growth of the vertebral column and spinal cord, the anterior and posterior roots of the spinal nerves below the first lumbar segment of the spinal cord descend within the vertebral canal until they reach their appropriate exits through the intervertebral foramina. Moreover, the pia mater, which attached the coccygeal end of the spinal cord to the coccyx, now extends down as a slender fibrous strand from the lower end of the cord to the coccyx and forms the **filum terminale**. The obliquely coursing anterior and posterior roots of the spinal nerves and the filum terminale, which now occupy the lower end of the vertebral canal, collectively form the **cauda equina**.

We now know how the cauda equina is enclosed within the subarachnoid space down as far as the level of the second sacral vertebra. In this region, below the level of the lower end of the spinal cord, a **lumbar puncture** can be performed (see p. 19).

As the result of the development of the limb buds during the fourth month and the additional sensory and motor neurons, the spinal cord becomes swollen in the cervical and lumbar regions to form the **cervical** and **lumbar enlargements**.

BRAIN

Once the neural tube has closed, the **three primary vesicles**—the **forebrain vesicle**, the **midbrain vesicle**, and the **hindbrain vesicle**—complete their development (Fig. 18-2). The forebrain vesicle will become the forebrain (**prosencephalon**), the midbrain vesicle will become the midbrain (**mesencephalon**), and the hindbrain vesicle will become the hindbrain (**rhombencephalon**).

By the fifth week, the forebrain and hindbrain vesicles divide into two secondary vesicles. The forebrain vesicle forms (1) the **telencephalon**, with its primitive cerebral hemispheres, and (2) the **diencephalon**, which develops optic vesicles. The hindbrain vesicle forms (1) the **metencephalon**, the future pons and cerebellum, and (2) the **myelencephalon**, or medulla oblongata (Table 18-1).

The basic pattern of the ventricular system is now established. The cavity in each cerebral hemisphere is known as the **lateral ventricle**. The cavity of the diencephalon is known as the **third ventricle**. With continued growth, the cavity of the midbrain vesicle becomes small and forms the **cerebral aqueduct** or **aqueduct of Sylvius**. The cavity of the hindbrain vesicle forms the **fourth ventricle**, which is continuous with the central canal of the spinal cord. The lateral ventricles communicate with the third ventricle through the **interventricular foramina**. The ventricular system and the central canal of the spinal cord are lined with ependyma and are filled with CSF. In the earliest stages, the CSF within the ventricular system is not continuous with that of the subarachnoid space.

Early in development, the embryo is a flat disc, and the neural tube is straight. Later, with the development of the head fold and tail fold, the neural tube becomes curved.

Medulla Oblongata (Myelencephalon)

The walls of the hindbrain vesicle initially show the typical organization seen in the neural tube, with the anterior thickenings, known as the **basal plates**, and the posterior thickenings, known as the **alar plates**, being separated by the **sulcus limitans** (Fig. 18-3). As development proceeds, the lateral walls are moved laterally (like an opening clamshell) at higher levels by the expanding fourth ventricle. As a result, the alar plates come to lie lateral to the basal plates. The neurons of the basal plate form the motor nuclei of cranial nerves (CNs) IX, X, XI, and XII and are situated in the floor of the fourth ventricle medial to the sulcus limitans. The neurons of the alar plate form the sensory nuclei of CNs V, VIII, IX, and X and the **gracile** and **cuneate nuclei**. Other cells of the alar plate migrate ventrolaterally and form the **olivary nuclei**.

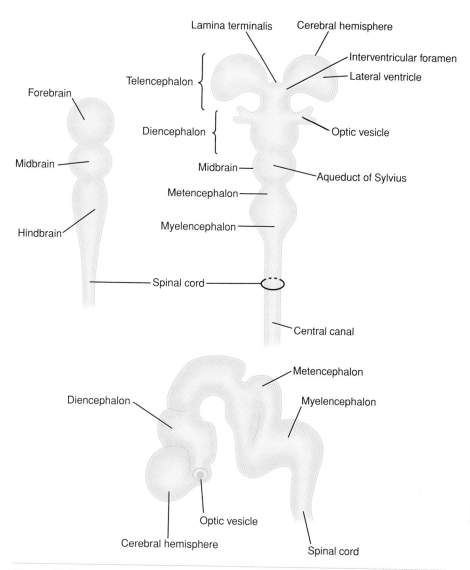

Figure 18-2   Division of the forebrain vesicle into the telencephalon and the diencephalon, and the hindbrain vesicle into the metencephalon and myelencephalon. Also shown is the way in which the cerebral hemisphere on each side develops as a diverticulum from the telencephalon.

Table 18-1   Primary Divisions of the Developing Brain

Primary Vesicle	Primary Division	Subdivision	Adult Structures
Forebrain vesicle	Prosencephalon (forebrain)	Telencephalon	Cerebral hemisphere, basal ganglia, hippocampus
		Diencephalon	Thalamus, hypothalamus, pineal body, infundibulum
Midbrain vesicle	Mesencephalon (midbrain)	Mesencephalon (midbrain)	Tectum, tegmentum, crus cerebri
Hindbrain vesicle	Rhombencephalon (hindbrain)	Metencephalon	Pons, cerebellum
		Myelencephalon	Medulla oblongata

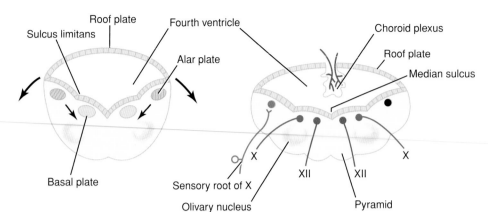

Figure 18-3 Development of the medulla oblongata (myelencephalon).

The roof plate becomes stretched into a thin layer of ependymal tissue. The vascular mesenchyme lying in contact with the outer surface of the roof plate forms the pia mater, and the two layers together form the **tela choroidea**. Vascular tufts of tela choroidea project into the cavity of the fourth ventricle to form the **choroid plexus**. Between the fourth and fifth months, local resorptions of the roof plate occur; forming paired lateral foramina, the **foramina of Luschka**, and a median foramen, the **foramen of Magendie**. These important foramina allow the escape of the CSF, which is produced in the ventricles, into the subarachnoid space (see p. 443).

The floor plate remains narrow and forms the region of the median sulcus. In the marginal layer on the anterior aspect of the medulla, descending axons from the neurons in the motor areas of the cerebral cortex (precentral gyrus) produce prominent swellings called the **pyramids**.

Pons (Ventral Part of Metencephalon)

The pons arises from the anterior part of the metencephalon (Fig. 18-4), but it also receives a cellular contribution from the alar part of the myelencephalon.

The neurons of the basal plates form the motor nuclei of CNs V, VI, and VII. The neurons of the ventromedial part of each alar plate form the main sensory nucleus of CN V, a sensory nucleus of CN VII, and the vestibular and cochlear nuclei of CN VIII; they also form the **pontine nuclei**. The axons of the pontine nuclei grow transversely to enter the developing cerebellum of the opposite side, thus forming the **transverse pontine fibers** and the **middle cerebellar peduncle**.

Cerebellum (Posterior Part of Metencephalon)

The cerebellum is formed from the posterior part of the alar plates of the metencephalon. On each side, the alar plates bend medially to form the **rhombic lips** (Fig. 18-5). As alar plates enlarge, the lips project caudally over the roof plate of the fourth ventricle and unite with each other in the midline to form the cerebellum (Fig. 18-6; also see Fig. 18-5). At the 12th week, a small midline portion, the **vermis**, and two lateral portions, the **cerebellar hemispheres**, may be recognized. At about the end of the fourth month, fissures develop on the surface of the cerebellum, and the characteristic folia of the adult cerebellum gradually develop.

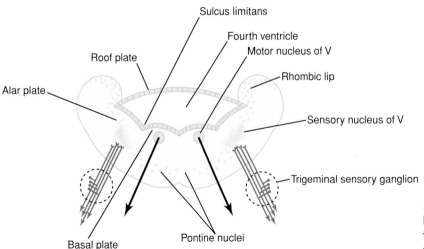

Figure 18-4 Development of the pons from the anterior part of the metencephalon.

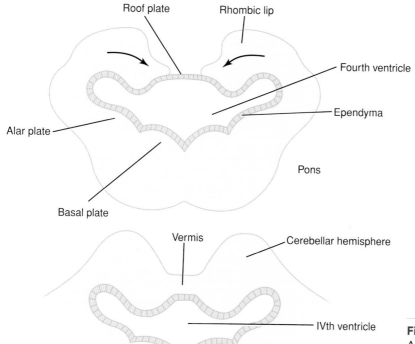

Figure 18-5 Development of the cerebellum. Also shown is the fusion of the rhombic lips in the midline to form the dumbbell-shaped cerebellum.

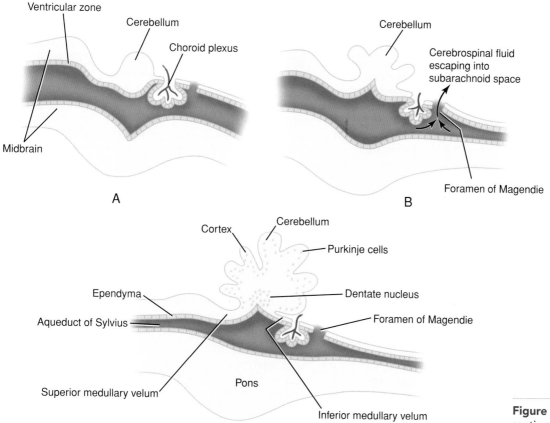

Figure 18-6 Sagittal sections of the developing cerebellum.

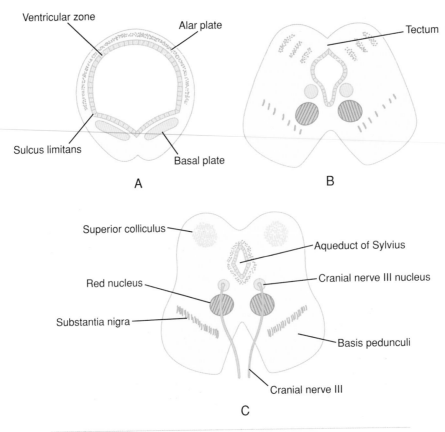

Figure 18-7 Successive stages in the development of the midbrain.

The neuroblasts derived from the matrix cells in the ventricular zone migrate toward the surface of the cerebellum and eventually give rise to the neurons forming the **cerebellar cortex**. Other neuroblasts remain close to the ventricular surface and differentiate into the **dentate** and other deep cerebellar nuclei. With further development, the axons of neurons forming these nuclei grow out into the mesencephalon (midbrain) to reach the forebrain, and these fibers will form the greater part of the superior cerebellar peduncle. Later, the growth of the axons of the pontocerebellar fibers and the corticopontine fibers will connect the cerebral cortex with the cerebellum, and so the middle cerebellar peduncle will be formed. The inferior cerebellar peduncle will be formed largely by the growth of sensory axons from the spinal cord, the vestibular nuclei, and olivary nuclei.

Midbrain (Mesencephalon)

The midbrain develops from the midbrain vesicle, the cavity of which becomes much reduced to form the **cerebral aqueduct** or **aqueduct of Sylvius** (Fig. 18-7). The sulcus limitans separates the alar plate from the basal plate on each side, as seen in the developing spinal cord. The neuroblasts in the basal plates will differentiate into the neurons forming the nuclei of **CNs III and IV** and possibly the **red nuclei**, the **substantia nigra**, and the **reticular formation**. The marginal zone of each basal plate enlarges considerably, thus forming

the **basis pedunculi** by the descent of nerve fibers from the cerebral cortex to the lower motor centers in the pons and spinal cord—that is, the **corticopontine, corticobulbar**, and **corticospinal tracts**.

The two alar plates and the original roof plate form the **tectum**. The neuroblasts in the alar plates differentiate into the sensory neurons of the **superior** and **inferior colliculi**. Four swellings representing the four colliculi appear on the posterior surface of the midbrain. The superior colliculi are associated with visual reflexes, and the inferior colliculi are associated with auditory reflexes.

With further development, the fibers of CN IV emerge on the posterior surface of the midbrain and decussate completely in the superior medullary velum. The fibers of CN III emerge on the anterior surface between the cerebral peduncles.

Forebrain (Prosencephalon)

The forebrain develops from the forebrain vesicle. The roof and floor plates remain thin, whereas the lateral walls become thick, as in the developing spinal cord. At an early stage, a lateral diverticulum called the **optic vesicle** appears on each side of the forebrain. That part of the forebrain that lies rostral to the optic vesicle is the telencephalon, and the remainder is the diencephalon (Fig. 18-8). The optic vesicle and stalk ultimately will form the retina and optic nerve.

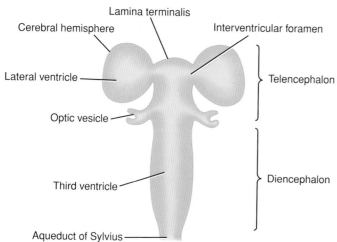

Figure 18-8   Division of the forebrain vesicle into the telencephalon and the diencephalon.

The telencephalon now develops a lateral diverticulum on each side of the cerebral hemisphere, and its cavity is known as the **lateral ventricle**. The anterior part of the third ventricle, therefore, is formed by the medial part of the telencephalon and ends at the **lamina terminalis**, which represents the rostral end of the neural tube. The opening into each lateral ventricle is the future **interventricular foramen**.

Diencephalon Fate

The cavity of the diencephalon forms the greater part of the third ventricle (see Fig. 18-8). Its roof shows a small diverticulum immediately anterior to the midbrain, which will form the **pineal body**. The remainder of the roof forms the **choroid plexus of the third ventricle** (Fig. 18-9). In the lateral wall of the third ventricle, the

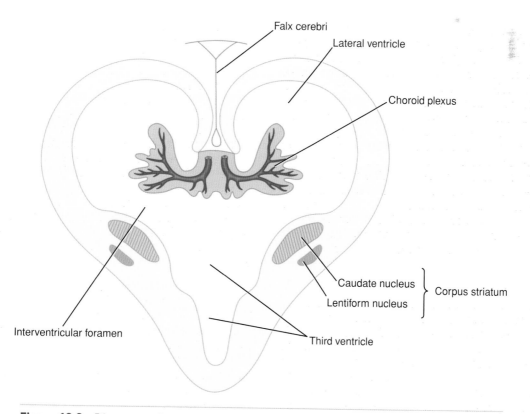

Figure 18-9   Diagrammatic representation of a coronal section of the cerebral hemispheres showing the developing choroid plexuses in the third and lateral ventricles.

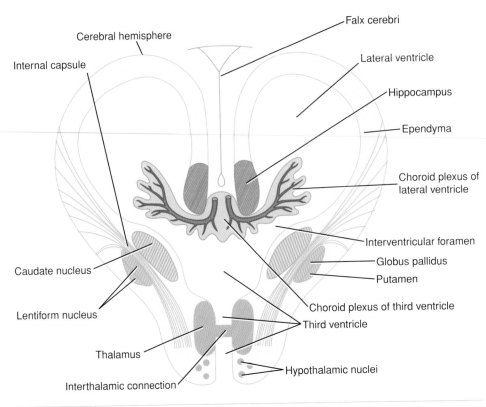

Figure 18-10 Diagrammatic representation of a coronal section of the cerebral hemispheres showing the choroid plexuses in the third and lateral ventricles. Also shown are the caudate and lentiform nuclei and the thalami. The ascending and descending nerve tracts can be seen passing between the masses of gray matter to form the internal capsule.

thalamus arises as a thickening of the alar plate on each side. Posterior to the thalamus, the **medial** and **lateral geniculate bodies** develop as solid buds. With the continued growth of the two thalami, the ventricular cavity becomes narrowed, and in some individuals, the two thalami may meet and fuse in the midline to form the **interthalamic connection** of gray matter that crosses the third ventricle (Fig. 18-10).

The lower part of the alar plate on each side will differentiate into a large number of **hypothalamic nuclei**. One of these becomes conspicuous on the inferior surface of the hypothalamus and forms a rounded swelling on each side of the midline called the **mammillary body**.

The **infundibulum** develops as a diverticulum from the floor of the diencephalon and from it will originate the **stalk** and **pars nervosa of the hypophysis**.

Telencephalon Fate

The telencephalon forms the anterior end of the third ventricle, which is closed by the lamina terminalis, while the diverticulum on either side forms the cerebral hemisphere.

Cerebral Hemispheres

Each cerebral hemisphere arises at the beginning of the fifth week of development. As it expands superiorly,

its walls thicken, and the interventricular foramen becomes reduced in size (see Figs. 18-8 to 18-10). The mesenchyme between each cerebral hemisphere condenses to form the **falx cerebri**. As development proceeds, the cerebral hemispheres grow and expand rapidly, first anteriorly to form the **frontal lobes**, then laterally and superiorly to form the **parietal lobes**, and finally posteriorly and inferiorly to produce the **occipital** and **temporal lobes**. As the result of this great expansion, the hemispheres cover the midbrain and hindbrain (Fig. 18-11).

The medial wall of the cerebral hemisphere remains thin and is formed by the ependymal cells. This area becomes invaginated by vascular mesoderm, which forms the **choroid plexus of the lateral ventricle** (see Fig. 18-10). The occipital lobe of the cerebral hemisphere is separated from the cerebellum by mesenchyme, which condenses to form the **tentorium cerebelli**.

Meanwhile, the matrix cells lining the floor of the forebrain vesicle proliferate, producing large numbers of neuroblasts. These collectively form a projection that encroaches on the cavity of the lateral ventricle and is known as the **corpus striatum** (see Fig. 18-9). Later, this differentiates into two parts: (1) the dorsomedial portion, the **caudate nucleus**, and (2) a ventrolateral part, the **lentiform nucleus**. The latter becomes subdivided

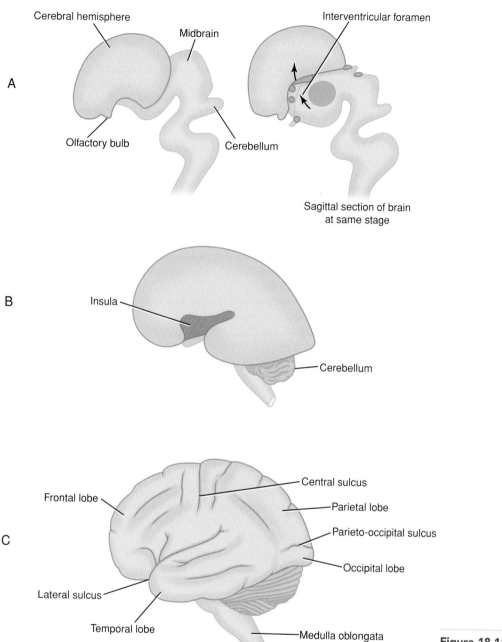

Figure 18-11 Successive stages in the development of the cerebral cortex.

into a lateral part, the **putamen**, and a medial part, the **globus pallidus** (see Fig. 18-10). As each hemisphere expands, its medial surface approaches the lateral surface of the diencephalon; thus, the caudate nucleus and thalamus come in close contact.

A further longitudinal thickening occurs in the wall of the forebrain vesicle, and the thickening protrudes into the lateral ventricle and forms the **hippocampus**.

While these various masses of gray matter are developing within each cerebral hemisphere, maturing neurons in different parts of the nervous system are sending axons either to or from the differentiating cortex. These axons form the large **ascending** and **descending tracts**, which, as they develop, are forced to pass between the

thalamus and caudate nucleus medially and the lentiform nucleus laterally. The compact bundle of ascending and descending tracts is known as the **internal capsule**. The **external capsule** consists of a few cortical projection fibers that pass lateral to the lentiform nucleus.

Cerebral Cortex

As each cerebral hemisphere rapidly expands, the **convolutions** or **gyri** separated by **fissures** or **sulci** become evident on its surface. The cortex covering the lentiform nucleus remains as a fixed area called the **insula** (see Fig. 18-11B). Later, this region becomes buried in the **lateral sulcus** as the result of overgrowth of the adjacent temporal, parietal, and frontal lobes.

The matrix cells lining the cavity of the cerebral hemisphere produce large numbers of neuroblasts and **neuroglial cells** that migrate out into the marginal zone. The remaining matrix cells ultimately will form the **ependyma**, which lines the lateral ventricle. In the 12th week, the cortex becomes very cellular because of the migration of large numbers of neuroblasts. At term, the neuroblasts have become differentiated and have assumed a stratified appearance as the result of the presence of incoming and outgoing fibers. Different areas of the cortex soon show specific cell types; thus, the motor cortex contains a large number of **pyramidal cells**, whereas the sensory areas are characterized mainly by **granular cells**.

Commissures

The **lamina terminalis**, which is the cephalic end of the neural tube, forms a bridge between the two cerebral hemispheres and enables nerve fibers to pass from one cerebral hemisphere to the other (see Fig. 18-8).

The **anterior commissure** is the first commissure to develop. It runs in the lamina terminalis and connects the olfactory bulb and the temporal lobe of the cortex on one side with the same structures of the opposite hemisphere.

The **fornix** is the second commissure to develop and connects the cortex of the hippocampus in each hemisphere.

The **corpus callosum**, the largest and most important commissure, is the third commissure to develop. Its first fibers connect the frontal lobes of both sides and, later, the parietal lobes. As the corpus callosum increases in size because of increased numbers of fibers, it arches back over the roof of the developing third ventricle.

The remains of the lamina terminalis, which lie between the corpus callosum and the fornix, become stretched out to form a thin septum, the **septum pellucidum**. The **optic chiasma** is formed in the inferior part of the lamina terminalis; it contains fibers from the medial halves of the retinae, which cross the midline to join the optic tract of the opposite side and so pass to the **lateral geniculate body** and the **superior colliculus**.

Myelination in the Central Nervous System

The myelin sheath in the central nervous system is formed and maintained by the oligodendrocytes of the neuroglia (see p. 54).

Myelination in the spinal cord begins first in the cervical region, and from here, the process extends caudally. The process of myelination begins within the cord at about the fourth month, and the sensory fibers are affected first. The last affected are the descending motor fibers.

Myelination in the brain begins at about the sixth month of fetal life but is restricted to the fibers of the basal ganglia. Later, the sensory fibers passing up from the spinal cord myelinate, but the progress is slow; therefore, at birth, the brain still is largely unmyelinated. Newborns have very little cerebral function; motor reactions such as respiration, sucking, and swallowing are essentially reflex. After birth, the corticobulbar, corticospinal, tectospinal, and corticopontocerebellar fibers begin to myelinate. This process of myelination is not haphazard but systematic, occurring in different nerve fibers at specific times. The corticospinal fibers, for example, start to myelinate at about 6 months after birth, and the process is largely complete by the end of the second year. It is believed that some nerve fibers in the brain and spinal cord do not complete myelination until puberty.

 Clinical Notes

Congenital Anomalies

Practically any part of the nervous system can show defects of development, and these produce a wide variety of clinical signs and symptoms. Only the common defects of the central nervous system are considered here. Spina bifida, hydrocephalus, and anencephaly each occur about 6 times/1,000 births and are therefore the more common congenital anomalies.

Spina Bifida

In spina bifida, the spines and arches of one or more adjacent vertebrae fail to develop (Fig. 18-12). The condition occurs most frequently in the lower thoracic, lumbar, and sacral regions. Beneath this defect, the meninges and spinal cord may or may not be involved in varying degrees. The condition is a result of failure of the mesenchyme, which grows in between the neural tube and the surface

ectoderm, to form the vertebral arches in the affected region. The types of spina bifida are as follows:

1. **Spina bifida occulta.** The spines and arches of one or more vertebrae, usually in the lumbar region, are absent, and the vertebral canal remains open posteriorly. The spinal cord and nerve roots usually are normal. The defect is covered by the postvertebral muscles and cannot be seen from the surface. A small tuft of hair or a fatty tumor may be present over the defect. Most cases are symptomless and are diagnosed by chance when the vertebral column is x-rayed.

2. **Meningocele.** The meninges project through the defect in the vertebral arches, forming a cystic swelling beneath the skin and containing CSF, which communicates with the subarachnoid space (Fig. 18-13; also see Fig. 18-12). The spinal cord and nerves usually are normal.

Spina bifida occulta

Meningocele

Meningomyelocele

Myelocele

Syringomyelocele

Figure 18-12   Different types of spina bifida.

3. **Meningomyelocele.** The normal spinal cord, or cauda equina, lies within the meningeal sac, which projects through the vertebral arch defect (see Fig. 18-12). The spinal cord or nerve roots are adherent to the inner wall of the sac.

4. **Myelocele.** The neural tube fails to close in the region of the defect. An oval raw area is found on the surface; this represents the neural groove whose lips are fused. The central canal discharges clear CSF onto the surface.

5. **Syringomyelocele.** This condition is rare. A meningomyelocele is present, and in addition, the central canal of the spinal cord at the level of the bony defect is grossly dilated.

Spina bifida occulta is the most common defect. The next most common defect is myelocele, and many afflicted infants are born dead. If the child is born alive, death from infection of the spinal cord may occur within a few days.

Figure 18-13   A meningocele in the lumbosacral region. (Courtesy Dr. L. Thompson.)

Most cases of spina bifida occulta require no treatment. A meningocele should be removed surgically within a few days of birth. Infants with meningomyelocele should also be treated surgically. The sac is opened, and the spinal cord or nerves are freed and carefully replaced in the vertebral canal. The meninges are sutured over the cord and the postvertebral muscles are approximated.

As the result of advances in medical and surgical care, many infants with the severe forms of spina bifida now survive. Unfortunately, these children are likely to have lifelong disabilities and psychosocial problems. The neurologic deficits alone may result in deformation of the limbs and spine and in bladder, bowel, and sexual dysfunction.

Hydrocephalus

Hydrocephalus is an abnormal increase in the volume of CSF within the skull. The condition may be associated with spina bifida and meningocele. Hydrocephalus alone may be caused by stenosis of the cerebral aqueduct or, more commonly, by the normal single channel being represented by many inadequate minute tubules. Another cause, which is progressive, is the overgrowth of neuroglia around the aqueduct. Inadequate development or failure of development of the interventricular foramen, or the foramina of Magendie and Luschka, may also be responsible.

In cases of hydrocephalus with spina bifida, the **Arnold–Chiari phenomenon** may occur. During development, the cephalic end of the spinal cord is fixed by virtue of the brain residing in the skull, and in the presence of spina bifida, the caudal end of the cord may also be fixed. The longitudinal growth of the vertebral column is more rapid and greater than that of the spinal cord, and this results in traction pulling the medulla and part of the cerebellum through the foramen magnum. This displacement of the hindbrain downward obstructs CSF flow through the foramina in the roof of the fourth ventricle.

Hydrocephalus may occur before birth and if it is advanced, it could obstruct labor. It usually is noticed during the first few months of life because of the enlarging head, which may attain a huge size, sometimes measur-

ing more than 30 in in diameter (Fig. 18-14). The cranial sutures are widely separated, and the anterior fontanelle is much enlarged. The veins of the scalp are distended, and the eyes look downward. CN paralyses are common. The ventricles of the brain become markedly dilated. This ventricular expansion occurs largely at the expense of the white matter, and the neurons of the cerebral cortex are mostly spared. This results in the preservation of cerebral function, but the destruction of the tracts, especially the corticobulbar and corticospinal tracts, produces a progressive loss of motor function.

If the condition is diagnosed by sonography while the fetus is in utero, it is possible to perform prenatal surgery with the introduction of a catheter into the ventricles of the brain and CSF drainage into the amniotic cavity. Should the diagnosis be delayed until after birth, a drainage tube fitted with a nonreturn valve can connect the ventricles to the internal jugular vein in the neck.

Anencephaly

In anencephaly, the greater part of the brain and the vault of the skull are absent (Fig. 18-15). The anomaly is caused by the failure of the rostral end of the neural tube to develop and as a consequence, its cavity remains open. In place of the normal neural tissue are thin-walled vascular channels resembling the choroid plexus and masses of neural tissue. Although the eyes are present, the optic nerves are absent. The condition commonly involves the spinal cord, and the neural tube remains open in the cervical region. The condition is commonly diagnosed before birth with sonography or x-ray studies. Most anencephalic infants are stillborn or die shortly after birth.

Neural Defect Prevention

The development and closure of the neural tube are normally completed within 28 days. In practical terms, this means that neural tube defects have occurred before many women are aware that they are pregnant.

Extensive clinical research has demonstrated that environmental and genetic factors have a joint role in the

Figure 18-14   Hydrocephalus. Note the large size of the head. (Courtesy Dr. G. Avery.)

causation of neural tube defects. The increased risk of neural defects in the lower socioeconomic groups suggests that poor nutrition may also be an important factor. More recent clinical research has demonstrated that the risk of recurrent neural defects is significantly reduced among women who take 4,000 mg of **folic acid** daily compared with women who do not. Further studies have shown that a daily dose that is 10 times lower is effective in preventing the defect. These findings have stimulated much new research to identify the genetic and biochemical bases of neural tube defects.

Because as many as 50% of pregnancies in the United States are unplanned and since the neural tube closes before most women know that they are pregnant, physicians should strongly urge women capable of becoming pregnant to consume at least 400 mg of folic acid per day, preferably as a multivitamin supplement.

Embryonic Stem Cell Treatment of Neurologic Diseases

Freed et al. (2001) reported treating patients with severe Parkinson disease by transplanting precursors of dopamine nerve cells in fragments of mesencephalon isolated from human fetuses 7 to 8 weeks after conception. The results showed that the transplants survived and produced some clinical benefit in younger but not in older patients. It was demonstrated that the cells survived and differentiated, as demonstrated by positron emission tomography or by histologic examination (see Fig. 10-9). In view of the large numbers of patients with Parkinson disease worldwide, it is unlikely that transplantation of embryonic fragments would be a practical therapy.

Embryonic stem cells have the unique property of being able to produce all adult cell types, including those of the nervous system. The successful transplantation of embryonic stem cells has been achieved in animal models of Parkinson disease, motor neuron disease, and spinal cord injury. The great promise of these results has stimulated the imagination of scientists and patients. The use of cell lines derived from human embryonic stem cells, however, poses profound ethical questions.

Embryonic stem cells are derived from the inner cell mass of the blastocyst, the stage at which the developing embryo is implanted into the uterus. Human embryonic stem cells were first successfully harvested by Thomson et al. in 1998. The isolated inner cell mass cells were then cultured in the laboratory. Although substantial advances have been made in this field, enormous efforts must now be devoted to this subject so that we can improve the health of patients with chronic debilitating neurologic diseases.

A

B

Figure 18-15 Example of anencephaly. Note that the greater part of the brain and the vault of the skull are absent. In the posterior view, the remainder of the brain is exposed. (Courtesy Dr. M. Platt.)

Key Concepts

Spinal Cord

- In early development, the neural tube dilates at the cephalic end to form the forebrain, midbrain, and hindbrain vesicles. The rest of the tube elongates to form the spinal cord.

- Matrix cells in the epithelial walls of the neural tube are referred to as the ventricular zone. Repeated divisions of the matrix cells result in increased length and diameter of the neural tube.

- Eventually, neuroblasts are formed and migrate to the intermediate zone to form the gray matter of the spinal cord.

- The cells of the intermediate zone grow fibers that extend and form a layer external to the intermediate zone, called the marginal zone. These fibers become myelinated and form the white matter of the spinal cord.

- Matrix cells will also give rise to astrocytes and oligodendrocytes. Microglial cells migrate in from the mesenchyme.

- The layers of the meninges are formed from the mesenchyme that surrounds the neural tube.

Brain

- Once the neural tube closes, the three primary vesicles complete their development.

- The forebrain vesicle forms the telencephalon, which matures into the cerebral hemisphere, basal ganglia, and hippocampus; and the diencephalon, which becomes the thalamus, hypothalamus, pineal body, and infundibulum.

- The midbrain vesicle forms the tectum, tegmentum, and crus cerebri components of the midbrain.

- The hindbrain vesicle forms the metencephalon, which includes the pons and cerebellum, and the myelencephalon, which includes the medulla oblongata.

? Clinical Problem Solving

1. A 10-year-old boy fell off his bicycle and hurt his back. Following a complete physical examination in the emergency department, nothing abnormal is found. An x-ray examination, however, reveals the complete absence of the spine and laminae of the fifth lumbar vertebra. How do you explain the presence of the bony defect?

2. A male child is delivered normally to a 20-year-old woman. A pediatrician examines the infant and finds a large swelling in the lower part of his back over the fourth and fifth lumbar vertebrae. On closer examination, the summit of the swelling has an oval raw area from which a clear fluid is discharging. The legs show hyperextension of the knees, and the feet are held in the position of talipes calcaneus. What is the

diagnosis? How do you explain the congenital defect on the back?

3. A 2-month-old girl is taken to a pediatrician because her mother is concerned about the size of her head. "She looks top-heavy," she says. Examination shows the head to be large and globular in shape. The anterior fontanelle is greatly enlarged and extends posteriorly to the enlarged posterior fontanelle. The enlarged head contrasts markedly with the small face. Neurologic examination reveals some evidence of optic atrophy on both sides, and tone is increased in the muscles of both lower limbs. What is the diagnosis? How do you explain this congenital anomaly? What is the prognosis if the patient is left untreated?

Answers and Explanations to Clinical Problem Solving

1. This patient has spina bifida occulta involving the fifth lumbar vertebra. The condition is a result of failure of the mesenchyme to grow between the neural tube and the surface ectoderm and form the vertebral arch; the vertebral canal remains open posteriorly. The defect, therefore, has existed since before birth and could not be seen or felt on physical examination because it was covered by the postvertebral muscles. The spinal cord and spinal nerve roots usually are normal. No treatment is required.

2. This child has a myelocele. In addition to the failure of the formation of the vertebral arches of the fourth and fifth lumbar vertebrae, the neural tube failed to close in this region. The oval raw area seen in this patient is the neural groove whose lips have not united. The central canal is discharging clear cerebrospinal fluid onto the skin surface. The deformities of the knee joints and feet are the result of the maldevelopment of the spinal cord in the lumbar region, with consequent interference with the innervation of certain muscle groups in the legs.

3. This child has hydrocephalus. A postmortem examination performed 1 year later showed that the cerebral aqueduct was not normally developed and consisted of a number of small tubules. This had resulted in the excessive accumulation of cerebrospinal fluid within the lateral and third ventricles of the brain. The distention of the ventricles, with the consequent enlargement of the brain and increased intracranial pressure, forced apart the bones of the cranial vault so that the head became greatly enlarged. The optic atrophy probably was caused by the stretching of the optic nerve on each side. The increased muscle tone of the lower limbs was almost certainly the result of destruction of the corticospinal and other descending tracts by the expanding lateral ventricles. Although in some cases the head ceases to enlarge spontaneously, in most patients the hydrocephalus is progressive, and death ultimately occurs. Surgical treatment of hydrocephalus may be attempted.

 Review Questions

Directions: Each of the numbered items in this section is followed by answers. Select the ONE lettered answer that is CORRECT.

1. The following statements concern the neural tube:
   (a) It is lined by stratified squamous cells.
   (b) The neuroblasts migrate medially to form the intermediate zone.
   (c) The repeated division of the matrix cells does not increase the length and diameter of the tube.
   (d) The ventricular zone will form the gray matter of the spinal cord.
   (e) The nerve fibers in the marginal zone become myelinated and form the white matter of the spinal cord.

2. The following statements concern the neural crest cells:
   (a) They are formed from the medial margin of the neural plate.
   (b) They give rise to the posterior root ganglia.
   (c) They do not form the neurons of the autonomic ganglia.
   (d) The Schwann cells of peripheral nerves are not formed from neural crest cells.
   (e) They form the cells of the suprarenal cortex.

3. The following statements concern the developing spinal cord:
   (a) The alar plates form the neurons in the anterior gray columns.
   (b) The nerve cells of the sympathetic outflow are not formed from the basal plates.
   (c) In the adult, the lower end of the spinal cord lies at the level of the lower border of the first lumbar vertebra.
   (d) At birth, the lower end of the spinal cord lies at the level of the third sacral vertebra.
   (e) The meninges surrounding the spinal cord are developed from the endoderm.

4. The following statements concern the development of the brainstem:
   (a) The cerebellum is formed from the dorsal part of the alar plates of the metencephalon.
   (b) The neurons of the deep cerebellar nuclei are derived from the matrix cells lining the cavity of the midbrain vesicle.
   (c) The neuroblasts in the dorsal plates will form the nuclei of the trochlear and oculomotor nerves.
   (d) The neuroblasts of the superior and inferior colliculi are also formed from the neurocytes in the basal plates.
   (e) The pons arises from the alar part of the metencephalon with cellular contributions from the alar part of the myelencephalon.

5. The following statements concern the fate of the forebrain vesicle:
   (a) The optic vesicle grows out of the midbrain vesicle.
   (b) The thalamus is formed from the alar plates in the medial walls of the diencephalon.
   (c) The lamina terminalis is formed from the rostral end of the diencephalon.
   (d) The pars nervosa of the hypophysis is formed from the floor of the diencephalon.
   (e) The hypothalamic nuclei are formed from the basal plates of the diencephalon.
6. The following statements concern the development of the cerebral hemispheres:
   (a) The corpus striatum is formed from the proliferation of the matrix cells lining the roof of the forebrain vesicle.
   (b) The interventricular foramen is formed by the cavity of the diencephalon.
   (c) The choroid plexus of the lateral ventricle is formed by vascular ectoderm covered by ependymal cells.
   (d) The internal capsule is formed by the developing ascending and descending tracts growing between the developing thalamus and caudate nucleus medially and the lentiform nucleus laterally.
   (e) The cortical neurons develop in situ and do not migrate out laterally from the matrix cells lining the cavity of the cerebral hemisphere.
7. The following statements concern the development of myelination in the brain:
   (a) Myelination begins at birth.
   (b) The sensory fibers are myelinated last.
   (c) The process of myelination is haphazard.
   (d) Myelination of the nerve tracts is largely complete by the fourth year of life.
   (e) Myelination is carried out by oligodendrocytes and not by neurons.
8. The following statements concern the condition of spina bifida:
   (a) It is one of the more common congenital anomalies of the central nervous system.

(b) The most common form of spina bifida is syringomyelocele.
(c) The condition occurs most often in the cervical and upper thoracic regions.
(d) In a myelocele, the neural tube closes in the region of the defect.
(e) Most cases of spina bifida occulta require explorative surgery.

Directions: Each case history is followed by questions. Read the case history, then select the ONE BEST lettered answer.

A 6-month-old girl was seen by the plastic surgeon because of the presence of a swelling at the root of the nose. The mother said that she had noticed the swelling when the child was born and that since then, it had gradually increased in size.

9. The surgeon examined the child and found the following likely signs except:
   (a) The swelling was situated at the root of the nose in the midline.
   (b) The swelling was located between the frontal and nasal bones.
   (c) The swelling was fluctuant and, on gentle pressure, could be reduced in size.
   (d) The swelling was pulsatile, and the pulse coincided with the heart rate.
   (e) The pulse did not coincide with the pulse felt over the anterior fontanelle of the skull.
10. The neurosurgeon was consulted, and the following possible additional findings were ascertained except:
    (a) A lateral radiograph of the skull revealed a defect in the membranous bones involving the nasal process of the frontal bone.
    (b) The defect in the membranous bones is known as cranioschisis.
    (c) The condition was associated with a cephalic meningocele.
    (d) There was a herniation of the meninges through the defect in the skull.
    (e) Brain tissue is never found within the hernia.

 Answers and Explanations to Review Questions

1. E is correct. The nerve fibers in the marginal zone of the developing neural tube become myelinated and form the white matter of the spinal cord. A. The wall of the neural tube is formed of a single layer of pseudostratified columnar epithelial cells (see Fig. 18-1). B. The neuroblasts migrate peripherally to form the intermediate zone (see Fig. 18-1). C. The repeated division of the matrix cells of the neural tube results in an increase in the length and diameter of the tube. D. The intermediate zone of the neural tube will form the gray matter of the spinal cord.
2. B is correct. The neural crest cells give rise to the posterior root ganglia (see Fig. 1-18). A. The neural crest cells are formed from the lateral margin of the neural plate (see Fig. 1-18). C. The neural crest cells form the neurons of the autonomic ganglia (see Fig. 1-18). D. The Schwann cells of peripheral nerves are formed from neural crest cells (see Fig. 1-18). E. The neural crest cells form the cells of the suprarenal medulla (see Fig. 1-18).
3. C is correct. In the adult, the lower end of the spinal cord lies at the level of the lower border of the first lumbar vertebra. A. The alar plates form the neurons in the posterior gray columns. B. The nerve cells of the sympathetic outflow are formed from the basal plates. D. At birth, the lower end of

the spinal cord lies at the level of the third lumbar vertebra. E. The meninges of the spinal cord are developed from the mesenchyme that surrounds the neural tube.

4. A is correct. The cerebellum is formed from the dorsal part of the alar plates of the metencephalon (see Fig. 18-6). B. The neurons of the deep cerebellar nuclei are derived from the matrix cells lining the cavity of the hindbrain vesicle. C. The neuroblasts in the basal plates will form the nuclei of the trochlear and oculomotor nerves. D. The neuroblasts of the superior and inferior colliculi are formed from the neurocytes in the alar plates (see Fig. 18-8). E. The pons arises from the anterior part of the metencephalon, with cellular contributions from the alar part of the myelencephalon.

5. D is correct. The pars nervosa of the hypophysis cerebri is formed from the floor of the diencephalon. A. The optic vesicle grows out of the forebrain vesicle (see Fig. 18-3). B. The thalamus is formed from the alar plates in the lateral walls of the diencephalon (see Fig. 18-10). C. The lamina terminalis is formed from the rostral end of the telencephalon. E. The hypothalamic nuclei are formed from the alar plates of the diencephalon.

6. D is correct. The internal capsule is formed by the developing ascending and descending tracts growing between the developing thalamus and caudate nucleus medially and the lentiform nucleus laterally (see Fig. 18-11). A. The corpus striatum is formed from the proliferation of the matrix cells lining the floor of the forebrain vesicle. B. The interventricular foramen is formed by the cavity of the telencephalon (see Fig. 18-11). C. The choroid plexus of the lateral ventricle is formed by vascular mesenchyme covered by ependymal cells. E. The neurons of the cerebral cortex develop from matrix cells lining the cavity of the cerebral hemisphere. These cells produce large numbers of neuroblasts that migrate out into the marginal zone.

7. E is correct. In the developing brain, myelination is carried out by oligodendrocytes and not by neurons. A. In the developing brain, myelination begins at about the sixth month of fetal life. B. In the developing brain, the sensory fibers are myelinated first. C. Myelination of the nerve tracts is not haphazard but systematic, occurring in different nerve fibers at specific times. D. Myelination of the nerve tracts is largely complete by the end of the second year.

8. A is correct. Spina bifida is one of the more common congenital anomalies of the central nervous system. B. The most common form of spina bifida is spina bifida occulta (see Fig. 18-13). C. Spina bifida occurs most often in the lower thoracic, lumbar, and sacral regions. D. In a myelocele, the neural tube fails to close in the region of the defect (see Fig. 18-13). E. Most cases of spina bifida occulta require no treatment.

9. E is the exception. In a cephalic meningocele, the cerebrospinal fluid (CSF) within the swelling is in direct communication with that in the subarachnoid space. The pulsation of the swelling is produced by the pulse wave of the cerebral arteries through the CSF. This pulse wave will coincide with the pulse felt over the anterior fontanelle of the skull.

10. E is the exception. Cranioschisis is characterized by a defect in the membranous bones of the skull through which meninges, or meninges and neural tissue may protrude. The defect usually occurs in the midline in the occipital region or between the frontal and nasal bones. The condition is probably the result of anomalous formation and separation of the neural tube from the surface ectoderm of the embryo.

Appendix

NEUROANATOMICAL DATA OF CLINICAL SIGNIFICANCE AND CLINICAL NEUROANATOMY TECHNIQUES

Baseline of the Skull

The baseline of the skull extends from the lower margin of the orbit backward through the upper margin of the external auditory meatus. The **cerebrum** lies entirely above the line, and the **cerebellum** lies in the posterior cranial fossa below the posterior third of the line (Fig. A-1).

Falx Cerebri, Superior Sagittal Sinus, and the Longitudinal Cerebral Fissure Between the Cerebral Hemispheres

The position of the falx cerebri, superior sagittal sinus, and the longitudinal cerebral fissure between the cerebral hemispheres can be indicated by passing a line over the vertex of the skull in the sagittal plane that joins the root of the nose to the external occipital protuberance.

Parietal Eminence

The parietal eminence is a raised area on the lateral surface of the parietal bone that can be felt about 2 in (5 cm) above the auricle. It lies close to the lower end of the **central cerebral sulcus of the brain**.

Pterion

The pterion is the point where the greater wing of the sphenoid bone meets the anteroinferior angle of the parietal bone. Lying 1½ in (4 cm) above the midpoint of the zygomatic arch, it is not marked by an eminence or a depression, but it is important since the **anterior branches of the middle meningeal artery and vein lie beneath it**.

Intracranial Hematoma Treatment

Cranial decompression is performed in a patient with a history of progressive neurologic deterioration and signs of brain herniation, despite adequate medical treatment. The presence of a hematoma should be confirmed by a computed tomography scan, if possible.

Temporal Burr Hole

1. The patient is placed in a supine position with the head rotated so that the side for the burr hole is uppermost. For example, in a patient with a right-sided fixed and dilated pupil, indicating herniation of the right uncus with pressure on the right oculomotor nerve, a hematoma on the right side must be presumed, and a burr hole is placed on the right side.
2. The temporal skin is shaved and prepared for surgery in the usual way.
3. A 3-cm vertical skin incision is made two fingerbreadths anterior to the tragus of the ear and three fingerbreadths above this level (Fig. A-2A).
4. The following structures are then incised:
   a. Skin.
   b. Superficial fascia containing small branches of the superficial temporal artery.
   c. Deep fascia covering the outer surface of the temporalis muscle.
   d. The temporalis muscle is then incised vertically down to the periosteum of the squamous part of the temporal bone.
   e. The temporalis muscle is elevated from its attachment to the skull, and a retractor is positioned (some muscular bleeding will be encountered).
   f. A small hole is then drilled through the outer and inner tables of the skull at right angles to the skull surface, and the hole is enlarged with a burr (unless a blood clot is present between the inner table and the endosteal layer of dura).
   g. The white meningeal layer of dura is flexible and slightly compresses with gentle pressure.
   h. The hole may be enlarged with a curette, and bleeding from the diploe may be controlled with bone wax.

The surgical wound is closed in layers with interrupted sutures placed in the temporalis muscle, the deep fascia covering the temporalis muscle, and the scalp.

Epidural Hematoma Burr Hole

Once the inner table of the squamous part of the temporal bone (or the anterior inferior angle of the parietal bone) is pierced with a small bit and enlarged with a burr, the dark red clotted blood beneath the endosteal layer of dura is usually easily recognized. However, bright red liquid blood means that the middle meningeal artery or one of its branches is bleeding. The meningeal artery is located deep to the clot and between the endosteal layer of dura and the meningeal layer of dura or in the substance of the endosteal layer of dura; or it may lie in a tunnel of bone.

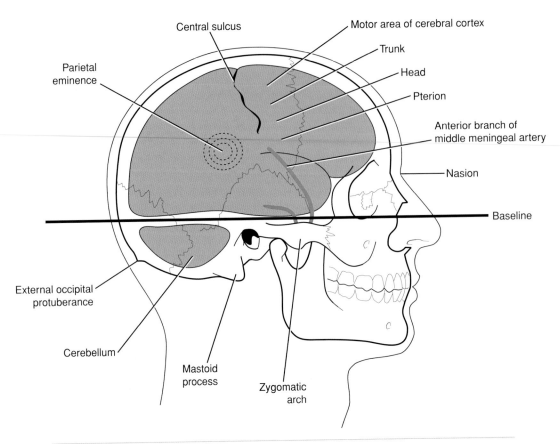

Figure A-1   Surface landmarks on the right side of the head. The relation of the middle meningeal artery and the brain to the surface of the skull is shown.

Subdural Hematoma Burr Hole

When the squamous part of the temporal bone is penetrated, as described earlier, the endosteal layer of dura will be exposed. In this case, there is no blood clot between the endosteal layer of dura and the meningeal layer of dura, but both fused layers of dura will be dark bluish. The dura (endosteal and meningeal layers) is gently incised to enter the space between the meningeal layer of dura and the arachnoid mater. The subdural blood usually gushes out, leaving the unprotected brain covered only by arachnoid and pia mater in the depths of the hole.

Ventriculostomy

Ventriculostomy is indicated in acute hydrocephalus, in which cerebrospinal fluid flow is suddenly obstructed.

Anatomy of the Technique

To perform a ventriculostomy, the needle is inserted into the lateral ventricle through either a frontal or parietal burr hole. The anatomy of these burr holes has been described previously. The needle is inserted through the burr hole using the following anatomical landmarks.

1. **Frontal Approach.** The needle is inserted through the frontal burr hole and is directed downward and forward in the direction of the inner canthus of the ipsilateral eye (Fig. A-3).

2. **Parietal Approach.** The needle is inserted through the parietal burr hole and is directed downward and forward in the direction of the pupil of the ipsilateral eye.

The needle is inserted to a depth of about 2 in (5.5 cm) from the skull opening; in cases of chronic hydrocephalus with gross dilatation of the ventricles, the depth of penetration to the ventricular cavity may be much less.

Vertebral Numbers and Spinal Cord Segments

Table A-1 relates which vertebral body is related to a particular spinal cord segment.

Segmental Innervation of Muscles

Test for the integrity of the segmental innervation of muscles by performing the following simple muscle reflexes.

Biceps brachii tendon reflex C5–C6 (flexion of the elbow joint by tapping the biceps tendon).
Triceps tendon reflex C6–C7 and C8 (extension of the elbow joint by tapping the triceps tendon).
Brachioradialis tendon reflex C5–C6 and C7 (supination of the radioulnar joints by tapping the insertion of the brachioradialis tendon).
Abdominal superficial reflexes (contraction of underlying abdominal muscles by stroking the skin). Upper

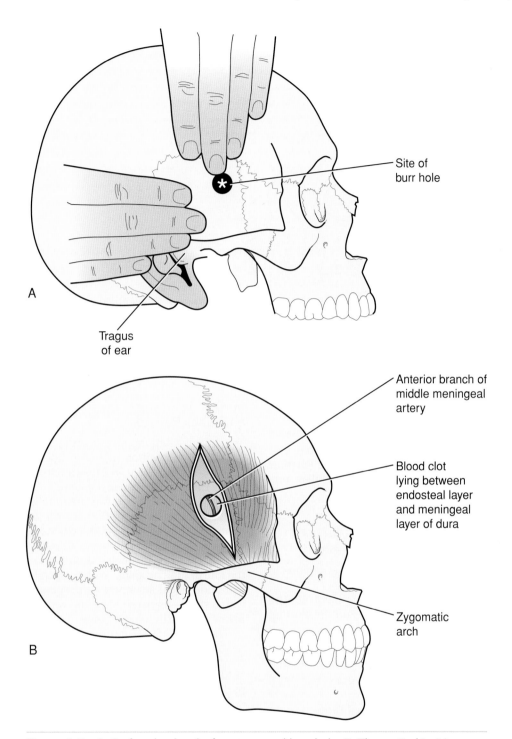

Figure A-2   A: Surface landmarks for a temporal burr hole. **B:** The vertical incision passes through the temporalis muscle down to bone. The middle meningeal artery lies between the endosteal and meningeal layers of dura and is embedded in the endosteal layer of dura or lies in a bony tunnel.

Figure A-3 Ventriculostomy. Needles passing through frontal or parietal burr holes to enter the lateral ventricle area are shown. The needle is inserted to a depth of about 2 in (5.5 cm) from the skull opening in order to enter the lateral ventricle.

abdominal skin T6–T7; middle abdominal skin T8–T9; lower abdominal skin T10–T12.

Patellar tendon reflex (knee jerk) L2, L3, and L4 (extension of knee joint on tapping the patellar tendon).

Achilles tendon reflex (ankle jerk) S1 and S2 (plantar flexion of ankle joint on tapping the Achilles tendon—tendo calcaneus).

Relationship Between Possible Intervertebral Disc Herniations and Spinal Nerve Roots

These are shown for the cervical and lumbar regions in Figure A-4.

A correlation between the nerve roots involved, the pain dermatome, the muscle weakness, and the missing or diminished reflex is shown in Table A-2.

Table A-1   Correlation of Vertebral Body With Spinal Cord Segment

Vertebra(e)	Spinal Segment(s)
Cervical vertebrae	Add 1
Upper thoracic vertebrae	Add 2
Lower thoracic vertebrae (7–9)	Add 3
Tenth thoracic vertebra	L1–L2 cord segments
Eleventh thoracic vertebra	L3–L4 cord segments
Twelfth thoracic vertebra	L5 cord segment
First lumbar vertebra	Sacral and coccygeal cord segments

Surface Landmarks for Performing a Lumbar Puncture

To perform a lumbar puncture, the patient is placed in the lateral prone position or in the upright sitting position. The trunk is then bent well forward to open up to the maximum, the space between adjoining laminae in the lumbar region. A groove runs down the middle of the back over the tips of the spines of the thoracic and the upper four lumbar vertebrae. The spines are made more prominent when the vertebral column is flexed. An imaginary line joining the highest points on the iliac crests passes over the fourth lumbar spine. With a careful aseptic technique and under local anesthesia, the spinal tap needle—fitted with a stylet—is passed into the vertebral canal above or below the fourth lumbar spine.

The following structures are pierced by the needle before it enters the subarachnoid space (Fig. A-5):

1. Skin
2. Superficial fascia
3. Supraspinous ligament
4. Interspinous ligament
5. Ligamentum flavum
6. Areolar tissue containing the internal vertebral venous plexus in the epidural space
7. Dura mater
8. Arachnoid mater

The **depth** to which the needle will have to pass will vary from an inch or less in children to as much as 4 in (10 cm) in obese adults.

The **pressure** of the cerebrospinal fluid in the lateral recumbent position is normally about 60 to 150 mm of water.

See Table 16-1 for physical characteristics and composition of the cerebrospinal fluid.

Figure A-4 A,B: Posterior views of vertebral bodies in the cervical and lumbar regions showing the relationship that might exist between herniated nucleus pulposus (pink) and spinal nerve roots. Note that there are eight cervical nerves and only seven cervical vertebrae. In the lumbar region, for example, the emerging L4 nerve roots pass out laterally close to the pedicles of the fourth lumbar vertebra and are not related to the intervertebral disc between the fourth and the fifth lumbar vertebrae. Pressure on the L5 motor nerve root produces weakness of plantar flexion of the ankle joint.

Table A-2   Correlation Between Nerve Roots, Pain Dermatome, Muscle Weakness, and Missing or Diminished Reflex

Root Injury	Dermatome Pain	Muscles Supplied	Movement Weakness	Reflex Involved
C5	Lower lateral aspect of upper arm	Deltoid and biceps	Shoulder abduction, elbow flexion	Biceps
C6	Lateral aspect of forearm	Extensor carpi radialis longus and brevis	Wrist extensors	Brachioradialis
C7	Middle finger	Triceps and flexor carpi radialis	Extension of elbow and flexion of wrist	Triceps
C8	Medial aspect of forearm	Flexor digitorum superficialis and profundus	Finger flexion	None
L1	Groin	Iliopsoas	Hip flexion	Cremaster
L2	Anterior aspect of thigh	Iliopsoas, sartorius, hip adductors	Hip flexion, hip adduction	Cremaster
L3	Medial aspect of knee	Iliopsoas, sartorius, quadriceps, hip adductors	Hip flexion, knee extension, hip adduction	Patellar
L4	Medial aspect of calf	Tibialis anterior, quadriceps	Foot inversion, knee extension	Patellar
L5	Lateral part of lower leg and dorsum of foot	Extensor hallucis longus, extensor digitorum longus	Toe extension, ankle dorsiflexion	None
S1	Lateral edge of foot	Gastrocnemius, soleus	Ankle plantar flexion	Ankle jerk
S2	Posterior part of thigh	Flexor digitorum longus, flexor hallucis longus	Ankle plantar flexion, toe flexion	None

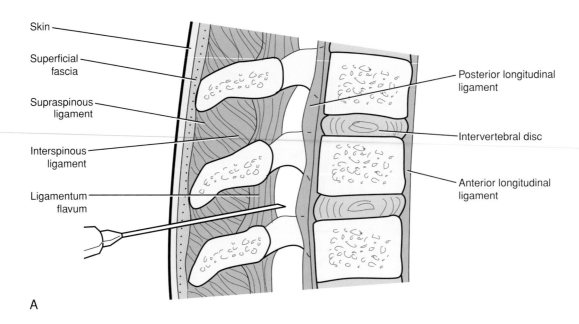

Skin

Superficial fascia

Supraspinous ligament

Interspinous ligament

Ligamentum flavum

Posterior longitudinal ligament

Intervertebral disc

Anterior longitudinal ligament

A

12th rib

Intercristal line (L4)

Iliac crest

B

Figure A-5   A: Structures penetrated by the spinal tap needle before it reaches the dura mater. **B:** Important anatomic landmarks when performing a spinal tap. Although this is usually performed with the patient in a lateral recumbent position with the vertebral column well flexed, the patient may be placed in the sitting position and bent well forward.

Index

Page numbers followed by "*f*" indicate figures. Page numbers followed by "*t*" indicate tables.

A

Abdominal aortic aneurysm, 479
Abdominal superficial reflexes, 100, 508–510
Abdominal systemic arteries, effect of autonomic system on, 397*t*
Abducens nerve, 204–205, 335, 336*f*, 351
  course, 336*f*, 337
  distribution, 336*f*
  nucleus, 335, 336*f*
  nucleus of, 205
Abnormal involuntary movements, 369
Absolute refractory period, 45
Accessory nerves, 204, 345, 353
  cranial root, 345, 346*f*
  distribution of, 347*f*
  function, 325*f*
  spinal root, 345–346, 346*f*
Accessory nucleus, 138
Accommodation reflex, 406
Acetylcholine (ACh), 54, 63, 94, 115, 301, 388, 392–393
  gated channels, 96
Acetylcholinesterase (AChE), 53*f*, 54, 96, 115
Achilles tendon reflex, 101, 510
Action potential (AP), 44–45
Acute esophagitis, 410
Acute labyrinthitis, 353
Adenosine triphosphate (ATP), 394
Adie tonic pupil syndrome, 408
Adiposogenital dystrophy syndrome, 267
Adrenergic endings, 393
Adrenergic receptor blockade, 394
Adult skull, 20
Afferent cerebellar pathways
  anterior spinocerebellar tract, 237–238, 238*t*
  from cerebral cortex, 236–237, 236*f*, 238*t*
  cerebro-olivocerebellar pathway, 236, 238*t*
  cerebroreticulocerebellar pathway, 236–237, 238*t*
  corticopontocerebellar pathway, 236, 238*t*
  cuneocerebellar tract, 238, 238*t*
  posterior spinocerebellar tract, 238, 238*t*
  from spinal cord, 237–238, 237*f*, 238*t*
  from vestibular nerve, 238, 238*t*
Afferent fibers, 12, 81, 234
Afferent nerve fibers, 312, 376–377, 378*f*, 378*t*, 388*f*, 390
Agranular type of cortex, 283
Agraphia, 291
Alar plate, 489–490
Albuterol, 393
Alcoholic headache, 429
Alexia, 291
Alpha (α) receptors, 393
Alpha rhythm, 292
Alveolar arch, 187
Alveolar process, 187
Alveus, 263, 303, 303*f*, 440
Alzheimer disease, 269–272
  cholinesterase inhibitors for, 272
  diagnosis of, 272
  signs for, 272
Amygdalohypothalamic fibers, 376

Amygdaloid complex destruction, 306
Amygdaloid nucleus, 261, 303, 311–312, 311*f*, 440
Amyotrophic lateral sclerosis (Lou Gehrig disease), 171
Anal canal involuntary internal sphincter, effect of autonomic system on, 397*t*, 402, 403*f*
Analgesic system, 146
Anencephaly, 500, 501*t*
Angular gyrus, lesions of, 291
Ankle jerk, 101
Annulus fibrosus, 135
Anorexia nervosa, 373
ANS. *See* Autonomic nervous system
Ansa lenticularis, 314
Anterior ascending ramus, 256
Anterior cerebral artery, 255, 465
  occlusion of, 472
Anterior cerebral vein, 470
Anterior clinoid process, 192
Anterior cochlear nuclei, 203, 207
Anterior columns of fornix, 254, 439
Anterior commissure, 254, 262, 498
Anterior communicating artery, 465
Anterior cord syndrome, 168, 169*f*
Anterior corticospinal tract, 155
Anterior cranial fossa, 191–192
Anterior external arcuate fibers, 196, 203
Anterior fontanelle, 191
Anterior gray column, 4, 138–139
Anterior gray commissure, 141
Anterior horizontal ramus, 256
Anterior horn of ventricles, 436, 439
  floor of, 439
  medial wall of, 439
  roof of, 439
Anterior inferior cerebellar artery, 468
Anterior intercavernous sinuses, 424
Anterior lobes of cerebellum, 229
Anterior longitudinal ligament, 135
Anterior median fissure of spinal cord, 196, 489, 489*f*
Anterior nerve cell groups, 138–139
Anterior neuropore, 15
Anterior or motor roots, 4
Anterior pituitary hormone, 380*t*
Anterior radicular artery, 472
Anterior ramus, 13
Anterior root, 12, 80
Anterior spinal artery, 466, 472
Anterior spinocerebellar tract, 149, 204, 208
Anterior spinothalamic tract, 146–147, 204
  injury, 163
Anterior temporal cortex, 289
Anterior thalamic nuclei, 365
Anterior white column, 4
Anterior white matter, 141
Anterograde amnesia, 305
Anterograde transport, 49
  fast, 49
  slow, 49
Anticholinesterases, 115

Aortic arch reflexes, 406
Appendicular pain, 410
Arachnoid granulations, 424*f*, 425, 450, 451*f*
Arachnoid mater, 4
  brain, 419*f*–420*f*, 422*f*, 424*f*–425*f*, 425
  spinal cord, 426, 426*f*
Arachnoid villi, 422, 425
Arbor vitae, 231, 234
Arcuate eminence, 194
Area postrema, 446
Area vestibuli, 205
Argyll Robertson pupil, 408
Arnold-Chiari phenomenon, 215, 215*f*, 500
Arrector pili muscle, effect of autonomic system on, 397*t*
Arterial lumen blockage, diseases resulting in, 473–474
Arterial wall disease, 473
Arteries of brain, 464–469
  anterior cerebral artery, 465
  anterior communicating artery, 465
  anterior inferior cerebellar artery, 468
  anterior spinal artery, 466
  basilar artery, 466–468
  central branches, 465, 468
  cerebral arteries
    areas supplied by, 467*f*
    nerve supply of, 468–469
  choroidal artery, 464–465
  circle of Willis, 464, 468
  cortical branches, 465, 468
  of inferior surface of brain, 466*f*
  internal carotid artery, 464–465, 465*f*
  labyrinthine artery, 467
  medullary arteries, 467
  meningeal branches, 466
  middle cerebral artery, 465, 468*f*
  ophthalmic artery, 464
  pontine arteries, 467
  posterior cerebral artery, 468
  posterior communicating artery, 464
  posterior inferior cerebellar artery, 466
  posterior spinal artery, 466
  to specific brain areas, 468
  superior cerebellar artery, 468
  vertebral artery, 466–468
Articular processes, 16, 133–135, 134*f*
Articular tubercle, 191
Ascending pathways, 150–151
Ascending tracts, 142–152
  anatomical organization, 142–152
  development of, 497
  functions
    ascending pathways, 150–151
    light touch and pressure pathways, 143*t*, 146–147, 147*f*
    muscle joint sense pathways, 143*t*, 147–150, 149*t*
    pain control, 146
    painful and thermal sensations, 142–145, 143*t*
    perception of pain, 145–146
    visceral sensory tracts, 149*t*, 151–152

Association cortex, 287–289
Association fibers, 264
Astereognosis, 291
Astrocytes, 488
    fibrous, 55
    functions, 55–58
    as phagocytes, 57
    processes of, 55
    protoplasmic, 55
    role in blood–brain barrier, 58
    storing of glycogen, 57
Ataxia, 241
Atherosclerotic parkinsonism, 317
Athetosis, 117, 167, 318
Atlanto-axial joints, 135
Atlanto-occipital joints, 135
Atonic bladder, 407
ATP. *See* Adenosine triphosphate
Atrophy, 267
Atropine, 63, 115, 394
Atropine methylnitrate, 457
Auditory afferents, 376
Auditory tube, 191
Automatic reflex bladder, 407
Autonomic ganglia, 15, 81
Autonomic ganglion, 390–391, 391*f*
Autonomic nerve plexuses, 390
Autonomic nervous system (ANS), 2, 83,
        387–410, 397*t*
    adrenergic receptor blockade, 394
    autonomic ganglia, 390–391, 391*f*
    causalgia, 410
    cholinergic receptor blockade, 394
    diseases to, 408
        Adie tonic pupil syndrome, 408
        Argyll Robertson pupil, 408
        caused by anticholinesterase agents, 409
        caused by black widow spider venom,
            408
        caused by botulinum toxin, 408
        diabetes mellitus, 408
        Frey syndrome, 408
        Hirschsprung disease, 408
        Horner syndrome, 408
    enteric nervous system, 394–395
    fast synaptic potentials, 392, 392*f*
    functions, 395
    ganglion-blocking agents, 392–393
    ganglion-stimulating agents, 392
    higher control, 394, 394*f*
    inhibitory synaptic potentials, 392, 392*f*
    injuries to, 406
        defecation, 407
        degeneration of autonomic nerves, 407
        ejaculation, 408
        erection, 407
        parasympathetic, 407
        regeneration of autonomic nerves, 407
        sympathetic, 406–407
        urinary bladder dysfunction, 407
    innervations, 396–405, 397*t*
    large autonomic plexuses, 390
    organization, 387–390
        parasympathetic part, 389*f*, 390
        sympathetic part, 388–390, 389*f*
    parasympathetic, 2
    physiologic reflexes, 406
    postganglionic nerve endings, 393
    postganglionic transmitters, 393–394, 393*f*
    preganglionic transmitters, 391*f*, 392, 392*f*
    referred visceral pain, 409–410, 409*f*
        appendicular pain, 410
        cardiac pain, 410
        gallbladder pain, 410
        stomach pain, 410
    slow synaptic potentials, 392, 392*f*
    sympathectomy
        hypertension, 409

        intermittent claudication, 409
        Raynaud disease, 409
    sympathetic, 2
    sympathetic *vs.* parasympathetic systems,
        395–396, 396*t*
Autonomic plexuses, 387
Autonomous bladder, 407
Axolemma, 48
Axonal reaction and axonal degeneration, 62
Axon hillock, 38, 48
Axonotmesis, 109
Axons, 2, 33, 48
    initial segment of, 48
    regeneration of, 108
    terminals of, 48
Axon transport, 49
Axoplasm, 48

B
Babinski sign, 166
Bacterial toxins, 115
Bainbridge right atrial reflex, 406
Band fiber, 106
Bands of Baillarger, 281
Barr body, 38
Basal nuclei (basal ganglia), 10, 260–262,
        310–318, 311*f*–312*f*, 314*f*
    amygdaloid nucleus, 311–312, 311*f*
    caudate nucleus, 311, 312*f*
    claustrum, 311, 311*f*, 312
    corpus striatum, 310–311, 311*f*
        afferent fibers, 312
        brainstem striatal fibers, 313*f*, 314
        caudate nucleus, 311, 312*f*
        connections, 312
        corticostriate fibers, 312, 313*f*
        efferent fibers, 313*f*, 314
        and globus pallidus, 312, 313*f*, 314
        lentiform nucleus, 311, 312*f*
        nigrostriate fibers, 313*f*, 314
        striatonigral fibers, 313*f*, 314
        striatopallidal fibers, 313*f*, 314
        thalamostriate fibers, 313*f*, 314
    disorders of, 267, 315
    functions, 314–315, 314*f*
    globus pallidus
        afferent fibers, 313*f*, 314
        connections, 312, 315
        efferent fibers, 314
        pallidofugal fibers, 314
        striatopallidal fibers, 313*f*, 314
    lentiform nucleus,corpus striatum, 311, 312*f*
    terminology used to describe, 310, 310*t*
Basal plates, 488, 490
Basal vein, 470
Baseline of skull, 507
Basilar artery, 466–468
Basilar groove, 204
Basis pedunculi, 154, 325
Basket cell, 231
Basolateral group, 303
Bell palsy, 352
Benedikt syndrome, 217, 218*f*
Benign fibroma, 112
Benzoquinonium, 115
Beta (β) receptors, 393
Beta rhythm, 292
Betz cells, 279, 282, 284
Biceps brachii tendon reflex, 100, 508
Bilateral anosmia, 349
Bilateral spastic paralysis, 170
Biliary ducts, effect of autonomic system on,
        397*t*, 401
Binocular vision neurons, 327–328, 328*f*
Biological clocks, reticular formation
            influence on, 301
Bipolar neurons, 34, 327
Bitemporal hemianopia, 349, 350*f*

Blood–brain barrier (BBB)
    brain trauma and, 457
    drugs and, 457
    in fetus and newborn, 457
    functional significance, 455
    in molecular terms, 453
    permeability of, 452
    structure of, 452–454, 453*f*
    tumors and, 457
Blood capillary of central nervous system
        (CNS), 453–454, 453*f*
Blood–cerebrospinal fluid barrier, 454
    functional significance, 455
    structure of, 454
Blood pressure
    blood viscosity, change in, 473
    carotid sinus syndrome, 473
    heart disease, 473
    physical shock, 473
    postural hypotension, 473
    psychological shock, 473
Blood supply to brain
    arteries, 464–469
    capillaries, 470
    cerebral circulation, 470–471
    veins, 469–470
Blood supply to spinal cord, 471–472
Blood viscosity changes, 473
Brachial plexus, 13, 83*f*, 111*t*
Brachioradialis tendon reflex, 100, 508
Bradykinin, 145
Brain, 4–11, 7*f*–8*f*
    arteries of, 464–469
    blood flow to, 470–471
        impairment of, 473–474
    capillaries, 470
    cerebrospinal fluid–brain interface,
        454–455, 455*f*
    computed tomography (CT) of, 24*f*, 270*f*
    coronal section of, 263*f*
    fetus with, 5*f*
    forebrain, 9–10
        cerebrum, 9–10
        diencephalon, 9–10
    hindbrain, 4–9
        cerebellum, 5
        medulla oblongata, 5
        pons, 5
    inferior view of, 259*f*
    magnetic resonance imaging (MRI) of, 25*f*,
        271*f*
    median sagittal section of, 9*f*
    meninges, 418–425
        arachnoid mater, 419*f*–420*f*, 422*f*,
            424*f*–425*f*, 425
        dura mater, 418–420, 419*f*–424*f*, 422–424
        pia mater, 419*f*, 425
    midbrain, 9
    primary divisions of developing, 15*t*
    structure, 10
    veins of, 469–470
    ventricular cavities of, 261*f*
    vesicles, 15
Brain development
    cerebellum (posterior part of
        metencephalon), 492–494
    cerebral cortex, 497–498
    cerebral hemispheres, 496–497
    commissures, 498
    diencephalon, 495–496
    forebrain (prosencephalon), 494–495
    medulla oblongata, 490–492
    midbrain (mesencephalon), 492
    myelination, in central nervous system, 498
    pons (ventral part of metencephalon), 492
    telencephalon, 496
    vesicles, 490, 491*t*
Brain injuries, 21–22

Brain lacerations, 21
Brain sand, 253
Brainstem, 4
    Arnold-Chiari phenomenon, 215, 215f
    cranial nerve nuclei, 204f
    cranial nerve nuclei in, 214f
    functions of, 195
    level inferior to pons, 204
    medulla oblongata, 4–5, 9, 194, 196–204,
        197f, 199t
        clinical significance of, 215
        cuneate nucleus, 197
        cuneate tubercle, 197
        decussation of lemnisci, 199, 199t, 201f
        decussation of pyramids, 198–199, 199t, 201f
        floor of fourth ventricle, 197
        gracile nucleus, 197
        internal structure, 197–204
        just inferior to pons, 199t, 203
        lateral medullary syndrome of
            Wallenberg, 215
        medial medullary syndrome, 215, 216f
        olives, 196, 199–203, 199t, 202f
        posterior cranial fossa, raised pressure
            of, 215
        posterior median sulcus, 197
        reticular formation, 204
        vascular disorders, 215
    midbrain
        Benedikt syndrome, 217, 218f
        cerebral aqueduct blockage in, 217
        clinical significance of, 217
        trauma of, 217
        vascular lesions, 217
        Weber syndrome, 217, 218f
    nucleus ambiguus, 203
    olivary nuclear complex, 199
    pons, 5, 9, 194
        anterior surface of, 204, 205f
        astrocytoma of, 216
        caudal part, 205–207, 206f
        clinical significance of, 215–217
        infarctions of, 217
        internal structure of, 205–209, 206f–208f
        level inferior to, 204
        posterior surface of, 205
        tumors of, 216–217
        posterior view, 196f
Brainstem striatal fibers, 313f, 314
Branchiomotor nerve fiber, 325
Branchiomotor nuclei, 325
Broca speech area, 284–285
    lesions of, 290–291
Brown-Séquard syndrome (cord
    hemisection), 169f–170f, 170

C
Calcar avis, 439
Calcarine sulcus, 256, 259, 439
Callosal sulcus, 259
Caloric tests, 353
Capillaries of brain, 470
Capsular cells, 81
Carbachol, 115
Carbamylcholine, 97
Cardiac pain, 410
Carotid canal, 191, 194
Carotid sinus reflexes, 406
Carotid sinus syndrome, 473
Catecholamines, 54
Cauda equina, 13, 447, 490
Caudal anesthesia, 20
Caudate nucleus, 10, 261, 439
    corpus striatum, 311, 312f
    tail of, 440
Causalgia, 410
Cauterization, thalamic surgical relief of pain
    by, 369

Cavernous sinuses, 424
Cavity of fourth ventricle, 196
Celiac plexus, 389
Cell body, 33
Cell coat, 43
Cells of Martinotti, 280, 282
Cells of suprarenal medulla, 15
Cell transport, 43
Central branches, 465, 468
Central canal, 4, 9, 141, 196, 436, 447, 489
Central cord syndrome, 168–170, 169f
Central gray matter, 210
Central nervous system (CNS), 1, 73, 79
    apparent recovery of, 112–113
    blood capillary of, 453–454, 453f
    brain, 1
    interior, 2
    major divisions, 2–11, 2f, 4t
    myelination of, 498
    neurons, 1
    pain control in, 146
    regeneration of axons, 108
    relationship between oligodendrocyte and
        myelinated nerve fibers, 74f
    spinal cord, 1. See also spinal cord
Central sulcus, 256
Centrioles, 43
Cerebellar cortex, 9, 231–233, 231f, 233f, 494
    afferent tracts
        from cerebral cortex, 236–237
        from spinal cord, 237–238
        from vestibular nerve, 237f, 238, 238t
    cellular organization of, 232f
    cerebellar efferent fibers, 239f
        dentothalamic pathway, 239–240, 240t
        fastigial reticular pathway, 240, 240t
        fastigial vestibular pathway, 240, 240t
        globose-emboliform-rubral pathway,
            239, 240t
    degeneration of, 267
    functional unit of, 235
    granular layer of cortex, 231, 233
    molecular layer of cortex, 231
    Purkinje cell layer of cortex, 231–232
Cerebellar efferent fibers, 239f
    dentothalamic pathway, 239–240, 240t
    fastigial reticular pathway, 240, 240t
    fastigial vestibular pathway, 240, 240t
    globose-emboliform-rubral pathway, 239,
        240t
Cerebellar hemisphere syndrome, 243
Cerebellar peduncles, 229, 235, 235f
    decussation of, 210, 239, 239f
    inferior, 9, 196, 203
    middle, 9, 204
    superior, 9, 205
        decussation of, 210, 239, 239f
Cerebelli, 195
Cerebellomedullary cistern, 447
Cerebellum, 5, 194, 204, 507
    arteries of, 468
    cerebellar cortical mechanisms, 234–235
    cerebellar cortical neurotransmitters,
        235
    cerebellar peduncles, 229, 235, 235f
    diseases involving
        cerebellar syndromes, 243
        common, 243
        gait, postural changes and alteration of,
            241
        ocular movement disturbances, 242
        reflexes, 242
        signs and symptoms of, 241–243
    functional areas, 233, 234f
    functions of, 240
    gross appearance, 229–231, 230f
    intermediate zone of cerebellar
        hemisphere, 233

        intracerebellar nuclei of, 233–234
        nuclear mechanism of, 235
    lobes of
        anterior, 229
        flocculonodular, 229
        middle, 229
    structures
        cerebellar cortex, 231–233, 231f, 233f
        cerebellar hemispheres, 229
        functional areas, 233
        gray matter of cortex, 231
        intracerebellar nuclei, 233–234
        white matter, 234
    veins of, 470
Cerebral aneurysms, 474
Cerebral angiography, 474–479, 475f–478f
Cerebral aqueduct (aqueduct of Sylvius), 9,
    209, 254, 436, 490, 494, 494f
Cerebral aqueduct of midbrain, 331, 332f
Cerebral artery, 466f–467f
    anterior, 465
    atheromatous degeneration of, 473
    middle, 465
    syndromes, 472
Cerebral circulation, 470–471
    impairment of cerebral blood flow,
        473–474
    interruption, 472–473
Cerebral commissures, 267–268
Cerebral cortex
    afferent cerebellar pathways of, 236–237,
        236f, 238t
    anatomical connections of, 284t
    cerebral dominance, 289–292
    cortical mechanisms, 283
    development of, 497–498, 497f
    function of, 290
    lesions, 290–291
    neuronal connections of, 281f
    structure
        cortical structure variations, 282–283
        layers, 281–282, 282f
        nerve cells, 279–280
        nerve fibers, 280–281
    types of neurons in, 280f
Cerebral cortical potentials, 292
Cerebral damage, 291–292
Cerebral dominance, 289–292
Cerebral edema, 64
Cerebral hemisphere lobes
    inferior surface, 259–260
    medial surface, 259–260
    superolateral surface, 258–259
Cerebral hemispheres, 23f, 255–256,
    255f–257f, 492
    amygdaloid nucleus, 261
    association fibers, 264
    basal nuclei (basal ganglia), 260–262
    claustrum, 262
    commissure fibers, 262–264
    corpus striatum, 261
    development of, 495f–496f, 496–497
    internal structure of, 260–266
    lateral ventricles, 260
    lateral view, 257f–258f
    medial view, 257f
    projection fibers, 264–265
    tela choroidea, 265
    venous drainage of, 469f
    white matter, 260, 262–265
Cerebral hemorrhage, 22, 429, 474
Cerebral ischemia, 472
Cerebral peduncles, 209–210, 210f
    crus cerebri of, 11f
    decussation of, 210
    superior, 9, 205, 208
        decussation of, 210, 239, 239f
    tegmentum of, 255

Cerebrospinal fluid (CSF), 1, 3f, 4, 9, 16, 436, 437f, 490
  absorption of, 450
  around optic nerve, 452f
  circulation of, 449–450, 450f
    blockage of, 456
  clinical measurement of, 456
  in disease, pressure/composition, 456–457
  expulsion of, 23
  formation of, 448–449, 449f
    excessive, 456
  functions of, 448, 449t
  glucose level in, 449, 456
  physical characteristics and composition, 448t
  pressure, 20, 22
Cerebrospinal fluid–brain interface, 454–455, 455f
Cerebrum, 9–10, 507
  cerebral hemisphere lobes
    inferior surface, 259–260
    medial surface, 259–260
    superolateral surface, 258–259
  cerebral hemispheres, 255–256, 255f–257f
    amygdaloid nucleus, 261
    association fibers, 264
    basal nuclei (basal ganglia), 260–262
    claustrum, 262
    commissure fibers, 262–264
    corpus striatum, 261
    internal structure of, 260–266
    lateral ventricles, 260
    lateral view, 257f–258f
    medial view, 257f
    projection fibers, 264–265
    tela choroidea, 265
    white matter, 260, 262–265
  diencephalon
    actual superior wall of, 250
    epithalamus, 253–254
    gross features, 249–250
    hypothalamic relations, 254
    hypothalamus, 250, 254
    inferior surface of, 251f, 254
    lateral surface of, 250
    mammillary bodies, 254–255
    medial surface of, 250, 251f
    optic chiasma, 254
    subthalamus, 253
    superior surface of, 249–250
    thalamus, 249–253, 252f
    third ventricle, 254–255
    tuber cinereum, 254
  subdivisions, 249
  sulci of
    calcarine sulcus, 256
    central sulcus, 256
    lateral sulcus, 256
    parieto-occipital sulcus, 256
Cervical disc herniations, 17–18
Cervical enlargement, 490
Cervical nerves, 12
Cervical plexus, 13
Cervical rib, 408
Cervical vertebrae, 12
Chemical synapses, 51–52
Chemoreceptors, 84
Chloramphenicol, 457
Cholinergic receptors, 393
  blockade of, 394
Cholinesterases, 115
Chorea, 167, 315
Choreiform movements, 117, 315
Choroidal artery, 464–465
Choroidal branch, 468
  of internal carotid, 265
Choroidal epithelial cells, 60
Choroidal fissure, 439

Choroidea of third ventricle, 250
Choroid plexus, 439, 442f, 492
  blood supply to, 441–443, 468
    from posterior inferior cerebellar arteries, 447
  function of, 440, 449
  of lateral ventricles, 440, 496
  of rhomboid fossa (floor), 447
  of third ventricle, 250, 441–443, 495
    calcification of, 267
Choroid vein, 470
Chromatolysis, 39, 106–107
Chromophobe adenoma, 267
Cingulate gyrus, 259
Cingulum, 264
Circle of Willis, 464, 468, 470f
Circumferential blindness, 349, 350f
Claustrum, 262, 311, 311f, 312
Climbing fibers, 234
Clostridium botulinum, 115
CNs. See Cranial nerves
Coccygeal nerve, 12
Cochlear nerve, 340–341, 340f
  descending auditory pathways, 341
  disturbances, 353
  nuclei, 340f, 341
Cochlear nuclei, 203, 207
Codeine, 164
Collateral eminence, 442
Collateral fissure, 442
Collateral sulcus, 259–260
Colliculus facialis, 335, 336f, 338
Colon, effect of autonomic system on, 397t, 400–401, 401f
Coma, 292
Commissure fibers, 262–264
Commissures
  anterior, 254, 262, 498
  anterior gray, 141
  cerebral, 267–268
  development of, 498
  of fornix, 264
  gray, 4, 141, 447
  habenular, 253–254, 264
  posterior, 253–254, 263
  posterior gray, 141
Communicating hydrocephalus, 456
Competitive blocking agents, 97
Compression of spinal cord
  clinical signs, 167
  extradural causes, 167
Computed tomography (CT), 23, 429
  cerebral ventricles, clinical investigation of, 456
  of cerebrovascular disease, 474
  structure of brain, 24f
Conduction velocity of nerve fiber, 46, 46t
Cones, visual system, 327
Congenital anomalies
  anencephaly, 500, 501t
  hydrocephalus, 500, 500f
  neural tube defects, 500–501
  spina bifida, 498–500
Consciousness, 292
  loss of, 306
  somatosensory pathways to, 143t
Consensual light reflexes, 406
Constrictor pupillae muscle, 329–330
Contralateral homonymous hemianopia, 349, 350f
Contrecoup injury, 22
Conus medullaris, 4
Convolutions, 497
Cord transection syndrome, complete, 168, 169f
Coronal suture, 187, 190
Corona radiata, 10, 146, 149, 154, 264, 325

Corpus callosum, 10, 255, 259, 262
  body of, 262
  development of, 498
  genu of, 262, 439
  radiation of, 262
  rostrum of, 262
  tapetum of, 439–440
Corpus striatum, 261, 310–311, 311f, 468, 496
  afferent fibers, 312
  brainstem striatal fibers, 313f, 314
  caudate nucleus, 311, 312f
  connections, 312
  corticostriate fibers, 312, 313f
  efferent fibers, 313f, 314
  and globus pallidus, 312, 313f, 314
  lentiform nucleus, 311, 312f
  nigrostriate fibers, 313f, 314
  striatonigral fibers, 313f, 314
  striatopallidal fibers, 313f, 314
  thalamostriate fibers, 313f, 314
Cortex, 9–10
  effect of autonomic system on, 397t
Cortical areas
  association cortex, 287–289
  frontal lobe, 283–285
    Broca speech area, 284–285
    frontal eye field, 284
    movement areas of body, 283–284
    posterior region, 283
    precentral area, 283
    premotor area, 284
    primary motor area, 283–284
    secondary motor area, 283
    supplementary motor area, 284
  insula, 287
  occipital lobe, 286–287
    macula lutea, 287
    occipital eye field, 287
    primary visual area (Brodmann area), 286–287
    secondary visual area (Brodmann areas), 287
    visual cortex, 287
  parietal lobe, 286
    outer layer of Baillarger, 286
    primary somesthetic area, 286
    secondary somesthetic area, 286
    somesthetic association area, 286
  prefrontal cortex, 285
  taste area, 287
  temporal lobe
    primary auditory area (Brodmann areas), 287
    secondary auditory area (auditory association cortex), 287
    sensory speech area of Wernicke, 287
  vestibular area, 287
Cortical branches, 465, 468
Cortical mechanisms, 283
Corticobulbar tract, 494
Corticohypothalamic fibers, 376
Corticomedial group, 303
Corticonuclear fibers, 214, 323, 325
Corticopontine fibers, 207, 214
Corticopontine tract, 494
Corticospinal fibers, 196, 214
Corticospinal tract (pyramidal tract), 154–156, 282, 494
  lesions, 166
  spinal cord
    anterior, 155
    lateral, 155
Corticostriate fibers, 312, 313f
Cranial cavity, 418, 422
  anterior cranial fossa, 191–192
  base of skull, 191, 192f
  mandible, 195
  middle cranial fossa, 192–195
  vault of skull, 191

Cranial nerve I
  olfactory bulb, 326f, 327
  olfactory nerves, 326–327, 326f
  olfactory tract, 326f, 327
Cranial nerve II, 327–331, 328f
  binocular vision neurons, 327–328, 328f
  lateral geniculate body, 327, 328f
  optic chiasma, 327, 328f
  optic radiation, 327, 328f
  optic tract, 327, 328f–329f
  visual pathway neurons, 327–328, 328f
  visual reflexes, 328–331, 329f
    accommodation reflex, 329–330, 329f
    consensual light reflex, 329, 329f
    corneal reflex, 330, 330f
    direct light reflex, 328, 329f
    pupillary skin reflex, 331
    visual body reflexes, 330–331, 330f
Cranial nerve III, 331, 332f, 494
  oculomotor nerve course, 331, 332f
  oculomotor nerve nuclei, 331, 332f
Cranial nerve IV, 331–332, 333f, 494
  trochlear nerve course, 331–332, 333f
  trochlear nerve nuclei, 331, 333f
Cranial nerve IX, 341
  course, 343, 343f
  distribution, 343f
  function, 325t
  nuclei, 341, 342f
    main motor nucleus, 341–342, 342f
    parasympathetic, 342, 342f
    sensory, 342, 342f
Cranial nerve nuclei, 323–353
  abducens nerve, 335, 336f
    course, 336f, 337
    nucleus, 335, 336f
  facial nerve, 337–339
    course, 338, 338f
    distribution, 338f, 339
    nuclei, 337–338, 337f
  general visceral motor nuclei, 325
  motor nuclei, 325
  oculomotor nerve, 331
    course, 331, 332f
    nuclei, 331, 332f
  olfactory nerves, 326–327, 326f
    olfactory bulb, 326f, 327
    olfactory tract, 326f, 327
  optic nerve, 327–331, 328f
    accommodation reflex, 329–330, 329f
    binocular vision neurons, 327–328, 328f
    consensual light reflex, 329, 329f
    corneal reflex, 330, 330f
    direct light reflex, 328, 329f
    lateral geniculate body, 327, 328f
    optic chiasma, 327, 328f
    optic radiation, 327, 328f
    optic tract, 327, 328f–329f
    pupillary skin reflex, 331
    visual body reflexes, 330–331, 330f
    visual pathway neurons, 327–328, 328f
    visual reflexes, 328–331, 329f
  organization, 323–326
  sensory nuclei of, 325–326
  somatic motor nucleus, 325
  trigeminal nerve, 332, 334f
    course, 335, 335f
    distribution of, 335f
    main sensory nucleus, 332–333, 334f
    mesencephalic nucleus, 333, 334f
    motor component, 334–335, 334f
    motor nucleus, 333, 334f
    nuclei, 332–333, 334f
    sensory components, 333–334, 334f
    spinal nucleus, 333, 334f
  trochlear nerve, 331
    course, 331–332, 333f
    nuclei, 331, 333f
Cranial nerves (CNs), 81, 82f, 323, 324t–325t
  branchiomotor nerve fiber of, 325
  functional components of, 324t
  general visceral motor nuclei of, 325
  motor nuclei of, 323, 325
  organization, 323–326
  sensory ganglia of, 15
  sensory nuclei of, 325–326
  somatic motor fiber of, 325
Cranial nerve V, 332, 334f
  distribution of, 335f
  main sensory nucleus, 332–333, 334f
  mesencephalic nucleus, 333, 334f
  motor component, 334–335, 334f
  motor nucleus, 333, 334f
  sensory components, 333–334, 334f
  spinal nucleus, 333, 334f
  trigeminal nerve course, 335, 335f
  trigeminal nerve nuclei, 332–333, 334f
Cranial nerve VI, 335, 336f
  abducens nerve course, 336f, 337
  abducens nerve nucleus, 335, 336f
Cranial nerve VII, 337–339
  course, 338, 338f
  distribution, 338f, 339
  nuclei, 337
    main motor, 337, 337f
    parasympathetic, 337, 337f
    sensory, 337–338, 337f
Cranial nerve VIII
  cochlear nerve, 340–341, 340f
  vestibulocochlear nerve, 339–341
Cranial nerve X, 343
  course, 344–345, 345f
  distribution of, 345f
  function, 325t
  nuclei, 343
    main motor, 343, 344f–345f
    parasympathetic, 343, 344f–345f
    sensory, 343–344, 344f–345f
Cranial nerve XI, 345
  cranial root, 345, 346f
  distribution of, 347f
  function, 325t
  spinal root, 345–346, 346f
Cranial nerve XII, 347
  course, 347f, 348, 348f
  function, 325t
  nucleus, 347–348, 347f–348f
Cranial part of accessory nerves, 204
Cranial root, 325t, 345, 346f
Craniopharyngioma, 267
Craniosacral outflow, 395
Cremasteric reflex, 166
Cribriform plate, 192
Crista galli, 192
Crossed extensor reflex, 161
Crossed homonymous hemianopia, 291
Crus cerebri, 210–211, 214
Cuneate nucleus, 197, 490
Cuneate tubercle, 197
Cuneatus of medulla oblongata, 149
Cuneocerebellar tract, 149–150
Cuneus, 259
Cutaneous nerves, 83
Cytoplasm, 38–43, 41f
Cytotoxic edema, 64

D
Decamethonium, 115
Decerebrate rigidity, 162
Decussation
  of cerebellar peduncles, 210, 239, 239f
  of lemnisci, 199, 199t, 201f
  in midbrain (mesencephalon), 210
  of pyramids, 154, 196, 198–199, 199t, 201f
  sensory, 149

Deep middle cerebral vein, 470
Defecation, 407
Degeneration of autonomic nerves, 407
Delta rhythm, 292
Dementia, 315
Dendrites, 33, 48
Dendritic spines, 48, 232, 280
Dentate, 494
Dentate gyrus, 303
Dentate nucleus of cerebellar nuclei, 9, 233
Dentothalamic pathway, 239–240, 240t
Dermatome, 98, 116
  dermatomal charts, 99f–100f
Descending autonomic fibers, 154, 159–160
Descending fibers, to brainstem, 377
Descending tracts, 152–160, 152f, 153t
  anatomical organization, 153
  descending autonomic fibers, 154, 159–160
  development of, 497
  functions, 153–160
  lesions of, 166
    clasp-knife reaction, 166
    exaggerated deep muscle reflexes, 166
    severe paralysis, 166
    spasticity or hypertonicity, 166
  olivospinal tract, 154, 159, 160f
  rubrospinal tract, 154, 157–158, 158f
  tectospinal tract, 154, 157, 157f
  vestibulospinal tract, 154, 158–159, 159f
Destructive lesions of frontal eye field, 290
Diabetes insipidus, 267, 382
Diabetes mellitus, 408
Diaphragma sellae, 254, 418, 419f, 420, 421f
Diencephalon, 9–10, 490, 495–496, 495f
  actual superior wall of, 250
  epithalamus, 253–254
  gross features, 249–250
  hypothalamic relations, 254
  hypothalamus, 250, 254
  inferior surface of, 251f, 254
  lateral surface of, 250
  mammillary bodies, 254
  medial surface of, 250, 251f
  optic chiasma, 254
  subthalamus, 253
  superior surface of, 249–250
  thalamus, 249–253, 252f
  third ventricle, 254–255
  tuber cinereum, 254
Diisopropylphosphorofluoridate (DPF), 63
Dimethyltubocurarine, 115
Diplegia, 166
Diploë, 185
Diploic veins, 422
Direct light reflexes, 406
Dopamine, 54, 391
Dorsal accessory olivary nuclei, 199
Dorsal motor nucleus, 325
Dorsal nucleus of vagus, 203
Dorsomedial nucleus, 365
Dorsum sellae, 194
D-tubocurarine, 97, 114
Dura mater, 4
  brain, 418–420, 419f–424f, 422–424
  spinal cord, 425–426, 426f–428f
Dysarthria, 243
Dysdiadochokinesia, 241–242
Dystonia, 167

E
Ectoderm, 14
Edema
  cerebral, 64
  cytotoxic, 64
  interstitial, 64
  vasogenic, 64
Edinger–Westphal nucleus, 213, 325, 329, 331

Effector endings
 cardiac muscular, neuromuscular
  junctions in, 98
 secretory cells of glands, nerve endings
  on, 98
 skeletal muscle, neuromuscular junctions
  in, 94–97, 94f
 skeletal muscle innervation, 93–94
 smooth muscle, neuromuscular junctions
  in, 97–98
Efferent fibers, 12, 80, 234
 corpus striatum, 313f, 314
Efferent nerve fibers, 377, 378f, 378t, 388–390,
  389f
 α efferents, 138
 Γ efferents, 138
Ehrlich, Paul, 452
Ejaculation, 408
 effect of autonomic system on, 397t, 403,
  404f
Electrical synapses, 54
Electrocorticograms, 292
Electroencephalogram, 292
Electromagnetic receptors, 84
Emaciation, 267
Emboliform nucleus of cerebellar nuclei,
  233–234
Embryonic stem cell treatment of neurologic
  diseases, 501
Emissary veins, 422
Emotional disorders, 382
Encapsulated receptors, 85–89
Encephalogram, 456
Endocrine nervous system control, 301
Endoneurium, 80
Endorphins, 146
Endosteal layer, 418
Endothelial cells of blood capillaries, 453
Endplate potential, 96
Enkephalins, 146
Enteric nervous system, 394–395
Entoderm, 14
Ependyma, 59–60, 141, 436, 498
Ependymal cells, 488
Ependymocytes, 59
Epidural hematoma burr hole, 507
Epidural (extradural) hemorrhage, 22, 429
Epilepsy, 292
Epineurium, 80
Epithalamus, 253–254
Epithelial cells, 59–60, 61f
Erectile tissue, effect of autonomic system
  on, 397t, 402–403, 404f
Erection, 407
 clitoral, 402–403
 penile, 402–403
Ethmoid, 187
Exocytosis, 96
Expressive aphasia, 290
External auditory meatus, 191
External band of Baillarger, 282
External capsule, 261–262, 497
External granular layer of cortex, 281–282
External medullary lamina, 363, 364f
External occipital protuberance, 188–190
External ophthalmoplegia, 351
External pyramidal layer of cortex, 282
Exteroceptive information, 142
Extracellular space, 60
Extrapyramidal tracts, 165
Eye, autonomic innervation of, 396–397, 397t
Eyeball, lateral rectus muscle of, 335, 336f,
  337
Eye field
 frontal, 284
  destructive lesions of, 290
  irritative lesions of, 290
 occipital, 287

F
Facial colliculus, 205, 445
Facial expression muscles control, 301
Facial nerve, 204, 337–339, 351–352
 course, 338, 338f
 distribution, 338f, 339
 function, 324t
 lesions, 351–352
 nuclei, 337
  main motor, 337, 337f
  parasympathetic, 337, 337f
  sensory, 337–338, 337f
Facial nucleus, 205
Falx cerebelli, 420
Falx cerebri, 10, 192, 255, 418, 419f, 421f, 496
Fasciculus cuneatus, 147–149, 198
 injury, 163–164
Fasciculus gracilis, 147–149, 198
 injury, 163–164
Fasciculus lenticularis, 314
Fastigial nucleus of cerebellar nuclei, 233–234
Fastigial reticular pathway, 240, 240t
Fastigial vestibular pathway, 240, 240t
Fast pain, 145–146
Feeder arteries, 472
Fibrous astrocytes, 55, 56f
Fifth cervical segment, spinal cord, 139f
Filum terminale, 4, 13, 13f, 490
Fimbria, 263, 303, 440
Fine-skilled voluntary movements, 166
First-order neuron, 142, 143t, 144, 146, 149t,
  153, 161, 325–326
Flaccid paralysis, 166
Flocculonodular lobes of cerebellum, 229
Folic acid, 501
Fontanelles, 191
Foramen cecum, 192
Foramen lacerum, 191, 194
Foramen magnum, 194
Foramen of Magendie, 443, 492
Foramen ovale, 191, 194
Foramen rotundum, 188, 193–194
Foramen spinosum, 191, 194, 422
Foramina of Luschka, 443, 446f, 492
Forceps major, 262, 439
Forceps minor, 262
Forebrain (prosencephalon)
 cerebrum, 9–10
 development of, 494–495
 diencephalon, 9–10
 vesicle, 15, 488, 490, 491f, 491t
Fornix, 249, 255, 263
 anterior column of, 439
 body of, 264, 302f, 303
 columns of, 304
 commissure of, 264, 303–304
 as crus of, 302f, 303
 development of, 498
 posterior column of, 440
 posterior columns of, 264
Fourth ventricle, 9, 197, 199t, 229, 234, 436,
  490
 cavity of, 141, 196
 floor of, 158, 197, 203, 454
 tumors of, 456–457
Free nerve endings, 84, 85f
Frey syndrome, 408
Frontal bone, 186–187
Frontal eye field, 284
 destructive lesions of, 290
 irritative lesions of, 290
Frontal leukotomy, 291
Frontal lobe, 256, 258, 496
 frontal eye field, 284
 movement areas of body, 283–284
 posterior region, 283
 precentral area, 283

premotor area, 284
 primary motor area, 283–284
 secondary motor area, 283
 supplementary motor area, 284
Frontal lobectomy, 291
Fronto-occipital fasciculus, 264
Fusiform cells, 280

G
Gag reflex, 353
Gait, postural changes and alteration of, 241
Gallamine, 115
Gallbladder
 effect of autonomic system on, 397t, 401
 pain, 410
Ganglia, 387
Ganglion
 basal nuclei, 310–318
 ciliary, 397
Ganglion-blocking agents, 392–393
Ganglion cells, 327–328
Ganglioneuroma, 62
Ganglionic layer (internal pyramidal layer) of
  cortex, 282
Ganglionic layer of retina, 327, 328f
Ganglion impar, 390
Ganglion-stimulating agents, 392
Gastrointestinal tract, effect of autonomic
  system on, 397t, 400–401, 401f
Gating, 47
Gating theory, 146
General visceral motor nuclei, 325
Geniculate ganglion, 338, 338f
Genital hypoplasia, 267
Genu of corpus callosum, 262, 264
Glands, effect of autonomic system on, 397t
Glial cells, 253
Gliotic scar, 63
Global aphasia, 291
Globose-emboliform-rubral pathway, 239,
  240t
Globose nucleus of cerebellar nuclei, 233–234
Globus pallidus, 496f, 497
 afferent fibers, 313f, 314
 connections, 312, 315
 efferent fibers, 314
 pallidofugal fibers, 314
 striatopallidal fibers, 313f, 314
Glossopharyngeal nerve, 341, 353
 accessory nerves, 204
 course, 343, 343f
 distribution, 343f
 function, 325t
 nuclei, 341, 342f
  main motor, 341–342, 342f
  parasympathetic, 342, 342f
  sensory, 342, 342f
Glutamate, 145
Glycocalyx, 43
Golgi complex, 39–41
Golgi tendon organs, 92–93
Golgi type II neurons, 34, 36f
Golgi type I neurons, 34, 35f–36f
Gracile nucleus, 197, 490
Granular cells, 327, 498
Granular layer of cortex, 231, 233, 283
Gray column, spinal cord
 accessory nucleus, 138
 anterior nerve cell groups, 138–139
 central canal, 141
 gray commissure, 141
 lateral nerve cell groups, 141
 lumbosacral nucleus, 138
 posterior nerve cell groups, 139–141
Gray commissure, 4, 141, 447
Gray matter, 2, 4
 central, 203–204
 interthalamic connection of, 496

Gray rami communicantes, 388
Great cerebral vein, 265, 423
Greater petrosal nerve, 194
Gyri, 10, 497
Gyrus rectus, 260

H
Habenular commissure, 253–254, 264
Habenular nucleus, 253, 264
Hair follicle receptors, 84–85, 86f–87f
Hand, thalamic, 369
Headache
    alcoholic, 429
    caused by cerebral tumors, 429
    due to diseases of teeth, paranasal sinuses,
        and eyes, 429
    meningeal, 429
    migraine, 429
Head Injuries
    acute cerebral injury, 21f
    skull fractures, 20–21
Heart, effect of autonomic system on, 397t,
    399, 400f
Hemiballismus, 167, 315
Hemiplegia, 166
Hemorrhage of pons, 217
Herniation of intervertebral discs, 16–17
Herpes simplex, 62
Herpes zoster, 62, 113
Heterotypical area of cortex, 282–283
Hexamethonium, 63
    block ganglia, 392
Hindbrain
    cerebellum, 5
    medulla oblongata, 5
    pons, 5
    vesicle, 15, 197, 488, 490, 491t
Hippocampohypothalamic fibers, 376
Hippocampus, 249, 301
    afferent connections of, 304–305, 305f
    efferent connections of, 305, 305f
Hirschsprung disease, 408
Histamine, 145
Homotypical area of cortex, 283
Homotypical cortex, 289
Homunculus, 154
Horizontal cells of Cajal, 280
Horizontal fissure, 229
Horner syndrome, 171, 408
Hunger center, 381
Huntingtin, 315
Huntington disease, 315, 316f
Hydrocephalus, 267, 455–456, 500, 500f
Hypalgesia, 116
Hyperesthesia, 116
Hyperkalemic paralysis, 115
Hyperkinetic disorders, 315
Hypertension, 409
Hyperthermia, 382
Hypertonia, 166
Hypertonicity, 166
Hypesthesia, 116
Hypoglossal canal, 191, 194
Hypoglossal nerves, 194, 204, 347, 353
    course, 347f, 348, 348f
    function, 325t
    nucleus, 347–348, 347f–348f
Hypoglossal nucleus, 203, 446
Hypoglossal triangle, 446
Hypokalemic periodic paralysis, 115
Hypokinetic disorders, 315
Hypophyseal portal system, 379–380, 380t
Hypophysis, 255
Hypophysis cerebri, 194, 254, 420
    connections with, 377–380, 379f, 380t
        hypophyseal portal system, 379–380,
            380t
        hypothalamohypophyseal tract, 377, 379

Hypotension, postural, 473
Hypothalamic nuclei, 375–376, 375f–376f
    lateral zone, 375–376
    lines of communication, 376–380
        afferent nervous connections, 376–377
        efferent nervous connections, 377
        hypophysis cerebri, connections with,
            377–380, 379f, 380t
        medial zone, 375–376
Hypothalamic regulatory hormone, 380t
Hypothalamic relations, 254
Hypothalamic sulcus, 250, 255
Hypothalamic syndromes, 267
Hypothalamohypophyseal tract, 377, 379
Hypothalamus, 9, 250, 254, 267, 373–382, 374f,
    454
    functions, 380–382, 380t
        autonomic control, 381, 381f
        circadian rhythms, control of, 382
        emotion and behavior, 381–382
        endocrine control, 381
        neurosecretion, 381
        regulation of food and water intake, 381
        temperature regulation, 381
    lesions, 382
    lines of communication, 376–380
        afferent nervous connections, 376–377,
            378t
        efferent nervous connections, 377, 378t
        hypophysis cerebri, connections with,
            377–380, 379f, 380t
    nuclei, 375–376, 375f–376f
        lateral zone, 375–376
        medial zone, 375–376
    parts of, 374f
    position, 374f
    structures, 373, 374f
Hypothermia, 382
Hypotonia, 166, 241

I
Iatrogenic parkinsonism, 317
Incisive fossa, 190
Incisures of Schmidt–Lanterman, 73
Indusium griseum, 303
Infarction of pons, 217
Inferior articular processes, 133
Inferior brachium, 209, 366
Inferior cerebellar peduncles, 9, 196, 203
Inferior colliculi/inferior colliculus, 210–213,
    211f–212f, 213t, 331, 333f, 494
Inferior conchae, 187
Inferior frontal gyrus, 258
Inferior frontal sulci, 258
Inferior horn of ventricles, 436, 440
    roof of, 440
Inferior longitudinal fasciculus, 264
Inferior medullary velum, 443, 445f
Inferior olivary nucleus, 196, 199
Inferior orbital fissure, 188
Inferior parietal lobule, 258
Inferior petrosal sinuses, 194, 424
Inferior quadrantic hemianopia, 291
Inferior sagittal sinus, 265, 419, 419f, 421f, 423
Inferior salivatory nucleus, 325
Inferior vertebral notch, 133
Inferior vestibular nucleus, 199
Infraorbital foramen, 187
Infratemporal crest, 188
Infratemporal fossa, 188
Infundibulum, 249, 254–255, 496
Inhibitory interneurons, 235
Inner band of Baillarger, 282
Inner glial limiting membranes, 55
Insula, 256, 287, 497
    lesions of, 291
Intermaxillary suture, 187
Intermittent claudication, 409

Internal acoustic meatus, 195
Internal arcuate fibers, 199
Internal capsule, 10, 146, 149, 154, 261, 327,
    497
    anterior limb, 264
    arteries of, 468
    auditory radiation of, 287
    lesions, 268–269
    posterior limb, 264
    of thalamus, 252
    of white matter, 250
Internal carotid artery, 424, 464–465
    occlusion of, 473
Internal carotid plexus, 331
Internal cerebral veins, 265
Internal granular layer of cortex, 282
Internal jugular vein, 195
Internal medullary lamina, 365f
Internal occipital crest, 195
Internal occipital protuberance, 195
Internal ophthalmoplegia, 351
Internal strabismus, 351
Internuclear ophthalmoplegia, 351
Internuncial neurons, 325
Interpeduncular cistern, 447
Interpeduncular fossa, 210, 331
Intersegmental spinal reflexes, 160
    crossed extensor reflex, 161
    influence of higher neuronal centers on,
        162
    monosynaptic reflex, 160, 161f
Intersegmental tracts, 160–162
Interspinous ligament, 135
Interstitial edema, 64
Interthalamic connection, 363, 364f
Intertransverse ligaments, 135
Interventricular foramen, 9, 260, 495
Interventricular foramina (foramina of
    Monro), 10, 254, 436, 490
Intervertebral foramen, 133
Intestine, effect of autonomic system on,
    397t, 400, 401f
Intracerebellar nuclei, 231
Intracranial hematoma treatment, 507–508
Intracranial hemorrhage, 22, 429, 474
    in infant, 429
Intracranial pneumography, 456
Intralaminar nuclei, 366
Intraparietal sulcus, 258
Intrinsic fibers, 234
Ipsilateral band of cutaneous anesthesia, 170
Ipsilateral lower motor neuron paralysis, 170
Ipsilateral spastic paralysis, 170
Iris, autonomic innervation of, 396–397, 397t,
    398f
Irritative lesions of frontal eye field, 290

J
Jacksonian epileptic seizure, 290
Jerk nystagmus, 242
Jugular foramen, 191, 194
Junctional folds, 96

K
Kidney, effect of autonomic system on, 397t,
    401, 402f
Kinesin-coated organelles, 43
K+ ions, 145
Klüver-Bucy syndrome, 306
Knee jerk, 101
    pendular, 242

L
Labyrinthine artery, 467
Lacrimal gland, autonomic innervation of,
    397–398, 397t, 399f
Lacrimal nuclei of facial nerve, 325
Lactic acid, 145

Lambdoid suture, 187–188
Laminae, 132
Lamina terminalis, 254, 262, 495, 498
Large autonomic plexuses, 390
Lateral corticospinal tract, 155, 198
Lateral dorsal nucleus, 366
Lateral geniculate body, 327–328, 328*f*, 366, 496, 498
Lateral gray column, 141
Lateral herniation, 18
Lateral lemniscus, 209, 211, 214, 341
Lateral medullary syndrome of Wallenberg, 215, 216*f*
Lateral nerve cell groups, 141
Lateral nucleus, 376
Lateral posterior nucleus, 366
Lateral pterygoid plate, 191
Lateral rectus muscle of eyeball, 335, 336*f*, 337
Lateral spinothalamic tract, 144–146, 204
    injury, 163
    terminations of, 146
Lateral sulcus, 256, 498
Lateral tuberal nuclei, 376
Lateral ventricles, 10, 260, 436–440, 441*f*, 468, 490
    anterior horn of, 436, 439
    body of, 436–439
    choroid plexus of, 439–440
    development of, 495
    disorders of, 267
    floor of, 439
    inferior horn of, 436, 440
    posterior horn of, 436, 439
    roof of, 439
Lateral vestibular nucleus, 240
Lateral white column, 4
Lateral white matter, 141
Law of reciprocal innervation, 161
L-dopa, 63, 457
Lenticulostriate artery, 22
Lentiform nucleus, 10, 261, 311, 312*f*, 496
Lesser petrosal nerve, 194
Lethargy, 292
Ligamentum denticulatum, 426, 490
Ligamentum flavum, 135
Ligamentum nuchae, 135
Light touch, 113
Limbic system, 301, 302*f*–305*f*, 303–306, 377
    alveus, 303, 303*f*
    amygdaloid nucleus, 303
    basolateral group, 303
    connecting pathways of, 303–304
    corticomedial group, 303
    dentate gyrus, 303–304
    fimbria, 303
    fornix, 302*f*, 303
    functions, 305
    hippocampal formation, 301, 302*f*–304*f*, 303
    hippocampal structure, 304
    hippocampus, 301
        afferent connections of, 304–305, 305*f*
        as crus of fornix, 302*f*, 303
        efferent connections of, 305, 305*f*
    indusium griseum, 303
    mammillary body, 304
    mammillothalamic tract, 304
    parahippocampal gyrus, 303
    pes hippocampus, 301
    septum pellucidum, 304
    striae, 303
    stria terminalis, 304
    uncus, 303
Lingual gyrus, 260
Lipofuscin, 43
Liver, effect of autonomic system on, 397*t*
Lobes, 10
    of cerebellum
        anterior, 229

flocculonodular, 229
        middle, 229
    of cerebral hemisphere
        inferior surface, 259–260
        medial surface, 259–260
        superolateral surface, 258–259
    frontal, 256, 258, 283–284, 496
    occipital, 256, 259, 286–287, 496
    parietal, 256, 258, 286, 496
    temporal, 193, 256, 258
Long association fibers, 264
Long ciliary nerves, 331, 397
Longitudinal cerebral fissure, 255
Longitudinal fissure, 10
Lower limb arteries, effect of autonomic system on, 397*t*, 405, 405*f*
Lower motor neurons, 152–153, 325
    cerebellum functions, influence on, 240
    inhibition, 162
    lesions, 166, 352*f*
    palsy, 217
    paralysis, 168, 170
    in progressive muscular atrophy, 171
    in syringomyelia, 170
Lumbar and sacral plexuses, 13
Lumbar disc herniations, 18–19
Lumbar enlargement, 490
Lumbar nerve, 12
Lumbar plexus, 13, 112*t*
Lumbar puncture, 490
    landmarks for performing, 510–512, 511*f*
Lumbosacral nucleus, 138
Lumbosacral root syndrome, 110*t*
Lung, effect of autonomic system on, 397*t*, 400, 400*f*
Lysosomes, 43

M
Macula, 327
Macula lutea, 287, 328
Magnetic resonance imaging (MRI), 23–26
    cerebral ventricles, clinical investigation of, 456
    of cerebrovascular disease, 474
    structure of brain, 25*f*
Main motor nucleus, 341–342, 342*f*
Major dense line, 73
Malignant sarcoma, 112
Mammillary bodies, 249, 255, 304, 496
Mammillotegmental tract, 377
Mammillothalamic tract, 304, 377
Mandible, 195
    angle of, 195
    body of, 195
Mandibular fossa, 191
Mastoid process, 187, 191
Maxillae, 187
Mechanoreceptors, 84
Meckel cave, 335
Medial accessory olivary nuclei, 199
Medial eminence, 205, 445
Medial geniculate body, 209, 366, 496
Medial lemniscus, 149, 203, 205, 211, 214
Medial longitudinal fasciculus, 157, 203, 205, 210, 213, 331, 333*f*
Medial medullary syndrome, 215, 216*f*
Medial occipitotemporal gyrus, 260
Medial pterygoid plate, 191
Medial vestibular nucleus, 199, 205
Medial wall, 439
Median eminence of tuber cinereum, 254
Median sulcus, 205, 445
Medulla, effect of autonomic system on, 397*t*
Medulla oblongata, 4–5, 9, 194, 196–204, 197*f*, 199*t*
    arteries of, 468
    clinical significance of, 215
    cuneate nucleus, 197

cuneate tubercle, 197
decussation
    of lemnisci, 199, 199*t*, 201*f*
    of pyramids, 198–199, 199*t*, 201*f*
development of, 490–492
floor of fourth ventricle, 197
gracile nucleus, 197
internal structure, 197–204
just inferior to pons, 199*t*, 203
lateral medullary syndrome of Wallenberg, 215, 216*f*
medial medullary syndrome, 215, 216*f*
olives, 196, 199–203, 199*t*, 202*f*
posterior cranial fossa, raised pressure of, 215
posterior median sulcus, 197
reticular formation, 204
vascular disorders, 215
veins of, 470
Medullary arteries, 467
    of Adamkiewicz, 472
Medullary reticulospinal tract, 156
Medulloblastoma of vermis, 243
Meissner corpuscles, 87–88, 87*f*–88*f*
Melanin granules, 43
Melanocytes, 15
Melatonin, 254
Ménière disease, 353
Meningeal artery and vein, middle, 188
Meningeal branches, 466
Meningeal headache, 429
Meningeal layer, 418, 419*f*–421*f*
Meningeal veins, 422, 423*f*
Meninges, 1, 418–430, 490
    brain, 418–425
        arachnoid mater, 419*f*–420*f*, 422*f*, 424*f*–425*f*, 425
        dural arterial supply, 422, 423*f*–424*f*
        dural nerve supply, 420, 422
        dural venous sinuses, 419*f*, 420, 421*f*–422*f*, 422–424
        dura mater, 418–420, 419*f*–424*f*, 422–424
        pia mater, 419*f*, 425
    excessive brain movement, 428–429
    functional significance, 428
    headaches, 429
    intracranial hemorrhage, 429
    intracranial hemorrhage in infant, 429
    spinal cord, 425–428
        arachnoid mater, 426, 426*f*
        dura mater, 425–426, 426*f*–428*f*
        pia mater, 426, 426*f*
Meningitis, 429
Meningocele, 498, 500*f*
Meningomyelocele, 499
Merkel cell, 84
Merkel discs, 84, 85*f*–86*f*
Mesaxon, 73, 79
Mesencephalon, 490
Mesoderm, 14
Metaproterenol, 393
Metencephalon. *See* cerebellum; midbrain (mesencephalon); pons
Methacholine chloride, 115
Metopic suture, 190
Microfilaments, 42
Microglia, 58–59
Microglial cells, 488
    reactions to injury, 63
Microtubules, 42, 42*f*
Midbrain, 209*f*, 490
    arteries of, 468
    basis pedunculi of, 154
    Benedikt syndrome, 217, 218*f*
    cerebral aqueduct of, 331, 332*f*–333*f*
        blockage in, 217
    cerebral peduncles, 209
    clinical significance of, 217

crus cerebri, 210–211, 214
  decussation in, 210
  development of, 492
  inferior brachium, 209
  inferior colliculus, 209–213, 211f–212f, 213t, 494
  medial geniculate body, 209
  reticular formation, 210
  substantia nigra, 210–211, 214
  superior brachium, 209
  superior colliculus of, 211f–213f, 213–214, 213f, 213t, 327, 329f, 494
  tectum, 364f
  trauma of, 217
  vascular lesions, 217
  veins of, 470
  Weber syndrome, 217, 218f
Midbrain vesicle, 15, 488, 490, 491t
Middle cerebellar peduncles, 9, 204, 492
Middle cerebral artery, 465
  occlusion of, 472–473
Middle conchae, 187
Middle cranial fossa, 192–195
Middle frontal gyrus, 258
Middle lobes of cerebellum, 229
Middle meningeal artery, 422
Middle meningeal vessels, 191
Middle temporal sulci, 258
Midline nuclei, 366
Migraine, 429
Minor dense line, 73
Mitochondria, 41
Mitral cell, 326f, 327
Modality of sensation, 113
Molecular layer (plexiform layer) of cortex, 231, 281
Monoplegia, 166
Monosynaptic reflex, 160, 161f
Morphine, 164
Mossy fibers, 235
Motor cortex, 282, 284, 286
  lesions of, 290
  precentral area, 283
  primary motor area, 153t, 154, 283–284
  secondary motor area, 153t, 154, 283
  supplementary motor area, 284
Motor endplate, 94, 95f–96f
  drugs and diseases affecting, 114t
  on stimulation of motor nerve, 97
Motor fibers, 12
Motor innervation of intrafusal fibers, 90
Motor nuclei/motor nucleus
  of cranial nerves, 323, 325
  dorsal, 325
  of facial nerve, 337, 337f, 338, 338f
  general visceral, 325
  of trigeminal nerve, 207, 333, 334f
Motor recovery, 109
Motor root, 204
Motor units, 93–94, 101–102
  components of, 101f
  skeletal muscle innervation, 93–94
Multiform layer (layer of polymorphic cells) of cortex, 282
Multiple sclerosis, 63–64, 171, 408
Multipolar neurons, 34
Muscarinic receptors, 392
Muscle action, 101–102
Muscle atrophy, 166
Muscle fatigue, 102
Muscle hypotonia, 243
Muscle joint sense pathways, 143t, 147–150, 149t
Muscles
  clinical observation of muscular activity, 117
  involuntary movement of, 117
  segmental innervation of, 100–101, 508–510
Muscle spasticity, 290
Muscle spindles, 101

Muscle systemic arteries, effect of autonomic system on, 397t
Muscle tone, 101–102, 116–117
  abnormal
    athetosis, 167
    chorea, 167
    dystonia, 167
    hemiballismus, 167
    hypertonia, 166
    hypotonia, 166
    myoclonus, 167
    spasms, 167
    tremors, 166
  skeletal, 116–117
  spinal cord, 165
Muscular contracture, 117, 166
Muscular coordination, 117
Muscular element of motor endplate, 94
Muscular fasciculation, 117, 166
Muscular power, 117
Myasthenia gravis, 115
Myelencephalon, 490
Myelinated nerve fibers, 71–73
  in peripheral nervous system, 75f
  relationship between oligodendrocyte and, 74f
Myelination in brain, 498
Myelin formation, 72–73
Myelin sheath, 72
Myelocele, 499
Myelography of vertebral column, 172, 173f–174f
Myoclonus, 117, 167

N

Nasal bone, 187
Neostigmine, 115
Nerve cell body, 34–37
  structures of, 39t
Nerve fibers, 2, 33
  afferent, 81, 84, 93
  autonomic, 97–98, 98f
  branching of, 81
  bundles of, 80–81
  myelinated, 71–73, 87, 92, 94
  nonmyelinated, 79
  peripheral, 80
  unmyelinated, 88–89
Nerve impulse, 44–45
Nerve of pterygoid canal, 194
Nerve plexuses, 13, 81
Nerve tracts, 71, 72f
Nerve transplantation, 110
Nervous system, early development of, 14–16
Nervus intermedius, 338
Neural crest, 14f, 15
Neural defect prevention, 500–501
Neural element of motor endplate, 94
Neural folds, 14, 14f
Neural groove, 14, 14f
Neural plate, 14, 14f
Neural tube, 15, 15f, 197
Neurilemmomas, 112
Neurites, 33
Neuroanatomy
  ascending tracts of spinal cord, 142–152, 143t, 147f
  autonomic nervous system, 387–410, 397t
  basal nuclei, 310–318
  cranial nerve nuclei, 323–353
  descending tracts of spinal cord, 152–160, 152f, 153t
  effector endings, 93–98
  hypothalamus, 373–382
  meninges of brain, spinal cord, 418–430
  motor units, 93–94, 101–102, 101f
  muscle fatigue, 102
  muscle tone, action, 101–102
  nerve fibers, 71–73, 79

neuroanatomical data of clinical significance, 507–512
neuroglia, 54–60
peripheral nerves, 81–83, 81f–83f, 109–110
receptor endings, 84–93
reticular formation, 299–301
segmental innervation
  of muscles, 100–101
  of skin, 98
spinal cord, 136–141
thalamus, 363–369
Neuroblastoma, 62
Neuroblasts, 488–490, 494
Neurofibrils, 42, 42f
Neurofilaments, 42, 42f
Neuroglia, 2, 4f, 54–60
  types of neuroglial cells
    astrocytes, 55–58
    ependyma, 59–60
    microglia, 58–59
    oligodendrocytes, 58, 58f
Neuroglial cells, 231, 498
  astrocytes, 55–58
  ependyma, 59–60
  microglia, 58–59
  oligodendrocytes, 58, 58f
  structural features, location, and functions of, 56t
Neuroglial reactions to injury, 63
Neurohypophysis, 254
Neurologic examination, 118
Neuroma, 107
Neuromodulators, 54, 54t
Neuromuscular blocking agents, 114–115
Neuromuscular junctions
  action of drugs on, 115–116
  in skeletal muscle, 94–97, 94f
  in smooth muscle, 97–98
Neuronal recovery, 107–108
Neuronal response to injury, 105–107
  apparent recovery of central nervous system function, 112–113
  of nerve cell body injury, 105
  of nerve cell process injury, 105–107
  nerve transplantation, 110
  neuronal degeneration associated with senescence, 109
  neuronal recovery, 107–108
  of peripheral nerve tumors, 110–112
  transneuronal degeneration, 108–109
  traumatic lesions of peripheral nerves, 109–110
Neurons, 1, 33, 40f, 325
  bipolar, 34
  classification, 35f, 37t, 78t
  fine structure of, 38f
  golgi type I and II, 34
  ionic and electrical changes, 44f, 46f
  multipolar, 34
  nerve cell body, 34–37
    cytoplasm, 38–43
    nucleus, 37–38
    structures of, 39t
  nerve cell processes, 48–49
    axon transport, 49
  neurofibrils with, 42f
  plasma membrane, 42–48
    depolarized, 45
    excitation and conduction, 44–47
    potassium channel, 47–48
    sodium channel, 47–48
  reactions to injury, 62
  synapses, 49–54
    chemical, 51–52
    electrical, 54
    neuromodulators, 54
    neurotransmitters, 52–54
  types, 33–34, 36f
  unipolar, 33

Neuron tumors, 62
Neurophysins, 377, 379f
Neuropraxia, 109
Neurotendinous spindles (Golgi tendon organs), 92–93
  functions, 93
Neurotmesis, 109
Neurotransmitters, 52–54, 54t
  cerebellar cortical, 235
  synapses, 52–54
  treatment of neurologic disease by manipulation of, 63
Nicotine, 63, 97, 392
Nicotinic receptors, 392
Nigrostriate fibers, 313f, 314
Nissl substance, 38–39
Nociceptors, 84
Nodes of Ranvier, 72–73, 75f–76f
Non-communicating hydrocephalus, 456
Nonencapsulated receptors, 84–85
Norepinephrine, 235, 457
Nterior ethmoidal nerve, 192
Nuclear envelope, 38
Nuclear pores, 38
Nuclei, 5
Nuclei gracilis, 149
Nucleus, 37–38, 37f
Nucleus ambiguus, 203
Nucleus cuneatus, 198–199
Nucleus dorsalis (Clarke column), 140, 149
Nucleus gracilis, 198–199
Nucleus of tractus solitarius, 203
Nucleus pulposus, 135
Nystagmus, 242

O
Obesity, 267, 382
Occipital bone, 187
Occipital condyles, 191
Occipital eye field, 287
Occipital lobe, 256, 259, 286–287, 496
  macula lutea, 287
  occipital eye field, 287
  primary visual area, 286–287
  secondary visual area, 287
  visual cortex, 287
Occipital sinus, 195, 420, 423–424
Occipitotemporal gyrus, 260
Occipitotemporal sulcus, 260
Ocular movement disturbances, 242
Oculomotor nerve, 331, 350–351
  course, 331, 332f
  distribution, 332f
  function, 324t
  nuclei, 331, 332f
Oculomotor nucleus, 213
Olfaction, 376
Olfactory aura, 306
Olfactory bulb, 192, 326f, 327
Olfactory hairs, 327
Olfactory nerves, 192, 326–327, 326f, 349–350
  distribution of, 326f
  fibers, 327
  function, 324t
  olfactory bulb, 326f, 327
  olfactory cells and neurons of olfactory bulb, connections between, 326f
  olfactory cells and neurons of olfactory system, connections between, 326f
  olfactory tract, 326f, 327
Olfactory receptor cells, 326–327
Olfactory sulcus, 260
Olfactory tract, 326f, 327
Oligodendrocytes, 58, 58f, 63, 72, 488
Olivary nuclear complex, 199
Olivary nuclei, 490
Olivospinal tract, 154, 159, 160f
Ophthalmic artery, 464

Optic canal, 193–194
Optic chiasma, 249, 254–255, 327, 328f, 366, 498
Optic disc, 327, 328f
Optic nerve, 254, 327–331, 328f, 455
  binocular vision neurons, 327–328, 328f
  function, 324t
  lateral geniculate body, 327, 328f
  optic chiasma, 327, 328f
  optic radiation, 327, 328f
  optic tract, 327, 328f–329f
  visual pathway neurons, 327–328, 328f
  visual reflexes, 328–331, 329f
    accommodation reflex, 329–330, 329f
    consensual light reflex, 329, 329f
    corneal reflex, 330, 330f
    direct light reflex, 328, 329f
    pupillary skin reflex, 331
    visual body reflexes, 330–331, 330f
Optic radiation, 265, 327, 328f, 439
Optic tract, 254, 327, 328f–329f
Orbital gyri, 260
Orbital margins, 187
Osmoreceptor, 379
Outer glial limiting membranes, 55
Outer layer of Baillarger, cerebral cortex, 286
Oxytocin hormones, 377

P
Pacinian corpuscles, 88, 88f–89f
Pain, 113–114
  acute, treatment of, 164
  chronic, treatment of, 164
  conduction in central nervous system, 145–146
  conduction to central nervous system, 145
  control in central nervous system (CNS), 146
  fast, 145–146
  pathways, 142–145, 143f–144f
  perception of, 145–146
  pressure, 114
  slow, 145–146
  somatic, 164
  thalamus, 369
  visceral, 164
Palatal processes of maxillae, 190
Palatine bones, horizontal plates of, 190
Palatine foramina, greater and lesser, 190
Pallidosubthalamic fibers, 314
Pallidotegmental fibers, 314
Pallidotomy, 318
Papilledema, 455
Paracentral lobule, 259
Parahippocampal gyrus, 260, 303
Parallel fibers, 233
Paralysis
  bilateral spastic, 170
  diplegia, 166
  flaccid, 166
  hemiplegia, 166
  ipsilateral spastic, 170
  monoplegia, 166
  paraplegia, 166
  quadriplegia, 166
  severe, 166
Paraplegia, 166
  in extension, 162
  in flexion, 162
Parasympathetic injuries, 407
Parasympathetic nucleus, 342, 342f
Paresthesia, 116
Parietal bones, 187
Parietal eminence, 507
Parietal lobe, 256, 258, 496
  outer layer of Baillarger, 286
  primary somesthetic area, 286
  secondary somesthetic area, 286
  somesthetic association area, 286

Parieto-occipital sulcus, 256
Parkinson disease, 171, 315, 316f–318f
  drug-induced, 318
  motor function in, 318, 318f
  symptoms, 317
  treatment of, 457
  types of, 317
Parkinsonism, 166
Parotid gland, autonomic innervation, 397t, 398–399, 399f
Patellar tendon reflex, 101, 510
Pedicles, 132
Peduncles, 9
  cerebellar, 229, 235, 235f
    inferior, 9, 196, 203
    middle, 9, 204
    superior, 9, 205, 210, 239, 239f
Pelvic colon, effect of autonomic system on, 397t, 400–401, 401f
Pendular knee jerk, 242
Pendular nystagmus, 242
Penicillin, 457
Perineurium, 80
Periosteum, 418
Peripheral nerves, 71, 77f
  autonomic ganglia, 81
  axons, regeneration of, 107–108
  blood vessels within, 112
  cranial nerves, 81, 82f
  endoneurial spaces within, 112
  injuries, clinical principles, 110
  local anesthetic action on nerve conduction, 112
  lymphatics within, 112
  peripheral nerve plexuses, 81–83
  plexuses, 81–83
  regeneration of, 109
  sensory ganglia, 81
  spinal nerves, 80–81, 82f–83f
  structure, 81f
  traumatic lesions of, 109–110
    motor changes, 109
    sensory changes, 109
    vasomotor, sudomotor, and trophic changes, 109
  tumors, 110–112
Peripheral nervous system (PNS), 1, 72, 79
  cranial and spinal nerves, 2
  cranial nerves, 12–13
  ganglia, 13–14
    autonomic ganglia, 14
    sensory ganglia, 14
  major divisions of, 12–14
  spinal nerves, 12–13
Pernicious anemia, 171–172
Persistent vegetative state, 292
Pes hippocampus, 301, 303, 440
Petit mal, 292
Phantom limb, 113–114
Phenothiazines, 63
Phenoxybenzamine, 116, 394
Phenylbutazone, 457
Phenylephrine, 393
Pheochromocytoma, 62
Physostigmine, 115
Pia mater, 4, 440, 443, 443f, 447, 450, 490, 492
  brain, 419f, 425
  spinal cord, 426, 426f
Pineal body, 254, 495
Pineal gland, 253–254
  functions, 253–254
  functions of, 267
Pinealocytes, 253
Pineal recess, 254
Pineal tumors, 267
Plasma membrane, 42–48
  depolarized, 45
  excitation and conduction, 44–47

potassium channel, 47–48
sodium channel, 47–48
summation of excitatory stimuli, 46
Pneumoencephalography, 267
Poliomyelitis, 62, 171
Polyneuropathy, 113
Pons, 5, 9, 194
anterior surface of, 204, 205f
arteries of, 468
astrocytoma of, 216
caudal part, 205–207, 206f
clinical significance of, 215–217
hemorrhage of, 217
infarctions of, 217
internal structure of, 205–209, 206f–208f
level inferior to, 204
posterior surface of, 205
tumors of, 216–217
veins of, 470
Pontine arteries, 467
Pontine cistern, 447
Pontine nuclei, 203, 207, 492
Pontine reticulospinal tract, 156
Positron emission tomography (PET), 26, 26f
of cerebrovascular disease, 474
Postencephalitic parkinsonism, 317
Posterior cerebral artery, 468
occlusion of, 473
Posterior clinoid processes, 194
Posterior cochlear nucleus, 203, 207
Posterior commissure, 253–254, 263
Posterior communicating artery, 464
Posterior external arcuate fibers, 149–150
Posterior fontanelle, 191
Posterior gray column, 4, 139–141
Posterior gray commissure, 141
Posterior horn of ventricles, 436, 439
bulb of, 439
median wall of, 439
roof of, 439
Posterior inferior cerebellar artery, 466
Posterior intercavernous sinuses, 424
Posterior longitudinal ligament, 135
Posterior median septum, 489
Posterior median sulcus, 197
Posterior nerve cell groups, 139–141
Posterior neuropore, 15
Posterior or sensory roots, 4
Posterior perforated substance, 210
Posterior radicular artery, 472
Posterior ramus, 13
Posterior root, 12, 80
Posterior root ganglion, 4, 12, 14–15, 34, 81, 142, 490
Posterior spinal arteries, 466, 471–472
Posterior spinocerebellar tract, 149
Posterior white column, 4
Posterior white matter, 141
Posterolateral tract of Lissauer, 144, 146
Postganglionic nerve endings, 393
Postganglionic transmitters, 393–394, 393f
Postsynaptic membranes, 51
Postural hypotension, 473
Postural sensibility, 114
Posture, 102
of individual, 117
Precentral area, cerebral cortex, 283
Precentral gyrus, 258
Precentral sulcus, 258
Precuneus, 259
Prefrontal cortex, 285, 289
tumors or traumatic destruction of, 291
Preganglionic transmitters, 391f, 392, 392f
Premotor area, cerebral cortex, 284
Preoptic area, 373, 375
Pressure pain, 114
Pretectal nucleus, 327, 329, 329f, 406

Pretectal nucleus, 213
Primary auditory area (Brodmann areas), 287
lesions of, 291
Primary fissure, 229
Primary lysosomes, 43
Primary motor area, cerebral cortex, 153t, 154, 283–284
Primary olfactory cortex, 327
Primary somesthetic area, cerebral cortex, 286
Primary visual area (Brodmann area), cerebral cortex, 286–287
lesions of, 291
Procaine, 63, 112
Programmed cell death, 16
Projection fibers, 264–265
Propranolol, 116, 394
Prosencephalon, 490
Protoplasmic astrocytes, 55, 57f
Pterion, 188, 507
Pterygoid hamulus, 191
Pterygomaxillary fissure, 188
Pterygopalatine fossa, 188
Pulvinar of thalamus, 327, 328f, 363, 364f, 366
Purkinje cells, 234–235, 239
in cortex, 231–232
Purkinje neuron, 235
Putamen, 497
Pyramidal cells, 279, 498
Pyramidal tracts, 154, 165
Pyramids, 165, 196, 203, 492
decussation of, 196, 198–199, 199t, 201f

Q

Quadriplegia, 166
Queckenstedt sign, 20, 456

R

Rabies, 62
Radial fibers, 280
Radicular arteries, 472
Rami, 187, 195
Ramus
anterior, 13
anterior ascending, 256
anterior horizontal, 256
posterior, 13
Rapid transport, 43
Raynaud disease, 409
Reaction of degeneration, 109, 166
Receptive aphasia, 290
Receptor endings, 84–93
anatomical receptor types, 84–89
encapsulated receptors, 85–89
free nerve endings, 84, 85f
hair follicle receptors, 84–85, 86f–87f
Meissner corpuscles, 87–88, 87f–88f
Merkel discs, 84, 85f–86f
nonencapsulated receptors, 84–85
Pacinian corpuscles, 88, 88f–89f
Ruffini corpuscles, 88–89
classification and comparison, 84t
cutaneous receptor functions, 89
joint receptors, 89
neuromuscular spindles, 89–90, 90f–91f
annulospiral endings, 89–90
extrafusal fibers, 89
flower-spray endings, 90
function, 90–92
intrafusal fiber control, 92
intrafusal fibers, 89
nuclear bag fibers, 89
nuclear chain fibers, 89
stretch reflex, 92
neurotendinous spindles (Golgi tendon organs), 92–93
sensory stimuli, transduction into nerve impulses, 89

Receptor potential, 89
Reciprocal inhibition, 92
Rectum, effect of autonomic system on, 397t, 400–401, 401f
Red nucleus, 157, 214, 253, 494
Reflex (es)
defined, 160
disturbances of, 242
Regeneration of autonomic nerves, 407
Relative refractory period, 46
Renal plexus, 389
Renshaw cells, 54, 63
lower motor neuron inhibition and, 162
Replacement gliosis, 57
Residual bodies, 43
Resting membrane potential, 44
Resting muscle fiber, 97
Reticular activating system, 301
Reticular alerting mechanism, 292
Reticular formation, 156, 299–301, 494
afferent projections, 300–301, 300f
arrangement, 299–300, 300f
autonomic nervous system control, 301
biological clocks, influence on, 301
efferent projections, 301
endocrine system control, 301
facial expression muscles control, 301
functions, 301
lateral column, 299, 300f
medial column, 299, 300f
median column, 299, 300f
reticular activating system, 301
skeletal muscle control, 301
somatic sensation control, 301
visceral sensation control, 301
Reticular nucleus, 366
Reticulospinal fibers, 157
Reticulospinal tract, 156–157, 156f
Retina, ganglionic layer of, 327, 328f
Retrograde degeneration, 106
Retrograde transneuronal degeneration, 109
Retrograde transport, 49
Rhinal sulci, 260
Rhombencephalon, 490
Rhombic lips, 492
Rods, visual system, 327
Rostrum of corpus callosum, 262
Rubrospinal tract, 154, 157–158, 158f, 199
Ruffini corpuscles, 88–89

S

Sacral nerve, 12
Sacral plexus, 13, 112t
Sacrum, 20f
Sagittal suture, 187, 190
Salivatory nucleus, 325
Saltatory conduction, 47
Satellite cells, 81, 490
Satiety center, 381
Schizophrenia, 291, 306
Schmidt–Lanterman incisures, 73, 78f
Schwann cell, 72, 79
cytoplasm, 73, 78f
Sciatica, 18
Scopolamine, 63, 115
Secondary auditory area (auditory association cortex), 287
lesions of, 291
Secondary lysosomes, 43
Secondary motor area, cerebral cortex, 153t, 154, 283
Secondary olfactory cortex, 327
Secondary somesthetic area, cerebral cortex, 286
Secondary visual area (Brodmann areas), cerebral cortex, 287
lesions of, 291

Second-order neurons, 142, 144–146, 149, 152–153, 325–326
Segmental innervation
of muscles, 100–101, 508–510
of skin, 98
Segmental spinal arteries, 472
Sella turcica, 194
Sensory cortex, 256, 291
primary, 286
lesions of, 291
secondary, 286
lesions of, 291
vertical units or columns of, 283
Sensory decussation, 149
Sensory fibers, 12, 81
Sensory ganglia, 14–15, 81
Sensory innervation of muscle spindles, 89
Sensory loss, 369
Sensory modality examination, 113–114
Sensory nuclei, 342, 342f
of cranial nerves, 325–326
Sensory perception abnormalities, 116
Sensory receptors and age, 113, 113t
Sensory recovery, 109
Sensory root, 204
Septum pellucidum, 262, 265, 304, 439, 498
Serotonin, 145–146, 235
Sexual disorders, 382
Shaken baby syndrome, 22–23
Shock, physical and psychologic, 473
Short association fibers, 264
Short ciliary nerves, 329, 397
Sigmoid sinus, 194–195
Sigmoid sinuses, 423
Skeletal muscle
anticholinesterases acting on, 115
control, 301
denervation supersensitivity of, 115
fiber contraction, 97
innervation, 93–94
motor unit, 93–94, 93f
sensory fibers, types of, 93
motor endplates, 96, 96f, 97
drugs and diseases affecting, 114t
motor nerve and, 115
nerve control, 115
nerve supply and blood supply to, 93
neuromuscular blocking agents acting on, 114–115
segmental innervation of muscles, 100–101, 508–510
Skeletal neuromuscular junctions, 94–97, 94f
action of drugs and other agents on, 114–115, 114t
anticholinesterases, action on, 115
bacterial toxins, action on, 115
Skin
effect of autonomic system on, 397t
segmental innervation of, 98
Skull anatomy
adult, 185–191, 189f
anterior view, 186–187, 186f
cranium, 186
external and internal tables, 185
facial bones, 186
inferior view, 190–191, 190f
lateral view, 187–188, 188f
posterior view, 188–190
superior view, 190
sutures, 185
neonatal, 191, 193f
openings in base of, 195t
Sleep, 292
disturbances, 267, 382
Slow pain, 145–146
Slow synaptic potentials, 392, 392f
Slow transport, 43

Small intensely fluorescent (SIF) cells, 391
Smooth endoplasmic reticulum (SER), 38f, 39, 40f
Sole plate, 94
Somatic afferents, 376
Somatic motor fiber, 325
Somatic pain, 164
Somatic sensation control, 301
Somatosensory pathways, 143, 143t
Somesthetic association area, cerebral cortex, 286
lesions of, 291
Space-occupying or expanding lesions within the skull, 23
Spasms, 167
Spasticity, 166
Speech disorders, 243
Sphenoid, greater wing of, 187
Sphenoid air sinuses, 193
Sphenoid bone, 193
Sphenopalatine foramen, 188
Spina bifida, 498–500, 499f
Spina bifida occulta, 498–500
Spinal cord, 1, 5f–7f, 15, 136–141
acute injuries, 167
amyotrophic lateral sclerosis (Lou Gehrig disease), 171
anatomical features, 163
organization of tracts, 164f
anterior and posterior nerve root lesions, 163
anterior gray column of, 37f, 41f
motor neuron, 49f
anterior median fissure of, 196
arteries of
anterior, 472
posterior, 471–472
segmental, 472
ascending tracts, 142–152
injury, 163–164
central canal of, 196, 436
clinical syndromes affecting, 169f
anterior cord syndrome, 168
Brown-Séquard syndrome (cord hemisection), 169f–170f, 170
central cord syndrome, 168–170, 169f
complete cord transection syndrome, 168
destructive spinal cord syndromes, 168–170
spinal shock syndrome, 167–168
compression of, chronic
clinical signs, 167
extradural causes, 167
corticospinal tract (pyramidal tract) lesions, 166
descending tracts, 152–160, 152f, 153t
anatomical organization, 153
descending autonomic fibers, 154, 159–160
functions, 153–160
lesions of, 166
olivospinal tract, 154, 159, 160f
rubrospinal tract, 154, 157–158, 158f
tectospinal tract, 154, 157, 157f
vestibulospinal tract, 154, 158–159, 159f
fetus with, 5f
gray column, 137f, 138–141, 139f–140f
accessory nucleus, 138
anterior nerve cell groups, 138–139
central canal, 141
gray commissure, 141
lateral nerve cell groups, 141
lumbosacral nucleus, 138
posterior nerve cell groups, 139–141
gray matter, 2, 4
anterior gray column or horn, 4

central canal, 4
posterior gray column or horn, 4
injuries, 16
intersegmental tracts, 160–162
lamination of ascending tracts, clinical significance, 163
lower motor neuron
inhibition, 162
lesions, 166
lumbar part of, 7f
meninges, 425–428
arachnoid mater, 426, 426f
dura mater, 425–426, 426f–428f
pia mater, 426, 426f
multiple sclerosis, 171
muscle tone, 165
athetosis, 167
chorea, 167
dystonia, 167
hemiballismus, 167
hypertonia, 166
hypotonia, 166
myoclonus, 167
spasms, 167
tremors, 167
muscular signs/symptoms, relationship to nervous system lesions, 166–167
neural tube, 15
oblique posterior view of, 13f
pain
acute, treatment of, 164
chronic, treatment of, 164
conduction in central nervous system, 145–146
conduction to central nervous system, 145
control in central nervous system (CNS), 146
fast, 145–146
pathways, 142–145, 143f–144f
perception of, 145–146
slow, 145–146
somatic, 164
visceral, 164
Parkinson disease, 171
pernicious anemia, 171–172
poliomyelitis, 171
posterior view of, 12f
protective covering of, 3f
reflex arcs, 160–161
Renshaw cells, 162
segments
vertebral numbers, 16
site of a syphilitic lesion on, 165f
spinal nerves, 12
structure, 4, 137–138, 138t
syringomyelia, 170–171, 171f
tabes dorsalis, 165
transverse section of, 139f–140f
upper motor neuron lesions, 165
veins, 472
vertebral column radiography of
computed tomography, 172, 172f
magnetic resonance imaging, 172, 173f
myelography, 172, 173f–174f
vertebral numbers and spinal cord segments, 510t
voluntary movement, 165
white matter, 2, 4, 137f, 141
Spinal cord development, 488–490
alar plate, 489
anterior roots of spinal nerves, 489
basal plates, 488
cervical and lumbar enlargements, 490
different stages, 489f
floor and roof plates, 488
forebrain vesicle, 488

hindbrain vesicle, 488
intermediate zone, 488
ligamentum denticulatum, 490
marginal zone, 488
meninges, 490
midbrain vesicle, 488
motor neurons, 489
neural tube development, 488
peripheral process and central process, 489–490
posterior roots of spinal nerves, 490
sensory neurons, in posterior gray matter, 489–490
subarachnoid space, 490
vertebral column, 490
Spinal cord ischemia
following abdominal aortic aneurysm, 479
signs and symptoms, 474–479, 479f
thoracic aortic dissection and, 479
Spinal lemnisci/spinal lemniscus, 145–146, 204, 209, 211, 214
Spinal nerve, 12
connection with spinal cord, 12, 12f
injuries, 109, 110t
posterior root of, 490
ramus
anterior, 13
posterior, 13
rootlets, 4
roots, 6f, 131, 135
anterior or motor, 4, 80–81
bundles of nerve fibers, 80–81
cervical and brachial plexuses, 13
lesions, 163
lumbar and sacral plexuses, 13
posterior or sensory, 4, 80–81
relationship between intervertebral disc herniations and, 510, 511t
Spinal nerve injuries
cervical disc herniations, 17–18
herniation of intervertebral discs, 16–17
lumbar disc herniations, 18–19
Spinal root, 325t, 345–346, 346f
Spinal stenosis, 172
Spinal tap (lumbar puncture), 19–20, 23
Spinal tract of trigeminal nerve, 199, 203
Spine, 132
Spine of sphenoid, 191
Spinocerebellar tract, 199
Spino-olivary tracts, 151, 199
Spinoreticular tract, 150–151
Spinotectal tracts, 150, 199, 204
Spinothalamic tracts, 199
Spinous process, 132
Splanchnic nerves, 389
Splenium, 262
Spontaneous intracerebral hemorrhage, 22
Squamotympanic fissure, 191
Stellate cells, 231, 280
Stereognosis, 114, 289
Stomach
effect of autonomic system on, 397t, 400, 401f
pain, 410
Straight sinus, 265, 419, 419f, 421f
Stratum zonale, 363, 364f
Striae, 303
Stria medullaris, 445
Stria medullaris thalami, 250, 250f, 255, 264
Stria of Gennari, 281
Striate cortex, 281
Stria terminalis, 304, 442
Striate vein, 470
Striatonigral fibers, 313f, 314
Striatopallidal fibers, 313f, 314
Stupor, 292
Styloid process, 187, 191

Stylomastoid foramen, 191
Subarachnoid cisterns, 447
Subarachnoid hemorrhage, 22, 429, 474
Subarachnoid space, 3f, 4, 9, 19, 19f, 426, 447, 448f
blockage, 456
development of, 490
extensions, 450
Subdural hematoma burr hole, 508
Subdural hemorrhage, 22, 429
Sublingual, submandibular salivary glands, autonomic innervation, 397t, 398–399, 398f
Substance P, 144–145
Substantia ferruginea, 205, 445
Substantia gelatinosa, 139, 199
Substantia nigra, 209, 211, 214, 253, 494
Subthalamic lesions, 267
Subthalamic nucleus, 253
Subthalamus, 253
Succinylcholine, 115
Sulci, 10, 497
Sulci of cerebrum
calcarine sulcus, 256
central sulcus, 256
lateral sulcus, 256
parieto-occipital sulcus, 256
Sulcus chiasmatis, 194
Sulcus limitans, 197, 205, 445, 489–490, 492f
Sulfonamide drugs, 457
Superciliary arches, 186
Superficial abdominal reflexes, 166
Superficial middle cerebral vein, 470
Superior articular processes, 133
Superior brachium, 209
Superior cerebellar artery, 468
Superior cerebellar peduncles, 9, 205, 208
decussation of, 210, 239, 239f
Superior cerebral veins, 423
Superior cerebral veins, 470
Superior colliculi/superior colliculus, 157, 211f–213f, 213–214, 213t, 327, 329f, 494, 498
Superior conchae, 187
Superior frontal gyrus, 258
Superior frontal sulci, 258
Superior longitudinal fasciculus, 264
Superior medullary velum, 443, 445f
Superior nuchal lines, 190
Superior orbital fissure, 193
Superior parietal lobule, 258
Superior petrosal sinuses, 195, 424
Superior quadrantic hemianopia, 291
Superior sagittal sinus, 191, 419, 419f, 421f, 422
Superior salivatory, 325
Superior semicircular canal, 194
Superior temporal sulci, 258
Superior vertebral notch, 133
Superior vestibular nucleus, 199
Supplementary motor area, cerebral cortex, 284
Suprachiasmatic nucleus, 376
Suprameatal crest, 191
Suprameatal spine, 191
Suprameatal triangle, 191
Supraoptic nucleus, 376
Supraorbital notch, 186
Suprarenal gland medulla, effect of autonomic system on, 397t, 401–402, 402f
Suprarenal medulla, 389
Supraspinous ligament, 135
Sutural ligaments, 418
Sydenham chorea, 315
Sympathetic and parasympathetic ganglia, 81
Sympathetic injuries, 406–407

Sympathetic nerve plexus, 424
Sympathetic trunks, 389f, 390
Symphysis menti, 191
Synaptic blocking agents, 62–63
Synaptic cleft, 96
Synaptic glomeruli, 327
Synaptic stripping, 107
Synaptic transmission, modification of, 63
Syringomyelia, 170–171, 171f, 408
Syringomyelocele, 499

T
Tabes dorsalis, 165
Tactile domes, 84
Tangential fibers, 281
Tanycytes, 59–60
Tapetum, 262
Taste area, 287
Tectospinal tract, 154, 157, 157f
Tectum, 494
Tegmental fibers, 377
Tegmentum, 205, 209
Tegmen tympani, 194
Tela choroidea, 265, 425, 492
Telencephalon, 490, 495f, 496
Temperature testing, 114
Temporal bone, 187
tympanic part of, 191
Temporal burr hole, 507, 509f
Temporal fossa, 188
Temporal lines, superior and inferior, 188
Temporal lobes, 193, 256, 258, 496
dysfunction, 306
primary auditory area (Brodmann areas), 287
secondary auditory area (auditory association cortex), 287
sensory speech area of Wernicke, 287
Temporomandibular joint, 195
Tendon spindles, 101
Tentorial notch, 419, 419f
Tentorium cerebelli, 192, 194, 256, 419, 419f, 421f, 496
Terminal ventricle, 141, 436, 447
Termor, 117
Tetanus toxin, 112
Tetracyclines, 457
Tetraethylammonium block ganglia, 393
Tetraethylammonium salts, 63
Thalamic hand, 369
Thalamohypothalamic fibers, 377
Thalamostriate fibers, 313f, 314
Thalamostriate vein, 470
Thalamus, 9, 249–254, 363–369, 364f, 496
abnormal involuntary movements, 369
activities of, 252
anterior end of, 252
arteries of, 468
brainstem, 364f
cauterization, surgical relief of pain by, 369
connections, 366, 367t, 368f
functions of, 367–368, 367t
general appearance, 363, 364f
internal capsule of, 252
interthalamic connection, 252, 363, 364f
lateral geniculate body, 252
lateral surface of, 252–253
lesions of, 267–272, 268f–271f, 369
medial surface of, 252
nuclei of, 252f
pain, 369
position and relations of, 364f
posterior end of, 252
posterior view of brainstem, 364f
pulvinar, 252, 327, 328f, 363, 364f
sensory loss, 369

Thalamus (*Continued*)
  subdivisions of, 252*f*, 253, 363–366, 364*f*
    anterior part, 365
    dorsal tier, nuclei, 366
    intralaminar nuclei, 366
    lateral part, 366
    medial part, 365
    midline nuclei, 366
    reticular nucleus, 366
    ventral tier, nuclei, 366
  superior surface of, 252
  thalamic hand, 369
Thecal sac, 172
Thermoreceptors, 84, 142–145, 143*f*–144*f*
Thiopental, 457
Third-order neuron, 325–326
Third-order neurons, 142, 145–146, 153
Third ventricle, 254–255, 490
  anterior wall of, 254
  choroid plexuses of, 255
  inferior wall or floor of, 255
  lateral wall of, 254–255
  optic recess of, 254
  posterior wall of, 254
  superior wall or roof of, 255
  tela choroidea of, 255
Thirst center, 381
Thoracic aortic dissection, 479
Thoracic nerve, 12
Thoracic outflow, 395
Tic, 117
Tinel sign, 109
Tonic spasm, 117
Total blindness of one eye, 349, 350*f*
Transneuronal degeneration, 108–109
Transverse fibers of pons, 207
Transverse pontine fibers, 492
Transverse pontocerebellar fibers, 154
Transverse process, 132, 135
Transverse sinus, 195, 419*f*, 420, 421*f*
Trapezoid body, 205, 207
Traumatic brain injury, 22
Tremors, 117, 166, 241
Triceps tendon reflex, 100, 508
Trigeminal ganglion, 194
Trigeminal lemnisci, 211, 214
Trigeminal nerve, 204, 332, 334*f*, 351
  course, 335, 335*f*
  distribution of, 335*f*
  motor component, 334–335, 334*f*
  motor nucleus of, 207
  nuclei, 332–333, 334*f*
    main sensory nucleus, 332–333, 334*f*
    mesencephalic nucleus, 333, 334*f*
    motor nucleus, 333, 334*f*
    spinal nucleus, 333, 334*f*
  principal sensory nucleus, 208
  principal sensory nucleus of, 208
  sensory components, 333–334, 334*f*
  spinal tract of, 199, 203
Trigeminal neuralgia, 351
Trochlear nerve, 209, 331, 351
  course, 331–332, 333*f*
  function, 324*t*
  nuclei, 331, 333*f*
Trochlear nucleus, 210
Tuber cinereum, 249, 254–255
Tuberomammillary nucleus, hypothalamus, 376
Tufted cells, 327
Tumors
  blood–brain barrier (BBB), 457
  fourth ventricle, 456–457
  neuron, 62
  peripheral nerve, 110–112
  peripheral nerves, 110–112
  pineal, 267

pons, 216–217
  prefrontal cortex, 291
Two-point tactile discrimination, 113
Tympanic plate, 191

U
Uncinate fasciculus, 264
Unconsciousness, 292
Uncus, 260, 303
Unilateral anosmia, 349
Unipolar neurons, 33
Upper lid, autonomic innervation of, 396, 397*t*, 398*f*
Upper limb arteries, effect of autonomic system on, 397*t*, 405, 405*f*
Upper motor neurons, 153
  disease, 171
  injury, 168
  lesions, 165–166, 317, 352*f*
  shock and response of, 168
Urinary bladder
  dysfunction, 407
  effect of autonomic system on, 397*t*, 402, 403*f*
Uterus, effect of autonomic system on, 397*t*, 403, 404*f*, 405
Uvulonodular fissures, 229

V
Vagal triangle, 446
Vagus accessory nerves, 204
Vagus nerve, 343, 353
  course, 344–345, 345*f*
  distribution of, 345*f*
  function, 325*t*
  nuclei, 343
    main motor, 343, 344*f*–345*f*
    parasympathetic, 343, 344*f*–345*f*
    sensory, 343–344, 344*f*–345*f*
Varicosities, 48
Vascular lesions of midbrain, 217
Vascular tela choroidea, 441
Vasoconstriction, 377
Vasogenic edema, 64
Vasopressin hormones, 377
Vault of cranium, 185
Veins of brain, 469–470
  anterior cerebral vein, 470
  basal vein, 470
  choroid vein, 470
  deep middle cerebral vein, 470
  external cerebral veins, 470
  internal cerebral veins, 470
  of specific brain areas, 470
  striate vein, 470
  superficial middle cerebral vein, 470
  superior cerebral veins, 470
  thalamostriate vein, 470
Venous lacunae, 423
Venous sinuses, 418, 419*f*
Ventral anterior nucleus, 366
Ventral lateral nucleus, 366
Ventral posterior nucleus, 366
Ventral posteromedial nucleus, 366
Ventricle, lateral, 10, 260, 436–440, 441*f*, 490
  anterior horn of, 436, 439
  body of, 436–439
  choroid plexus of, 439–440
  development of, 495
  disorders of, 267
  floor of, 439
  inferior horn of, 436, 440
  posterior horn of, 436, 439
  roof of, 439
Ventricular system
  central canal, 447

cerebral aqueduct (aqueduct of Sylvius), 443
  fourth ventricle, 443, 444*f*–445*f*
  lateral boundaries, 443
  lateral ventricles, 436–440
    anterior horn of, 436, 439
    body of, 436–439
    choroid plexus of, 439–440
    floor of, 439
    inferior horn of, 436, 440
    posterior horn of, 436, 439
    roof of, 439
  posterior wall (roof), 443
  rhomboid fossa (floor), 445–447
  third ventricle, 440–443
    choroid plexuses, 441–443
Ventricular zone, spinal cord, 488
Ventriculogram, 456
Ventriculography, 267, 456
Ventriculostomy, 510*f*
  technique, 508
Ventrolateral nucleus of thalamus, 239–240
Vermis, 9, 492
Vermis syndrome, 243
Vertebral arch, 132
Vertebral artery, 466–468
Vertebral canal, 4
Vertebral column
  composition, 132–135
  joints, 134, 134*f*
    innervation of, 135*f*
    intervertebral discs, 134–135
    ligaments, 135
    nerve supply, 135
    between two vertebral arches, 135
  lateral view, 133*f*
  ligaments, 135
  posterior view, 132*f*
  typical vertebra, 132
  vertebrae, 132–134, 133*f*
  vertebral arch, 132
  vertebral foramen, 132
Vertebral foramen, 132
Vertebral joint nerve supply, 135
Vertebrobasilar artery occlusion, 473
Vestibular area, 287, 445
Vestibular nerve, 339, 339*f*
  function, 325*t*
  vestibular nuclear complex, 339–340, 339*f*
Vestibular nuclear complex, 199–203, 339–340, 339*f*
Vestibular nuclei, 158–159
  medial and inferior, 203
Vestibulocochlear nerve, 204, 339–341, 352–353
  course, 341, 341*f*
  distribution, 341*f*
  disturbances of, 353
  function, 325*t*
Vestibulospinal tract, 154, 158–159, 159*f*, 199, 240, 340
Visceral afferent nucleus, 140
Visceral afferents, 376
Visceral pain, 164
Visceral sensation control, 301
Visceral sensory tracts, 149*t*, 151–152
Visual acuity, 349
Visual afferents, 376
Visual cortex, 327
Visual fields, 349
Visual pathway lesions, 349
Visual pathway neurons, 327–328, 328*f*
Visual reflexes, 328–331, 329*f*
  accommodation reflex, 329–330, 329*f*
  consensual light reflex, 329, 329*f*
  corneal reflex, 330, 330*f*
  direct light reflex, 328, 329*f*

pupillary skin reflex, 331
visual body reflexes, 330–331, 330*f*
Vomer, 190

W

Wallerian degeneration, 105
Wasting, 382
    muscle, 117
Weber syndrome, 217, 218*f*
Wernicke area, 287, 288*f*
    lesions of, 290–291
White column
    anterior, 4, 141, 155, 157–158, 160, 164*f*,
        198–199

lateral, 4, 141, 149–150, 154, 159–160,
    164*f*, 170–171, 172, 199, 237–238
posterior, 4, 141–142, 147–149, 160, 164*f*,
    167–168, 170, 172
White matter, 2, 4, 137*f*, 141, 260, 262–265
    anterior, lateral, and posterior, 141
    association fibers, 264
    commissure fibers, 262–264
    internal capsule of, 250
    nerve fiber tract arrangement, 141, 141*f*
    posterior, 147–149
    projection fibers, 264–265
    white columns, anterior, lateral, and
        posterior, 4, 7*f*

White rami communicantes, 331,
    388
Winding up phenomenon, 145

X

Xanthochromia, 456

Y

Young child's skull, 20

Z

Zygomatic arch, 187
Zygomatic bone, 187
Zygomatic process, 187